Butterworths International Medical Reviews

Neurology 3

Cerebral Vascular Disease

Butterworths International Medical Reviews

Neurology

Published in this Series

Volume 1   *Clinical Neurophysiology*
Edited by E. Stålberg and R. R. Young

Volume 2   *Movement Disorders*
Edited by C. D. Marsden and S. Fahn

Next Volume in the Series

Peripheral Nerves

Butterworths
International
Medical
Reviews

Neurology 3

Cerebral Vascular Disease

Edited by

M. J. G. Harrison, DM, FRCP
Consultant Neurologist
The Middlesex Hospital;
Director of Research
Institute of Neurological Studies
The Middlesex Hospital Medical School
London, UK

and

Mark L. Dyken, MD, FACP
Professor and Chairman
Department of Neurology
University of Indiana School of Medicine
Indianapolis
Indiana, USA

Butterworths
London Boston Durban
Singapore Sydney Toronto Wellington

First published 1983

© Butterworth & Co. (Publishers) Ltd. 1983

British Library Cataloguing in Publication Data

Cerebral vascular disease. – Butterworths
  international medical reviews. Neurology
  ISSN 0260 – 0137; 3
  1. Cerebrovascular disease
  I. Harrison, M. J. G.   II. Dyken, Mark L.
  616.8′1   RC388.5

  ISBN 0-407-02296-1

Photoset by Butterworths Litho Preparation Department
Printed and bound in England by Robert Hartnoll Ltd, Bodmin, Cornwall

Preface

Cerebrovascular disease has emerged from its place as the Cinderella of medical research into one of the most rapidly expanding fields. Such is the specialization within the subject that basic scientists and clinical investigators have difficulty in keeping an up-to-date overall view of the subject. As the new techniques are applied there is a need to maintain a clinical perspective, and clinicians are called upon to refine their definitions and revise their ideas of pathological processes.

We have set out in this book to review the fundamental concepts necessary for an understanding of the processes occurring in patients with cerebrovascular diseases, and to describe current medical practice relating it wherever possible to the latest laboratory discoveries.

At a time when large multicentre trials are grappling with the problem of identifying therapeutic regimes that influence prognosis, that very soil is found to be moving beneath our feet with a changing natural history. We have therefore attempted to define the current state of the art and provide the reader with the background against which to see the developments of the next few years.

Michael Harrison
Mark Dyken

List of Contributors

Charles R. A. Clarke, MB, MRCP
Consultant Neurologist, St Bartholomew's Hospital, London, UK

Randall D. Cebul, MD
Assistant Professor, Section of General Medicine, Department of Medicine,
University of Pennsylvania School of Medicine, Philadelphia, Pennsylvania, USA

Mark L. Dyken, MD, FACP
Professor and Chairman, Department of Neurology, Indiana University Medical
School, Indianapolis, Indiana, USA

Myron D. Ginsberg, MD
Professor of Neurology and Director, Cerebral Vascular Disease Research Center,
University of Miami School of Medicine, Miami, Florida, USA

R. J. Greenwood, MD, MRCP
Senior Registrar in Neurology, St Bartholomew's Hospital, London, UK

M. J. G. Harrison, DM, FRCP
Consultant Neurologist, The Middlesex Hospital, and Director of Research,
Institute of Neurological Studies, The Middlesex Hospital Medical School,
London, UK

P. R. D. Humphrey, DM, MRCP
Senior Registrar, St Bartholomew's Hospital, London, UK

John F. Kurtzke, MD, FACP
Professor and Vice-Chairman, Department of Neurology, and Professor,
Department of Community Medicine, Georgetown University School of Medicine;
and Chief, Neurology Service, Veterans Administration Medical Center,
Washington DC, USA

Lawrence C. McHenry, Jr, MD
Professor of Neurology, Bowman Gray School of Medicine of Wake Forest
University, Winston-Salem, North Carolina, USA

J. R. A. Mitchell, MD, DPhil, FRCP
Professor of Medicine, University Hospital, Queen's Medical Centre,
Nottingham, UK

Sean Moore, MB, FRCP(C)
Professor of Pathology, McMaster University, Hamilton, Ontario, Canada

H. R. Müller, MD
Professor of Neurology, University Clinic of Neurology, Kantonsspital, Basel,
Switzerland

E. W. Radu, MD
Senior Registrar, University Clinic of Neurology, Kantonsspital, Basel,
Switzerland

Martin Reivich, MD
Professor of Neurology and Radiology, Director of the Cerebrovascular Research
Center, School of Medicine, University of Pennsylvania, Philadelphia, USA

R. W. Ross Russell
National Hospital, London, UK

A. L. Sahs, MD
Professor Emeritus, Neurology, University of Iowa, Iowa, USA

Thoralf M. Sundt, Jr, MD
Professor and Chairman, Department of Neurologic Surgery, Mayo Clinic,
Rochester, Minnesota, USA

Contents

Part 1
Fundamental concepts

1
Atheroma

Sean Moore

The importance of atheromatous involvement of the carotid and vertebral arteries in the causation of ischemic disease of the brain is well established and will be explored in detail in subsequent chapters of this book. The events which develop in association with atheroma of these vessels and which lead to clinically recognizable episodes or syndromes do not differ from those which occur in other vascular territories. However, study of the clinical events associated with the lesions in the carotid–vertebral system has led to the development of concepts about the nature of the events and the progression of the disease which have illuminated these mechanisms in other vascular territories. Attempts to modify or ameliorate the process of atheroma formation must rest on an understanding of the mechanisms involved in atherogenesis, progression and regression of the disease. We are a long way from any comprehensive understanding of these events. However, in the last decade some significant changes have occurred in our thinking about the factors involved. More correctly, some long held views, especially related to the part played by formed elements of the blood and thrombosis in plaque development, have derived renewed support from experimental and clinical observations. These, together with new knowledge about plaque development, permit a synthesis between the lipid hypothesis and the concept of atheroma development as a response to injury.

In this chapter this new knowledge will be reviewed to provide a basis for understanding the manner in which environmental or risk factors may modify the process.

THE LESIONS OF ATHEROSCLEROSIS

It is generally accepted that there are three main lesions of atherosclerosis, the fatty dot or streak, the fibrous plaque and the complicated lesion[84].

Fatty dots and streaks are apparent as yellow lesions, slightly raised above the intimal surface. The streaks are usually oriented in a longitudinal fashion, that is, with their long axis parallel to the direction of blood flow[45]. Microscopically they show lipid droplets in smooth muscle cells. In larger lesions there may also be lipid in the interstitial tissue and the cells may be so filled with lipid (foam cells) that the cell type is no longer recognizable.

Fibrous plaques are variably elevated above the intimal surface and appear as pearly white or grey in colour. They are of varying size, but in general their long axis is parallel to the direction of blood flow. Microscopically there is abundant interstitial tissue composed of collagen, elastica and proteoglycans. This tissue usually separates the smooth muscle cells rather widely. The cells themselves are often small, appearing as thin straps, with relatively little cytoplasm in proportion to the nucleus, which is also small. There is a variable amount and distribution of lipid. Usually there is a finely dispersed lipid appearing as granules in the interstitium. There may also be intracellular lipid droplets. In the thicker, i.e. more elevated lesions, there is often a basally placed central lipid pool. If the lesion is markedly elevated it may be referred to as atheroma. Calcium may be present in the lesion.

Complicated lesions are similar to fibrous plques but in addition show surface ulceration and thrombus formation. Often the process has extended into the media and may have replaced much of the arterial wall. If this process is extensive aneurysm formation may occur. Usually there is abundant calcification in the lesion and there may be bone formation. A central lipid pool or a number of lipid pools at various levels of the lesion is a usual feature. Lipid may also be present in smooth muscle cells, and foam cells, whose histogenesis is uncertain, may be prominent.

As these lesions occur at different points in the human life span many assume that there is a progression of lesions. Thus, fatty streaks are considered as early lesions, fibrous plaques develop later and evolve to complicated lesions. This sequence however is inferred rather than being known to occur. One problem is that fatty streaks seen in infants, children and during early adult life may not be present later[49]. In some populations, where more advanced lesions do not occur, fatty streaks may be the principal lesion observed[67]. Whether or not fatty streaks evolve to become fibrous plaques is also unclear, though there is some evidence supporting the transition[114]. Some authors consider gelatinous or insudative lesions and mural microthrombi as early lesions, being precursors to the other types[45].

All of these lesions can be reproduced experimentally by various techniques, although some of these techniques cause lesions of only one type and some of the lesions produced do not closely resemble the lesions seen in human arteries. The lesions induced by dietary hyperlipemia may be associated with more accumulation of macrophages[20, 35] than is commonly seen in human disease. In lesions induced by intimal or endothelial injury, smooth muscle cell proliferation appears to form the major component and therefore these lesions resemble the human lesions[82].

ARTERIAL WALL INJURY

The thrombogenic theory

Rokitansky's concept[95] that atheroma developed from incorporation of elements of the blood mass into the vessel wall was modified in this century by Duguid[22, 23] who proposed that the lesion developed in response to thrombus deposition and was essentially derived from organization of the thrombotic mass. However, attempts to reproduce the disease by inducing arterial thrombosis were frustrated by the absence of lipid in the plaque which formed when the thrombus was organized[74, 88]. With few exceptions, the lesions were composed of smooth muscle cells forming an intimal thickening or plaque which was negative for lipid stains[124].

It was therefore surprising when, in the course of experiments designed to examine the effect of aggregates of platelets in the renal microcirculation, raised lipid-rich lesions were constantly produced in association with an indwelling plastic catheter left in the rabbit aorta[72, 73]. The catheters were placed by way of an arteriotomy in a femoral artery and extended to the upper thoracic aorta. At points when there appeared to be catheter–wall contact, raised yellow lesions were seen.

On histological examination these seemed to be identical to human atheromata. The lesions usually showed platelet–fibrin thrombus on their surface and were composed of smooth muscle cells, many containing lipid droplets in their cytoplasm (*Figure 1.1*). Other cells were so lipid-laden that they could not be identified

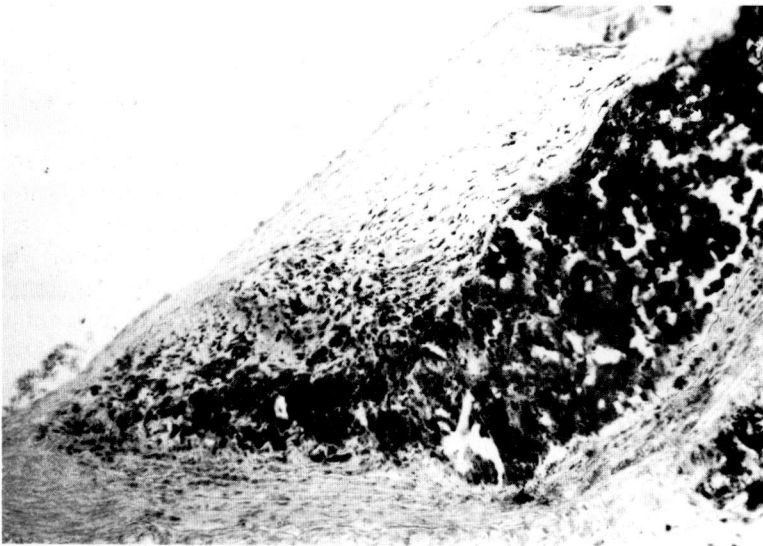

Figure 1.1 Photomicrograph of edge of a type 1 lesion showing a raised lesion with abundant lipid appearing as black. Oil red-O stained frozen section. Enlarged approximately 2.6× from original magnificantion ×400

although in early lesions lipid-containing macrophages were identified in relation to thrombus. At the base of the lesion there was often a large pool of lipid. Calcification and even ossification occurred in the lesions. Other lesions were also formed. For several weeks after placement of the catheters, lipid-filled smooth muscle cells and foam cells were found in focally thickened intima. These closely resembled human fatty streaks or dots[81]. Occasionally oedematous (gelatinous) lesions were observed. In areas where the catheter appeared to be non-mobile, or was actually incorporated into the wall, intimal thickenings composed of smooth muscle cells, i.e. lesions resembling organized thrombus, were seen. These appeared to be covered by endothelium and lacked stainable lipid. Thus, the main types of lesions seen in human atherosclerosis, viz. raised lipid containing lesions, fibrous intimal thickenings without lipid and fatty streaks, were observed in response to continuing or repeated mechanical damage to the aortic intima. Lipid analysis of the raised lesions showed substantial increases in free cholesterol and cholesteryl ester[18]. The rise in cholesteryl ester content was particularly striking, being 35-fold greater than that of intimal medial tissue from normal aorta at four months after catheter insertion. Metabolic studies of fatty acid incorporation into cholesteryl ester showed more incorporation of oleic than linoleic acid, indicating that synthesis of cholesteryl ester was occurring[18].

In a subsequent experiment it was found that repeated injury caused by injecting lymphocytotoxic human serum into a temporarily isolated segment of rabbit carotid artery every week for four weeks resulted in the development of lipid-rich, raised, atheromatous lesions[29]. Human serum which had no lymphocytotoxic activity, autologous rabbit serum, lymphocytotoxic human serum absorbed against rabbit buffy coat cells or physiological saline caused no raised, lipid-rich lesions. Occasionally oedematous intimal thickening or fatty streaks were observed following two or three exposures to lymphocytotoxic serum.

These experiments indicated that injury to the intimal lining of large arteries caused a proliferation of smooth muscle cells to form a neointima and that if the injury was repetitive lipid appeared in the lesions even though the animals were maintained on a diet which had no added lipid supplement.

Because injury to the intima leads to thrombus formation these experiments left unanswered the question of whether injury or the thrombosis accompanying injury leads to the development of lesions; further, whether repeated injury or repeated deposition of thrombus lead to the accumlation of lipid in the raised lesions. One clue to the latter was the observation of lipid around the cavity containing the polyethylene catheter. This occurred where it had become embedded in the vessel wall, when thrombus was also present. When the neointimal tissue was tightly attached to the catheter, excluding thrombus, there was no lipid in the tissue.

The report by Ross *et al.* of a platelet-derived growth factor (PDGF) which stimulated the proliferation of smooth muscle cells in tissue culture indicated a role for platelets in the proliferative response[96]. To examine this in an *in vivo* setting, severe thrombocytopenia was induced by injecting antiplatelet serum repeatedly into rabbits which had an intra-aortic catheter inserted. The development of raised lipid-containing lesions was markedly inhibited and in some cases entirely prevented[78, 80]. If the serum was given after catheter placement, no inhibition was achieved. This indicated that the stimulus to the vessel wall by material released from platelets was delivered in a very short time frame. Platelet factor 4, a 7800 dalton polypeptide, which, like the platelet-derived growth factor is contained in the α-granules of the platelet, has been shown to permeate the vessel wall within minutes of platelet attachment to the site of endothelial injury and has disappeared after four hours[37].

One of the first events observed following endothelial damage or removal is migration of smooth muscle cells from the media to the intima where they subsequently proliferate[110].

This has been examined by studying migration of smooth muscle cells across a polycarbonate filter of $8.0\,\mu$ pore size in a modified Boyden chamber. Cells plated on the upper side of the filter migrated across to the lower side when disrupted platelets or platelets reacted with thrombin or collagen were placed in the lower chamber[54]. Agents such as sulfinpyrazone or indomethacin which inhibits the platelet cyclo-oxygenase pathway failed to block the release of the factor which stimulated the migration of smooth muscle cells. This platelet-derived chemotactic factor (PDCF) is probably the same material as the platelet-derived growth factor[52] but differs from it in its lack of requirement for a co-factor or factors in serum or plasma. Migration did not occur if the filters were not coated with gelatin. Similarly, Grotendorst et al.[39] have shown a requirement for collagen coating of the filters for migration to occur. The platelet-derived chemotactic factor is similar to the platelet-derived growth factor in its physical properties and in the lack of effect of inhibitors of the cyclo-oxygenase pathway in preventing its release when platelets are exposed to thrombin or large concentrations of collagen[53]. It is therefore unlikely that drugs such as aspirin, indomethacin or sulfinpyrazone, which block the formation of products of arachidonic acid metabolism, would block the release of PDGF or PDCF from platelets which have adhered to the vessel wall and released their granule contents[52]. Although dipyridamole also fails to block the release of PDGF from platelets exposed to thrombin or collagen[52], it may have some action in inhibiting the adherence of platelets to collagen and the damaged vessel wall[59]. Aspirin and dipyridamole in combination inhibit intimal thickening in coronary artery venous bypass grafts in dogs[69] and veno-arterial grafts in monkeys[66].

Other factors influencing smooth muscle cell proliferation

Although the materials released from platelets play an important and probably essential part in smooth muscle cell proliferation, other factors also influence the process. There seems to be a clear requirement for another factor or factors present in serum or plasma. Serum from platelet rich plasma or whole blood stimulates growth as does a mixture of material released from washed platelets and platelet poor plasma. Either of these alone do not stimulate growth. If the concentration of the material released from platelets is kept constant in the growth medium in the presence of increasing concentrations of platelet poor serum, a dose response effect can be demonstrated[53]. Similarly, an increasing concentration of material released from platelets in the presence of a fixed concentration of platelet poor plasma serum causes increased stimulation of growth. Similar requirements have been shown for BALB/C 3T3 cells to grow in culture[12, 87]. PDGF makes cells quiescent in culture competent to respond to factors in platelet poor plasma serum, termed progression factors[120]. Somatomedin-C and other factors present in Somatomedin-C deficient plasma are required[12].

Since the discovery of the important part played by PDGF in neointimal proliferation, the role of other growth factors has been explored. Two of these are of potential importance in atherogenesis. Endothelium derived growth factor (EDGF) is formed by endothelial cells in culture, whether these are proliferating or in a stationary phase[33]. Because it can be produced in serum free medium it may be important in modulating the proliferation of smooth muscle cells under the regenerated endothelium of the neointima formed in response to injury. Peritoneal macrophages or monocytes stimulated by endotoxin or Concanavalin A release a factor which stimulates smooth muscle cell as well as fibroblast proliferation[36]. It is attractive to speculate that, since macrophages are numerous in the surface areas of organizing thrombi, they may stimulate the proliferation of smooth muscle cells which organize the mass. In this they would then play a part analogous to their stimulation of fibroblast proliferation in granulation tissue[19].

Another factor which may have a role in intimal proliferation is Factor VIII-von Willebrand factor. The mechanism which may inhibit plaque formation in hemophiliacs is decreased adherence of platelets to the subendothelium[10, 32]. Segments of rabbit aorta, denuded of endothelium and everted on glass rods in a perfusion chamber, accumulate fewer platelets when the system is exposed to blood from patients with von Willebrand's disease[116]. The adhesion is flow dependent with fewer platelets adhering at higher shear rates. It has been reported that pigs with von Willebrand's disease are resistant to diet-induced atherosclerosis[32]. The significance of this finding in relation to human disease is debatable. In general, autopsy studies have not shown any sparing of the vessels of hemophiliac patients by the atherosclerotic process[15].

The response to selective endothelial injury

One might suppose that damage or destruction of the endothelium would lead to thrombus formation. However, the response to removal of the endothelial layer with a Fogarty balloon catheter differs greatly from that seen with the more severe forms of injury induced by a polyethylene catheter or immunological injury. Possibly with these forms of injury a deeper lesion is induced and elements of the coagulation process are recruited in addition to platelet adherence and aggregation. Selective endothelial injury has been studied extensively[3, 4, 40, 76, 83, 90, 100, 110] since the original description by Baumgartner and Studer[5]. Another approach to selective endothelial injury has been to cause air drying of the endothelium of the rat carotid artery[27].

The sequence of events has been well described by a number of workers and the findings are entirely reproducible and similar in different species of animals. The balloon removes the endothelium and presumably any myointimal cells which might be present in the intima. In rabbits myointimal cells are few and in some arterial segments are absent. This exposes the basement membrane, some fragments of collagen and the microfibrils of the elastica. Examination of the surface 10 minutes after endothelial denudation shows a monolayer of platelets interrupted at intervals by small aggregates of platelets. It is probable that the latter occur in relation to fibrils of collagen. However, the aggregates rapidly disappear, presumably being swept away in the blood stream. The remaining carpet of platelets spread themselves over the surface and appear to degranulate.

The kinetics of the platelet–vessel wall interaction have been examined using ^{51}Cr-labelled platelets[40]. The initial carpeting of the aortic wall by platelets involves 0.5 % of the circulating platelets. There is little further uptake and the initially adherent platelets begin to detach from the surface. By four days there is an incomplete cover and by seven days only occasional platelets are seen. The development of a technique to examine 2 cm lengths of the rabbit aorta by scanning electron microscopy[92] has revealed that following balloon removal of the endothelium there is an area distal to the origin of branch vessels where very few or no platelets adhere to the surface[93]. On the distal rim of the vessel orifice platelet–fibrin thrombus is seen. A second balloon injury two weeks following the first results in a different pattern of formed element accumulation. Platelet–fibrin thrombi, arranged in linear ridges in the long axis of the vessel, are seen on a background of adherent platelets. The thrombi extend within and beyond the areas where endothelium had regenerated after the first balloon injury. Again, a ridge of platelet–fibrin thrombus occurs on the rim of the flow divider and a 'bare area' distal to this. These findings indicate that the reaction of the neointima in response to balloon removal of the surface layers differs from the reaction following the first removal of the endothelium. Fibrin formation is prominent and platelet consumption is increased. The latter is prevented by pretreatment with heparin[41]. The change in the surface appears not to be related to whether or not it has been covered by regenerated endothelium. Rather, it is flow dependent. Presumably the 'bare area' represents the effect of high shear. Thus the reaction of the neointima, whether covered by regenerated endothelium or not, is distinctly different from the reaction to the first removal of the endothelial layer. The difference relates to fibrin formation when the neointima is damaged.

Progression and regression of lesions induced by injury

The raised lipid-rich lesions which develop in response to injury caused by an indwelling aortic catheter and those which result from repeated immunological injury appear to regress rapidly when the injury stimulus is removed or is no longer active[30, 81]. The regression involves decrease in size, decrease and eventual loss of stainable lipid and calcium. During regression, increasing numbers of fatty streaks are observed. These are short lived and the final form of the lesions appears to be a fibro-musculo-elastic plaque without lipid being evident.

These findings indicate that this type of injury which is associated with repeated or continuing deposition of platelet–fibrin thrombus has the characteristics of undergoing marked regression when endothelial regeneration is permitted to occur.

The sequence of events which follows from selective injury to the endothelium is very different (*Figure 1.2*). Paradoxically this lesser injury, associated with much less thrombus deposition, is characterized by progression in both the number of

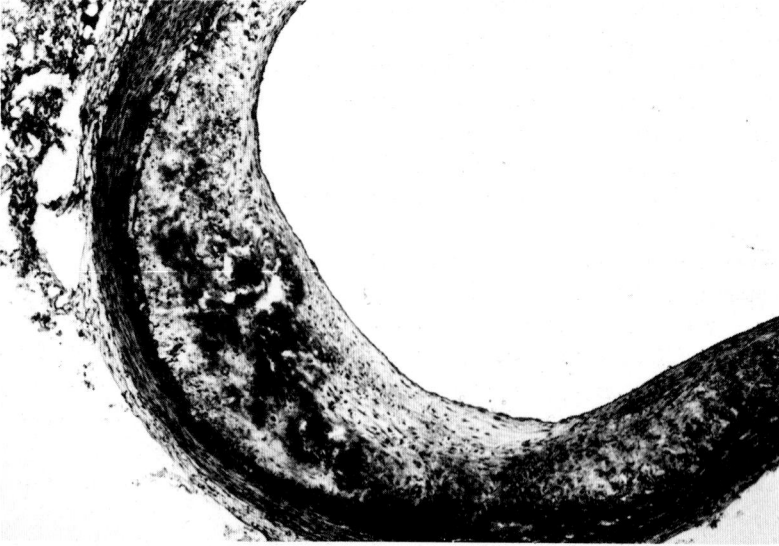

Figure 1.2 Photomicrograph of a type 2 lesion. The black material in the thickened neointima is lipid. Oil red-O stained frozen section. Enlarged approximately 2.6× from original magnification ×250

smooth muscle cells in the neointima and in the amount of lipid deposited in the tissue. At first the lesions resulting from balloon damage to the endothelium were studied in the context of repeated or multiple injuries based on the experience with the indwelling aortic catheter and repeated immunological injury in the carotid artery. In these settings continued or repeated injury had been needed for the production of raised lipid-filled lesions. When the aortas were examined at various intervals from one week to six months following six balloon removals, carried out at intervals of two weeks, lipid-rich plaques were formed in areas, mainly around branch vessels, where endothelial regeneration had occurred[76, 82]. These areas are conveniently outlined by their exclusion of Evans blue dye injected intravenously half an hour before killing the animal. The areas which remain uncovered by endothelium stain blue. When samples of the wall in white areas (covered by regenerated endothelium) and blue areas (not covered by endothelium) were stained with oil red-O, much more lipid was found in the white areas. In fact lipid, if present in the blue areas at all, which was rare, was seen in trace amounts, often confined to staining of the internal elastic lamina.

These lesions progressed over time, showing larger amounts of intra- and extracellular lipid. Eventually cholesterol clefts were seen. Because of a report showing the development of atheroma-like lesions in a small number of rabbits, two years after a single balloon removal of the endothelium and our observation of lesions with lipid in animals which did not have the full regimen of six endothelial removals, a further experiment was done. In this lesion development was compared in groups of animals examined at the same intervals after balloon removal of the endothelium whether they had one or six removals of the endothelium[79]. As estimated morphologically, lipid accumulation was similar in amount at the same time intervals following the first balloon removal of the endothelium in those which had had multiple removals as those which had had only one removal. Lesions were thicker in animals with multiple compared to those with a single balloon removal. In both groups there was, as before, much more lipid in areas of endothelial regeneration than in areas where endothelium had not regrown. White areas were also thicker than blue areas. Lesions of the abdominal aorta were thicker than those of the thoracic aorta. This finding is in keeping with kinetic studies showing greater incorporation of ^{3}H-thymidine into abdominal than into thoracic neointima following de-endothelialization of the rabbit aorta[38].

There also appeared to be a relationship between the amount of lipid accumulation in the vessel wall and the serum cholesterol level.

Although platelets adhere to the vessel wall for only a brief period following de-endothelialization, the stimulus to smooth muscle cell migration and proliferation is sustained. The requirement for platelets has been demonstrated by using purified anti-platelet serum given before balloon de-endothelialization to cause a profound thrombocytopenia. This either markedly inhibits or prevents the development of a neointima[31]. The rate of endothelial regeneration was not affected by treatment with antiplatelet serum, suggesting that platelets are not involved in the stimulus to endothelial cell replication.

The lesions following removal of the endothelial layer are progressive in terms of the deposition of lipid and the thickness of the neointima which continues to increase for 62 weeks after de-endothelialization.

There is therefore a striking difference in the evolution and development of lesions in response to mechanical or immunological injury and those which result from a simple removal of the endothelial layer. This apparently paradoxical situation, in which the more severe injury associated with abundant and continuing platelet–fibrin thrombus formation readily regresses when the injury stimulus is removed, whereas the lesser injury of endothelial removal associated with a short-lived adhesion of platelets, progresses in terms of cell proliferation and lipid accumulation raises some interesting questions.

These concern the mechanisms of the continuing stimulus to smooth muscle cell proliferation which is especially marked in the areas beneath regenerated endothelium and the mechanism of lipid accumulation which also occurs preferentially in these locations. A possible explanation for the greater thickness of the neointima covered by regenerated endothelium is the release from endothelial cells of EDGF which may modulate the process[33].

Lipid accumulation in lesions induced by injury

The accumulation of lipid in lesions induced by injury in the presence of hypercholesterolemia is well known and has been extensively documented[71]. Any type of vessel wall injury, whether it is physical, chemical, immunologically mediated or caused by virus interaction with the vessel wall, can act synergistically with hypercholesterolemia to produce lipid containing intimal plaques. Except for immunologically mediated injury the two influences must be present simultaneously. Plaques which develop in association with immune complex mediated injury can accumulate lipid if hypercholesterolemia is induced by diet after the plaques have formed. The development of lipid-rich lesions by the combination of dietary hyperlipemia and injury is not surprising. Most forms of significant arterial wall injury result in endothelial damage with the resultant migration and proliferation of smooth muscle cells to form a plaque in the intima[75]. It is perhaps not widely appreciated that dietary hypercholesterolemia causes intimal changes which precede the deposition of lipid[21]. This was clearly stated in many of the early reports of atherosclerosis induced by diet[20]. Attention was also drawn to necrosis of medial smooth muscle cells and more recently it has been shown that oxidation products of cholesterol cause vessel wall damage[55]. Increased replication of endothelial cells has been reported in association with dietary hyperlipemia and the changes are reversed when animals are returned to a normal diet[101]. Evidence of endothelial injury in association with diet-induced hyperlipemia has been sought[17, 63, 64, 85, 97, 113, 121, 125].

More recently, the possible effects of hyperlipemia on endothelial cell function and integrity have been explored in tissue culture[26, 46–48]. Low density lipoprotein (LDL) has been reported to produce progressive injury of human endothelial cells in primary culture. The injury was inhibited by the addition of high density lipoprotein (HDL). LDL may also inhibit the production of prostacyclin (PGI$_2$) by endothelial cells[86].

It appears that lipid accumulates in injury-induced lesions in normally fed rabbits in relation to regeneration of endothelium. This is particularly relevant to the accumulation of lipid in the endothelium covered neointima which develops following balloon removal of the endothelium. The mechanisms involved in the process have been the subject of much recent interest. Vlodavsky *et al.* observed that noncontact-inhibited endothelial cells bound, internalized and broke down more low density lipoprotein than confluent, contact-inhibited endothelium[119]. Newly regenerated endothelium might thus take up more lipoprotein than stable contact inhibited endothelium. Fielding proposes that endothelial cells have a receptor for chylomicrons that is not down-regulated by increasing concentration[28]. The presence of regenerated endothelium in some way modifies the lipid metabolism of the neointima. Lipid accumulation is seen consistently 11 weeks following removal of the endothelial layer and in some rabbits occurs in a matter of a few weeks. This suggests that at increased uptake by receptors or increased permeability associated with newly regenerated endothelium is not as critical as a change in the neointimal tissue, although this is probably modulated by the endothelium. One possibility is a 'reverse barrier function' of the endothelium such that low density lipoprotein which normally enters, and is to some extent concentrated in the intima[104], may not escape back into the blood stream by way of the now mature and contact inhibited endothelial layer. A relative decrease in acid cholesteryl esterase has been shown in re-endothelialized areas of rabbit aorta compared to areas remaining uncovered by endothelium[42]. Another possible mechanism contributing to the accumulation might be the synthesis of lipid in the lesions[18].

One of the striking differences between the neointima covered by regenerated endothelium and the areas which remain uncovered is the concentration of glycosaminoglycans (GAGs). This has been demonstrated histochemically,

chemically[122], and by morphometric study of granules positively stained by ruthenium red on electron microscopy[94]. Ruthenium red stains the glycosamino-glycan units of the proteoglycan molecules. Two types of granules are observed: small granules (20 nm) occur mainly in the subendothelial basement membrane and large granules (20–50 nm) occur in the intercellular matrix of the neointima and in the media of the normal vessel wall. The small granules are thought to represent heparan sulphate and may have an important role in regulating permeability[58]. The large granules are chondroitin and/or dermatan sulphate. These GAGs can bind low density lipoproteins to form complexes[8, 9, 56, 57].

Compared to normal aortas there was an increase in large granule content in the re-endothelialized areas and a decrease in large and small granules in the non-endothelialized areas. This is consistent with the concept that LDL which enters the intima is trapped, presumably at first in the interstitial tissue and later in the smooth muscle cells. In *in vitro* studies the formation of GAG–LDL complexes is inhibited and complexes already formed are dissociated by the addition of high density lipoprotein[8]. Since LDL is normally in somewhat higher levels in the intima than plasma[105], indicating a concentration mechanism, the loss of endothelial cover possibly allows for egress of this material from the vessel wall to the blood stream. Possibly GAG formed in the neointima uncovered by endothelium may more readily diffuse into the blood stream, carrying with it LDL that may have entered from the blood[11]. The complexes of LDL and GAG would then be presumably removed by the reticulo-endothelial system.

Areas of the aorta of white Carneau pigeons which spontaneously develop atherosclerosis show a selective increase in chondroitin 4-sulphate[14]. GAG–LDL complexes have been found in extracts of human atheromatous aortas[16, 34, 106, 107, 123] and in dietarily induced atheroma in monkeys and rats[89, 118]. Increase in GAG content paralleled the accumulation of lipid. Thus, it seems that in most types of spontaneously occurring atherosclerosis or those induced by diet or injury there are GAG–LDL complexes. An exception is the reported decrease in glycosaminoglycans in advanced human disease[111]. Future research should determine whether increase in GAG concentration precedes, accompanies or follows lipid accumulation in lesions in the various experimental settings.

Recently we have explored these relationships in an experiment employing an indwelling polyethylene catheter in the rabbit aorta[83]. In this system raised lipid-rich lesions develop quickly and regress when the catheter is withdrawn. Stainable lipid disappears from the lesions so that the final form is an intimal thickening, covered by endothelium and composed of smooth muscle cells and connective tissue. Catheters were left in place in rabbit aortas for three weeks and then withdrawn. Animals were killed at this time, and at four and eight weeks after catheter removal. Tissues from various types of lesions were taken from the perfusion-fixed aortas and processed for electron microscopy, the sections being stained with ruthenium red. In early lesions associated with organizing thrombus there was little or no GAG in association with lipid containing macrophages in the surface part of the lesions. Deeper, around smooth muscle cells, there was an increased content of GAG. In later lesions, characterized by lipid in the interstitium and in the smooth muscle cells, the GAG content of the intercellular space was markedly increased. When lesions had regressed to non-lipid containing plaques their content of GAG was reduced below normal. These findings again show the close association between GAG content and lipid accumulation extra-cellularly and in smooth muscle cells. They are consistent with the notion that GAG may act to trap LDL but do not prove that GAG accumulation is causative.

More research on this aspect of lipid accumulation in the vessel wall is needed. Perhaps the relationship can be explored in a controlled fashion, using tissue culture, addressing the question of possible modulation of smooth muscle cell synthetic activity in the presence of endothelium or endothelial cell conditioned media. Experiments such as those recently reported by Merilees and Scott[69] may provide further insight into the mechanisms involved. They found that co-cultivation of aortic endothelial cells and smooth muscle cells resulted in marked increase in hyaluronic acid levels and a lesser increase in sulphated GAG levels compared with separate culture of the two cell types. Culture of smooth muscle cells in aortic endothelial cell conditioned medium produced similar changes; smooth muscle cell conditioned medium had no effect on the GAG production by endothelial cells. This suggests that endothelial cells have a regulating influence on GAG production by smooth muscle cells and provides an explanation for the increased GAG production in the endothelium covered neointima which may then trap LDL leading to progressive lipid accumulation.

Two types of response of the arterial wall to injury

As described above there are two types of reaction of the arterial wall to injury (*Figure 1.3*). Although these have many similarities, viz. smooth muscle cell proliferation, lipid accumulation and interactions of platelets with the denuded vessel wall, there are also striking differences. One occurs only in response to a

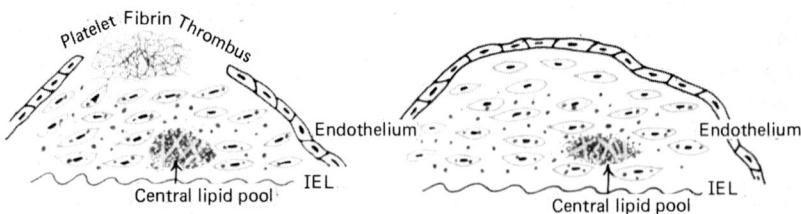

Figure 1.3 Diagram of type 1 (*left*) and type 2 lesions

continuing or repeated injury, is characterized by the formation of platelet–fibrin thrombus, the rapid development of raised lipid filled lesions and rapid regression when the injury stimulus is withdrawn.

The other occurs as a result of selective damage to only the endothelial layer, is characterized by a slight and transitory interaction of platelets with the vessel wall, by a slow development and progressive deposition of lipid. Both lesions can be inhibited or prevented by the removal of most of the circulating platelets[31, 78, 80].

Both lesions show some increase in free cholesterol and marked increases in cholesteryl ester. While some element of lipid synthesis is present in both lesions, a possibly more significant mechanism may be binding of LDL to GAG in the interstitium of the neointima. If this is so, the reasons why GAG persists in one type of lesion while decreasing below normal levels in the other type need further investigation.

An understanding of the mechanisms of development of these two types of lesions is important in understanding the progression of atherosclerosis. Leaving aside the question of whether injury mechanisms play a key part in the genesis of lesions, the reaction to established lesions may be better understood by appreciating the response to formed platelet–fibrin thrombus in the one instance and reaction to the deposition of a small number of platelets, and in the case of repeated injury of some fibrin in the other. Morphological studies have strongly indicated that one way that established atheromatous lesions grow is by incorporation of thrombus into the plaque[75].

From what we know of organizing thrombus and from study of the type of lesion that develops in response to continuing or repeated injury associated with thrombus formation, it is possible to speculate that this increase in the mass of the plaque might be associated with lipid deposition only in the early phase of the reaction, with later loss of lipid from the new or superficial portion of the thickened intima. This might account for the often observed presence of a thick fibrous cap in human atheromas with a very deeply placed central lipid pool[115], the latter presumably related to the early development of the lesion.

Similarly, in the lesion developing from an injury or from injuries mainly involving the endothelial layer, lipid accumulation would persist as in the human fibrous plaque. If, in the course of time, such a lesion were to disrupt superficially thus inducing abundant thrombus formation, lipid might be seen near the surface of the plaque shortly after the event, but would be lost later, resulting again in the development of a fibrous cap. Various combinations of events could then explain why some atheromas show several strata of fibrous material and lipid.

A better understanding of these events is clearly of importance in deciding on the possible or probable outcomes of therapy directed to preventing the development of a completed stroke and the possible sequelae of surgical attack on atheromatous lesions of the carotid arterial system. The occurrence of amaurosis fugax or transient ischemic attacks in association with atheromatous disease of the carotid arteries is well established[60]. It is also known that these clinical events presage a definable risk for the development of a brain infarct. Since it is known that amaurosis fugax and transient ischemic attacks are associated with embolism of platelet aggregates and atheromatous debris and brain infarcts with embolism of formed platelet–fibrin thrombus, the kind of thrombus formation occurring on the surface of a plaque may determine the outcome. Stroke may occur in the absence of premonitory embolism of platelet aggregates.

The precursor to embolism from a carotid atheroma is probably disruption of the plaque with exposure of the plaque contents to the flowing blood. This may be followed by blood dissecting into the plaque, thus enlarging its volume and thus further narrowing or blocking the lumen. Exposure of collagen in the fibrous cap causes platelets to aggregate and undergo the release reaction. Thromboxane A_2 released from the forming platelet or thrombus mass may cause spasm of the vessel[24]. Possibly thromboxane A_2 released from platelet masses which have embolized into the microcirculation of the brain may cause spasm of the small arteries. Lodgement of a large embolus composed of platelet–fibrin thrombus in a supplying vessel such as the middle cerebral artery or one of its branches may cause brain infarct. Removal of some or all of the atheroma inevitably exposes the flowing blood to thrombogenic materials in the plaque or in the arterial wall, especially collagen[3, 4, 50, 51]. This may mean that therapy directed to modifying the thrombotic process may be useful.

Human examples of atheroma developing in response to injury

Attempts to modify the initial stages and progression of the disease will depend on better understanding of the biological reactions of the vessel wall to injury. This pre-supposes that injury is a key player in atherogenesis. So far, in this chapter, experimental evidence for this has been explored. There are a number of clinical observations which support the idea that injury may be an important factor.

Individuals who suffer from homocystinemia develop precocious and extensive thrombosis in arteries and veins and rapidly develop atherosclerosis. This relationship has been explored experimentally by Harker *et al.*, who demonstrated multifocal areas of endothelial denudation in the large arterial vessels in baboons receiving chronic intravenous infusions of homocystine[43]. This was associated with a decrease in platelet survival, restored by treatment with dipyridamole, which also inhibited the development of proliferative lesions occurring in response to endothelial injury.

Arterial intimal thickenings, rich in foam cells, are seen in the late rejection of transplanted organs[70]. In the case of heart transplantation there is evidence that their occurrence does not relate closely to the presence or absence of hypercholesterolemia[6]. Alonso, Starek and Minick have shown the development of severe atherosclerosis in cardiac allografts of hypercholesterolemic rabbits[1]. Sharma and Geer have shown that early aortic lesions in rabbits due to serum sickness are characterized by endothelial damage, presumably induced by antigen–antibody complexes, followed by platelet deposition[102].

There is evidence from old autopsy studies that atherosclerosis is more severe in autopsy material from subjects who die following infections or with immunologically mediated diseases such as rheumatic fever[98, 99, 126]. The association of tertiary syphilis with advanced atherosclerotic disease of the proximal aorta is well known[99]. Similarly, the premature development of atherosclerosis in association with lupus erythematosus has been recorded[91].

Diabetes mellitus provides a number of insights into mechanisms which may favour the development of atherosclerosis in response to injury[77]. Antibodies to insulin might facilitate endothelial injury by antigen–antibody complexes.

Ledet has shown that serum from juvenile diabetics is more stimulatory to smooth muscle cell proliferation than serum from age-matched controls[61]. The factor which causes this is probably growth hormone[62]. There is also some evidence that insulin may facilitate smooth muscle cell proliferation as well as the synthesis of cholesterol and other lipids by arterial wall tissue[112]. In relation to trapping of LDL by glycosaminoglycans previously discussed, there is evidence of alteration of glycosaminoglycan metabolism in the arterial wall in diabetes. In the coronary arteries of diabetic dogs dermatan sulphate, which has a high binding activity for LDL, is increased in relation to other glycosaminoglycans[103]. There is an extensive literature on increased platelet reactivity in diabetics[13].

Further evidence comes from experience with various surgical procedures on vessels. Veins transplanted into arterial systems develop intimal thickenings and in some of these the accumulation of lipid results in lesions described as atheromatous[2, 7, 25]. This is seen in transplants into peripheral vessels and in aorto–coronary venous bypass grafts. Plaques which significantly narrow the lumen may develop in the artery at the point of venous–arterial anastomosis[65]. It is not clear why the lesion is more severe in the arterial than in the venous segment. Undoubtedly the surgical procedure and the resulting hemodynamic influences cause or promote endothelial injury at and close to the point of anastomosis in the artery. Possibly the larger population of smooth muscle cells in the arterial wall provides a larger pool of cells available to migrate and proliferate than are available in the vein wall.

Atherosclerotic changes also develop in the vein wall at the site of insertion of arterio–venous dialysis shunts[108, 109]. There is a large build-up of platelet–fibrin thrombus which may occlude the channel requiring shunt revision. Examination of venous segments removed at shunt revision show marked intimal thickening with luminal thrombus. Oil red-O stains of frozen sections reveal abundant lipid in the intimal plaques. Foam cells are often seen and, more rarely, cholesterol clefts. The lesions are similar to those produced experimentally[77].

In neonatal intensive care units catheters are frequently placed in the aorta by way of an umbilical artery to monitor blood gases. Lesions produced in the arterial wall resemble the range of lesions that we have observed following the intra-aortic placement of catheters in rabbits[117].

Thus, there seems to be good evidence that injury to the endothelium of chemical, immunological or mechanical nature produces atheroma-like lesions in human arteries.

Implications of the injury hypothesis of atherogenesis for atherosclerosis in man

The evidence from animal experimentation and from certain clinical settings in which vascular injury occurs make it clear that endothelial and/or intimal injury could serve as initiators of atherosclerosis or lead to progression of established disease. This still leaves uncertainty as to what agent or agents could cause the injury in man. There is no lack of candidates. Viruses, antigen–antibody complexes, anti-endothelial antibodies, 'toxic' damage to endothelium from chemical agents, hyperlipidemia and possibly other agents, now not recognized as being injurious may act singly or in combination. The experimental techniques which damage large areas of the endothelial lining and are not completely specific or selective for endothelial cells may have no counterpart in the early lesions of the human disease. It has been shown that very small areas of injury involving an area encompassing several endothelial cells can heal readily by cell spreading or by a combination of cell spreading and replication within a very short period of time[44]. Because, presumably, smooth muscle cells have not migrated into the small focus of injury, no plaque develops. One would therefore have to think in terms of repeated injury as an appropriate stimulus.

However, the situation may differ in the case of established atheromatous lesions where it is possible that, for example, plaque disruption could cause loss of endothelial cover over a large territory. From what we know about the differing responses to injury outlined above, it would be likely that such an event would be associated with the formation of abundant platelet–fibrin thrombus, carrying with it not only the danger of embolization of forming or formed thrombus, but also the capability of resolution by organization.

SUMMARY AND CONCLUSIONS

Recent experimental work and thinking on the problem of atherogenesis supports the concept that injury and the thrombosis associated with injury play a key part in initiation and progression of lesions. Recent work on the mechanism of lipid accumulation in lesions provides, as a working hypothesis, that the neointima covered by regenerated endothelium serves as a trap or sink for lipid deposition. Changes in enzyme activity of the cells of the neointima and in the concentration of proteoglycans in the ground substance may be important in the process. Specifically, binding of low density lipoproteins to the glycosaminoglycan moieties of the proteoglycan molecules suggests a relationship between injury and hyperlipemia in lesion progression. It also provides an explanation for the benefit of an increase in circulating high density lipoprotein in relation to low density lipoprotein. Lastly, the recognition of two types of response of the arterial wall to injury gives insight into progression and regression of lesions.

References

1 ALONSO, D. R., STAREK, P. K. and MINICK, C. R. Studies on the pathogenesis of atheroarteriosclerosis induced in rabbit cardiac allografts by the synergy of graft rejection and hypercholesterolemia. *American Journal of Pathology*, **87**, 415–422 (1977)

2 BARBORIAK, J. J., PINTAR, K. and KORNS, M. F. Atherosclerosis in aortocoronary vein grafts. *Lancet*, **2**, 621–627 (1974)

3 BAUMGARTNER, H. R. Platelet interaction with collagen. 1. Reaction of human platelets with α-chymotrypsin-digested subendothelium. *Thrombosis and Haemostasis*, **37**, 1–16 (1977)

4 BAUMGARTNER, H. R. Platelet interaction with vascular structures. *Thrombosis and Haemostasis*, **51**, (Suppl.) 161–176 (1972)

5 BAUMGARTNER, H. R. and STUDER, A. Gezielte uberdehung der aorta abdominalis am normo und hypercholesterinaemischen kanninchen. *Pathologie et Microbiologie* (Basel) **26**, 129–148 (1963)

6 BIEBER, C. P., STINSON, E. B., SHUMWAY, N. E., PAYNE, R. and KOSEK, J. Cardiac transplantation in man: cardiac allograft pathology. *Circulation*, **41**, 753–772 (1970)

7 BEBBE, H. G., CLARK, W. F. and DeWEESE, J. A. Atherosclerotic change occurring in an autogenous vein arterial graft. *Archives of Surgery*, **101**, 85–88 (1970)

8 BIHARI-VARGA, M. Influence of serum high density lipoproteins on the low density lipoprotein–aortic glycosaminoglycan interactions. *Artery*, **4**, 504–511 (1978)

9 BIHARI-VARGA, M. and VEGH, M. Quantitative studies on the complexes formed between aortic mucopolysaccharides and serum lipoproteins. *Biochimica Biophysica Acta*, **144**, 202–210 (1967)

10 BOWIE, E. J. W., FUSTER, V., FASS, D. N. and OWEN, C. A. Jr. The role of Willebrand factor in platelet–blood vessel interaction, including a discussion of resistance to atherosclerosis in pigs with von Willebrand's disease. *Philosophical Transactions of the Royal Society London, Series B*, **294**, 267–279 (1981)

11 CAPURSO, A., PACE, L., RESTA, F., RISO, V., DiMONTE, D. and BONOMA, L. Possible role of glycosaminoglycans in reducing the uptake of human lipoproteins by the arterial wall. *Pharmacological Research Communications*, **11**, 311–322 (1979)

12 CLEMMONS, D. R., VAN WYCK, J. J. and PLEDGER, W. J. Sequential addition of platelet factor and plasma to BALB/C-3T3 fibroblast cultures stimulates somatomedin-C binding early in cell cycle. *Proceedings of the National Academy of Science USA*, **77**, 6644–6648 (1980)

13 COLWELL, J. A., HALUSHKA, P. V., SARJI, K. E. and SAGEL, J. Platelet function and diabetes mellitus. *Medical Clinics of North America*, **62**, 757–760 (1978)

14 CURWEN, K. D. and SMITH, S. C. Aortic glycosaminoglycans in atherosclerosis susceptible and resistant pigeons. *Experimental and Molecular Pathology*, **27**, 121–133 (1977)

15 DALDORF, F. C., TAYLOR, R. E. and BLATT, P. M. Arteriosclerosis in severe hemophilia: a postmortem study. *Archives of Pathology and Laboratory Medicine*, **105**, 652–654 (1981)

16 DALFERES, E. R. Jr, RUIZ, H., KUMAR, V., RADAKRISHNAMURTHY, B. and BERENSON, G. S. Acid mucopolysaccharides of fatty streaks in young human male aortas. *Atherosclerosis*, **13**, 121–131 (1971)

17 DAVIES, P. F., REIDY, M. A., GOODE, T. B. and BOWYER, D. E. Scanning electron microscopy in the evaluation of endothelial integrity of fatty lesions in atherosclerosis. *Atherosclerosis*, **25**, 125–130 (1976)

18 DAY, A. J., BELL, F. P., MOORE, S. and FRIEDMAN, R. J. Lipid composition and metabolism of thrombo-atherosclerotic lesions produced by continued endothelial damage in normal rabbits. *Circulation Research*, **34**, 467–476 (1974)

19 De LUSTRO, F., SHERER, G. K. and LEROY, E. C. Human monocyte stimulation of fibroblast growth by a soluble mediator(s). *Journal of the Reticuloendothelial Society*, **28**, 519–532 (1980)

20 DUFF, G. I.. Experimental cholesterol atherosclerosis and its relationship to human atherosclerosis. *Archives of Pathology and Laboratory Medicine*, **20**, 80–124, 259–304 (1935)

21 DUFF, G. L., McMILLAN, G. C. and RITCHIE, A. C. The morphology of early atherosclerotic lesions of the aorta demonstrated by the surface technique in rabbits fed cholesterol. *American Journal of Pathology*, **33**, 845–874 (1957)

22 DUGUID, J. B. Thrombosis as a factor in the pathogenesis of coronary atherosclerosis. *Journal of Pathology and Bacteriology*, **58**, 207–212 (1946)

23 DUGUID, J. B. Thrombosis as a factor in the pathogenesis of aortic atherosclerosis. *Journal of Pathology and Bacteriology*, **60**, 57–61 (1948)

24 ELLIS, E. F., NIES, A. S. and OATES, J. A. Cerebral arterial smooth muscle cell contraction by thromboxane A_2. *Stroke*, **8**, 480–483 (1977)

25 ERJUP, B., MERTON, T. and MOBERG, A. Atheromatous changes in autogenous vein grafts. Functional and anatomic aspects: case report. *Acta Chirurgica Scandinavica*, **121**, 211–218 (1977)

26 EVENSEN, S. A. Injury to cultured endothelial cells: the role of lipoproteins and thrombo-active agents. *Haemostasis*, **8**, 203–210 (1979)

27 FISHMAN, J. A., RYAN, G. B. and KARNOVSKY, M. J. Endothelial regeneration in the rat carotid artery and the significance of endothelial denudation in the pathogenesis of myo-intimal thickening. *Laboratory Investigation*, **32**, 339–351 (1975)

28 FIELDING, C. J. Metabolism of cholesterol-rich chylomicrons. Mechanism of binding and uptake of cholesteryl esters by the vascular bed of the perfused heart. *Journal of Clinical Investigation*, **62**, 141–151 (1978)

29 FRIEDMAN, R. J., MOORE, S. and SINGAL, D. P. Repeated endothelial injury and induction of atherosclerosis in normolipemic rabbits. *Laboratory Investigation*, **30**, 404–415 (1975)

30 FRIEDMAN, R. J., MOORE, S., SINGAL, D. P. and GENT, M. Regression injury-induced atheromatous lesions in rabbits. *Archives of Pathology and Laboratory Medicine*, **100**, 185–195 (1976)

31 FRIEDMAN, R. J., STEMERMAN, M. B., WENZ, B., MOORE, S., GAULDIE, J., GENT, M., TIELL, M. L. and SPAET, T. H. The effect of thrombocytopenia on experimental arteriosclerotic lesion formation in rabbits. 1. Smooth muscle cell proliferation and re-endothelialization. *Journal of Clinical Investigation*, **60**, 1191–1201 (1977)

32 FUSTER, V., BOWIE, E. J. W., LEWIS, J. C., FASS, D. N. and OWEN, C. A. Jr. Resistance to arteriosclerosis in pigs with von Willebrand's disease: spontaneous and high cholesterol diet-induced arteriosclerosis. *Journal of Clinical Investigation*, **61**, 722–730 (1978)

33 GAJDUSEK, C., DiCORLETO, P., ROSS, R. and SCHWARTZ, S. An endothelial–cell derived growth factor. *Journal of Cell Biology*, **85**, 467–472 (1980)

34 GERO, S., GERGELY, J., DEVENYI, T., JAKAB, L., SZEKELY, J. and VIRAG, S. Role of mucoid substances of the aorta in the deposition of lipids. *Nature*, **187**, 152–153 (1960)

35 GERRITY, R. G. The role of the monocyte in atherogenesis. 1. Transition of blood borne monocytes into foam cells in fatty lesions. *American Journal of Pathology*, **103**, 181–190 (1981)

36 GLENN, K. and ROSS, R. Human monocyte-derived growth factor(s) for mesenchymal cells: activation of secretion by endotoxin and Concanavalin A (Con A). *Cell*, **25**, 603–615 (1981)

37 GOLDBERG, I. D., STEMERMAN, M. B. and HANDIN, R. I. Vascular permeation of platelet factor-4 after endothelial injury. *Science*, **209**, 611–612 (1980)

38 GOLDBERG, I. D., STEMERMAN, M. B., RANSIL, B. J. and FUHRO, R. L. *In vivo* aortic muscle cell growth kinetics: differences between thoracic and abdominal segments after intimal injury in the rabbit. *Circulation Research*, **47**, 182–189 (1980)

39 GROTENDORST, G. R., SEPPA, H. E. J., KLEINMAN, H. K. and MARTIN, G. R. Attachment of smooth muscle cells to collagen and their migration toward platelet derived growth factor. *Proceedings of the National Academy of Science USA*, **78**, 3669–3672 (1981)

40 GROVES, H. M., KINLOUGH-RATHBONE, R. L., RICHARDSON, M., MOORE, S. and MUSTARD, J. F. Platelet interaction with damaged rabbit aorta. *Laboratory Investigation*, **40**, 194–200 (1979)

41 GROVES, H. M., KINLOUGH-RATHBONE, R. L., RICHARDSON, M., JORGENSEN, L., MOORE, S. and MUSTARD, J. F. Thrombin generation and fibrin formation following injury to rabbit neointima: studies of vessel wall reactivity and platelet survival. *Laboratory Investigation*, **46**, 603–612 (1982)

42 HAJJAR, D. P., FALCONE, D. J., FOWLER, S. and MINICK, C. R. Endothelium modifies the altered metabolism of the injured aortic wall. *American Journal of Pathology*, **102**, 28–39 (1981)

43 HARKER, L. A., ROSS, R., SLICHTER, J. and SCOTT, C. R. Homocystine induced arteriosclerosis. *Journal of Clinical Investigation*, **58**, 763–741 (1976)

44 HAUDENSCHILD, C. C. and SCHWARTZ, S. M. Endothelial regeneration. II. Restitution of endothelial continuity. *Laboratory Investigation*, **41**, 407–418 (1979)

45 HAUST, M. D. The morphogenesis and fate of potential and early atherosclerotic lesions in man. *Human Pathology*, **2**, 1–29 (1971)

46 HENDRIKSEN, T., EVENSEN, S. A. and CARLANDER, B. Injury to human endothelial cells in culture induced by low density lipoproteins. *Scandinavian Journal of Clinical and Laboratory Investigation*, **39**, 361–368 (1979)

47 HENDRIKSEN, T., EVENSEN, S. A. and CARLANDER, B. Injury to cultured endothelial cells induced by low density lipoproteins – protection by high density lipoproteins. *Scandinavian Journal of Clinical and Laboratory Investigation*, **39**, 369–375 (1979)

48 HESSLER, J. R., ROBERTSON, A. L. and CHISOLM, G. M. LDL-induced cytotoxicity and its inhibition by HDL in human vascular smooth muscle and endothelial cells in culture. *Atherosclerosis*, **32**, 219–229 (1979)

49 HOLMAN, R. L., McGILL, H. C., STRONG, J. P. and GEER, J. C. The natural history of atherosclerosis. The early aortic lesions as seen in New Orleans in the middle of the 20th Century. *American Journal of Pathology*, **34**, 209–235 (1958)

50 HOVIG, T. Aggregation of rabbit blood platelets produced *in vitro* by saline 'extract' of tendons. *Thrombosis et Diathesis Haemorrhagica*, **9**, 248–263 (1963)

51 HUGUES, J. Accolement des plaquettes aux structures conjonctives perivasculaires. *Thombosis Diath. Haemorrhag*, **8**, 141–255 (1962)

52 IHNATOWYCZ, I. O., CAZENAVE, J. P., MUSTARD, J. F. and MOORE, S. Effect of indometha-cin, sulfinpyrazone and dipyridamole on the release of the platelet derived growth factor. *Thrombosis Research*, **14**, 311–321 (1979)

53 IHNATOWYCZ, I. O., CAZENAVE, J. P., MUSTARD, J. F. and MOORE, S. The effect of a platelet derived growth factor on the proliferation of rabbit arterial smooth muscle cells in tissue culture. *Thombosis Research*, **14**, 477–487 (1979)

54 IHNATOWYCZ, I. O., WINOCOUR, P. D. and MOORE, S. A platelet-derived factor chemo-tactic for rabbit arterial smooth muscle cells in culture. *Artery*, **9**, 316–327 (1981)

55 IMAI, H., WERTHESSEN, N. T., TAYLOR, B. and LEE, K. T. Angiotoxicity and arterioscler-osis due to contaminants of USP-grade cholesterol. *Archives of Pathology and Laboratory Medicine*, **100**, 565–572 (1976)

56 IVERIUS, P. H. The interaction between human plasma lipoproteins and connective tissue glycosaminoglycans. *Journal of Biological Chemistry*, **247**, 2607–2613 (1972)

57 IVERIUS, P. H. Possible role of glycosaminoglycans in the genesis of atheroscler-osis. In *Atherogenesis: Initiating Factors*. Ciba Symposium, 12, Amsterdam, Elsevier, North Holland Co (1973)

58 KANWAR, Y. S. and FARQHAR, M. G. Isolation of glycosaminoglycans (heparan sulphate) from glomerular basement membranes. *Proceedings of the National Academy of Science USA*, **76**, 4493–4497 (1979)

59 KINLOUGH-RATHBONE, R. L., GROVES, H. M., CAZENAVE, J. P., RICHARDSON, M. and MUSTARD, J. F. Effect of dipyridamole and aspirin on platelet adherence to damaged rabbit aorta. *Federation Proceedings*, **37**, 260 (1978) (abstract)

60 KISHORE, P. S. The significance of the ulcerative plaque. *Radiology Clinics of North America*, **12**, 343–352 (1974)

61 LEDET, T. Growth of rabbit aortic smooth muscle cells in serum from patients with juvenile diabetes. *Acta Pathologica et Microbiologica Scandinavica Section A*, **84**, 508–516 (1976)

62 LEDET, T. Diabetic macroangiopathy and growth hormone. *Diabetes*, **30** (Suppl. 2) 14–17 (1981)

63 LEWIS, J. C. and KOTTKE, B. A. Endothelial damage and thrombocyte adhesion in pigeon atherosclerosis. *Science*, **196**, 1007–1009 (1977)

64 MACA, R. D. and HOAK, J. C. Endothelial injury and platelet aggregation associated with acute lipid mobilization. *Laboratory Investigation*, **30**, 589–595 (1974)

65 MADRAS, P. N., WARD, C. A., JOHNSON, W. R. and SINGH, P. I. Anastomotic hyperplasia. *Surgery*, **90**, 922–923 (1981)

66 McCANN, R. L., HAGEN, P. O. and FUCHS, J. C. A. Aspirin and dipyridamole decrease intimal hyperplasia in experimental vein grafts. *Annals of Surgery*, **191**, 238–243 (1980)

67 McGILL, H. C. In *The Geographic Pathology of Atherosclerosis*, edited by H. C. McGill. The Williams and Wilkins Co., Baltimore, Md. (1968)

68 MERRILEES, M. J. and SCOTT, L. Interaction of aortic, endothelial and smooth muscle cells in culture: effect on glycosaminoglycan levels. *Atherosclerosis*, **39**, 147–161 (1981)

69 METKE, M. P., LIE, J. T., FUSTED, V., JOSA, M. and KAYE, M. P. Reduction of intimal thickening in canine coronary bypass vein grafts with dipyridamole and aspirin. *American Journal of Cardiology*, **43**, 1144–1148 (1979)

70 MINICK, C. R. Immunologic arterial injury in atherogenesis. *Annals of the New York Academy of Science*, **275**, 210–227 (1976)

71 MINICK, C. R. Synergy of arterial injury and hypercholesterolemia in atherogenesis. In *Injury Mechanisms in Atherosclerosis*, edited by S. Moore. Marcel Dekker, New York (1981)

72 MOORE, S. Plaque lipid: an expression of endothelial damage. *Circulation*, **44–II**, 23 (1971) (abstract)

73 MOORE, S. Thromboatherosclerosis in normolipemic rabbits: a result of continued endothelial damage. *Laboratory Investigation*, **29**, 478–487 (1973)

74 MOORE, S. Thrombosis and atherosclerosis. *Thrombosis and Haemostasis*, **60** (Suppl.) 205–212 (1974)

75 MOORE, S. Atherosclerosis. In *Animal Models of Thrombosis and Hemorrhagic Diseases*. Department of Health, Education and Welfare Publication No. (N.I.H.)72–962. Washington, D.C. USA (1976)

76 MOORE, S. Endothelial injury and atherosclerosis. *Experimental and Molecular Pathology*, **31**, 182–190 (1979)

77 MOORE, S. Responses of the arterial wall to injury. *Diabetes*, **30** (Suppl.) 8–13 (1981)

78 MOORE, S., BELBECK, L. W. and GAULDIE, J. Thrombocytopenia induced by Busulphan and antiplatelet serum inhibits aortic lesions caused by injury. *Circulation*, **56–III**, 120 (1977)

79 MOORE, S., BELBECK, L. W., RICHARDSON, M. and TAYLOR, W. Lipid accumulation in the neointima formed in normal-fed rabbits in response to one or six removals of the aortic endothelium. *Laboratory Investigation*, **47**, 32–42 (1982)

80 MOORE, S., FRIEDMAN, R. J., SINGAL, D. P., GAULDIE, J., BLAJCHAMN, M. A. and ROBERTS, R. J. Inhibition of injury-induced thromboatherosclerotic lesions by antiplatelet serum in rabbits. *Thrombosis and Haemostasis*, **35**, 70–81 (1976)

81 MOORE, S., FRIEDMAN, R. J. and GENT, M. Resolution of lipid-containing atherosclerotic lesions induced by injury. *Blood Vessels*, **14**, 193–203 (1977)

82 MOORE, S. and IHNATOWYCZ, I. O. Vessel injury and atherosclerosis. In *Thrombosis: Animal and Clinical Models*, edited by H. James Day, Basil A. Molony, Edward E. Nishizawa and Ronald H. Rynbrant. Plenum Publishing Corporation, New York (1978)

83 MOORE, S. and RICHARDSON, M. Glycosaminoglycan (GAG) distribution in catheter induced lesions in rabbit aortae in relation to lipid accumulation. *Thrombosis and Haemostasis*, **478**, 221 (1981) (abstract 696)

84 NATIONAL INSTITUTES OF HEALTH. Arteriosclerosis: a report by the National Heart and Lung Institute Task Force on Arteriosclerosis. Vol. 2. Department of Health, Education and Welfare Publication No. 72–219. Government Printing Office, Washington, D.C. (1971)

85 NELSON, E., GETZ, S. D., RENNELS, M. L., FORBES, M. S., KAHN, M. A., HEALD, F. P. and EARL, F. L. Endothelial lesions in the aorta of egg yolk-fed miniature swine: a study by

scanning and transmission electron microscopy. *Experimental and Molecular Pathology*, **25**, 208–220 (1976)

86 NORDOY, A. The interaction of lipids, platelets and endothelial cells in thrombogenesis. *Acta Medica Scandinavica*, **642** (Suppl.) 113–120 (1980)

87 PLEDGER, W. J., STILES, C. D., ANTONIADES, H. N. and SCHER, C. D. Induction of DNA synthesis in BALB/C-3T3 cells by serum components: re-evaluation of the commitment process. *Proceedings of the National Academy of Science USA*, **74**, 4481–4485 (1977)

88 PRATHAP, P. The morphology of two-year healed platelet-rich thrombi in femoral arteries of normocholesterolaemic monkeys: light and electron microscopic observations. *Journal of Pathology*, **110**, 145–151 (1973)

89 RADAKRISHNAMURTHY, B., RUIZ, M. A., DALFERES, E. R., VESSELINOVITCH, D., WISSLER, R. W. and BERENSON, G. S. The effect of various dietary regimes and cholesterylamine on aortic glycosaminoglycans during regression of atherosclerotic lesions in rhesus monkeys. *Atherosclerosis*, **33**, 17–28 (1979)

90 RATLIFF, N. B., GERRARD, J. G. and WHITE, J. G. Platelet–leukocyte interactions following arterial endothelial injury. *American Journal of Pathology*, **96**, 567–580 (1979)

91 RICH, A. R. and GREGORY, J. L. Experimental anaphylactic lesions of the coronary arteries of the sclerotic type commonly associated with rheumatic fever and disseminated lupus erythematous. *Bulletin of Johns Hopkins Hospital*, **81**, 312–324 (1947)

92 RICHARDSON, M. and MOORE, S. Preparation of large curved biological surfaces for SEM. *Artery*, **6,** 409–417 (1980)

93 RICHARDSON, M. and MOORE, S. Formed element accumulation on rabbit aortic wall after a second balloon stripping of the endothelium. *Federation Proceedings*, **39**, 774 (1980) (abstract)

94 RICHARDSON, M., IHNATOWYCZ, I. and MOORE, S. Glycosaminoglycan distribution in rabbit aortic wall following balloon catheter de-endothelialization: an ultrastructural study. *Laboratory Investigation*, **43**, 509–516 (1980)

95 ROKITANSKY, K. *Handbuch der pathologischen anatomie*. Braumuller und Seidel, Vienna (1852)

96 ROSS, R., GLOMSET, J. A., KARIYA, B. and HARKER, L. A. A platelet dependent serum factor that stimulates the proliferation of arterial smooth muscle cells *in vitro*. *Proceedings of the National Academy of Sciences of the USA*, **71**, 1207–1210 (1974)

97 ROSS, R. and HARKER, L. Hyperlipidemia and atherosclerosis. *Science*, **193**, 1094–1100 (1976)

98 SAPHIR, O. and GORE, I. Evidence for an inflammatory basis for coronary atherosclerosis in the young. *Archives of Pathology*, **49**, 418–426 (1950)

99 SAPHIR, O., OHRINGER, L. and WONG, R. Changes in the intramural coronary branches in coronary arteriosclerosis. *Archives of Pathology*, **62**, 159–170 (1965)

100 SCHWARTZ, S. M., STEMERMAN, M. B. and BENDITT, E. P. The aortic intima. II. Repair of the aortic lining after mechanical denudation. *American Journal of Pathology*, **81**, 15–42 (1975)

101 SCOTT, R. F., THOMAS, W. A., FLORENTIN, R. A. and REINER, J. M. Population dynamics of arterial cells during atherogenesis. XII. Reversal of endothelial cell loss over atherosclerotic lesions in swine changed to normolipidemic-regression diet. *Experimental Molecular Pathology*, **35**, 163–169 (1981)

102 SHARMA, H. M. and GEER, J. C. Experimental aortic lesions of acute serum sickness in rabbits. *American Journal of Pathology*, **88**, 255–266 (1977)

103 SIREK, O. V., SIREK, A. and CUKERMAN, E. Arterial glycosaminoglycans in diabetic dogs. *Blood Vessels*, **17**, 271–275 (1980)

104 SMITH, E. B. The relationship between plasma and tissue lipids in human atherosclerosis. *Advances in Lipid Research*, **12**, 1–49 (1974)

105 SMITH, E. B. Molecular interactions in human atherosclerotic plaques. *American Journal of Pathology*, **86**, 665–674 (1977)

106 SRINAVASAN, S. R., DOLAN, P., RADAKRISHNAMURTHY, B. and BERENSON, G. Isolation of lipoprotein-acid mucopolysaccharide complexes from fatty streaks of the human aorta. *Atherosclerosis*, **16**, 95–104 (1972)

107 SRINAVASAN, S. R., DOLAN, P., RADAKRISHNAMURTHY, B., PARAGAONKAR, P. S. and BERENSON, G. S. Lipoprotein-acid mucopolysaccharide complexes of human atherosclerotic lesions. *Biochimica et Biophysica Acta*, **388**, 58–70 (1975)

108 STEHBENS, W. E. and KARMODY, A. M. Venous atherosclerosis associated with arteriovenous fistulas for hemodialysis. *Archives of Surgery*, **110**, 176–180 (1975)

109 STEHBENS, W. E. Blood vessel changes in chronic experimental arterio-venous fistulas. *Surgery, Gynecology and Obstetrics*, **127**, 327–338 (1968)

110 STEMERMAN, M. B. and ROSS, R. Experimental arteriosclerosis. I. Fibrous plaque formation in primates, an electron microscopic study. *Journal of Experimental Medicine*, **136**, 769–789 (1972)

111 STEVEN, R. L., COLOMBO, M., GONZALES, J. J., HOLLANDER, W. and SCHMID, K. The glycosaminoglycans of the human artery and their changes in atherosclerosis. *Journal of Clinical Investigation*, **58**, 470–478 (1976)

112 STOUT, R. W., BIERMAN, E. L. and ROSS, R. The effect of insulin on the proliferation of cultured primate arterial smooth muscle cells. *Circulation Research*, **36**, 319–327 (1975)

113 SVENDSEN, E. Focal endothelial cell injury in rabbit aorta: aggravation of injury by 2 days of cholesterol feeding. *Acta Pathologica et Microbiologica Scandinavica*, **87**, 123–130 (1979)

114 TRACY, R. E. and TOCA, V. Relationship of raised atherosclerotic lesions to fatty streaks in 19 location-race groups. *Atherosclerosis*, **21**, 21–36 (1975)

115 TRACY, R. E., STRONG, J. P., TOCA, V. T. and LOPEZ, C. R. Atheronecrosis and its fibroproliferative base and cap in the thoracic aorta. *Laboratory Investigation*, **41**, 546–552 (1979)

116 TSCHOPP, T. B., WEISS, H. J. and BAUMGARTNER, H. R. Decreased adhesion of platelets and subendothelium in von Willebrand's disease. *Journal of Laboratory and Clinical Medicine*, **83**, 196–300 (1974)

117 TYSON, J. E, DeSA, D. J. and MOORE, S. Thromboatheromatous complications of umbilical arterial catheterization in the newborn period. Clinico-pathological study. *Archives of Diseases in Childhood*, **51**, 744–754 (1976)

118 VIJAYDKUMAR, S. T., LEELAMMA, S. and KURUP, P. A. Changes in aortic glycosamino-glycans and lipoprotein lipase activity in rats with age and atheroma. *Athero-sclerosis*, **21**, 1–14 (1975)

119 VLODAVSKY, I., FIELDING, P. E., FIELDING, C. J. and GOSPODAROWICZ, D. Role of contact inhibition in the regulation of receptor-mediated uptake of low density lipopro-tein in cultured vascular endothelial cells. *Proceedings of the National Academy of Science USA*, **75**, 356–360 (1978)

120 VOGEL, A., RAINES, E., KARIYA, B., RIVERST, M. J. and ROSS, R. Co-ordinate control of 3T3 cell proliferation by platelet-derived growth factor and plasma components. *Proceedings of National Academy of Science USA*, **75**, 2810–2814 (1978)

121 WEBER, G., FABBRINI, P. and RESI, L. Scanning and transmission electron microscopy observations on the surface lining of aortic intimal plaques in rabbits on a hypercholesterolic diet. *Virchows Archives of Pathology and Anatomy A*, **364**, 325–331 (1974)

122 WIGHT, T. N., CURWEN, K. D., HOMAN, W. and MINICK, C. R. Effect of regenerated endothelium on glycosaminoglycan accumulation in the arterial wall. *Federation Proceedings*, **38**, 1075 (1979) (abstract)

123 WOODWARD, J. F., SRINIVASAN, S. R., ZIMMY, M. L., RADAKRISHNAMURTHY, B. and BEREN-SON, G. S. Electron microscopic features of lipoprotein-glycosaminoglycan com-plexes from human atherosclerotic plaques. *Laboratory Investigation*, **34**, 516–521 (1976)

124 WOOLF, N. J., BRADLEY, J. W. P., CRAWFORD, T. and CARSTAIRS, K. C. Experimental mural thrombi in the pig aorta: the early natural history. *British Journal of Experimental Pathology*, **44**, 257–264 (1968)

125 WU, K. K., ARMSTRONG, M. L., HOAK, J. C. and MEGAN, M. B. Platelet aggregates in hpercholesterolemic rhesus monkeys. *Thombosis Research*, **7**, 917–924 (1975)

126 ZEEK, P. Studies in atherosclerosis. *American Journal of Medical Science*, **184**, 350–355 (1932)

2
Epidemiology and risk factors in thrombotic brain infarction

John F. Kurtzke

INTRODUCTION

In order to consider the risk factors in stroke we need first to define two aspects of the problem: what are the characteristics of stroke and what is meant by risk. Both aspects, in fact, emerge out of epidemiology.

Epidemiology

The science of clinical medicine, when properly defined, is little more than applied epidemiology[46]. And one useful definition of epidemiology is that it is the discipline concerned with the study of the natural history of disease, based upon the original roots of the word: *logos*, from *legein*, study; *epi*, [what is] upon; *demos*, the people.

Essential to all of epidemiology is the definition of the disease in view, since the epidemiological unit of study is the affected person. After diagnosis, the next question is the frequency of the disorder. The most valid measures of frequency are those which relate a numerator (the cases) to its true denominator (the population at risk). Such ratios, with the addition of the time factor to which they pertain, are referred to as rates. The population-based rates in common use are the *incidence rate*, the *mortality rate*, and the *prevalence rate*, which are all ordinarily expressed in unit-population values. For example, 10 cases among a community of 20 000 represents a rate of 50 per 100 000 population or 0.5 per 1000 population.

The *incidence* or *attack rate* is defined as the number of new cases of the disease beginning in a unit of time within the specified population. This is usually given as an annual incidence rate in cases per 100 000 population per year. The date of onset of clinical symptoms ordinarily decides the time of accession, though occasionally the date of first diagnosis is used.

The *mortality* or *death rate* refers to the number of deaths with this disease as the underlying cause of death occurring within a unit time and population, and thus an annual death rate per 100 000 population. The *case fatality ratio* refers to the proportion of the affected who die from the disease.

The *point prevalence rate* is more properly a ratio, and refers to the number of the affected at one point in time within the community, again expressed per unit of population. If there is no change in case fatality ratios over time and no change in annual incidence rates (and no migration), then the average annual incidence rate times the average duration of illness in years equals the point prevalence rate. Both incidence and prevalence rates are derived from surveys for the disease in question as it occurs within circumscribed populations. Mortality rates come from official published sources.

Stroke epidemiology

There is a large body of literature dealing with the epidemiology of cerebrovascular disease (CVD). Several recent overviews are those of Kannel[37], Kuller[42], Kurtzke[45], Dawber[10], Ostfeld[59] and Schoenberg[73].

For epidemiological purposes, disease classification must be kept as simple as possible. For stroke, one may then consider the principal anatomic types as: acute brain infarct; brain ('cerebral') hemorrhage; subarachnoid hemorrhage; and a class of 'other' or 'unspecified'. Acute brain infarct may be subdivided into embolic and thrombotic – and the latter could be further specified as to arterial or venous.

Transient ischemic attacks (TIA) and cerebral arteriosclerosis are ordinarily excluded from the corpus of acute CVD. Spinal cord vascular disease has little impact on the overall stroke problem.

Population-based surveys defining the incidence of stroke provide our best estimates as to the relative frequency by type. Overall at present, about one in eight strokes are diagnosed as brain hemorrhage, one in twelve as subarachnoid hemorrhage, and three in four as acute brain infarct[45].

As to actual frequency, reasonable estimates for Whites of the Occident would seem to be about 150 per 100 000 population per year as annual incidence rate; about 600 per 100 000 population as point prevalence rate, and thus an average duration of some four years for stroke; and about 70 per 100 000 as an annual mortality rate[45].

One aspect of stroke epidemiology of considerable recent interest is the evidence for a declining frequency of stroke. This was first based on mortality data[21], but more recently has had solid support from morbidity surveys[18,81]. The decline holds for brain hemorrhage[16,81] and brain infarct[19] but not for subarachnoid hemorrhage[68]. The data available extend no further back than the 1940s at best, however.

But if we can trust mortality data, in the United States at least, a decreasing stroke death rate has been a feature for as long as there are records available. By 1977, the age adjusted annual death rates for Whites had declined to less than half the levels of 1915–1920. The decrease applied to males and females, and to nonWhites as well as Whites. On an arithmetic scale the decrease appeared linear over these 60 years[45].

If this decline has truly occurred evenly over this interval, one would be hard pressed to attribute the improvement to any recent dietary or socioeconomic changes, or to medical interventions. When plotted on a logarithmic scale, the death rate decline appeared greater in the last few years of observation. This was the interpretation of Ostfeld[59], who measured the decrease between 1975 and 1977 at 4–5% a year, as opposed to 1.5% (between 1951 and 1974) or 1.0% (between 1900 and 1950). Further data, though, are required to define whether there has truly been an inflection in the curve of stroke incidence or mortality – and when it occurred.

RISK

According to Fox *et al*[15]: 'The basic premise of epidemiology is that disease does not occur randomly but in patterns which reflect the operation of the underlying causes . . . that knowledge of these patterns is not only of predictive value with respect to future disease occurrence, but also constitutes a major key to understanding causation . . .'. The 'patterns' mentioned are those which comprise the 'risk factors' for a disease. To consider risk factors, we must first define risk.

Take, for example, a group or cohort of 1000 healthy people – over a given interval they will incur a certain number of events, such as strokes. If 10 strokes occur in one year in that cohort, its annual frequency is 1%. Thus the experience of a population cohort followed over time provides a measure of the cumulative frequency of the event over time, i.e. the chances or probability of the event. This is risk, and for this defined group it is the *absolute risk* of the event. The experience in one cohort is then extrapolated to the experience of other cohorts, such as the general population. If our study group indeed represented the general population, we would decide that the absolute risk of stroke in one year is 1%, based on the experience of this cohort.

Risk is measured by the frequency of later events in a population defined at the start of the period of observation. Incidence and mortality rates are based on counts of events over time within the average population during the interval. In real life the distinction is trivial, and an annual absolute risk of stroke is very well approximated by the annual incidence rate of stroke.

Events which alter the expected absolute risk or probability of disease are referred to as risk factors. We know that the likelihood of stroke increases markedly with age, and therefore age is clearly a risk factor for stroke.

When we speak of risk factors, there is no implication of cause or pathogenesis. In one sense they are mathematical abstractions: events which are associated with a significant alteration in the frequency of disease, regardless of reason. It is the function of the clinical scientist to ascertain reasons, for among the myriad of risk factors for any disease will be the cause(s) and major precipitant(s) of the disease.

If we know the absolute risk (or the incidence rate) in two population subgroups which differ as to the presence of a factor, then the ratio of the risk in those with the factor to those without is a measure of the *relative risk* for that factor. If the incidence rate of disease is 8 per 100 000 for those with factor X and 4 per 100 000 for those without factor X, then for factor X the relative risk is 2. In situations where true incidence rates are unknown, prospective studies of comparable groups, one with and one without the factor, will also provide relative risk ratios. If twice as many with the factor develop the disease as do those without the factor, then again the relative risk is 2.

Relative risk, therefore, is the ratio of the rate in the 'exposed' to the rate in the standard ('unexposed'). The higher this ratio, the more likely is this factor to be directly related to the cause or precipitation of the disease in question.

In retrospective comparisons if a group of the affected differs from a group of matched controls on a given factor this too provides a measure of relative risk. In such case-control comparisons it is defined as ad/bc in *Table 2.1*[52].

Table 2.1

Factor	Case	Control	Total
+	a	b	a+b
−	c	d	c+d
Total	a+c	b+d	

It is the quotent of 'hits' over 'misses' in this circumstance.

The excess of the rate of occurrence of disease in those 'exposed' to a factor beyond the rate in the 'standard' not exposed to the factor provides a measure of the amount of disease blamed on or attributed to this factor, and this excess is called the *attributable* risk. It is the quantitative amount of disease that one could hope to avoid by removal of the risk factor in question.

An example of both kinds of risk may clarify the distinctions. If we look at smoking habits in deaths from two diseases, bronchogenic carcinoma and coronary thrombosis, the data in *Table 2.2* emerge[52].

Table 2.2

Cause of death	Death rate per 100 000 Non-smoker	Heavy smoker	Smoking as risk factor Attributable risk	Relative risk
	(a)	(b)	(b−a)	(b/a)
Lung carcinoma	7	166	159	23.7
Coronary thrombosis	422	599	177	1.4

Smoking is clearly more 'important' in the pathogenesis of lung carcinoma (CA) than in coronary artery disease (CAD), according to relative risk ratios. However, as to the numbers of deaths 'blamed' on smoking, then CAD has caused more than CA, from the attributable risk data.

Neither attributable nor relative risk speak to the 'sensitivity' of the risk factor. For example, if in the above example 50% of the population were heavy smokers, then despite the relative risk of 24 the absolute annual risk of death from CA in that group would be only 0.3% – for every 1000 with the risk factor, only three would be affected that year. It is important to remember this aspect if we hope to affect disease frequency by altering risk factors; at some point we need to consider a 'cost-benefit' ratio.

THROMBOTIC BRAIN INFARCT RISK FACTORS

The limited space available precludes consideration here of risk factors for each type of stroke, so we shall concentrate on that type which provides the bulk of acute CVD. Although some attention to these factors is provided in the appropriate chapters of this book, a few points on other types are raised here.

The risk factors for *brain hemorrhage* are by and large qualitatively not dissimilar to those considered here for brain infarct.

For *cerebral embolism*, while the major cause (valvular heart disease) is of less importance in the United States with the decrease of rheumatic heart disease, this is not the case in other parts of the world. We have considered most of our current cases to be attributable to acute mural thrombi or acute arrhythmias. The Framingham experience, though, raises the real possibility that chronic atrial fibrillation is a major cause of cerebral emboli[87]. Another recent contributor may well be prolapsed mitral valve[5].

For *subarachnoid hemorrhage* age is much less of a factor than for other strokes. However, hypertension plays a role. Of interest is the contention of Hillbom and Kaste[30, 32] that alcohol intoxication is a precipitant of subarachnoid hemorrhage. An early indication that contraceptive pills were a risk factor has not been borne out in a larger study[34]. Petitti and Wingerd[66], with only 11 cases in past or present users, still contend a relative risk of 6 for the pill; for pill + smoking the relative risk was 22. The difference, with smoking controlled, was not statistically significant.

As to *thrombotic brain infarcts* these comprise such a large proportion of stroke that any discernible risk factors for CVD as a whole will reflect acute brain infarction (ABI); conversely, major risk factors for ABI will affect greatly the frequency of all strokes. ABI actually means thromboembolic brain infarct, but again, the vast majority of these cases are thrombotic and thus it is really to this class that the risk factors refer.

Age and sex

For deaths from stroke or from acute brain infarct, there is a logarithmic increase in the age-specific death rates with increasing age. Comparable age-specific incidence rates follow the same pattern except for a lessening of the rate of increase in the more elderly[45].

For stroke as a whole, and for ABI, there is a modest male excess. Average annual age-adjusted incidence rates show a 1.3 to 1 male to female ratio. By age, there is a slightly greater male preponderance in the younger adult years and a lessening, or even a reversal, of the sex ratio in the elderly[45].

Race and geography

The consensus is that in the United States stroke as a whole is more commonly reported as a cause of death in Blacks than in Whites. This racial difference is supported by a modest number of morbidity surveys[12, 28, 60, 64, 65] where the age-adjusted annual incidence rates were generally about twice as high in Blacks as in Whites.

Japan has long been noted to have reported death rates from stroke, and in particular for cerebral hemorrhage, far above those of other countries. Annual age-adjusted incidence rates from community surveys in Japan fall within a range of some 200–400 per 100 000 population[17, 25, 40, 78, 81]. The higher rates and those with higher proportions attributed to cerebral hemorrhage arise principally from cases without autopsy or computerized tomography (CT) confirmation. It is my impression that cerebral hemorrhage is not in excess in Japan[44, 45], while cerebral thrombosis may well be more frequent than in the occident, perhaps up to twice as common[45].

On Hawaii, though, stroke incidence rates for Japanese residents appeared similar to those of occidental Whites[35, 45]. However, Brust[7] claims that Hawaiian Japanese show the same predilection for intracranial (vs extracerebral) involvement as do those in Japan. Regardless of that point, if the incidence of ABI truly differs between Japan and Hawaii among Japanese, then there would be an important geographic, or geographically related, risk factor in ABI.

In the United States, there is also some degree of geographic variation, with strokes more common in the southeastern 'cotton belt' states than in the northern midwest regardless of sex or color[43, 56, 57]. In Scandinavia stroke rates are moderately higher in Finland than in the other lands, and similarly in Scotland, rates are higher than in the rest of Great Britain[45].

Blood pressure

It hardly needs mentioning that *hypertension* is not only a risk factor in stroke, but also the major one aside from age. This is documented in all the studies noted above, east or west, Black or White, male or female, and also specifically for acute brain infarction. Hypertension was the single most powerful risk factor for cerebral infarct in Rochester, Minnesota, with a relative risk of 6.0[74], and in ex-college students it was the strongest predictor of nonfatal stroke[62]. In Framingham there was no clean dichotomy between 'normal' blood pressure and 'hypertension', but rather the risk increased progressively with increasing levels even from well into the 'normotensive' range. Further, systolic hypertension alone was associated with a 2–4-fold increase in stroke in that survey[39].

A most important study was that reported by the multi-centered Hypertension Detection and Follow-up Program Cooperative Group[33]. This was a community-based, randomized, controlled clinical trial of 'systematic stepped care therapy' (SC) compared with 'referred care' (RC) in hypertensives. The former were actively treated, while the latter were referred back to their own physicians, the implication being that most would not have remained in treatment in the RC group. The 5-year stroke incidence rates were 1.9% in SC vs 2.9% in RC. Annual mortality rates from stroke were 1.06 per 1000 population aged between 35 and 74 (SC) and 1.91 per 1000 (RC) – against the recorded total US rate of 0.83 per 1000 between the ages of 35 and 74.

Hypotension

This also appears to be a precipitant of ischemic stroke. In an autopsy study, Mitchinson[55] attributed 40% of fatal strokes in the elderly '. . . to acute hypotension caused by such extracranial events as heart-failure, occult haemorrhage, or multiple pulmonary emboli.' In a study of patients who had been resuscitated after cardiac arrest and then succumbed, 7 (5%) brains had recent infarcts with no (4 patients) or only moderate (3 patients) cerebral atherosclerosis[80]. It was their inference that hypotension was not relevant here because of a lack of correlation with atherosclerosis. It seems more likely to me that this study indicates that hypotension *per se* can, in fact, cause focal brain infarcts.

Coronary artery disease

The principal underlying cause of thrombotic brain infarction is atherosclerosis. It is not surprising, therefore, that atherosclerotic heart disease is a precursor of ischemic stroke. It is, in fact, rather unexpected that CAD and CVD deaths in the United States have rather different geographic patterns, and the rare occurrence of CAD in Japan has been contrasted with their stroke frequencies[44].

However, in formal prospective surveys, there is no question that CAD, no matter how measured, is a significant risk factor in acute brain infarct. This applies to clinical CAD, including angina and myocardial infarction, to electrocardiograph (EKG) changes of an appropriate nature, and to congestive heart failure *per se*. In Framingham, for example, each of these factors is a predictor of acute brain infarct: EKG changes of left ventricular hypertrophy increase the risk 10-fold; nonspecific ST and T wave changes by 4-fold; and congestive heart failure, 9-fold. These all remain risk factors regardless of the level of blood pressure[86]. Hypertensive and valvular heart disease also had a relative risk of 2 for ischemic stroke in Rochester, Minnesota[74].

McAllen and Marshall[54] contested the importance of myocardial infarction, since only 4% of a series of 260 survivors of MI had a completed stroke in 5 years. However, the median age of the cases was about 56 years. A 5-year incidence at age 55–64 would be about 1500 per 100 000[45], so that the 4% would seem to provide a relative risk in excess of 2, even in this clinical series.

Atherosclerosis

Extracranial cerebral vessel disease

This is considered a major cause of acute brain infarct. Whether many or few of these strokes are artery-to-artery emboli, as opposed to thrombotic or hypoperfusion events in the brain, is irrelevant to the pragmatic determination of stroke risk factors.

Asymptomatic carotid bruits

These are one index of atherosclerosis. In Framingham, Wolf et al.[88] found an equal frequency of such bruits by sex but, of course, an increasing frequency with age: 3.5% age 44–54, 3.9% age 55–64, and 7.0% age 65–79. Both hypertension and diabetes were risk factors for bruit. Ischemic stroke developed in 14 of 171 such patients in 2 years, an annual incidence of 4%. Relative risk ratios for stroke were about 2. However, the relative risks for myocardial infarction and for overall mortality were in similar excess, and only 6 of 14 cerebral infarcts had occurred within the territory of the vessel with the bruit.

Extracranial artery disease can also be measured by ultrasonic techniques. In one such study, 33% of surgical patients with major aortic or iliac disease had evidence of carotid stenosis, as opposed to 6% of patients with CAD or 'high risk' patients with neither[26].

Occluded carotid arteries

Patients with occluded carotid arteries who had presented with TIA had a 30% chance of a completed infarct within 5 years in one study, with no significant difference in outcome when middle cerebral anastomosis had been performed. There was also no significant difference in survival: 20% were dead within 5 years – 80% of cardiac disease[50].

Peripheral vascular disease

This had a relative risk for ischemic stroke of only 1.4 in Rochester[74], and thus would seem of less predictive value than major vessel disease warranting surgery (*see above*).

Retinal artery disease

Savino et al.[72]. followed 86 patients with retinal artery occlusion alone (37) or with visible emboli with or without occlusion (49). Survivorship was decreased, primarily due to the poor prognosis of the latter group. Again, though, the principal cause of death was cardiac. The stroke mortality rate was estimated to be 4–5 times expectation. Arteriosclerotic retinal vessel changes were also a significant risk factor for ischemic stroke in a prospective survey in Japan[3,4].

Systemic arteriosclerosis

Another index of systemic arteriosclerosis might be 'dizzy spells'. Heyman et al.[29] reported that among patients later hospitalized for stroke, 2.3% had previously recorded this complaint on questionnaire, as opposed to 1.1% without stroke, a relative risk of 2.

Diabetes mellitus

Another widely accepted risk factor for stroke as a whole, and particularly for ischemic brain infarct, is diabetes mellitus. This is true in Framingham, where it was the sixth most important predictive factor, after blood pressure, age, cholesterol, cigarettes and EKG changes[37]. In Mexico, it followed hypertension and heart disease[58]. For college students also it followed hypertension and CAD[63], with a stroke prevalence in diabetics 3 times that in nondiabetics. The relative risk for ischemic stroke in diabetes was 3 in Rochester, Minnesota[74].

The contraceptive pill

There is considerable literature on the adverse effects of contraceptive medication, which has recently been summarized by Stadel[77]. Based primarily on British experience, he estimated for CVD a relative risk of 5 and an annual attributable risk of 37 cases per 100 000 users[49]. This was for stroke as a whole. One of his sources had reported relative risks of death from stroke as 4 for SAH, 2 for 'other stroke' for current users, 3 for 'other stroke' in former users. All numbers were very small. However, Vessey et al.[82] were Stadel's major resource. They had reported a 'standardized first event rate' of 0.45 cases per 1000 women-years for stroke in pill users vs 0.09 per 1000 in non-pill contraceptive users; respective numbers of cases were 10 and 3. For SAH, there were 2 in each group, pill users and not. The 2 cerebral emboli patients were pill users; 1 had cardiomyopathy, the other mitral stenosis. Three of the six thrombotic strokes were classed as 'ill-defined' and 5 of these 6 were pill users. In their 1977 report, Vessey et al.[84] had recorded only 2 CVD deaths (1 SAH, 1 brain infarct) in pill users. This number was unchanged by 1981, when they had also recorded 1 SAH death in a non-pill user[83].

Another prospective study cited by Stadel was actually not confirmatory of any increase in ABI. Petitti et al.[67] had found no effect of the pill on the frequency of stroke, aside from SAH, when smoking was controlled. Even in that instance, SAH in current users was not significantly increased (*see above*).

In Rochester, Minnesota, the average annual incidence of stroke for females between the ages of 15 and 49 had declined to 12.9 per 100 000 when the pill was in use from the immediately preceding period when it was 23.3 per 100 000[75]. This last argument is admittedly tenuous in view of the decreasing stroke incidence throughout that population, as discussed above. However, the frequency of surgical menopause in women of Framingham who had suffered a stroke was the same (26%) as in the unaffected population (30%)[37]. In Australia, Shearman[76] was unable to find any excess of any vascular deaths, whether cardiac or cerebral, both of which have been steadily declining there. We may be returning to an earlier conclusion (*see* p. 87 of ref. 44), that the pill has no important role in the genesis of stroke, at least of thrombotic stroke.

Cholesterol and lipids

Claims as to the role of lipids in stroke have also been conflicting. Farid and Anderson[14] described hyperlipoproteinemia, mostly type IV, in a small series of patients. Mathew *et al.*[53] confirmed the excess in both intracranial and extracranial disease in referral patients with transient or completed strokes. Similar excess in TIA and completed stroke were reported for type IV lipoprotein, triglycerides and cholesterol[48]. Serum cholesterol levels were directly, but modestly, related to CVD death rates, and then in only two out of three prospective Chicago epidemiological studies[11]. Plasma high-density lipoproteins (HDL) are inversely related to cholesterol levels and to CAD deaths[13, 89]. In Framingham 'the association of blood lipids with ABI . . . is considerably weaker than for coronary heart disease . . .'[37]. Ostfeld[59] reviewed a number of studies and concluded there was a '. . . weak and uncertain relationship between lipids and stroke.' If at all related, they seemed associated with an increased risk only under age 50 – in Framingham.

Transient ischemic attacks

It is perhaps a matter of semantics whether TIAs are considered a precursor or a manifestation of stroke. They have their own risk factors which, in essence, are also age, hypertension, cardiac disease, diabetes and evidence of carotid artery disease. The increase with age is far less striking than that for brain infarction, but the effect of the sex ratio on the incidence rates is similar, with only a slight male preponderance[45]. Barnett *et al.*[5] have called attention to prolapsed mitral valve as a cause of TIA – and of completed stroke. The situation of reversible ischemic neurologic deficit (RIND) seems even more clearly part of ischemic stroke.

Schoenberg *et al.*[74] claim differential risk factors between brain infarct and TIA, in that relative risk ratios for diabetes and angina differed between the two states. It seems more likely to me that we are seeing only chance variations between rather small numbers in that survey.

As to TIA *per se* as a risk factor for completed stroke, in Rochester the relative risk ratio was 4.6; only hypertension (RR 6.0) was higher[74].

'By and large, one might expect that after two to four years, one out of six patients with TIA will have suffered a thrombotic stroke and one out of four will have died. By 15 years over ⅓ will have had a stroke and some ⅔ will be dead . . . [but] at least half the deaths at any stage of follow-up . . . are cardiac in origin'[47].

Although it is clear that TIA is a highly significant risk factor, Ostfeld[59] indicates it has little impact on the overall stroke problem because 'only about one in 10 [patients] had TIA before the stroke'. Average annual incidence of TIA is about 30 per 100 000, as opposed to some 120 for brain infarct[45]. They are therefore common enough to be considered worthy of treatment as a stroke preventive.

Smoking

Ostfeld[59] also questions whether smoking has 'an important effect' in stroke. Some evidence to this point was presented earlier, and it was concluded that a 'low-order positive relationship between cigarette smoking and CVD deaths does seem to be present'[44]. Paffenbarger and Williams[61] found this to be one of their major risk factors for later occlusive stroke deaths in college students, with over twice as many smokers affected as in the controls. In Framingham men – but not women – who smoked cigarettes heavily had three times the risk of brain infarction as non-smokers. The effect was greatest at younger ages, paralleled the number of cigarettes smoked, and 'in multivariate analysis had a significant independent effect taking other factors into account'[37]. Recall above, where smoking may have been the confounding variable in the assessments of stroke and the contraceptive pill.

Other risk factors

Socioeconomic status

In England there was a weak and irregular direct correlation between CVD incidence and social class, the rates in (high) classes I and II being 102 and 106 vs 61 in class V[1]. The same first author, however, found exactly the opposite in the United States, where 'the men dying of stroke were evidently poorer than the controls'[2].

Season and climate

Stroke deaths in the US were at a low when temperature was in the 60 and 70 degrees Fahrenheit and rose sharply at higher temperatures – and also during snowfalls[71]. In Britain, which climatically does not approach the semitropical parts of the US, there was also a seasonal variation, with stroke deaths highest in spring and winter and lowest in late summer[22]. Bull[8] found a negative correlation between ambient temperature and stroke admissions or deaths in the UK. Knox[41] thought this was related more to levels of air pollution than to the temperature itself – but there was no strong relation to respiratory illness *per se*.

In general, there seems to be somewhat of a U-shaped relation between the frequency of stroke deaths, with maxima at the extremes of temperature. Whether the incidence varies in a similar way or if this is a reflection of case fatality ratios remains unclear.

Obesity

A positive relation between excess body weight and stroke was claimed by Heyden *et al.*[27]. Obesity was weakly related to ABI incidence, at least in women, in Framingham[37]. In ex-college students 36% of occlusive stroke death patients had had a (low) ponderal index, less than 12.9, as opposed to 25% of controls[6]. (In two medical dictionaries ponderal index is cube root of weight divided by height times 100. However, other usage has been height over cube root of weight and the latter seems to have been the one employed here.) Excess weight though does not in most series appear to be a major stroke risk factor[44, 59].

Ethanol

It is possible that cigarette smoking as a stroke risk factor might, at least in part, reflect drinking habits, or *vice versa*. Hillbom and Kaste[31] noted alcohol intoxication shortly preceded the onset of acute brain infarct in 10/23 patients under age 40 in Helsinki. They pointed out that the daily frequency curve for all stroke onsets followed by one day the curve for alcohol consumption. Of the 23 patients, 13 were smokers and several also had at least one of the other aforementioned risk factors. Seven of the 23 stroke patients were smokers + drinkers, 3 were non-smoking drinkers, and 6 were non-drinking smokers. The 10 drinkers were not chronic alcoholics, and only one was considered a 'heavy drinker'.

In Framingham, alcohol consumption showed no relation to ABI occurrence in women. There was a trend toward increased frequency with increasing alcohol consumption in men, but this was considered statistically insignificant[37]. However, numbers in Framingham would seem small for either sex at the higher amounts of alcohol intake, and certainly a real relationship cannot be ruled out. Kagan *et al.*[36] in Hawaii found a correlation of hemorrhagic stroke (but not ABI) with alcohol consumption which, however, was largely attributable to hypertension and smoking[6]. A striking linear correlation between alcohol consumption and blood pressure was found in Australia[9], independent of age, weight or smoking. It is possible, therefore, that even alcohol might reflect little more than hypertension, but further work is needed.

Hemoglobin

It has long been accepted that polycythemia may result in brain infarction. Thomas *et al.*[79] pointed out that cerebral blood flow was decreased in polycythemia vera, even after hematocrit levels had been reduced to 46–52%. In Framingham, within the normal range of hemoglobin, the risk of brain infarct 'was found to be proportional to the blood hemoglobin concentration in both sexes'[38]. However, when corrected for blood pressure and smoking 'hemoglobin level had only a modest residual effect, no longer statistically significant'. Harrison *et al.*[23] found a direct correlation, though, between hemoglobin levels and the size of brain infarcts in England, attributing the adverse effects to decreased collateral flow with increased viscosity.

Sickle cell disease

This is a stroke risk factor. In one hospital series, 17% of hemoglobin SS patients had one or more 'cerebrovascular accident' episodes; their age-range was 2–55 years with a mean of 10 years. In SC disease 1 in 20 and in AS trait 4 in 227 patients had had strokes in that same series[69].

Familial factors

In the Danish national twin study of Harvald and Hauge[24], 25% of monozygotic (MZ) affected twins were found at follow-up to be concordant for hypertension, i.e. both twins of the set were so diagnosed. The concordance frequencies in MZ twins were 22% for stroke and 20% for CAD. In CAD, concordance did not differ significantly between MZ and same-sexed dizygous (DZ_1) twins, who had a rate of 15%. However, for hypertension and for CVD, the MZ concordance ratios were significantly elevated: DZ_1 concordances were 9% for hypertension vs 25% (MZ), and 11% for stroke vs 22% (*see* pp. 86–87 of ref. 44).

Gifford[20] had reported that parents of stroke patients had stroke recorded as underlying cause of death four times as often as expected. In the Paffenbarger and Williams[61] study of stroke precursors in college students, parents of occlusive stroke-death subjects had died of a 'cardiovascular renal cause' at a frequency (16%) much greater than that in the controls (2%). Therefore, there does seem to be considerable evidence for a heredofamilial predisposition in stroke, and some evidence that this predisposition is indeed genetic.

Prior stroke

In the National Survey of Stroke[85], Robins and Baum[70] calculated an annual incidence of recurrent stroke that was 30–50 times the incidence of hospitalized first strokes, using as the population at risk those who had suffered a stroke. This can be redefined as a risk of recurrent stroke of 4–7% per annum (for perhaps 3 years or so). Their observed annual incidence rates were 142 per 100 000 for first strokes and 56 for subsequent strokes. Leonberg and Elliott[51] state that the 5-year recurrence rate for strokes is reported to range from 20–40%. In their own series, with intensive management of multiple risk factors in 88 survivors of ABI, their 5-year stroke recurrence rate was 16% (and fatality rate 17%). If validated, this would prove to be a highly important study.

Multiple risk factors

Admittedly, the most important risk factor for ischemic stroke is that for which we desire no change, i.e. age. But the main purpose of identifying CVD risk factors is to see if stroke can be prevented. We therefore need to know not only what are the (modifiable) risk factors, but also which of them are the most important for the individual (relative risk) or for society (attributable risk). In addition, we need to know whether the factors are independent of each other, whether one relies upon another, and whether they interact, positively or negatively, with one another.

The Framingham group has put together a set of elegant tables which demon-strate the additive nature of most of the previously discussed correctible risk factors. The precision of the estimates can well be questioned, there being few cases in a number of the cells when more than one or two factors were considered.

However, by taking five risk factors, a 'stroke risk profile' was devised, with which 'one-tenth of the asymptomatic population can be identified from which about half the ABIs will emerge' (*see* p. 17 of ref. 37). These factors were systolic blood pressure, serum cholesterol, glucose tolerance, cigarette smoking, and EKG-LVH (left ventricular hypertrophy). By decile of risk there was an increasing rate of the increasing probability of ABI for this combination.

Paffenbarger and Williams[61], using smoking, systolic blood pressure and (low) ponderal index, found a markedly increasing stroke mortality ratio with combinations of any of these three, reaching a ratio of 8 (vs 1) when all three were present. By using three others (body height, a parent dead and not a varsity athlete), the mortality ratio increased from 1 to 4 with all these three factors. Of the six, the highest single ratio was that due to blood pressure.

Ostfeld, while acknowledging the Framingham stroke profile, concludes: 'For stroke, the predominant factor is HBP [high blood pressure] and it is doubtful that serum cholesterol and cigarette smoking have an important effect' (*see* p. 147 of ref. 59).

Summary

The most important risk factor in thrombotic brain infarction is age, and next come hypertension and evidence of atherosclerotic vascular disease, in particular that of the heart. Diabetes is a risk factor for atherosclerosis, which in turn is a risk factor for stroke. Transient ischemic attacks can be regarded in a similar light. Smoking appears to be a risk factor of modest importance, whose mechanism is not clear. Further study should be directed to alcohol and to genetic factors in stroke.

Accepting a racial difference in susceptibility, with a higher frequency in Blacks, this difference may still be explicable by some or all of the aforementioned risk factors. A modest excess in Japan, and some geographical patterning elsewhere, would indicate some environmental precipitants, but even here they may be microclimatic (in the individual) rather than macroclimatic. I do not believe that body weight, cholesterol or lipids, the contraceptive pill, diet, climate, weather, wind and water have separately or together any important influence on the development of acute thrombotic brain infarction.

References

1 ACHESON, R. M. and FAIRBAIRN, A. S. Record linkage in studies of cerebrovascular disease in Oxford, England. *Stroke*, **2**, 48–57 (1971)

2 ACHESON, R. M., HEYMAN, A. and NEFZGER, M. D. Mortality from stroke among US veterans in Georgia and five western states. III. Hypertension and demographic characteristics. *Journal of Chronic Diseases*, **26**, 417–429 (1973)

3 AOKI, N. Epidemiological evaluation of funduscopic findings in cerebrovascular diseases. I. Funduscopic findings as risk factors for cerebrovascular diseases. *Japanese Circulation Journal*, **39**, 257–269 (1975a)

4 AOKI, N. Epidemiological evaluation of funduscopic findings in cerebrovascular diseases. II. A multivariate analysis of funduscopic findings. *Japanese Circulation Journal*, **39**, 271–282 (1975b)

5 BARNETT, H. J. M., JONES, M. W., BOUGHNER, D. R. and KOSTUCK, W. J. Cerebral ischemic events associated with prolapsed mitral valve. *Archives of Neurology*, **33**, 777–782 (1976)

6 BLACKWELDER, W. C., YANO, K., RHOADS, G. G., KAGAN, A., GORDON, T and PALESCH, Y. Alcohol and mortality: the Honolulu Heart Study. *American Journal of Medicine*, **68**, 164–169 (1980)

7 BRUST, R. W., Jr. Patterns of cerebrovascular disease in Japanese and other population groups in Hawaii: an angiographical study. *Stroke*, **6**, 539–542 (1975)

8 BULL, G. M. Meteorological correlates with myocardial and cerebral infarction and respiratory disease. *British Journal of Preventive and Social Medicine*, **27**, 108–113 (1973)

9 COOKE, K. M., FROST, G. W., THORNELL, I. R. and STOKES, G. S. Alcohol consumption and blood pressure. Survey of the relationship at a health-screening clinic. *Medical Journal of Australia*, **1**, 65–69 (1982)

10 DAWBER, T. R. *The Framingham Study. The Epidemiology of Atherosclerotic Disease*. Cambridge, Mass., Harvard University Press (1980)

11 DYER, A. R., STAMLER, J., OGLESBY, P., SHEKELLE, R. B., SCHOENBERGER, J. A., BERKSON, D. M., LEPPER, M., COLLETTE, P., SHEKELLE, S. and LINDBERG, H. A. Serum cholesterol and risk of death from cancer and other causes in three Chicago epidemiological studies. *Journal of Chronic Diseases*, **34**, 249–260 (1981)

12 ECKSTROM, P. T., BRAND, F. R., EDLAVITCH, S. A. and PARRISH, H. M. Epidemiology of stroke in a rural area. *Public Health Reports*, **84**, 878–882 (1969)

13 EDITORIAL. High-density lipoprotein. *Lancet*, **1**, 478–480 (1981)

14 FARID, N. R. and ANDERSON, J. Cerebrovascular disease and hyperlipoproteinaemia. *Lancet*, **1**, 1398–1399 (1972)

15 FOX, J. P., HALL, C. E. and ELVEBACK, L. R. *Epidemiology. Man and Disease*, pp. 185, 339. London, Macmillan (1970)

16 FURLAN, A. J., WHISNANT, J. P. and ELVEBACK, L. R. The decreasing incidence of primary intracerebral hemorrhage: a population study. *Annals of Neurology*, **5**, 367–373 (1979)

17 FUSA, K. An epidemiological study of hypertension. A prospective study of incidence of cerebrovascular disease and myocardial infarction in an area in Tohoku District of Japan. *Journal of the Japanese Society of Internal Medicine*, **63**, 630–642 (1974)

18 GARRAWAY, W. M., WHISNANT, J. P., FURLAN, A. J., PHILLIPS, L. H. II, KURLAND, L. T. and O'FALLON, W. M. The declining incidence of stroke. *New England Journal of Medicine*, **300**, 449–452 (1979a)

19 GARRAWAY, W. M., WHISNANT, J. P., KURLAND, L. T. and O'FALLON, W. M. Changing pattern of cerebral infarction: 1945–1974. *Stroke*, **10**, 657–663 (1979b)

20 GIFFORD, A. J. An epidemiological study of cerebrovascular disease. *American Journal of Public Health*, **56**, 452–461 (1966)

21 HABERMAN, S., CAPILDEO, R. and ROSE, F. C. The changing mortality of cerebrovascular disease. *Quarterly Journal of Medicine*, **47**, 71–88 (1978)

22 HABERMAN, S., CAPILDEO, R. and ROSE, F. C. The seasonal variation in mortality from cerebrovascular disease. *Journal of Neurological Science*, **52**, 25–36 (1981)

23 HARRISON, M. J. G., POLLOCK, S., KENDALL, B. E. and MARSHALL, J. Effect of haematocrit on carotid stenosis and cerebral infarction. *Lancet*, **2**, 114–115 (1981)

24 HARVALD, B. and HAUGE, M. Hereditary factors elucidated by twin studies. In *Genetics and the Epidemiology of Chronic Diseases,* edited by J. V. Neel, M. W. Shaw and W. J. Schull, pp. 61–76. Washington, Government Printing Office (Public Health Service Publication No. 1163) (1965)

25 HATANO, S. Experience from a multicentre stroke register; a preliminary report. *Bulletin of the World Health Organization*, **54**, 541–553 (1976)

26 HENNERICI, M., AULICH, A., SANDMANN, W. and FREUND, H. J. Incidence of asymptomatic extracranial arterial disease. *Stroke*, **12**, 750–758 (1981)

27 HEYDEN, S., HAMES, C. G., BARTEL, A., CASSEL, J. C., TRYOLER, H. A. and CORONI, J. C. Weight and weight history in relation to cerebrovascular and ischemic heart disease. *Archives of Internal Medicine*, **128**, 956–960 (1971)

28 HEYMAN, A., KARP, H. R., HEYDEN, S., BARTEL, A., CASSEL, J. C., TRYOLER, H. A. and HAMES, C. G. Cerebrovascular disease in the biracial population of Evans County, Georgia. *Archives of Internal Medicine*, **128**, 949–955 (1971)

29 HEYMAN, A., WILKINSON, W., PFEFFER, R. and VOGT, T. 'Dizzy spells' in the elderly – a predictor of stroke? *Transactions of the American Neurological Association*, **105**, 169–171 (1980)

30 HILLBOM, M. and KASTE, M. Does alcohol intoxication precipitate subarachnoid haemorrhage? *Journal of Neurology, Neurosurgery and Psychiatry*, **44**, 523–526 (1981a)

31 HILLBOM, M. and KASTE, M. Ethanol intoxication: a risk factor for ischemic brain infarction in adolescents and young adults. *Stroke*, **12**, 422–425 (1981b)

32 HILLBOM, M. and KASTE, M. Alcohol intoxication: a risk factor for primary subarachnoid hemorrhage. *Neurology*, **32**, 706–711 (1982)

33 HYPERTENSION DETECTION AND FOLLOW-UP PROGRAM COOPERATIVE GROUP. Five-year findings of the Hypertension Detection and Follow-up Program. III. Reduction in stroke incidence among persons with high blood pressure. *Journal of the American Medical Association,* **247**, 633–638 (1982)

34 INMAN, W. H. W. Oral contraceptives and fatal subarachnoid haemorrhage. *British Medical Journal*, **2**, 1468–1470 (1979)

35 KAGAN, A., POPPER, J. S. and RHOADS, G. G. Factors related to stroke incidence in Hawaiian Japanese men. The Honolulu Heart Study. *Stroke*, **11**, 14–21 (1980)

36 KAGAN, A., YANO, K., RHOADS, G. G. and McGEE, D. L. Alcohol and cardiovascular disease: the Hawaiian experience. *Circulation*, **64** (Suppl. III), III-27–III-31 (1981)

37 KANNEL, W. B. Epidemiology of cerebrovascular disease. In *Cerebral Arterial Disease,* edited by R. W. R. Russell, pp. 1–23. Edinburgh, Churchill Livingstone (1976)

38 KANNEL, W. B., GORDON, T., WOLF, P. A. and McNAMARA, P. Hemoglobin and the risk of cerebral infarction: the Framingham study. *Stroke*, **3**, 409–420 (1972)

39 KANNEL, W. B., WOLF, P. A., McGEE, D. L., DAWBER, T. R., McNAMARA, P. and CASTELLI, W. P. Systolic blood pressure, arterial rigidity, and risk of stroke. The Framingham study. *Journal of the American Medical Association*, **245**, 1225–1229 (1981)

40 KATSUKI, S., HIROTA, Y., AKAZOME, T., TAKEYA, S., OMAE, T. and TAKANO, S. Epidemiological studies in Hisayama, Kyushu Island, Japan. *Japanese Heart Journal*, **5**, 12–36 (1964)

41 KNOX, E. G. Meteorological associations of cerebrovascular disease mortality in England and Wales. *Journal of Epidemiology and Community Health*, **35**, 220–223 (1981)

42 KULLER, L. H. Epidemiology of stroke. *Advances in Neurology*, **19**, 281–310 (1978)

43 KULLER, L., ANDERSON, H., PETERSON, D., CASSEL, J., SPIERS, P., CURRY, H., PAEGEL, B., SASLAW, M., SISK, C., WILBER, J., MILLWARD, D., WINKELSTEIN, W., Jr., LILIENFELD, A. and SELTSER, R. Nationwide cerebrovascular disease morbidity study. *Stroke*, **1**, 86–99 (1970)

44 KURTZKE, J. F. *Epidemiology of Cerebrovascular Disease*. Berlin, Springer Verlag (1969)

45 KURTZKE, J. F. Epidemiology of cerebrovascular disease. In *Cerebrovascular Survey Report for Joint Council Subcommittee on Cerebrovascular Disease*. National Institute of Neurological and Communicative Disorders and Stroke and National Heart and Lung Institute (Revised) January 1980, pp. 135–176. Rochester, MN, Whiting Press (1980)

46 KURTZKE, J. F. An introduction to neuroepidemiology. In *Atti del Secundo Convegno Nazionale di Neuroepidemiologia, Milano, 12–13 dicembre 1980*, edited by R. Boeri and G. Filippini, pp. 1–14. Milan, Officini Grafiche Sabaini (1981)

47 KURTZKE, J. F. Review of clinical trials. Surgical treatment in cerebrovascular disease. *Neuroepidemiology* (in press)

48 LADURNER, G., DORNAUER, U., OTT, E., ILIFF, L. D., KÖRNER, E. and LECHNER, H. Gefässbund und Lipide bei ischämischer Hirnerkrankung. *Psychiatria et Neurologia (Thessalonika)*, **1**, 1–8 (1978)

49 LAYDE, P. M., BERAL, V. and KAY, C. R. Further analyses of mortality in oral contraceptive users. (Royal College of General Practitioners' Oral Contraceptive Study). *Lancet*, **1**, 541–546 (1981)

50 LEE, M. C., PARK, S. H., LOEWENSON, R. B., KLASSEN, A. C. and RESCH, J. A. Long-term effect of internal carotid artery occlusion with or without STA–MCA anastomosis. *Transactions of the American Neurological Association*, **105**, 171–174 (1980)

51 LEONBERG, S. C. and ELLIOTT, F. A. Prevention of recurrent stroke. *Stroke*, **12**, 731–735 (1981)

52 MacMAHON, B. Epidemiologic methods. In *Preventive Medicine*, edited by D. W. Clark and B. MacMahon, pp. 81–104. Boston, Little, Brown & Co. (1967)

53 MATHEW, N. T., DAVIS, D., MEYER, J. S. and CHANDAR, K. Hyperlipoproteinemia in occlusive cerebrovascular disease. *Journal of the American Medical Association*, **232**, 262–266 (1975)

54 McALLEN, P. M. and MARSHALL, J. Cerebrovascular incidents after myocardial infarction. *Journal of Neurology, Neurosurgery and Psychiatry*, **40**, 951–955 (1977)

55 MITCHINSON, M. J. The hypotensive stroke. *Lancet*, **1**, 244–246 (1980)

56 NEFZGER, M. D., HEYMAN, A. and ACHESON, R. M. Stroke, geography and blood pressure. *Journal of Chronic Diseases*, **26**, 389–391 (1973a)

57 NEFZGER, M. D., ACHESON, R. M. and HEYMAN, A. Mortality from stroke among US veterans in Georgia and 5 western states. I. Study plan and death rates. *Journal of Chronic Diseases*, **26**, 393–404 (1973b)

58 OLIVARES, L., CASTAÑEDA, E., GRIFÉ, A. and ALTER, M. Risk factors in stroke: a clinical study in Mexican patients. *Stroke*, **4**, 773–781 (1973)

59 OSTFELD, A. M. A review of stroke epidemiology. *Epidemiologic Reviews*, **2**, 136–152 (1980)

60 OSTFELD, A. M., SHEKELLE, R. B., KLAWANS, H. and TUFO, H. M. Epidemiology of stroke in an elderly welfare population. *American Journal of Public Health*, **64**, 450–458 (1974)

61 PAFFENBARGER, R. S., Jr. and WILLIAMS, J. L. Chronic disease in former college students. V. Early precursors of fatal stroke. *American Journal of Public Health*, **57**, 1290–1299 (1967)

62 PAFFENBARGER, R. S., Jr. and WING, A. L. Characteristics in youth predisposing to fatal stroke in later years. *Lancet*, **1**, 753–754 (1967)

63 PAFFENBARGER, R. S., Jr. and WING, A. L. Chronic disease in former college students. XI. Early precursors of nonfatal stroke. *American Journal of Epidemiology*, **94**, 524–530 (1971)

64 PARRISH, H. M., PAYNE, G. H., ALLEN, W. C., GOLDNER, J. C. and SAUER, H. I. Mid-Missouri stroke survey: a preliminary report. *Missouri Medicine*, **63**, 816–821 (1966)

65 PEACOCK, P. B., RILEY, C. P., LAMPTON, T. D., RAFFEL, S. S. and WALKER, J. S. The Birmingham stroke, epidemiology and rehabilitation study. In *Trends in Epidemiology. Application to Health Service Research and Training*, edited by G. T. Stewart, pp. 231–345. Springfield, Illinois, Charles C. Thomas (1972)

66 PETITTI, D. B. and WINGERD, J. Use of oral contraceptives, cigarette smoking, and risk of subarachnoid haemorrhage. *Lancet*, **2**, 234–236 (1978)

67 PETITTI, D. B., WINGERD, J., PELLEGRIN, F. and RAMCHARAN, S. Risk of vascular disease in women. Smoking, oral contraceptives, noncontraceptive estrogens, and other factors. *Journal of the American Medical Association*, **242**, 1150–1154 (1979)

68 PHILLIPS, L. H. II, WHISNANT, J. P., O'FALLON, W. M. and SUNDT, T. M. The unchanging pattern of subarachnoid hemorrhage in a community. *Neurology*, **30**, 1034–1040 (1980)

69 PORTNOY, B. A. and HERION, J. C. Neurological manifestations in sickle-cell disease with a review of the literature and emphasis on the prevalance of hemiplegia. *Annals of Internal Medicine*, **76**, 643–652 (1972)

70 ROBINS, M. and BAUM, H. M. National survey of stroke. Incidence. *Stroke*, **12** (Suppl. 1), I-45–I-57 (1981)

71 ROGOT, E. and PADGETT, S. J. Associations of coronary and stroke mortality with temperature and snowfall in selected areas of the United States, 1962–1966. *American Journal of Epidemiology*, **103**, 565–575 (1976)

72 SAVINO, P. J., GLASER, J. S. and CASSADY, J. Retinal stroke. Is the patient at risk? *Archives of Ophthalmology*, **95**, 1185–1189 (1977)

73 SCHOENBERG, B. S. Risk factors for cerebrovascular disease. In *Clinical Neuroepidemiology*, edited by F. C. Rose, pp. 151–162. Tunbridge Wells, UK, Pitman Medical (1980).

74 SCHOENBERG, B. S., SCHOENBERG, D. G., PRITCHARD, D. A., LILIENFELD, A. M. and WHISNANT, J. P. Differential risk factors for completed stroke and transient ischemic attacks (TIA): study of vascular diseases (hypertension, cardiac disease, peripheral vascular disease) and diabetes mellitus. *Transactions of the American Neurological Association*, **105**, 165–167 (1980)

75 SCHOENBERG, B. S., WHISNANT, J. P., TAYLOR, W. F. and KEMPERS, R. D. Strokes in women of childbearing age. *Neurology*, **20**, 181–189 (1970)

76 SHEARMAN, R. P. Oral contraceptives: where are the excess deaths? *Medical Journal of Australia*, **1**, 698–700 (1981)

77 STADEL, B. V. Oral contraceptives and cardiovascular disease. *New England Journal of Medicine*, **305**, 612–618, 672–677 (1981)

78 TANAKA, H., UEDA, Y., HAYASHI, M., DATE, C., BABA, T., YAMASHITA, H., SHOJI, H., TANAKA, Y., OWADA, K. and DETELS, R. Risk factors for cerebral hemorrhage and cerebral infarction in a Japanese rural community. *Stroke*, **13**, 62–73 (1982)

79 THOMAS, D. J., duBOULAY, G. H., MARSHALL, J., PEARSON, T. C., RUSSELL, R. W. R., SYMON, L., WETHERLEY-MEIN, G. and ZILKHA, E. Cerebral blood-flow in polycythaemia. *Lancet*, **2**, 161–163 (1977)

80 TORVIK, A. and SKULLERUD, K. How often are brain infarcts caused by hypotensive episodes? *Stroke*, **7**, 255–257 (1976)

81 UEDA, K., OMAE, T., HIROTA, Y., TAKESHITA, M., KATSUKI, S., TANAKA, K. and ENJOJI, M. Decreasing trend in incidence and mortality from stroke in Hisayama residents, Japan. *Stroke*, **12**, 154–160 (1981)

82 VESSEY, M., DOLL, R., PETO, R., JOHNSON, B. and WIGGINS, P. A long-term follow-up study of women using different methods of contraception – an interim report. *Journal of Biosocial Science*, **8**, 373–427 (1976)

83 VESSEY, M. P., McPHERSON, K. and YEATES, D. Mortality in oral contraceptive users. *Lancet*, **1**, 549–550 (1981)

84 VESSEY, M. P., McPHERSON, K. and JOHNSON, B. Mortality among women participating in the Oxford/Family Planning Association contraceptive study. *Lancet*, **2**, 731–733 (1977)

85 WEINFELD, F. D. (ed). The National Survey of Stroke. (National Institute of Neurological and Communicative Disorders and Stroke). *Stroke*, **12** (Suppl. 1), I-1–I-91 (1981)

86 WOLF, P. A., DAWBER, T. R. and KANNEL, W. B. Heart disease as a precursor of stroke. *Advances in Neurology*, **19**, 567–577 (1978a)

87 WOLF, P. A., DAWBER, T. R., THOMAS, H. E., Jr. and KANNEL, W. B. Epidemiologic assessment of chronic atrial fibrillation and risk of stroke: the Framingham study. *Neurology*, **28**, 973–977 (1978b)

88 WOLF, P. A., KANNEL, W. B., SORLIE, P. and McNAMARA, P. Asymptomatic carotid bruit and risk of stroke. The Framingham study. *Journal of the American Medical Association*, **245**, 1442–1445 (1981)

89 YAARI, S., GOLDBOURT, U., EVEN-ZOHAR, S. and NEUFELD, H. N. Associations of serum high density lipoprotein and total cholesterol with total, cardiovascular, and cancer mortality in a 7-year prospective study of 10,000 men. *Lancet*, **1**, 1011–1015 (1981)

3
Hypertension and stroke

J. R. A. Mitchell

'The heart was larger than ordinary, especially the walls of the left ventricle, which were as thick as the breadth of two fingers. When I opened his head I found in the cavity of the right ventricle of the brain, an extravasation of about two pints of black clotted blood which was the cause of his apoplexy and death.'

(Baglivi[5], describing the autopsy on Malpighi, 1694)

'Statistics show that the expectation of life shortens as the blood pressure is higher. The possibility of cerebral haemorrhage and coronary thrombosis introduces the chief elements of uncertainty into the prognosis'.

(Lewis 1942)[26]

INTRODUCTION

The centuries spanned by these observations saw the early suspicions that the heart and circulation contributed to apoplexy clinched beyond all doubt. As in every field, it has been the availability of appropriate techniques which has determined the pace of progress. Until the early 1900s, when systemic arterial pressure could first be reliably and simply measured by the cuff technique, clinicians had only been able to guess at the arterial pressure by feeling the pulse, or by noting heart size at necropsy. When they began to measure blood pressure, confusion and chaos resulted because most of them were literate but not numerate. They had lived in an era where diseases were either present or they were not, so that a simple *qualitative* division had sufficed to separate diseased patients from the normal population. This led them to believe that hypertension was a similar disease entity and that patients with it could be separated from 'normotensive' individuals by erecting an arbitrary boundary. The major advance in our understanding of the relationship between blood pressure and health was the demolition of this boundary by Pickering[32]. He fought the entrenched authorities of the day and showed that blood pressure had to be treated as a continuous *quantitative* variable. The third step forward was the realization that retrospective and case-control studies could only create hypotheses. Long-term prospective, natural history studies were then required to assess the contribution made by a variety of characteristics to end-points, such as stroke or heart attack.

Our ability to measure blood pressure, to use the figures themselves rather than trying to force them into a disease/normality framework and our recognition of the need to invest time, money and effort into following the fate of well individuals for many years has yielded the knowledge set out in the preceding chapter which shows that there is a correlation between a subject's systemic arterial pressure and his risk of death, especially from heart attack, stroke and heart failure. What then remains for us to do which will be recognized next century as an advance similar in magnitude to the three set out above?

First, we need better and more widely available methods for distinguishing between the different diseases which present with sudden neurological deficit and which are labelled as 'strokes'. Only then can we separate pseudostrokes from vascular events and assign the latter to the diametrically opposed processes of bleeding and infarction. The links between hypertension and cerebral haemorrhage may be very different from the links between hypertension and cerebral infarction and this may imply a difference in our ability to modify the processes by prophylactic measures. We thus need more precise ways of categorizing strokes which can be used under field conditions in long-term trials.

Second, we need to determine where on the curve which correlates stroke risk with systemic blood pressure we should intervene. None of the agents used are free from side effects and potential hazards, so it has been said that 'operational hypertension' begins at the level above which detection, investigation and treatment do more good than harm[13].

Our goals for the future should therefore be the more accurate diagnosis of stroke-like illnesses, the clarification of the way in which hypertension contributes to risk in each of the subcategories thus revealed, and the determination of the operational levels at which good rather than harm results from treatment in men and women of different ages and of different racial groups. This chapter examines the starting points from which each of these advances must begin.

LIKE MUST BE COMPARED WITH LIKE

The first requirement in any study is homogeneity in the groups under scrutiny. One would make little progress in studying anaemia by collecting pale people and even if one ensured that their pallor was due to a low haemoglobin, a trial comparing the value of treatment with iron, folic acid and vitamin B_{12} would produce nothing but confusion until bleeders and haemolysers had been removed and the remainder had been characterized by examining at least a blood film and measuring red cell size. To carry accuracy still further, blood levels of the haematinics under test and bone marrow examination would be needed, so the search for precision is accompanied by an increase in the complexity and invasiveness of the tests which may make them unacceptable or non-available under field conditions. So too with stroke, where clinical diagnosis is about as meaningful as using pallor to indicate anaemia. Increasing precision comes when it is too late (at necropsy) or from techniques such as computerized axial tomography (CAT) scanning which are not applicable to the majority of the 240 000 stroke victims each year in England and Wales.

The need for increased precision is shown in *Table 3.1*[34] which reveals that 41% of the certificates issued for fatal strokes in England and Wales are ill-defined (the last three categories). Moreover, the certificates which do contain diagnoses are at

Table 3.1 Deaths attributed to cerebrovascular disease (England and Wales 1973)[34]

Group	ICD* code	Total deaths
Cerebrovascular disease	430–438	80 583
Subarachnoid haemorrhage	430	4 066
Cerebral haemorrhage	431	15 380
Occlusion of precerebral arteries	432	464
Cerebral thrombosis	433	27 020
Cerebral embolism	434	310
Transient cerebral ischaemia	435	14
Acute but ill-defined cerebrovascular disease	436	20 828
Generalized ischaemic cerebrovascular disease	437	11 099
Other and ill-defined cerebrovascular disease	438	1 404

* International Classification of Disease

variance with studies specifically mounted to clarify the nature of stroke; for example, only 0.4% of the death certificates attributed the fatal stroke to embolization, whereas at least 50% of cerebral infarcts have been shown to be embolic in nature[1]. Even where special studies have been mounted, unclassifiable strokes still loom large; in the Danish Stroke Register, where particular attention was given to classification, 2.7% were attributed to subarachnoid haemorrhage, 13.6% to intracerebral haemorrhage, 32.1% to cerebral infarction and 51.6% could only be labelled as 'unspecified stroke'[27].

Until we can end this uncertainty we should avoid the use of falsely precise labels which conceal our diagnostic confusion. For example, the Framingham project, which produced immaculate documentation of its subjects on entry, chose to use a totally misleading descriptor as an end-point[16]; 'atherothrombotic brain infarction' or 'ABI' ought to imply a specific pathological process. If it did, one could then search for risk factors linked with the thrombotic or embolic occlusion which had produced ischaemic brain death. Unhappily, their apparently precise 'ABI' is really stroke without blood in the cerebrospinal fluid, so this category could contain patients with intra-cerebral haemorrhages which had not broken through into the ventricles. It seems likely that until we can confidently match the opposing processes of infarction and bleeding with the on-entry characteristics of patients in studies such as Framingham, we shall make little progress in dissecting out the precise mechanisms by which hypertension mediates its harmful effects. This implies that all such studies should have necropsy or CAT-scan endpoints rather than bedside labels; if not, the generic term 'stroke' should be used because it is less misleading than spuriously accurate pseudopathological labels.

HOW MIGHT HYPERTENSION PRODUCE CEREBRAL HAEMORRHAGE?

When Wepfer described haemorrhagic apoplexy in 1655[48] he was puzzled by the source of the bleeding: 'the ventricles laid open I found them all filled up with blood . . . there was nothing further to observe and I was able to find no ruptured artery or vein'. The source of such massive bleeding continued to puzzle pathologists for two centuries but in 1850 Paget described a fat washerwoman of 47 who had died of cerebral haemorrhage and observed that 'some, also, of the small blood vessels presented with well marked partial dilatations, like aneurysmal pouches, or like more extended varicose enlargements of their walls'[32]. These aneurysms were shown by Heschl in 1865 to have the same age distribution as the apoplexy[32], but the link was not clarified until 1866 when Charcot and Bouchard[32] observed 'while studying an apoplectic focus, we saw, after careful cleansing of its walls, two small spherical masses, each attached to a vascular filament. They represented two small aneurysms, one of which had ruptured'. They then studied 60 patients with cerebral haemorrhage and found these miliary aneurysms in all of them. They stressed the distinction between the miliary aneurysms and atheroma, noting that 'miliary aneurysms may be present and are frequently found in considerable numbers independently of any atheromatous lesion of the arteries of the base, or the arteries that are distributed to the meninges. The opposite is also true, namely that quite often the most marked atheromas are encountered, and still no single aneurysm is found in the brain'. They found no difficulty in accounting for this discrepancy because Virchow was teaching[47] that atheroma was an inflammation of the inner layers of an artery (endarteritis deformans) whereas they thought that their aneurysms resulted from a different process whereby the outer layers were weakened by periarteritis. Charcot struggled unsuccessfully to get the aneurysms recognized but pedantic terminology defeated him. At that time, a 'true' aneurysm was one which arose by an outpouching of all the three layers of the vessel wall, whereas a 'false' aneurysm was one in which the inner layers were in their normal place but the outer layers had given way (as in a dissecting aortic aneurysm). Ellis and Pick in 1909 and 1910 regarded the Charcot-Bouchard lesions as being periarterial or intra-arterial haematomas[32] and described what they saw as 'false' or 'spurious' aneurysms. This may have been medically correct, but colloquial usage attached a different meaning to 'false' or 'spurious' so medical opinion swung to an acceptance that the aneurysms were not there at all or that, if they were, they were an artefact of preparation.

In 1963 Russell[40] used injection techniques to reaffirm that the lesions were real, that they were aneurysms and that they showed two very important correlations – first, their anatomical distribution coincided with the common sites of intracerebral haemorrhage, and second, their prevalence depended on the levels of blood pressure recorded in life (*Table 3.2*). These observations were confirmed and extended by Cole and Yates[8], who showed that aneurysm formation was strongly age dependent but that this age pattern was distorted by the presence of hypertension (the youngest 'normotensive' subject with aneurysms was 66 but for the 'hypertensives' aneurysms began at 44). This poses two crucial questions: first, if aneurysm formation is an inevitable consequence of arterial ageing[30] but can be

Table 3.2 Prevalence of intracerebral aneurysms[40]

	Number of patients with stated number of aneurysms			
	None	*1–5*	*6–10*	*More than 10*
Control group	25	7	2	1
Hypertensive group	1	5	5	4

accelerated by hypertension, then would the detection and treatment of high blood pressure delay aneurysm formation? Second, are the factors which produce aneurysms the same as those which allow them to rupture or bleed massively once they do rupture? If the factors are different, then the treatment of hypertension once aneurysms have developed may not prevent their rupture.

WHAT CAUSES BLEEDING OUTSIDE THE BRAIN?

If we accept that Charcot-Bouchard aneurysms only begin to arise in middle life and that their development is accelerated by hypertension then the situation seems totally different from the picture of subarachnoid haemorrhage which is cherished by medical students and therefore by most doctors. Despite its persistence, this picture is a classic example of misinformation being transmitted from the notes of the teacher to the notes of the student without entering the mind of either (what Trotter called the 'mysterious viability of the false')[44]. Most people believe that subarachnoid haemorrhage arises from congenital aneurysms on the Circle of Willis, but if this were true then the aneurysms would be present from birth, and would be seen at post-mortem in children and young adults. When the rarity of such aneurysms is pointed out, the next suggestion is that the congenital anomaly is a 'weakness of the vessels' so that although the lesions only develop in later life, they do so against a background of congenital abnormality. If one compares an artery, with its medial and adventitial muscular and fibrous tissue, to a wire-covered hose-pipe, then the armouring for a single tube must divide into two at a junction, thereby creating a less well supported area. It is thus the basic design which is at fault rather than a weakness which 'abnormals' have and 'normals' do not. As Alphonso of Castile observed 'If I had been present at the Creation I could have given some useful hints for the better management of the Universe'. Crompton points out that the facts about berry aneurysms have been known since the early years of the century[9]. He emphasizes that 'all the arteries of the body have a defect or gap in the media at the apex of their bifurcation or branchings . . . age, arterial hypertension and atheroma, all of which are inter-related, are associated with disruption of the internal elastic lamina. It might then be expected that berry aneurysms would form in the second half of life. This is indeed the case. The aneurysms themselves are not congenital; the congenital feature (which is not an abnormality) is the arterial medial defect, present in most of the cerebral arteries of all individuals'.

Why is this shift of emphasis so important? It is because 'congenital aneurysms' or 'congenital weaknesses' like 'idiopathic' diseases or 'essential' hypertension, imply that the patient's destiny is fore-ordained so that nothing can be done. If, however, berry aneurysms form part of a package with the miliary, intracerebral Charcot-Bouchard lesions, then the combination of age and hypertension is crucial to their development and rupture. The former is untreatable but the latter is not, so a shift of emphasis could take us from defeatism to optimism about the likely value of prophylactic treatment.

DOES IGNORANCE INHIBIT PROGRESS?

Most students could assemble a list of stroke-types which would include cerebral infarction, intracerebral haemorrhage and subarachnoid haemorrhage, but they would not have heard of 'état lacunaire' or 'lacunes'. And yet the existence of mysterious holes in the brain was noted in 1843 and was fully described by Marie in 1901[11]. As with the Charcot-Bouchard aneurysms for a time, lacunes were the poor relations of cerebral arterial disease. This is no longer the case[15]. Lacunes 'are small infarcts . . . when of recent origin they show liquefaction necrosis . . . The dimensions of lacunes range from 0.5 to 15 mm'. They are common (11% of a consecutive post-mortem series in a general hospital had lacunes) and their importance in the present context lies in their close association with systemic arterial pressure (in one series 111 out of 114 patients with lacunes had documented hypertension; in another, the prevalence was 38% in hypertensives and 10% in normotensives. Their presence seems to be at least as strongly correlated with a risk of intracerebral haemorrhage as with infarction. (In Marie's series of 50 lacunar brains there were haemorrhages in 16 and infarcts in 7, while in Fisher's series of 114 affected brains 35% also had haemorrhage and 26% infarcts.)[15]

It has been said[15] that 'some medical terms, like clothes, fall in and out of fashion for variable periods of time. Most clinicians who attend necropsies, and all pathologists, are familiar with lacunes but many of the clinicians at least may not recognize what they are, for it is a term that nowadays is rarely used. Undoubtedly the last word has not been said on lacunes'.

HOW COULD HYPERTENSION ENHANCE THE RISK OF CEREBRAL INFARCTION?

So far, we have seen that measuring blood pressure enables the risk of primary intracerebral bleeding, subarachnoid haemorrhage and lacunar disease to be predicted. Moreover, one can conceive of ways in which mechanical damage to the vessel walls could lead to these pathological processes. In cerebral infarction, the link is less easy to understand for, as we shall see, the critical process in infarction is luminal occlusion, in the shape of thrombosis or embolization. It is easy to see how hypertension could link with the vessel wall disease we call atheroma, but it is less easy to link it with the process by which blood solidifies in the lumen. The two processes therefore need separate scrutiny.

Hypertension and atheroma

In 1915 Turnbull showed that plaques of 'atheroma' occurred in pulmonary arteries of patients with severe mitral stenosis and attributed this to their high right-sided pressures[31]. When one moves to the systemic side of the circulation the position is much more complex for if blood pressure rises with age and atheroma increases in severity with age, then a spurious correlation between blood pressure and disease will be observed. Moreover, many studies have lumped together flat fatty streaks and raised, stenosing, ulcerated and thrombosing lesions[37].

In our Oxford necropsy survey[31], where we made planimetric measurements of the areas of the great vessels covered by the different types of plaque, we found that adding in-life diastolic pressure into our multivariate analysis increased the predictive power of the equation for raised fatty and fibrous lesions in men and raised fatty lesions in women but not for the other types of lesion. This lack of correlation with advanced or complicated lesions may indicate that once a lesion is produced, its subsequent natural history is unrelated to any original initiating factors such as hypertension. Prophylactic measures may therefore only be of value at an early stage of plaque evolution so that treatment in the elderly would not be expected to affect outcome.

A massive study of the geographical pathology of vascular disease[38] revealed very similar results for the aorta and extended the measurements to the coronary arteries (*Table 3.3*). The authors commented 'persons with hypertension or diabetes mellitus consistently have more atherosclerosis in the coronary arteries and abdominal aorta than persons without hypertension and diabetes, regardless of sex, age, race and geographic location. Hypertension and diabetes do not appear to

Table 3.3 Mean percentage of arterial surface affected by raised lesions in subjects with and without hypertension[38]

Site	Sex	Age (years)	Hypertension	No Hypertension
Aorta	Male	35–44	27	14
		45–54	36	25
		55–64	47	34
	Female	35–44	22	10
		45–54	34	19
		55–64	44	31
Coronary	Male	35–44	26	11
		45–54	33	18
		55–64	36	24
	Female	35–44	13	4
		45–54	24	10
		55–64	30	16

be primary causes of atherosclerosis . . . However the findings indicate that hypertension and diabetes, when present, accelerate the natural progression of atherosclerosis'.

It is not too difficult to visualize mechanisms which link high pressure in the lumen, and the increased stress it places upon the walls, with wall disease. Whether one believes in endothelial breaches, in lipid insudation, in inaccurate cell replication or in the proliferation and disruption of smooth muscle cells allowing them to accumulate lipid, a mechanistic view seems appropriate. Our hope must be that the damage which hypertension does to the artery walls can be prevented or minimized, if not necessarily reversed, by the detection and treatment of high blood pressure.

Hypertension and thrombosis

As the distribution of cerebral infarction is more directly related to the presence of occluding thrombi or emboli in the subtending arteries than to the severity of atheroma in those arteries[28], how do alterations of pressure trigger thrombo-embolism?

The most obvious, and therefore probably incorrect, explanation would be that the hypertension-enhanced atheroma initiated thrombosis. Many theoretical mechanisms have been adduced to account for such a relationship. In the past the loss of endothelium, and the consequent exposure of basement membranes and contact-activating lipids, was held to be responsible whereas the current speculation is that insufficient antithrombotic prostacyclin (PGI_2) is formed by atheromatous vessels, leaving the thromboxane A_2 (TXA_2) produced by the platelets to operate unchecked and produce platelet aggregation[29]. This argument is crucial to the selection of an appropriate dose of aspirin to use in stroke trials, which will figure in other chapters, because doses in excess of 40 mg every third day block the formation of the 'good' PGI_2 as well as the 'bad' TXA_2[17], which may account for the confusing results obtained with traditional doses.

Whatever the mechanism, if thrombosis is directly triggered by atheroma, as Virchow thought[47], then the treatment of hypertension should automatically affect thrombotic risk. However, many workers have been reluctant to accept the view that atheroma causes thrombosis and some, such as Rokitansky[39], have suggested that it is mural thrombi which give rise to atheromatous plaques. If thrombosis is a process in its own right and not just the passive vassal of atheroma, then how might arterial hypertension affect it? An arterial thrombus consists of fibrin, platelets and leucocytes and there is no hint, as yet, of a direct link between hypertension and the clotting cascade, or platelet and white cell behaviour. However, red cells play a crucial role in platelet activity and therefore perhaps in thrombosis. Hellem showed that platelets were not naturally 'sticky' but only became so in the presence of red cells[21]. Adenosine diphosphate (ADP), which is present in red cells, stimulates platelets to aggregate and when ADP-removing enzyme systems are used, this enhancing effect of red cells on platelet behaviour is abolished[18]. The relevance of this is that although no clues to a link between fibrin, platelets, leucocytes and hypertension can yet be perceived, there is an abundance of evidence linking red cell numbers and behaviour to high blood pressure and stroke. It is well known that the height of the haematocrit, even within the normal range, is a predictive risk factor for stroke[24] and that it correlates inversely with cerebral blood flow. It is also known that 'polycythaemia' and its corresponding increase in blood viscosity correlates not only with hypertension but also with obesity and serum urate levels, thus forming a 'risk package' of considerable predictive power in cardiovascular disease. Over the next few years we must try to disentangle this package and decide whether a direct attack on haematocrit, by venesection for example, might offer more to thrombotic risk than we can offer by attacking fibrin formation with anticoagulants and platelet activity with aspirin, dipyridamole, sulphinpyrazone, thromboxane and prostacyclin manipulators. Finally, when we try to link red cells with thrombosis we should note that intrinsic abnormalities of their membranes in respect of ion fluxes are now being claimed in patients with hypertension, the pattern differing between 'essential' and 'secondary' hypertensives[7, 14]. Such abnormalities could well affect the ability of the red cells to make ADP available at sites of disturbed flow, or alternatively the membrane abnormality may also be present in the platelets, conferring altered reactivity and providing a more direct link with thrombotic behaviour.

The final way in which hypertension could affect thromboembolic risk is again an obvious one. If some 60% of 'cerebral thrombi' are really emboli, and if many of these originate in the heart, then linking mechanisms can be readily perceived (hypertension enhances the risk of myocardial infarction and infarcts give rise to mural thrombi which then embolize; ischaemic hearts develop atrial fibrillation which increases the risk of embolic stroke 5-fold). This re-emphasizes the unity of vascular disease but a note of caution should be sounded; the relative importance of different risk factors suggests that although there may be a common multi-factorial stem of causation, the brain, heart and limb vessels must have other properties which relate in different degrees to these common factors (for example, although hypertension, smoking, serum cholesterol, ECG abnormalities and glucose intolerance all contribute to the risk of disease in the head, heart and legs, the contribution of hypertension to stroke risk is maximal while cigarette smoking makes little contribution). This paradox of unity but diversity is emphasized by racial studies, which show that at given pressure levels black Americans and West Indians[10] show more strokes and less heart disease than corresponding white populations, and by secular studies, which show that the patterns of stroke and coronary disease in a given community do not follow the same trends. Anderson[3] has pointed out that these observations 'challenge the simplistic idea that both are the automatic end-result of a single pathological process'.

While the debates continue about the relative importance of atheroma or thrombosis and the mechanisms involved, hypertension clearly serves as a major risk marker for future stroke. Osler's motto, adapted from Thomas Carlyle, is therefore very relevant to today's dilemma: 'Our main business is not to see what lies dimly at a distance but to do what lies clearly at hand'. What, then, is the evidence that treating high blood pressure reduces stroke morbidity and mortality?

EFFECT OF TREATING HYPERTENSION ON STROKE

At what pressure level does treatment confer benefit?

When ganglion blocking agents became available in the 1950s we were able, for the first time, to manipulate arterial pressure, but unpleasant side effects led clinicians to restrict their use to patients with malignant hypertension. Untreated, such patients had died within months from the consequences of fibrinoid arteriolar necrosis such as renal failure, so stroke was not a significant end-point in these early studies. As treatment regimes became less unpleasant, the debate about their efficacy switched to patients with severe, but not malignant hypertension, then to moderate and finally to mild hypertension.

Severe hypertension

A pioneering study was mounted by the Veterans Administration in the United States[45]. The nature of the institutions concerned creates problems in attempting to extrapolate from them to the general community in that all the subjects were men, over half were black and many of them already had evidence of vascular problems and of other complicating diseases. Another point of difference from routine clinical practice was that the subjects were admitted to hospital for assessment and were only entered into the trial if their diastolic pressures on the fourth to the sixth in-patient day lay between 90 and 129 mmHg and if their subsequent pretrial out-patient pressures averaged 115 to 129 mmHg. They also had to be compliant, as shown by their pretrial consumption of a riboflavin marked placebo which could be checked by urine fluorescence. The regimes used were placebo ($n = 70$) or a combination of hydrochlorothiazide, reserpine and hydralazine ($n = 73$). After an average period of observation of some 18 months, 4 placebo patients and no active-treatment patients had died; the numbers developing non-fatal end points were 23 and 2 respectively. As one would expect, the number of strokes was too small to allow any separate conclusion to be drawn (4 and 1 respectively).

Moderate hypertension

Again the Veterans led the way[46]; a similar protocol was followed so all the subjects were men who were admitted to hospital and excluded if their 4th to 6th day pressures fell outside the 90–129 mmHg diastolic range. Back in the out-patient clinic they had to prove their compliance and show average pre-entry blood pressure levels of 90 to 114 mmHg. Of 194 placebo patients, 21 died, while of 186 actively-treated patients, 10 died. There were 20 fatal and non-fatal strokes in the placebo and 5 in the active group. All should then be clear, in that treating pressures from 90 to 114 mmHg diastolic pressure appears to have altered mortality and morbidity. However, in addition to the problems posed by the groups studied and by their pretrial handling, there were some other internal puzzles (*Table 3.4*) in

Table 3.4 Percentage of patients with morbid events in Veterans Administration Study[41]

Pre-randomization BP	% with events
Diastolic 90–104 mmHg	16.3
Diastolic 105–114 mmHg	8.0
Systolic under 165 mmHg	9.3
Systolic 165 mmHg and over	15.4

that patients treated for diastolic pressures of 105–114 mmHg appeared to fare better than those treated for pressures of 90–104 mmHg. For systolic pressures, on the other hand, the lower the entry pressure the more favourable the treated outcome and we shall return to this systolic–diastolic discrepancy later. In respect of diastolic pressure, these findings raise the possibility that in some subjects lowering an already low blood pressure may actually be harmful, whereas at higher pressure levels benefit will outweigh harm.

Mild hypertension

As one moves down the pressure scale the problems inherent in trials become greater. (1) The morbid event rate will be lower so the numbers needed to prove or refute benefit become larger and the follow-up period increases. (2) Compliance becomes a limiting factor because all current drugs produce side-effects whereas the longer-term consequences of discontinuing them do not immediately become apparent. This is in sharp contrast to oral contraceptives where the peril of non-compliance readily becomes obvious so that women are prepared to tolerate minor breast and leg discomfort, plus a known, albeit low, risk of vascular disease, in order to reap the self-evident benefits. If stopping hypotensive tablets produces immediate symptomatic improvement but no obvious harm, we must ask ourselves 'What kind of people are prepared to take life-long, symptom-producing treatment to prevent a condition such as stroke which they may not want to know about and which may never happen to them anyway?'

Three studies in mild hypertension have been reported and a fourth is awaited with interest.

THE HYPERTENSION DETECTION AND FOLLOW-UP PROGRAMME (HDFP)[22, 23]
In this study they recruited 10 940 men and women aged between 30 and 69 years and randomly allocated them to a systematic and tightly supervised treatment programme (stepped-care, SC) or referred them to their own community medical services (referred-care, RC). What was being compared was not just the effect of different intensities of treatment but of all the other confounding variables introduced when one compares two entirely different systems of health-care delivery. The diastolic pressures used were Phase V (disappearance) so any

conclusions reached need to be corrected by doctors who use Phase IV (muffling) since Phase IV end-points are approximately 10 mmHg higher than Phase V (so 90–104 mmHg in HDFP roughly equals 100–114 mmHg for any Phase IV-based doctor). As with the VA studies, the HDFP used drugs which would not now form the front-line treatment regimes for physicians who are unfettered by the FDA. Step 1 was chlorthalidone plus triamterene or spironolactone where necessary; Step 2 was the addition of reserpine or methyldopa; Step 3, the addition of hydralazine; Step 4 the addition or substitution of guanethidine and Step 5 the addition or substitution of any drug thought to be useful. I will contrast this with an acceptable stepped-care regime later.

Table 3.5 shows total mortality, expressed in life-table terms: unlike the VA trial, the greatest apparent difference between the regimes lay in the lowest BP stratum.

Table 3.5 Death rates per 100 in HDFP Study[22]

Diastolic Blood Pressure	Stepped-care group	Referred-care group
90–104 mmHg	5.9	7.4
105–114 mmHg	6.7	7.4
115+ mmHg	9.0	9.7

However, as the comparison was not between treatment and no treatment group, but between patients treated in two different ways, the authors wondered whether higher-pressure subjects had been treated more efficiently by their routine services, unlike the lower strata who had aroused less concern. In respect of strokes the total deaths were 29 out of the 5485 SC patients and 52 out of the 5455 RC patients. To produce a total difference in stroke deaths of 23, 158 906 subjects had been screened and 10 940 had been studied; we will return to the cost-benefit or 'over-kill' problem which such an approach produces later. For patients in the 90–105 blood pressure stratum the figures were 17 strokes out of 3903 SC and 31 out of 3922 RC.

Patients with Phase V pressures of 90–104 mmHg thus fared better when they were supervised in special clinics than when they were referred to their own doctors. While this may, in part, have been due to better pressure control (mean diastolic pressures for the total groups at year five were 84.1 mmHg for SC and 89.1 mmHg for RC) there could also have been important differences in the general health-care advice given to the two groups in respect of smoking, alcohol, weight and physical activity. 'Suggestive, but not proven and using yesterday's drugs' must therefore be the verdict on HDFP.

AUSTRALIAN THERAPEUTIC TRIAL IN MILD HYPERTENSION[35]

In Australia, mass miniature X-ray is compulsory, so BP screening units were set up next to the radiographic units to attract subjects aged between 30 and 69 years as they emerged from their compulsory X-rays. It should be noted that even under this system compliance was not 100%, younger men being particularly likely to slip

Table 3.6 Events in Australian National Blood Pressure Study[35]

	Active (n = 1721)	Placebo (n = 1706)
CVS deaths	8	18
Non CVS deaths	17	17
Total deaths	25	35
Non fatal end points	113	133
Total end points	138	168
Fatal stroke	3	6
Non fatal stroke	14	25
Total stroke	17	31

out sideways between the X-ray and BP check. From 104 171 screened subjects they identified 3931 who had Phase V diastolic pressures between 95 and 110 mmHg (provided that the systolic pressure was below 200 mmHg) and who were free from overt cardiovascular or general disease. In 504, their diastolic pressure fell below the qualifying threshold before the trial began, so 3427 subjects (3.3% of those screened) entered the randomized phase which compared active treatment with matching placebos. Step 1 in the active group was chlorothiazide 500 mg per day, Step 2 was 500 mg twice daily or the addition of methyldopa, propranolol or pindolol, and Step 3 was the addition of hydralazine or clonidine. Target pressure was initially 90 mmHg or less but after 2 years this was reduced to 80 mmHg.

Table 3.6 shows the outcome when analyzed by the initial intention-to-treat categories which is the only way to approach a massive community problem such as this. Although there were consistent trends between the groups, the differences in total deaths and nonfatal end-points fell short of conventional significance. If we look at the results in respect of strokes (*Table 3.7*) we see that 17 events occurred despite active treatment, so that these subjects had taken drugs unnecessarily. If we subtract them from the 31 subjects who got strokes in the placebo group and from

Table 3.7 How much benefit at how much cost in the Australian National Study[35]

	Active group (n = 1721)		Placebo group (n = 1706)
Strokes despite therapy	17		
Strokes on placebo			31
Potential strokes prevented		14	
Patients treated to attain this	1704		
Patients remaining stroke free despite no therapy			1675

the total numbers actively treated we can see that to prevent 14 strokes (31−17) 1704 subjects (1721−17) had taken drugs for 4 years. In the placebo group, on the other hand, 1675 (1706−31) subjects who had taken no drugs still remained stroke-free, so they would have been treated unnecessarily had they been randomized to active treatment. To achieve these 'benefits', 104 171 subjects were screened and it seems likely that a campaign against smoking, alcohol, obesity and bad driving would have benefited the Australian community more. Society and not medicine must, however, decide this.

OSLO STUDY[20]

Men and women aged between 40 and 49 years with systolic pressures between 150 and 174 mmHg and diastolic pressures below 110 mmHg were randomly allocated to placebo or to active treatment for which the basic regimen was a thiazide diuretic. Of 785 subjects, seven in the placebo group and none in the treated group developed strokes, but in contrast the apparent effect of treatment on heart attacks was to increase them (13 placebo; 20 active). The trial is, of course, far too small to answer such questions, but it touches on two crucial issues which we shall re-examine later; the possibility that hypotensive therapy might affect stroke and heart attacks differently, and the possibility that hidden harm from some treatment regimes might negate their beneficial hypotensive effect.

MEDICAL RESEARCH COUNCIL MILD HYPERTENSION TRIAL[36]

A screening system has been set up in selected general practices to recruit subjects aged between 35 and 64 years of either sex and with Phase V diastolic pressures of 90–109 mmHg. They are then allocated to placebo or to one of two active regimes (in the first, the primary agent is a thiazide, supplemented where necessary by propranolol or methyldopa; in the second, the primary agent is propranolol, supplemented by a thiazide or by guanethidine). Whatever the results of the trial, several serious problems will arise when we decide how to interpret them for the benefit of the total community.

Firstly, do the findings of a study based on a screening mode of entry apply to patients who are identified by their doctors in the course of their routine practice (the case-finding mode)? We know that if all doctors recorded blood pressure at every patient contact, then over a 2-year period the yield of hypertensives would be almost as great as for the more expensive screening-mode method[6]. Case-found patients may also show different attitudes to the advice given and different compliance patterns from screened subjects because of differences in the doctor–patient relationship in the two modes.

Secondly, does the method of lowering blood pressure affect outcome?[12, 37] Thiazide diuretics raise serum urate and renin, increase carbohydrate intolerance and reduce serum potassium so their beneficial effect on blood pressure may be negated by adverse effects on other risk factors. β-blockers elevate triglycerides and reduce high density lipoprotein (HDL) cholesterol so there may be a balance between their favourable effects on blood pressure and unfavourable effects on other risk factors. Ideally the MRC trial should have been able to answer two questions: does blood pressure reduction confer benefit and does the method of lowering pressure matter? The use of the supplementary drug schedules may make it impossible to answer both questions.

Finally, as with the VA and HDFP studies, the active regimes studied are 'yesterday's drugs' in that propranolol is not an ideal hypotensive agent (it is nonselective in its action and variable in its dose-response pattern so that carefully titrated multi-dose regimes may be needed) and few practising physicians would now use guanethidine in patients with symptomless mild hypertension.

WHAT OTHER QUESTIONS NEED ANSWERING?

What about women?

The VA subjects were all male, and the Australian study had too few events to allow separate analyses for men and women. There is considerable background evidence that women withstand given pressure levels better than men[32], so it is of interest that in HDFP[22, 23] the patients who showed no benefit from supervized care were the white women (*Table 3.8*). I therefore know of no evidence which allows

Table 3.8 Death rates per 100 in HDFP study[22, 23]

Group	Stepped-care group	Referred-care group
Black men	10.6	13.0
Black women	5.2	7.2
White men	5.8	6.8
White women	4.9	4.8

physicians to decide on a blood pressure level in women above which prophylactic therapy for mild or moderate hypertension will confer proven benefit. The lung cancer and coronary heart disease mortality patterns ensure that there is a considerable excess of women in the age groups who consult general practitioners and who are therefore likely to be found to be hypertensive, so the contribution of the MRC trial to this crucial question is therefore awaited.

What about the elderly?

Although the results of the European Working Party on Hypertension in the Elderly (EWHPE)[2] should soon be known, only one randomized study has so far been reported[42]. In this, subjects whose mean age was 81 years and who had a casual Phase IV diastolic pressure of 100 mmHg or more were randomized to no treatment or to treatment with α-methyldopa. No significant difference in mortality was observed over a 7-year period; if anything, the treated group fared slightly worse at most phases of the follow-up. When the screened patients whose casual blood pressures had not qualified them for the trial (i.e. their diastolic had been under 100 mmHg) were compared with the hypertensive trialists, no difference in outcome could be detected. Unlike younger subjects, it therefore appeared that in this very elderly group, mild to moderate hypertension, whether treated or not, was not a risk predictor. The identification of an age-level at which hypertension and its treatment makes no difference to outcome is vital since the majority of primary care consultations which would result in the detection of hypertension on a case-finding mode occur in the elderly and not in the young.

Have we become obsessed with diastolic pressure?

Diastolic pressure is notoriously difficult to measure accurately and even doctors in the same institution, to say nothing of doctors in different countries, cannot agree on whether to use Phase IV or Phase V. Systolic pressure is much easier to measure but has been ignored until relatively recently. Rabkin *et al.*[33] studied the relationship between blood pressure and stroke incidence and survival in 3983 subjects and on multivariate analysis concluded that 'systolic blood pressure was the best predictor of short-term mortality'. In their younger men, diastolic pressure correlated better with coronary disease but in the older groups, ischaemic heart disease joined stroke in being more strongly linked with systolic pressure. The authors concluded that 'in middle-aged men the general concept that diastolic is more important than systolic is not justified for cerebrovascular disease or for ischaemic heart disease'. Similar findings emerged from the Framingham study[25]; they pointed out that the very strong correlation between diastolic and systolic pressure made interpretation difficult but that 'systolic pressure is actually the more potent contributor to cardiovascular sequelae. Even isolated systolic pressure elevation is associated with an excess cardiovascular mortality'. It was particularly 'ominous in the elderly in whom it is highly prevalent'.

Anderson[4] has re-examined the Framingham data by 'unsmoothing' the 'smoothed' curves which are usually presented and which have been accepted as showing a progressive rise in risk for both systolic and diastolic pressures. This has led to the therapeutic concept that 'the lower the pressure the better', but he has suggested that the diastolic risk-pattern bottoms out at 90 mmHg so that detecting and treating such pressures would not be expected to confer benefit. Systolic pressure, however, shows a 'no-threshold' pattern, risk being proportional to pressure across the whole range.

Most trialists and practising clinicians have ignored systolic pressure; suppose a patient presents with an initial pressure of 240/115 mmHg and attains a pressure of 180/110 mmHg on treatment. This would be called a diastolic 'treatment-failure' and the patient would then receive unpleasant supplementary drugs or be withdrawn for failing to reach a target diastolic. And yet he has shed 60 mmHg off his systolic pressure, so might this not modify the genesis and rupture of Charcot-Bouchard aneurysms, the incidence of heart failure or the cracking of atheromatous plaques which may stimulate thrombi to form? Might the *mean* pressure perceived by an artery over its owner's life-time determine risk and should we not use systolic and mean pressures as well as diastolic levels in controlling hypertension and in reporting the results of trials?

LESSONS FOR THE FUTURE

Every time a patient is given treatment it is in reality an experiment, but it is usually an uncontrolled and ill-recorded one. In a common condition such as hypertension and in common sub-groups in our society such as women and the elderly it is an appalling indictment of our health care systems that we have no factual evidence on which we can base rational prescribing policy. To paraphrase Finagle's Third Law 'What we have is not what we want; what we want is not what we need; what we need is not what we can obtain'. What we need is information on the blood pressure levels above which treatment does more good than harm for women, for the elderly and for men in the diastolic pressure stratum below 105 mmHg. At 105 mmHg and above in young and middle-aged men the evidence that treatment confers benefit is strong although it is difficult to extrapolate directly from the VA subjects to the general population or from their treatment schedules to the ones currently in use. In symptomless mild and moderate hypertension the key to success is compliance and the key to compliance is simplicity and freedom from side effects[19]. The stepped care and alternative drug regimes used in the trials set out above fail dismally on these counts which is why I referred to them as 'yesterday's drugs'. On present evidence an optimal stepped-care regime in practice or in new trials should be the following.

Step 1 Begin with a once-daily thiazide (such as bendrofluazide 5 mg) or a once-daily cardioselective β-blocker (such as atenolol 100 mg or metoprolol 200 mg)[49, 50]. In choosing which to use first, either toss a coin or add up the pros and cons (for thiazides – cheapness, freedom from immediate and perceived side effects; against thiazides – silent metabolic changes which may increase cardiovascular risk, such as in serum urate and blood glucose; for β-blockers – modification of post-infarction mortality rate; against β-blockers – cost, cold extremities, fatigue, relatively poor effect in black subjects and elevations of blood lipids).

Step 2 Add the thiazide and β-blocker together.

Step 3 Withdraw the patient from a trial, or if in routine practice, refer for further investigation and for consideration of the use of vasodilators or angiotensin-manipulating drugs such as captopril.

Having simplified our regimes we must then ask ourselves whether our community wishes to be offered life-long medication in exchange for a given level of risk reduction? If so, are they prepared to pay the personal and financial price of intervention? This question was addressed in a study to assess whether the treatment of hypertension is an efficient use of health resources[43]. This was carried out in 1977 so the absolute figures need to be updated appropriately, but the sentiments are timeless. The authors concluded that '$4850 for an additional year of quality-adjusted life expectancy for patients with diastolic blood pressures above 105 mmHg and $9880 for those with diastolic blood pressures between 95 and 104 mmHg seem like reasonable prices to pay. When the problem of patient adherence is introduced, however, these figures rise to $10 500 and $20 400. Are these still reasonable prices to pay? In the absence of comparable analyses for other uses of health care resources the answer to this question depends solely on the subjective valuation that one wants to place on a year of life'.

But is death the only arbiter? 'It seems to me most strange that men should fear, seeing that death, a necessary end, will come when it will come'.[43] Disability on the other hand, imposes a burden of illness on the individual, the family and on the community, so that if one was looking to a hypertension detection and treatment programme to reduce the burden of illness in society, one might wish to invest more in regimes which reduced disability by preventing stroke than in ones which merely reduced death by preventing myocardial infarction.

CONCLUSION

Having demonstrated the link between hypertension and stroke but having reviewed a mass of information that falls tantalizingly short of proof in respect of who we should treat to prevent stroke and how we should treat them, we can see the wisdom of the excellent definition[13] of hypertension alluded to earlier: 'In an operational sense, hypertension should be defined in terms of a blood pressure level above which investigation and treatment do more good than harm. Probably this critical level will vary with age and sex and it will certainly be affected by the medical facilities available and by personal and cultural assessments of good and harm'. The task for medicine is now to define a series of levels which will allow society and individuals to decide how much benefit accrues from how much cost and then delineate their personal and cultural definitions of good and harm.

References

1 ADAMS, R. D. and VAN DER EECKEN, H. M. Vascular diseases of the brain. *Annual Review of Medicine*, **4**, 213–252 (1953)

2 AMERY, A. and DE SCHAEPARIJVER, A. European Working Party on High Blood Pressure in the Elderly (EWPHE): organisation of a double blind multicentre trial on antihypertensive therapy in elderly patients. *Clinical Science and Molecular Medicine*, **45**, 71S–73S (1973)

3 ANDERSON, T. W. Cerebral infarction and myocardial infarction. *Lancet*, **2**, 205–206 (1978)

4 ANDERSON, T. W. Re-examination of some of the Framingham blood pressure data. *Lancet*, **2**, 1139–1141 (1978)

5 BAGLIVI, G. *The Practice of Physick*. London: Bell (1704)

6 BARBER, J. H., BEEVERS, D. G., FIFE, R., HAWTHORNE, V. M., McKENZIE, H. M., SINCLAIR, R. G., SIMPSON, R. J., STEWART, G. M. and WILLIAMS, D. I. Blood pressure screening and supervision in general practice. *British Medical Journal*, **1**, 843–846 (1979)

7 CANESSA, M., ADRAGNA, N., SOLOMON, H. S., CONNOLLY, T. M. and TOSTESON, D. C. Increased sodium-lithium countertransport in red cells of patients with essential hypertension. *New England Journal of Medicine*, **302**, 772–776 (1980)

8 COLE, F. M. and YATES, P. O. The occurrence and significance of intra-cerebral micro-aneurysms. *Journal of Pathology and Bacteriology*, **93**, 393–411 (1967)

9 CROMPTON, M. R. Pathology of degenerative cerebral arterial disease. In *Cerebral Arterial Disease*, edited by R. W. Ross Russell. Edinburgh: Churchill Livingstone (1976)

10 CRUICKSHANK, J. K., BEEVERS, D. G., OSBOURNE, V. L., HAYNES, R. A., CORLETT, J. C. R. and SELBY, S. Heart attack, stroke, diabetes and hypertension in West Indians, Asians and Whites in Birmingham, England. *British Medical Journal*, **281**, 1108 (1980)

11 EDITORIAL. Lacunes. *British Medical Journal*, **1**, 251 (1970)

12 EDITORIAL. Which drug for hypertension? *British Medical Journal*, **2**, 75–76 (1978)

13 EVANS, J. G. and ROSE, G. A. Hypertension. *British Medical Bulletin*, **27**, 37–42 (1971)

14 GARAY, R. P., ELGHOLZL, J.-L., DAGHER, G. and MEYER, P. Laboratory distinction between essential and secondary hypertension by measurement of erythrocyte cation fluxes. *New England Journal of Medicine*, **302**, 769–771 (1980)

15 GAUTIER, J. C. Cerebral ischaemia in hypertension. In *Cerebral Arterial Disease*, edited by R. W. Ross Russell. Edinburgh: Churchill Livingstone (1976)

16 GORDON, T. and KANNEL, W. B. Predisposition to atherosclerosis in the head, heart and legs. *Journal of the American Medical Association*, **221**, 661–666 (1972)

17 HANLEY, S. P., BEVAN, J., COCKBILL, S. R. and HEPTINSTALL, S. Differential inhibition by low-dose aspirin of human venous prostacyclin synthesis and platelet thromboxane synthesis. *Lancet*, **1**, 969–971 (1981)

18 HARRISON, M. J. G. and MITCHELL, J. R. A. The influence of red blood-cells on platelet adhesiveness. *Lancet*, **2**, 1163–1164 (1966)

19 HAYNES, R. B., SACKETT, D. L., TAYLOR, D. W., ROBERTS, R. S. and JOHNSON, A. L. Manipulation of the therapeutic regimen to improve compliance: conceptions and misconceptions. *Clinical Pharmacology and Therapeutics*, **22**, 125–130 (1977)

20 HELGELAND, A. Treatment of mild hypertension: a five-year controlled drug trial – the Oslo study. *American Journal of Medicine*, **69**, 725–732 (1980)

21 HELLEM, A. J. The adhesiveness of human blood platelets *in vitro*. *Scandinavian Journal of Clinical and Laboratory Investigations*, **12** (Suppl. 51), 1–117 (1960)

22 HYPERTENSION DETECTION AND FOLLOW-UP PROGRAM CO-OPERATIVE GROUP. Five year findings of the hypertension detection and follow-up program. I. Reduction in mortality of persons with high blood pressure including mild hypertension. *Journal of the American Medical Association*, **242**, 2562–2571 (1979)

23 HYPERTENSION DETECTION AND FOLLOW-UP PROGRAM CO-OPERATIVE GROUP. Five-year findings of the hypertension detection and follow-up program. II. Mortality by race sex and age. *Journal of the American Medical Association*, **242**, 2572–2577 (1979)

24 KANNEL, W. B. Epidemiology of cerebrovascular disease. In *Cerebral Arterial Disease*, edited by R. W. Ross Russell. Edinburgh: Churchill Livingstone (1976)

25 KANNEL, W. B., DAWBER, T. R. and McGEE, D. L. Perspectives on systolic hypertension. The Framingham study. *Circulation*, **61**, 1179–1182 (1980)

26 LEWIS, T. *Diseases of the Heart*, 3rd edition. London: Macmillan (1942)

27 MARQUARDSEN, J. An epidemiologic study of stroke in a Danish urban community. In *Stroke*, edited by F. J. Gillingham, C. Mawdsley and A. E. Williams. Edinburgh: Churchill Livingstone (1976)

28 MITCHELL, J. R. A. Has our basic knowledge of cerebro-vascular disease led to effective and rational treatment? In *Stroke*, edited by F. J. Gillingham, C. Mawdsley and A. E. Williams. Edinburgh: Churchill Livingstone (1976)

29 MITCHELL, J. R. A. Prostaglandins in vascular disease: a seminal approach. *British Medical Journal*, **282**, 590–594 (1981)

30 MITCHELL, J. R. A. and ADAMS, J. H. Aortic size and aortic calcification: a necropsy study. *Atherosclerosis*, **27**, 437–446 (1977)

31 MITCHELL, J. R. A. and SCHWARTZ, C. J. *Arterial Disease*. Oxford: Blackwell Scientific (1965)

32 PICKERING, G. W. *High Blood Pressure*, 2nd edition. London: Churchill (1968)

33 RABKIN, S. W., MATHEWSON, F. A. L. and TATE, R. B. The relation of blood pressure to stroke prognosis. *Annals of Internal Medicine*, **89**, 15–20 (1978)

34 REGISTRAR GENERAL. *Statistical Review of England and Wales for the Year 1973*. Part 1A Tables, medical. London: Her Majesty's Stationery Office (1975)

35 REPORT BY THE MANAGEMENT COMMITTEE. The Australian Therapeutic Trial in mild hypertension. *Lancet*, **1**, 1261–1267 (1980)

36 REPORT OF MEDICAL RESEARCH COUNCIL WORKING PARTY ON MILD TO MODERATE HYPERTENSION. Randomised controlled trial of treatment for mild hypertension; design and pilot trial. *British Medical Journal*, **1**, 1437–1440 (1977)

37 REPORT OF MEDICAL RESEARCH COUNCIL WORKING PARTY ON MILD TO MODERATE HYPERTENSION. Adverse reactions to bendrofluazide and propranolol for the treatment of mild hypertension. *Lancet*, **2**, 539–543 (1981)

38 ROBERTSON, W. B. and STRONG, J. P. Atherosclerosis in persons with hypertension and diabetes mellitus. *Laboratory Investigation*, **18**, 538–551 (1968)

39 ROKITANSKY, C. *Handbuch der pathologischen Anatomie*. Translated by W. E. Swaine and G. E. Day. London: New Sydenham Society (1852)

40 RUSSELL, R. W. R. Observations on intracerebral aneurysms. *Brain*, **86**, 425–442 (1963)

41 SHAKESPEARE, W. *Julius Caesar*, Act II Scene 2. London: Oxford University Press

42 SPRACKLING, M. E., MITCHELL, J. R. A. and WATT, G. Blood pressure reduction in the elderly: a randomised controlled trial of methyldopa. *British Medical Journal*, **283**, 1151–1153 (1981)

43 STASON, W. B. and WEINSTEIN, M. C. Allocation of resources to manage hypertension. *New England Journal of Medicine*, **296**, 732–739 (1977)

44 TROTTER, W. R. *The Collected Papers of Wilfred Trotter*. London: Oxford University Press (1941)

45 VETERANS ADMINISTRATION CO-OPERATIVE STUDY GROUP ON ANTI-HYPERTENSIVE AGENTS. I. Effects of treatment on morbidity in hypertension; results in patients

with diastolic blood pressures averaging 115 through 129 mmHg. *Journal of the American Medical Association*, **202,** 1028–1034 (1967)

46 VETERANS ADMINISTRATION CO-OPERATIVE STUDY GROUP ON ANTI-HYPERTENSIVE AGENTS. Effects of treatment on morbidity in hypertension. II. Results in patients with diastolic blood pressure averaging 90 through 114 mmHg. *Journal of the American Medical Association*, **213,** 1143–1152 (1970)

47 VIRCHOW, R. Phlogose und Thrombose in Gefäss-System. In *Gessamelte Abhandlungen zur wissenschaftlichen Medicin.* Frankfurt: Meidinger Sohn (1856)

48 WEPFER, J. J. *Historiae Apoplecticorum.* Amsterdam: Jassonio-Waesbergios (1724)

49 WILCOX, R. G. Randomised study of six β-blockers and a thiazide diuretic in essential hypertension. *British Medical Journal*, **2,** 383–385 (1978)

50 WILCOX, R. G. and MITCHELL, J. R. A. Contribution of atenolol, bendrofluazide and hydrallazine to management of severe hypertension. *British Medical Journal*, **2,** 547–550 (1977)

4
Cerebral blood flow and metabolism
Lawrence C. McHenry, Jr

The human brain with its complex vascular network may be viewed as a 'three pound biological computer' that is composed of billions of cells and circuits that make it the most sophisticated organism in the universe that we know of. While the brain is most efficient, it only utilizes the energy equivalent to that of a small light bulb, and although it represents only approximately 2% of the total body weight, it demands 15% of the resting cardiac output and at rest utilizes 25% of the total body inspired oxygen.

HISTORY OF THE STUDY OF THE CEREBRAL CIRCULATION

Since the late 18th century when Alexander Monro[295] put forth his notions on intracranial circulation, it has been accepted that the control of blood flow through the brain differs from that of other organs. George Burrows[53] first demonstrated that the amount of blood in the brain can vary and that this may be responsible for clinical signs. Sir Astley Cooper[70] was the first to show that loss of consciousness could be experimentally induced by producing anemia in the brain. Donders[89] first observed and studied the cerebral circulation in the living animal by observation of the pial vessels through a sealed glass window in the calvarium. Mosso[296] recorded changes in the volume of intracranial contents by sealing a tambour system within the scalps of patients with cranial defects and continuously recording the alterations produced under varying physiological conditions.

Although a great deal of information was obtained during the 19th century on a physiology of the cerebral circulation, the first truly scientific studies were carried out by Charles Roy and Charles Sherrington at Cambridge University. Using a delicate recording apparatus, Roy and Sherrington[370] measured changes in the vertical diameter of the brain in the open cranium. They found that under many experimental conditions the blood supply of the brain varied directly with the blood pressure in the systemic arteries. They also observed that during asphyxia and following the intravenous infusion of strong acids, a marked expansion of the brain occurred which was independent of the arterial blood pressure. From their many studies, they concluded that the variation in caliber of the cerebral vessels was regulated by

> . . . the chemical products of cerebral metabolism contained in the lymph which bathes the walls of the arterioles of the brain . . . In this reaction the brain possesses an intrinsic mechanism by which its vascular supply can be varied locally in correspondence with local variations of functional activity.

This fundamental concept of Roy and Sherrington was subsequently shown to be the basis of the regulation of the cerebral circulation. This was challenged by Leonard Hill[156] and William Bayliss[20], who, from their experiments, proposed that 'the cerebral circulation passively follows a change in general arterial and venous pressure.'

Modern studies of the human cerebral circulation were made much less difficult by an innovative technique introduced by Myerson[303] who showed that cerebral venous blood could be obtained safely and easily through the insertion of a needle into the internal jugular vein. Using this technique, changes in cerebral blood flow were estimated by Lennox and Gibbs[241] by measuring cerebral arteriovenous oxygen, glucose and carbon dioxide difference.

The recent era of the study of cerebral blood flow began in the mid 1940s. Prior to this qualitative, or at best, semiquantitative methods such as the pial window technique in the skull, were developed but were only applicable to animal experimentation. In man the methods for studying cerebral circulation were the following:

(1) Direct observations of the retinal circulation.
(2) Thermocouple measurements of the temperature of the exposed surface of the brain or of the blood in the internal jugular vein.
(3) Determination of the cerebral arteriovenous difference.
(4) Measurement of the displacement of cerebral spinal fluid during obstruction of the internal jugular vein.

None of these methods would permit quantitative measurement of cerebral blood flow and all, except the cerebral arteriovenous difference, had theoretical and practical limitations for even the qualitative evaluation of changes of the cerebral circulation in man. In spite of this a number of investigators, including Harold Forbes[117] and Morgens Fog[113, 114, 115] continued investigating cerebral vascular physiology through a variety of techniques. This period was, nevertheless, productive since many physiological and pathological observations on the cerebral circulation were made.

The real milestone in the development of techniques for studying the human cerebral blood flow was the nitrous oxide inert gas method developed by Kety and Schmidt[204, 205]. It was based on the Fick principle[100] and was of particular value because it allowed one to measure cerebral metabolism as well as cerebral blood flow by utilizing cerebral arteriovenous differences. This invasive quantitative measurement of global or average portion of cerebral blood flow was modified by a number of investigators. The krypton-85 saturation method of Lassen and Munck[239, 298] and the krypton-desaturation method of McHenry[256] were used by a number of investigators, particularly Dyken[93]. Lassen and Klee[237] compared the saturation and desaturation methods. The hydrogen clearance method was introduced by Gotoh and Meyer[136]. The argon desaturation with mass spectrometry was utilized by Hass[149] and others[392].

During the early 1960s, Lassen and Ingvar[182, 183, 184, 235] pioneered the development of the invasive quantitative measurement of regional cerebral blood flow by the intra-arterial injection of radioactive inert gases. The γ-camera, introduced by Heiss[152] as a substitute for multiple detectors, was extensively used by Mathew and Meyer[268] among others. A variety of important studies were carried out by the Kety-Schmidt and the xenon injection techniques.

While the invasive intracarotid injection method was being utilized, it was the goal of a number of scientists to develop a noninvasive method for measuring regional cerebral blood flow. This was first done by Mallett and Veall[262, 263, 442, 443] and Glass and Harper[145] and subsequently perfected by Obrist *et al.*[319, 320, 322]. The intravenous injection of radio-isotopes in place of inhalation was utilized by Agnoli[5] and Austin[14]. A number of techniques for the computer analysis of clearance curves and methods of data handling have become more and more sophisticated.

Other quantitative methods of both research and clinical interest include those of sequential scinti photography by Heiss, Prosenz and Roszucky (1972)[152], intravenous technetium angiography by Planiol *et al.* (1971)[335a]. The use of stable xenon and CT scanning for the measurement of cerebral blood flow and cerebral blood volume has been used extensively by Meyer *et al.*[281]. The most sophisticated methods yet to be introduced, positron emission tomography (PET) and nuclear magnetic resonance (NMR), are currently opening a new era for the investigation of cerebral blood flow and metabolism.

METHODS FOR CEREBRAL BLOOD FLOW MEASUREMENT

The Kety-Schmidt method and its modification for average portion of cerebral blood flow measurement

The original Kety-Schmidt method[204, 205] is based on the Fick principle which is a restatement of the law of the conservation of matter. In its simplest form, the Fick principle states that the quantity of a given substance taken up by an organ in a given time from the arterial blood equals the amount of the substance carried to the organ by the arterial blood minus the amount removed by the venous blood during the same time or $Q = QA - QV$, where Q is the total quantity of the substance, and A and V are its content in arterial and venous blood respectively. In the case of the brain, however, none of these quantities can be determined for any substance without knowing the blood flow. Thus $Q_B = TF(A - V)$ where Q_B equals the quantity of substance taken up by the brain and TF equals the blood flow; $A - V$ is the difference in concentration of the substance in the arterial and venous blood. If cerebral blood flow is to be determined TF = Q_B A−V. By determining the difference between integrated values of the concentration of inert gas in the arterial and cerebral venous blood and knowing the value of the partition coefficient of that gas as well as concentration of the inert gas in the venous blood at specific times, the blood flow per unit volume of brain can be calculated. This information was obtained in the original Kety-Schmidt method.

Certain modifications of the Kety-Schmidt technique have been developed in the past 25 years. Scheinberg and Stead[377] modified the original technique by taking continuous samples of arterial and jugular venous blood during the 10 minute period. This technique allows for physical integration of the arteriovenous nitrous oxide difference and was extensively used by Fazekas[99], Bernsmeier and Siemons[24] and others. Kennedy and Sokoloff[199] developed a microanalytic method that could be used in children. Lewis et al.[245] using krypton-79, a high energy, γ-emitting tracer, compared the indirect Fick method with their direct Fick method, i.e. by directly measuring the concentration in the brain with an external probe while simultaneously obtaining arteriovenous differences. By both the direct and indirect Fick methods, mean cerebral blood flow values were similar.

In 1955, Lassen and Munck[239, 298] substituted the radioactive inert tracer, kryptron-85, for nitrous oxide. Krypton-85 in air was administered via inhalation, and blood samples were obtained for analysis in specially constructed cuvettes. In addition to extending the period of saturation to fifteen minutes, Lassen and Munck introduced extrapolation of the arteriovenous krypton curves to infinity. This was based on the experimental observation that after 6–8 minutes of krypton inhalation, the arterial concentration was almost constant, and the venous concentration curve approaches the arterial in a manner that can be approximated by a simple monoexponential function. Lassen and Lane[238] found the calculated 'infinity' cerebral blood flow value to be 6.8% less than the 16 minute value which was in turn 8.5% less than the ten minute value. Lassen pointed out that extrapolation to infinity would eliminate the systematic error of incomplete saturation, and the lack of equilibrium between the cerebral venous blood and brain tissue at the end of ten minutes.

The Kety-Schmidt nitrous oxide and the krypton-85 saturation methods were used by a number of investigators and several modifications improved the application of the original techniques for a variety of studies of cerebral blood flow and metabolism in man. For example, Alexander et al.[6] developed equations to calculate whole brain inert gas uptake during periods of stable cerebral blood flow. In addition to the direct and indirect saturation methods for measuring cerebral blood flow, a krypton-85 desaturation technique was developed by McHenry[256].

The Kety-Schmidt technique and its modifications provided information only on an average fraction of total cerebral blood flow, and hence could not be used to study focal or regional alterations in circulation or true total cerebral blood flow. Local changes in blood flow may not be reflected in an average blood flow value for the whole brain. In areas of the brain that are devoid of blood supply from infarction or hemorrhage, a portion of the brain is essentially removed from the circulation, and theoretically it would be possible to obtain a normal cerebral blood flow. The Kety-Schmidt method has best been applied when cerebral blood flow and cerebral metabolism are studied in diffuse abnormalities of brain function. In order to carry quantitative studies of the cerebral circulation beyond merely measuring an average fraction of total cerebral blood flow, new techniques were developed to measure total and regional cerebral blood flow.

Regional cerebral blood flow

Most cerebral diseases begin with focal involvement of the brain or are regional in character, particularly cerebrovascular diasease. To study such regional alterations in brain circulation, as well as focal differences in blood circulation in the normal brain, methods were developed that would specifically measure regional cerebral blood flow.

The theoretical basis for the measurement of regional cerebral blood flow was developed by Kety and was first employed for autoradiographic studies in animals by him[200, 202, 203]. Data obtained from autoradiographic studies, however, were not applicable to studies in man. Methods which permit observations on the human subject and through the intact skull were thus developed to study alterations in regional cerebral blood flow in man. Several techniques were advocated for the study of human regional cerebral blood flow that were based on the intravenous, intra-arterial injection or inhalation of biologically inert radioactive substances. Two fundamentally different types of tracers were used, namely, nondiffusible indicators, which remain within the vascular system, and diffusible tracers, which move freely across the blood–brain barrier. Radiological monitoring of the isotopes was made over different regions of the skull or over the carotid and jugular vessels in the neck. The methods that use nondiffusible isotopes will not quantitatively measure regional cerebral blood flow, but only measure cerebral circulation time[321].

The intra-carotid xenon-133 injection method for regional cerebral blood measurement

The application of diffusible indicators to the quantitative determination of regional cerebral blood flow in man was first employed by Lassen and Ingvar[182, 183, 235]. They applied this method by injecting krypton-85 or xenon-133 into the carotid artery and following the clearance of the tracer from the brain by external scintillation detectors. Suitable collimation was used to obtain measurement of a circumscribed area of cerebral circulation, and Ingvar *et al.*[181b] performed the first studies in normal healthy male volunteers. Their results were in good agreement with values obtained by the Kety-Schmidt method and its modifications. The theoretical basis of this method was reviewed by Hoedt-Rasmussen *et al.*[161–164] and the mathematical equations for this method were first formulated by Zierler[468]. Sveinsdottir[421] devised a computer program for analysis of the regional cerebral blood flow data obtained by the intra-carotid xenon injection method.

Several techniques or methods were developed for analysis of the clearance curves obtained from the intracarotid method, as well as the noninvasive inhalation method (described below). By the *stochastic method*, which is based on the Fick principle, regional cerebral blood flow is calculated by the height of the clearance curve divided by the area under the curve after multiplying by the tissue-blood solubility coefficient[164, 234].

Two-compartment analysis is a more sophisticated method and allows one to separate grey matter flow from white matter flow[162]. Reivich *et al.*[361] has shown that normal brain blood flow fits a bimodal Gaussian distribution which is closely predicted by a two exponential model. By graphic means of curve fitting, two exponential values can be derived from nearly any washout curve. Values are obtained for the zero time intercepts and for the half-time of each component. From these, one may calculate the relative weights of a rapidly clearing component and a more slowly clearing component equated respectively with grey and white matter under each probe. The absolute flow through each compartment was derived as well as mean flow in each region[163, 164].

There are qualitative features in cerebral clearance curves in addition to the quantitative data revealed by mathematical analysis. In the initial portion of the curve, one may occasionally see peaks or areas of rapid shunting. The most frequent site where normal peaks are seen is over the carotid siphon. This is a very brief peak lasting five to six seconds. It may also occasionally be found over the Sylvian fissure. Abnormal brief arterial peaks are seen over arteriovenous malformations and very vascular tumors. These may be recognized by their abnormal size and location away from the carotid siphon. The nature of the lesion can be confirmed angiographically. Less rapid clearing peaks, called 'tissue peaks' or super-fast components, may be seen over areas of hyperemia so called 'luxury perfusion' of Lassen in diseased tissue[163, 231]. They are usually associated with angiographically recognizable blushes or early filling veins. These peaks represent abnormal perfusion at a precapillary or capillary level and are probably associated with hypoxia in the involved vascular territory.

The initial-slope index ISI_{10} or the two-minute flow index (TMFI) was described by Hutten and Brock[179] and Olesen, Paulson and Lassen[327], and Risberg *et al.*[362]. It has been noted that the initial portion of the cerebral clearance curve declines almost monoexponentially when plotted on semilogarithmic paper. If one takes the logarithmic slope during the first minute as percent of a decade and multiplies it by two, the result is an estimate of flow which is remarkably close in many cases to the ten minute regional cerebral blood flow value.

There is no doubt that the xenon injection method is the most sophisticated method available to study brain circulation, but it is not easily implemented, and it is traumatic in that it requires carotid artery puncture and catheterization. In patients with cerebral vascular disease, particularly extracranial vascular disease, there is a potential risk in this method. During catheterization of the internal carotid artery via the common carotid artery, emboli can be dislodged from a stenotic lesion at the carotid bifurcation. Although few complications of this method have been reported[185], this remains a potential hazard in the use of the technique. Another drawback is that the carotid catheterization should be carried out under fluoroscopic guidance to establish the fact that the carotid bifurcation is patent, and that the catheter has indeed passed into the internal carotid artery rather than into the external carotid artery. Further, in order to carry out serial or repeated studies, repeated carotid artery puncture and catheterization of the internal carotid artery must be done.

The xenon-133 inhalation method for regional cerebral blood flow measurement

In order to overcome the necessity for use of the traumatic method of carotid artery puncture, an atraumatic cerebral blood flow method was developed largely through the work of Veall and Obrist *et al*. The xenon inhalation method has become of great value for the study of regional cerebral blood flow in man because it is atraumatic and hence can be repeated at frequent intervals. Since the method has been shown to yield reproducible quantitative data, it has greater potential for on-line clinical use than any of the methods for cerebral blood flow measurement that have yet been devised. In 1967 Obrist *et al*.[320] reported the first results obtained from xenon inhalation cerebral blood flow measurements in 15 normal subjects age 20–30 years.

In the analysis of his data, Obrist found that consistently negative values occurred for the time displacement between the head and expired air curves, indicating that the best computer fits were obtained when expired air recording led curves by an average of 7.6 seconds. Obrist also showed that comparing arterial isotope sampling with expired air sampling, that although the two curves were of similar shape, the arterial data consistently lagged behind the expired air data by about 10 seconds. The arterial curve thus also lagged the expired air curve as well as the head curve. Differences in lung to brain circulation time (plus a small delay in arterial blood sampling) probably account for this displacement or delay. Providing this information is considered in mathematical analysis of the data, end-expiratory air is a reasonable substitute for arterial blood.

Another factor in the xenon inhalation method examined by Obrist *et al*.[322] was the additional input to the brain by isotope recirculation. This was the factor accounting for the slower clearance rates of inhalation curves, in contrast to the xenon injection method where recirculation is negligible. Hence, in the xenon inhalation method, it is necessary to correct for recirculation. As Obrist points out, its influence is apparent from the shape of the head curve which contains a 'recirculation hump', that is, counts continue to rise after the cessation of isotope inhalation. This primarily affects the fast component of the clearance curve. After subtraction of the second and third components, and correcting for recirculation, a monoexponential delay curve can be demonstrated. In this instance, the clearance rate is the same for the curve with or without correction for recirculation. Obrist emphasizes that 'although recirculation can safely be neglected in the second and third components from later portions of the curve, it is nevertheless necessary to assess its effect on these components at earlier times in order to make an accurate estimate of the first component.'

Obrist *et al.* (1971)[321] then reported a simplified procedure for determining *fast component regional CBF* by xenon inhalation. This was done to overcome the influence of extracerebral contamination and the undesirability of long periods of monitoring. The theoretical possibility of extracting fast component 'grey' matter flow can be performed when curve analysis is restricted to the early part of the washout curve. Obrist demonstrated that the combined slow cerebral and extra-cerebral components approximate a single exponential when (1) the difference in their decay constants is small; and (2) when the analysis interval is relatively short to their half times. In such analysis only the first compartment can provide meaningful estimates of cerebral blood flow. The second compartment is 'less meaningful' because of extracerebral components.

Since the short two-compartment method is limited to grey matter flow, Obrist explored the possibility of eliminating extracerebral contamination and obtaining information on white matter flow. In order to accomplish this, one must separate slower cerebral and extracerebral components. One approach, the spectrum subtraction technique, was proposed by Oldendorf and Fisaka[324] and tested by Crawley and Veall (1971)[74] and used by Obrist *et al.*[319]. The *spectrum subtraction technique* makes use of the differences in tissue absorption between X-rays and γ-rays of different energies. After equating counting efficiencies for the two energy levels, it was possible to obtain different curves that selectively reflect xenon-133 clearance in the deeper structures, that is the brain as opposed to the extracerebral tissue.

In 1975 Obrist *et al.*[322] described their method for estimating the clearance rate and *fractional flow* of the fast (grey matter) compartment of the brain from the first 10 minutes of the xenon clearance curve following one-minute inhalation. Compu-ter simulated data were used to test the adequacy of the two-compartment model employed, and to evaluate the stability of the parameters in the presence of random noise. Obrist also made a comparison between this approach and the previously reported three-compartment analysis.

As has been pointed out, one advantage of the noninvasive xenon inhalation method is the opportunity to acquire adequate normal control data that can serve as a baseline for the interpretation of patient findings. Another advantage is the ability to perform serial bilateral studies, thus making it possible to assess changes in regional cerebral blood flow related to the natural history of a disorder or to therapeutic intervention.

Nondiffusible methods for cerebral blood flow measurement

Total or average portion CBF can be measured using poorly diffusible or non-diffusible indicators[117a, 316, 385]. These are substances that do not leave the cerebral blood vessels in appreciable amounts to enter cerebral tissue. Measurements can be made of regional cerebral blood volume but not of regional cerebral blood flow. Measurements of cerebral circulation time may be obtained with radiopaque nondiffusible indicators such as those used for cerebral angiography. An index of the speed of cerebral circulation or the circulation time is obtained by measuring the interval between maximal filling of the carotid siphon and maximal filling of the parietal veins. Using this method intracranial and extracranial vascular patterns can be demonstrated if the surface of the brain is exposed. Similar information, including details of laminar flow, can be obtained by photographically recording the passage of fluorescein or other indicators through cerebral vessels[78, 151, 369].

Using such nondiffusible radioactive indicators, as sodium pertechnetate containing technetium-99, which are injected intravenously or inhaled, their passages through the cerebral blood vessels can be monitored with scintigraphic scanning techniques. Scintillation methods have the advantage in that carotid artery puncture is not necessary and gross obstructions to the passage of an indicator are evident. These methods have been useful for screening patients with cerebrovascular disease and detecting gross disturbances of the cerebral circulation.

Another aspect of these methods is that in theory blood flow through individual cerebral vessels can be calculated from time-concentration curves of an indicator for two points along an unbranched segment of a vessel of known caliber. The difference between the mean transit times at the two points multiplied by the distance between the points and the cross-sectional area of the vessel gives the volume flow of the indicator. If the indicator is fully dispersed, this is equivalent to blood flow. The difficulties in measuring cerebral vessel caliber and the indicator concentration put practical limitations to this method.

Total cerebral blood flow measurement

The determination of total cerebral blood flow was first performed in man by Gibbs, Maxwell and Gibbs[124] by injecting Evans blue dye into the carotid artery and sampling from the jugular vein. This method, based on the Stewart-Hamilton principle, was used in a more accurate way by Shenkin, Harmel and Kety[385], Nylin et al.[316] and Reinmuth, Scheinberg and Bourne[356]. A variable in this method is the assumption that the internal jugular blood represents mixed cerebral venous blood. However, as pointed out previously, extra-cerebral contamination is minimal (usually 3%), and Lassen and Lane[238] have shown that examples of contamination are relatively rare. In contrast to methods using the Stewart-Hamilton principle to determine total cerebral blood flow, those depending upon external γ detection and the Fick technique may not measure all blood flow through all parts of the brain as they are dependent upon the amount of brain tissue 'seen' by the scintillation detectors.

Positron emission tomography and cerebral blood flow and metabolism

Positron emission tomography (PET) is a computerized imaging technique which utilizes diffusible radiopharmaceuticals to obtain quantitative information about regional cerebral blood flow, regional cerebral blood volume and regional cerebral metabolism. Both invasive and noninvasive methods are used employing

short-lived positron emitting isotopes produced by a high energy particle accelera-
tor, usually a cyclotron. These isotopes include oxygen-15, carbon-11 and
nitrogen-13[17, 192, 335, 339, 341, 343, 430–432].

Positron emission tomography utilizes the unique properties of the annihilation
of radiation generated when positrons are absorbed. Image reconstruction from the
radioactive counting data gives an accurate representation of the spatial distribution of the radionucleotide in the chosen section or plane. The resulting data makes
it possible to calculate values for parameters of physiological and biological
significance when using appropriate mathematical models. PET scanning is analogous to quantitative tissue autoradiography with the added advantage of *in vivo*
studies. Positron emission tomography offers unparalleled opportunities for the
investigation of the relationship between regional cerebral metabolism and brain
function[57, 139, 178, 223, 227, 417].

According to Ackerman[2], PET scanning of the brain has the best potential at
present for providing the physiological data needed for the development of therapy
for acute ischemic stroke. Treatment which might be appropriate for one phase of
tissue alteration might be irrelevant or even detrimental for another. The utilization of PET scanning for the therapeutic evaluation of the stroke patient is of value
in the following ways:

(1) positron emission tomography can detect physiological changes that anticipate
    rather than follow structural changes;
(2) following an ischemic stroke, changes in cerebral blood flow evolve in a
    patchwork, heterogeneous fashion in contrast to a more uniform response of
    oxygen metabolism in the area of tissue ischemia;
(3) cerebral blood flow findings themselves are of limited value without data on
    cerebral oxygen metabolism;
(4) the increase or decrease in oxygen metabolism relative to cerebral blood flow is
    a prognostic value regarding tissue viability; and
(5) two phases of non-nutritional flow can be identified. The first is that it occurs
    acutely and is prominent for 10 to 20 days and may be best characterized as a
    luxury profusion syndrome. The second phase of non-nutritional flow is related
    to the patho-anatomic evolution of cerebral infarction.

Nuclear magnetic resonance

The phenomena of nuclear magnetic resonance was demonstrated in 1946 by
Purcell and Pound[337] and Bloch *et al.*[32], and in 1952 Purcell and Bloch received the
Nobel Prize for their discovery. It had been a continual aspiration of physiologists
to have the capability to monitor biochemical reactions as they occurred in living
tissues, and to do so quantitatively, repeatedly, noninvasively and nondestructive-
ly. Also, it became clear that methods needed to be developed to track fluids within
the body without making any contact to the body or disturbing or disrupting the
subject at any matter[13, 48, 457].

Nuclear magnetic resonance depends on the measurement of specific radio frequency emissions elicited in a strong magnetic field from molecules containing nuclei with magnetic properties. The nucleus of the hydrogen atom is a single proton which possesses both a positive charge and an intrinsic angular momentum or spin. The result of this is that the hydrogen atom has a magnetic diapole moment and can be treated like a small bar magnet. An NMR image depicts the signal obtained from a very large number of similar magnetic nuclei in each resolved volume of tissue when they are suitably disturbed. Their measurement and detection are possible when a large number of such spin magnets are placed in an external magnetic field and the majority lie in the direction of the field.

The relaxation time (T) is a term which describes the measurement of the amount of time required for an unstable proton to return to a realignment after being out of alignment. There are two relaxation timers used: (1) the spin-lattice relaxation time (T_1); and (2) the spin-spin relaxation time (T_2). Both depend on the motion of the hydrogen nuclei, the regional temperature and viscosity of the tissue and the magnetic effects of nearby nuclei. The relaxation time gives information about local tissue condition and can be measured at each point of an image.

Two distinct approaches[98] to human *in vivo* NMR studies have developed. First, proton imaging involves the generation of NMR images that reflect the spatial distribution of nuclear density. The proton images are used in studying internal anatomy with the aim of describing normal anatomy and detecting various disease states. The second use of NMR, called *in vivo* spectroscopy, is that of obtaining specific chemical information from selected regions of the organ through the application of localized chemical shift spectroscopy. This involves the use of phosphorus nuclear magnetic resonance. Localized phosphorus spectra provide metabolic information which directly reflects the state of health of the tissue. This is of particular interest because of the ability to measure certain phosphorus-containing metabolites of living cells. These include adenosine triphosphate (ATP) and creatine phosphate. From the NMR signal of inorganic phosphate, intracellular pH can also be calculated with accuracy. NMR may be said to employ both imaging and high resolution spectroscopy to the human body or an individual organ[177, 457].

NMR imaging of the brain

The most remarkable feature of NMR brain images is the striking grey–white matter differentiation seen with the inversion–recovery sequence. White matter is seen from the central region of the brain to the subcortical level with the clarity quite unequalled by CT. The central grey matter, incuding the basal ganglia and thalamus, are defined by the surrounding white matter and the cerebral spinal fluid[51].

Cerebral infarction is characterized by a loss of grey–white matter contrast. This change has been seen in the area where no abnormality has been detected by the CT image. The margins of the loss of contrast define the boundaries of the area infarction. In cases where this change is seen on CT, the correspondence with NMR is excellent. From initial reports the NMR image of brain ischemia shows a higher contrast than that achieved by CT after injection of contrast material[90, 150, 457].

Nuclear magnetic resonance as applied to cerebral blood flow

Two areas where NMR has limitations, at the present time, are the measurement of permeability changes in the blood–brain barrier and the measurement of regional cerebral blood flow. Some possibilities exist, however; for example, following injection of magnesium ion, a disruption in the blood–brain barrier is obtained by noting a change in the t−1 parameter.

An additional feature is the observation that nuclear magnetic resonance provides approaches to the measurement of blood flow along with the capability of characterization of tissue constituents of the diseased vessel wall. Of primary importance is in atherosclerosis where NMR shows disruption in the architecture of the arteries. Based on further developments, it is expected that NMR will detect the early processes of atherosclerosis, even before intraluminal protrusion of a plaque occurs.

Currently NMR can give large vessel flow measurements, but does not yet have the capability of measuring tissue blood flow[18, 19]. The first major investigation of blood flow measurement utilizing NMR has been carried out by Singer *et al*.[396, 396a]. The simplest method of obtaining NMR flow information has been termed the 'Qualitative Measurement Procedure'. Early studies have led these investigators to the establishment of a sound basis for the development of a clinical blood flow imaging system. The implementation developed has been the utilization of focusing of the magnetic field to a specific region and carrying out the blood flow measurement in that region. The region of interest can thus be localized by successive scanning of the regions in the neighborhood of the blood flow region. The exact localization of the specific region of interest will clearly stand out by virtue of the measurement of flow parameters developed by Singer. With certain procedural modifications, blood flow measurements within small regions may be developed particularly with regional selection by setting the plane focus using a static magnetic field gradient, to bring a specific slice of tissue containing the flow vessel of interest into resonance.

Nuclear magnetic resonance (NMR) in the measurement of cerebral metabolism

Since cellular and organ metabolism reflects the physiological state of the tissue, NMR measurements have the potential for establishing changes in cerebral metabolism. The following metabolic parameters can be obtained:

(1) Quantitation of interest of cellular phosphorylated substrates. This will give important biochemical information on cellular energy production and utilization. This is particularly true of compounds capable of yielding free energy that maintain cellular function.
(2) Intracellular pH. This will provide information on tissue ischemia and hypoxia.
(3) Direct measurement of enzyme kinetics. This will provide information about cellular energetics and the compartmentalization of substrates and enzymes within tissue[60].

Metabolic NMR measurements are thus noninvasive and are done *in vivo* and have the potential for:

(1) the clinical diagnosis of disease states such as cerebral infarction or hemorrhage;
(2) observing the progression of tissue metabolic alterations such as in cerebral hypoxia and ischemia; and
(3) the assessment of drug or other therapies on the changes in abnormal metabolic states, as well as the restoration of normal metabolic function.

CEREBRAL METABOLISM

As pointed out in the introduction to this chapter, it was Sherrington[370] who first showed the fundamental importance of cerebral metabolism as the primary factor in the regulation of the cerebral circulation. Changes in the functional activity of the brain, whether they be mental activity or transient focal vascular insufficiency, are reflected in changes in cerebral metabolism. Recent studies of cerebral metabolism show that such changes occur in a variety of physiological, as well as pathophysiological, circumstances. For example, one may demonstrate an increase in regional cerebral blood flow in the occipital cortex by retinal light stimulation; regional metabolism in the precentral motor cortex will increase with exercise of the opposite extremity; somatosensory stimuli will increase metabolism in the postcentral gyrus and changes in speech and mental activity produce a variety of changes in regional cerebral metabolism. All of these studies have been carried out in man[212, 236, 326, 363].

The brain may be considered to be 'obligatory aerobe', that is, it derives all of its energy from the metabolism of oxygen and glucose[158]. The brain uses about 25% of the total body oxygen consumption per minute and in quantitative terms it consumes 45–55 ml of oxygen and 60 ml of glucose per minute. In order to maintain the oxidative metabolism of glucose, oxygen must be present and of sufficiently high concentration in the brain tissue.

Cerebral metabolism on a tissue level is based in many ways on capillary densities in the brain which vary from one location to another as do the distances from one capillary to another. The boundaries of brain tissue supplied by a capillary are assumed to be cylindrical and are referred to as the Krogh cylinder. In the human brain, the radius of the Krogh cylinder has been calculated to be approximately 30 micrometre. A level of 'critical oxygen tension' has been defined as that oxygen tension below which cerebral oxygen consumption is reduced. This may vary from one area to the other, but in humans consciousness is usually lost at an arterial oxygen tension of 30 mmHg or a critical venous oxygen tension of about 18 mmHg. Normal atmospheric oxygen tension of 150 mmHg results in an alveolar oxygen tension of 100 mmHg and, theoretically, of similar arterial oxygen tension. In practice, however, arterial oxygen tension usually varies between 80 and 90 mmHg depending on the patient's age and pulmonary status. Venous oxygen tension is usually about 40 mmHg. The complexities of capillary circulation have made it difficult to determine average capillary oxygen tension. The oxygen tension in the capillary is not an average of the arterial and venous oxygen tension and in fact it is approximately 60 mmHg.

A relatively high arterial oxygen tension in the blood is mandatory for the maintenance of oxygen tension above the critical value of 1 to 2 mmHg in cells furthest from the capillary. It has been assumed by some investigators that the glial cells play some role in oxygen transfer from the blood to the nerve cells. Others seem to accept that the oxygen is supplied to the tissue by diffusion alone and is not energy dependent on the glial cells. Investigation in this area using newer methods of measurement is under way, particularly as related to cerebral ischemia[51, 91, 167, 169, 243, 309].

Early studies of cerebral metabolism were carried out by using the arteriovenous oxygen difference method originally described by Lennox and Gibbs[241]. This is still a valuable tool under certain circumstances to study total cerebral metabolism. Overall cerebral metabolism can be studied by this method and calculated as an average value for the brain if the average cerebral blood flow and the arterial venous difference for oxygen or glucose are known. Cerebral metabolic rate (CMR) is the product of the difference between the concentration of the metabolite (that is, oxygen or glucose or lactic acid) in the arterial and venous blood multiplied by the cerebral blood flow. When the cerebral blood flow is assumed to be essentially in a steady state, changes in cerebral metabolism are reflected by changes in arterial venous differences of the metabolite. Since the cerebral blood flow is reported as ml/100 g of brain/min, the cerebral metabolic rate is referred to in a similar manner, that is ml of oxygen per 100 g of brain per minute. Regional or focal changes in cerebral metabolism cannot be detected by this method which will determine only overall or gross changes in metabolism. The cerebral metabolic rate for oxygen ($CMRO_2$) is approximately 3.0–3.5 ml/100 g of brain per minute, representing an overall oxygen consumption of 50 ml/min for the total brain. This is approximately 20–25% of the total body utilization of oxygen at rest. Since the respiratory quotient of the brain is approximately 1, the oxygen consumption is equal to carbon dioxide production[158]. Using similar arterial–venous difference measurements for glucose, the cerebral metabolic rate of glucose is approximately 4.5–5.5 mg/100 g of brain per minute or about 80 mg/min for the entire brain. The cerebral metabolic rate for lactate is 2.3 mol/100 g of brain per minute under normal circumstances. The cerebral metabolic rate for lactate increases during hypoxia and cerebral ischemia[187].

Cerebral energy metabolism of the human brain takes place in the mitochondrion of the cells. Its lipid membrane serves three separate functions: (1) the membrane carries the enzyme that catalyzes ATP synthesis by oxidative phosphorylation; (2) it serves as a barrier that permits the generation of an electrochemical-proton gradient; and (3) proteins and coenzymes that transmit electrons from reduced nicotinomide (NADH) to oxygen are embedded in the membrane. In the metabolism of glucose each molecule is split via glycolysis or the Embden-Meyerhof pathway into two molecules of pyruvic acid and yields two molecules of ATP per molecule of glucose that is split. From an energy standpoint, this sequence of reactions is inefficient and, in theory, 36 molecules of ATP should be released.

The Krebs or citric acid cycle is the more efficient source of energy metabolism. Via this cycle, the majority of the ATP needed by the brain is generated by the metabolism of pyruvic acid to carbon dioxide and water. Through the action of a series of coenzymes, pyruvic acid yields 10 hydrogen atoms during each cycle. Eight of these hydrogen atoms are enzymatically added to nicotinamide adenine dinucleotide (NAD+) to give the reduced form of the coenzyme NADH. This in turn reduces the next coenzyme in the respiratory chain. In the electron transfer system hydrogen atoms are separated into electrons and protons, the latter being ejected outside of the mitochondrion. During their passage along the respiratory chain the electrons generate still more protons that are also ejected outside of the membrane. In the meantime, the electrons proceed from coenzyme to coenzyme until finally they are reduced to oxygen and then into water.

In the oxidative metabolism of glucose the hydrogen ions are thus oxidized to generate ATP. This overall process is called oxidative phosphorylization and efficiently generates the majority of the ATP synthesized per gram of tissue per second. The brain actually oxidizes from between 90 and 100% of the glucose taken up which is reflected by the oxygen–glucose index of essentially 1. Normally there is sufficient oxygen to take up all electrons but during hypoxia or ischemia the electron flow slows and levels of reduced coenzymes increase along with other chemical changes. The studies by Reivich, Raichle, Siesjo and others on cerebral metabolism have been particularly valuable[340, 342, 357, 358, 360, 373, 381, 389].

The metabolic protection of the brain by hyperventilation or anesthesia, especially barbiturates, has been the clinically useful application of these observations[69, 288, 333, 400, 406, 465].

The most sophisticated studies of cerebral metabolism have been carried out by positron emission tomography[16b, 17, 340, 342, 437]. Positron brain scans are obtained during the continuous inhalation of $C^{15}O_2$ and $^{15}O_2$. The $C^{15}O_2$ instantaneously labels stable water and during the continuous inhalation of $^{15}O_2$ body tissues extract oxygen from the blood in proportion to local cerebral metabolic needs. Positron emission tomography allows one to determine the distribution of blood flow. Local cerebral oxygen consumption can be calculated when the arterial oxygen content is known. In addition to measuring regional oxygen consumption, a method has been developed utilizing the PET scanner to determine regional cerebral glucose metabolism using C-11 glucose. It has been shown that it is possible to calculate regional glucose consumption within a core of tissue that is seen by a scintillation detector. This method has been validated in animal experiments and preliminary reports suggest that one may be able to use positron emission tomography to determine the local glucose metabolism. A method has been developed to measure local glucose consumption in various structures of the brain using (F-18)-2-deoxy-2-fluoro-D-glucose as an exchange of the glucose between plasma and the brain and its phosphorylation by hexokinase in tissue[360].

REGULATION OF CEREBRAL CIRCULATION

The regulation of cerebral circulation is based on a concept of 'cerebral autoregulation' which, basically, is the intrinsic tendency of the brain to maintain a constant blood flow despite changes in arterial perfusion pressure. The following three theories have been developed to explain autoregulation:

(1) the existence of pressure of tissue fluid on the low pressure vessels;
(2) an intrinsic mechanism in the smooth muscle cells of the arteries or arterioles that responds to an increase in internal pressure or tension in the wall by contraction (Bayliss effect); and
(3) the metabolic hypothesis.

In the normal brain it is not likely that the pressure of tissue fluid has much effect on local cerebral blood flow. Tissue perfusion pressure can be a profound influence on blood flow in areas of cerebral edema. Still, the fact that the ability of the brain to autoregulate until a critical intracranial pressure has been attained indicates that this mechanism is not significant in normal tissue.

The classical work on cerebral autoregulation was done by Rapela and Green[344] who believed that the metabolic hypothesis is the most logical explanation for cerebral autoregulation. This is directly related to alterations in arterial carbon dioxide tension. Others, including Lassen[232] and Skinhoj[398], concluded that the main factor controlling cerebral blood flow at the cellular level is the brain extracellular pH. This hypothesis, however, which was originally suggested as early as 1890 by Sherrington[370], has not found uniform acceptance. There is now increasing interest in the search for specific agents that might couple metabolic activity to vascular dilatation.

The maintenance of an adequate perfusion pressure at the origin of the penetrating vessel from the cortical conducting vessel is probably accomplished through the Bayliss effect. This is modulated by the sympathetic nervous system. Although this hypothesis remains unproved it is certainly not disproved. It is consistent with anatomical findings and some physiological studies[56, 233, 270, 415, 416].

This buffer function is an energy dependent system whose function is impaired in areas of cerebral ischemia. In the peripheral vascular system, the effector organ with its functional α- or β-adrenergic ending is sensitized to circulating catecholamines following end-organ sympathectomy. Such an effect may occur in the brain following transient early focal cerebral ischemia. The homeostatic function of the cerebral autonomic nervous system in the modulation of the myogenic tone of the conducting vessels would permit appropriate responses to both altered perfusion pressure and distal circulatory demands. The synchronous response of these vessels to alterations in the arterial carbon dioxide tension permits them to function in harmony with the penetrating vessel. If one accepts the theory regarding the role of the conducting system then focal autoregulation is at the level of the penetrating vessels. This places the regional or true metabolic blood flow couple at the arteriolar level, where, according to anatomical studies, it should reside.

Neuronal function and blood flow regulation

An increase in CBF occurs in appropriate regions of the brain under a variety of stimuli and is coupled to neuronal activity and metabolism: direct cortical electrical excitation, seizures, flashing lights, mental activity, and motor function (hand movement) all increase CBF. Conversely, CBF falls in states of depressed cerebral activity and barbiturate anesthesia. Kety was the first to document the parallel decrease in CBF and the rate of oxygen utilization by the brain in comatose and stuporous patients. Evidence supporting the close relationship between neuronal activity and blood flow is now overwhelming; however, it is still unknown how this relationship functions[12, 252, 269].

Cerebral perfusion pressure

Perfusion pressure is defined as the difference between cerebral arterial pressure and the cerebral venous pressure. The venous pressure is normally low (except in cases with increased intracranial pressure) and is negative in the erect posture, which partly compensates for a relative decrease in the arterial perfusion pressure in this position. A relatively normal cerebral blood flow is maintained over a wide perfusion pressure range by cerebral autoregulation. In hypertensive subjects, CBF remains normal if autoregulation is functional, with a compensatory increase in the vascular resistance to offset the increase in the perfusion pressure. This is of more than academic interest because stump pressures or the degree of backflow varies with the peripheral vascular resistance and cannot be equated with CBF in patients undergoing carotid endarterectomy. In normal animals that are hypotensive, flow is maintained at near normal levels until mean arterial pressure drops below 50–70 mmHg. Therefore, it seems unlikely that local changes in perfusion pressure in patients with normal autoregulation produce variations in regional flow. It is important to note, however, the primary importance of perfusion pressure in regions of the brain with paralyzed autoregulation. The upper and lower limits of autoregulation are shifted upwards in hypertensive individuals[415, 416] in whom modest reductions in blood pressure may provoke significant falls in CBF.

Oxygen tension

Moderate fluctuations in oxygen tension above or below normal levels do not affect cerebral blood flow, and significant elevations produce only a modest decrease in cerebral blood flow. However, hypoxia is associated with an increase in cerebral blood flow probably as a result of increased anaerobic metabolism and lactic acid production. The normal CBF response to hypoxia is preserved following section of the 9th and 10th cranial nerves. It should be noted that a paradoxical systemic hypotensive response occurs from hypoxia after section of these nerves, indicating importance of the carotid bodies and sinuses. Overall, it seems unlikely that local changes in oxygen availability play much of a role in the regulation of normal regional brain blood flow[218].

Carbon dioxide tension

The profound effect of alterations in the tension of blood carbon dioxide on CBF has been documented repeatedly[147]. Carbon dioxide is by far the most-potent vasodilator. An increase in $Paco_2$ of 1 mmHg produces about 1 ml/100 g/min increase in CBF within the range of 20–60 mmHg. Although some workers reported that minor fluctuations in $Paco_2$ were not associated with changes in cerebral blood flow, the evidence favors a parallel response.

It was formerly believed that carbon dioxide directly affected either the cerebral arteriole or the smooth muscle. However, it is now considered that this effect is primarily, although not exclusively, mediated by the extracellular pH. It is known that CO_2 diffuses freely across the blood–brain barrier, but hydrogen ions and bicarbonate ions do not. Gotoh[137] and Lassen[232] view the arterioles as Pco_2 electrodes that respond to the intracellular pH of smooth-muscle fibers. It is known that glial cells are rich in carbonic anhydrase, and it has been proposed that CO_2 is a local transmitter from neuronal to extra-arteriolar, extracellular fluid through glial cells. The glial cells would have the theoretical role of facilitating the hydrogen ion CO_2 equilibrium at both the neuronal and arteriolar sensor sites. There is, therefore, considerable indirect evidence for the coupling of metabolism and blood flow through CO_2 production, but there is no proof[383, 400].

Lactic acid and extracellular pH

Lassen[232] proposed that neuronal metabolism is coupled to blood flow by lactic acid production. According to this theory, extracellular pH drops as lactic acid accumulates. The reduction in pH, in turn, produces a vascular dilatation by alteration in membrane permeability or by changes in the responsiveness of membrane receptors. Until recently, this was widely accepted as the most likely explanation for autoregulation, and it still remains a viable theory[394].

Neurogenic reflexes

The existence of nerve fibers innervating cerebral vessels has been known since the work of Scarpa in the 18th century and their role has been studied by many investigators[67, 113–115, 117, 146, 154, 195, 282, 283, 286, 334, 367, 439] in the last 200 years. In spite of this, the neurogenic factors regulating cerebral blood flow still remain somewhat of an enigma.

As pointed out above, the sympathetic nervous system possibly modulates myogenic tone in the conducting or epicerebral vessels and protects these vessels from the effects of circulating catecholamines. This hypothesis is consistent with studies of isolated vessel preparations[82]. α-Blocking agents alter the constriction of the basilar and vertebral arteries to changes in $Paco_2$. This implies that in the conducting vessels the effects of $Paco_2$ are mediated through a neuronal reflex. However, this does not settle the dispute regarding a reflex center in the brain stem that modulates myogenic tone, because the blockade at the neuromuscular junction would be effective against a direct local action of CO_2 or an indirect neuronal reflex. As discussed previously, there is also evidence that the brain stem, through the locus ceruleus and the ascending intrinsic adrenergic nervous system, may alter cerebral blood flow. Although this supports earlier work dealing with general cerebral blood flow responses to brain stem lesions and CO_2 stimulation, there is no substantial evidence linking the local changes in blood flow from metabolic activity to neuronal reflexes. Nevertheless, this also remains a viable hypothesis, and, undoubtedly, total cerebral blood flow, distinct from local or regional cerebral blood flow, is modulated by a brain stem center.

Coupling agents

Using deoxyglucose labelled with radioactive carbon, Sokoloff[408] recently showed that the brain metabolism of normal monkeys varies from one region to another. For example, he found that specific motor activity altered metabolism in the appropriate anatomical structures of the brain. However, the mechanism for coupling increased metabolic activity to increased blood flow is unresolved. The search continues for a specific coupling agent, with adenosine receiving considerable attention. It causes pial vascular dilatation in physiological concentrations and increases in the extracellular space following electrical stimulation, hypoxia, and hypotension. The presence of α- and β-adrenergic receptors is well documented. However, these may be unrelated to responses of cerebral vessels to neuronal metabolic activity, and more than one type of receptor may be involved with vascular activity. The increase in levels of cAMP when physiological concentrations of adenosine are added to the bathing solutions of isolated strips of vascular smooth muscle, suggests that adenosine is capable of functioning as a coupling agent.

CEREBRAL BLOOD FLOW CHANGES IN CEREBROVASCULAR DISEASE

During the last 30 years many studies have been performed in patients with cerebrovascular disease, using the Kety-Schmidt method and intra-arterial method of Lassen and Ingvar to study cerebral blood flow. Recently the atraumatic xenon inhalation method has been used in a more effective way in these patients, particularly those with transient ischemic attacks. This subject will be discussed in detail in the following chapter.

Acknowledgements

I wish to thank Mrs. Sherry Holland for her assistance in preparation of the manuscript of this chapter.

References

The combined references for Chapters 4 and 5 can be found on pp. 106–135.

5
Pathophysiology of cerebral ischemia
Martin Reivich

Cerebrovascular disease is associated with significant alterations in cerebral blood flow and metabolism. A large body of information is available concerning these alterations in humans. This has been possible because of the development of various techniques for measuring cerebral blood flow and metabolism in man which can be traced back to the work of Kety and Schmidt in 1945[204]. At that time the inert gas technique for the measurement of average cerebral blood flow and metabolism in humans was first developed. Since then several techniques for the measurement of average, total and regional cerebral blood flow, glucose metabolism and oxygen metabolism have been developed (*see* Chapter 4). With the use of these techniques much has been learned about the normal regulation of cerebral blood flow and metabolism in man and the derangements that occur in cerebrovascular disorders. This knowledge has been amplified by studies in animal models of ischemia. Here we shall consider the pathophysiological aspects of cerebral hemodynamics and metabolism as they apply to cerebrovascular disease.

PATHOPHYSIOLOGY OF CEREBRAL CIRCULATION

Hemodynamic abnormalities

The effects of cerebrovascular disease on cerebral hemodynamics and metabolism have been studied both in patients and in animal models. In most patients with acute strokes there is an average reduction in perfusion rates in the involved hemisphere. There may also be a transient reduction in flow in the contralateral hemisphere postulated to be due to a transneuronal depression of metabolism[160, 197, 284, 397, 401]. This remote effect of injury has been termed diaschisis[444]. Within the ischemic hemisphere there may be an increased variability of perfusion rates among various regions[105]. There may be focal areas of decreased flow or focal areas of hyperemia[75, 181a]. The latter has been termed the 'luxury perfusion' syndrome[163, 231] and has been postulated to be due to local metabolic acidosis within the brain. Lactic acidosis has been demonstrated in animal models of ischemia[277] and in patients with stroke[325]. In this syndrome the local blood flow is in excess of the metabolic demands of the tissue. Normally the metabolic requirements of a region of the brain and the tissue perfusion of that region are tightly coupled[73, 186, 407]. This coupling is generally thought to depend mainly upon the regional production of CO_2[201]. In ischemic regions in which blood flow is no longer regulated by the requirements of the metabolically depressed area a pathological condition of hyperoxygenation in relation to the metabolic requirements can occur. Therefore, the oxygen content of the venous blood draining this region is higher than normal, resulting in some cases in red local venous blood. The latter has been observed during experimental occlusion of the middle cerebral artery[418, 446, 447, 449]. Increased venous oxygen tension may also be observed when the metabolic requirements of the tissue are depressed and oxygen utilization is decreased. In areas of hyperemia early filling of veins with contrast material may be seen on arteriography.

The areas of decreased flow seem to correspond to the site of infarction while the hyperemic areas may more often be observed at the periphery of the infarct. This has been observed in patients with occlusion of the middle cerebral artery[331]. Similar hemodynamic changes have been observed in animal models and tend to confirm the location of focal ischemic and hyperemic regions in relation to the infarct[420, 450, 464]. Oxygen tension in the area of infarction is reduced while in the periphery of the infarction it may be increased[278]. Infarction occurs when flow to that region falls below the critical level needed to maintain tissue viability. Below a flow of approximately 20–25 ml/100 g/min the EEG gradually disappears. In the range of 15 ml 100 g/min cortical evoked responses disappear. When flow drops to 5–6 ml/100 g/min a massive release of potassium from cells occurs[11, 38]. Cellular viability most likely cannot be maintained at this lower level of flow. Neurons may remain structurally intact but non functional between flow levels of 6–20 ml/100 g/min[175, 247, 328, 426].

Derangements of the control of cerebral circulation have also been demonstrated to be present in occlusive cerebrovascular disorders. The normal autoregulatory ability of the cerebral circulation, by which flow is maintained relatively constant in spite of large changes in perfusion pressure[230], is often lost following acute infarction. CBF may become pressure-dependent at all levels of perfusion pressure. This has been demonstrated both in human[105] and animal studies[446]. In addition, animal studies have shown that oxygen tension in the infarction falls when blood pressure is lowered[278]. The normal autoregulatory mechanism may recover days to weeks after the ischemic event.

The normal responsiveness of the cerebral vasculature to carbon dioxide may also be reduced or lost, or in fact paradoxical responses may occur following infarction[102, 105]. Thus, a reduction in flow in response to CO_2 inhalation has been documented in ischemic regions as well as an increase in flow with hypocarbia. It is postulated that the ischemic areas are no longer responsive to CO_2 because of the accumulation of acid metabolites, mainly lactic acid, and the presence of hypoxia. The more normal surrounding regions are still reactive to CO_2. Thus with hypercarbia the vessels in the perifocal area dilate, causing a reduction in cerebrovascular resistance and in local perfusion pressure[39, 382, 423]. This, in turn, produces a decrease in flow through the vessels of the ischemic area whose resistance does not change any further[102]. This has been termed the intracerebral steal syndrome. Conversely, hypocarbia causes an increase in resistance and in local perfusion pressure, resulting in an increase of flow through the vessels of the infarct which remain dilated. Attempts to improve the outcome in patients with ischemic infarction by means of hyperventilation, however, have been unsuccessful. In addition to these clinical observations, paradoxical effects of CO_2 have been produced experimentally[39, 424]. Experimental studies have also shown that in the area of an infarct the expected increase in oxygen tension during hypercarbia and the decrease during hypocarbia may not occur[142].

The incidence of hyperemic foci is highest during the first few days following an acute stroke[76, 77, 105, 163, 332]. Angiography may show early filling of regional veins and a capillary blush in these cases. Hyperemic foci appear to be more often seen in cases in which complete arterial occlusion is not present. They have been produced experimentally by reopening a previously occluded middle cerebral artery[103]. Oxygen availability also increases to higher than normal levels in this circumstance with a dilation of pial vessels and red blood in the local veins[418, 420, 447].

Acute strokes due to occlusion of a vessel more often show foci of decreased flow, sometimes with hyperemic perifocal regions. If flow is re-established either spontaneously, as in the case of an embolic occlusion, or following endarterectomy the anemic infarct may be converted into a hemorrhagic one[50, 106, 135, 463]. Similar observations have been made in animal studies[103]. Experimental occlusion of the middle cerebral artery combined with hypertension has also been reported to produce hemorrhagic infarction[88, 275].

In some acute strokes flow is reduced not only in the ischemic focus but in the entire hemisphere[102, 104, 331, 332]. Furthermore, a reduction in blood flow has been observed in the contralateral hemisphere[160]. This may be due to a general depression of mental activity and level of consciousness in these patients with a reduced cerebral metabolic rate or due to the phenomenon of diaschisis[401]. In this situation a global loss of autoregulation may occur in the affected hemisphere[331, 332] and even in the contralateral hemisphere[333]. In these patients the responsiveness to CO_2 was normal and the autoregulation could be restored by hypocapnia[333]. The restoration of autoregulation by hypocapnia has also been observed experimentally in animals during hypoxia[140]. This has been postulated to be due to the correction of tissue acidosis which has produced the defect in autoregulation[333].

Regional losses of CO_2 responsiveness or of autoregulation can occur independently of each other, that is, a region may show loss of autoregulation and still be responsive to CO_2 or vice versa[101]. The former, however, is more frequently observed.

A focal paradoxical response to an increase in blood pressure consisting of a fall in regional blood flow has been reported in some cases with global loss of autoregulation[332]. This may be due to an increase in intracranial pressure associated with the rise in blood pressure, causing an increase in cerebrovascular resistance in the focal area of the infarct and, consequently, a reduction in flow.

In patients with transient ischemic attacks disturbances of regional cerebral blood flow and its regulation have been observed for a few hours after the attack[399]. When determination of regional flow in 'white' and 'grey' matter and the relative weight of 'white' and 'grey' matter is made in patients with transient ischemic attacks, focal abnormalities in these parameters have persisted for several weeks after the last episode[346]. In a few cases the focal CO_2 responsiveness was also abnormal.

In patients with acute strokes without arterial occlusion, abnormalities of regional cerebral blood flow and its regulation have been observed for two weeks following the ictus[4]. In acute strokes due to occlusion of the middle cerebral artery abnormalities of flow and its regulation may be present for several months[331]. There is some evidence to indicate that autoregulatory abnormalities may recover before abnormal CO_2 responsiveness[4, 102].

Microcirculatory abnormalities

The effects of ischemia on the cerebral microcirculation have been studied in animal models. Until the work of Denny-Brown and Meyer[87, 276, 277] there were no adequate animal models of focal cerebral ischemia secondary to arterial occlusion. These investigators produced focal changes in the superficial cortical microvasculature by occlusion of the middle cerebral artery or its branches. Sundt and Waltz[419] refined this model using a retro-orbital approach to the middle cerebral artery with minimal trauma to the brain. In distinction to the studies of Denny-Brown and Meyer, in which severe and irreversible changes could be produced only by interfering with collateral circulation either by occlusion of collateral channels or by the production of systemic hypotension, Waltz and Sundt[449] found that severe microvascular changes occurred even though the collateral circulation to the area supplied by the middle cerebral artery was not compromised.

Normally the walls of small blood vessels are transparent. In vessels as small as precapillary arterioles, axial streaming and laminar flow are present[366]. Flow velocity is fastest in arterial vessels, less in veins and least in capillaries. Flow in arterial vessels is usually in only one direction. In large veins flow is unidirectional, but in cortical venules (and, rarely, small arterioles) flow may stop or reverse.

The microcirculatory changes that have been seen in a region of ischemia consist of slowing of the velocity of blood flow, darkening of venous blood and aggregation of the formed elements of the blood. This is followed by cortical pallor, vasoconstriction, the development of platelet thrombi in veins, the appearance of red venous blood, collapse of vessels, perivenous hemorrhages and cerebral edema[87, 275, 449]. White thrombi, composed of platelets, may appear. Local edema may be minimal or marked; there may be swelling of perivascular glial elements. Later, there may be focal reddening of venous blood indicating abnormally high oxygen saturation. This may be due to regional increases of cerebral blood flow in or near the ischemic zone (hyperemia) or to failure of ischemic neurones to utilize all the oxygen made available to them. Dilatation or proliferation of small vessels may occur near the edge of ischemic zones[274]. It is felt that similar microvascular changes occur during the process of cerebral infarction in man.

It has been postulated that following an ischemic insult astrocytic foot swelling, endothelial blebs and capillary collapse occur which prevent reperfusion, i.e. the 'no-reflow phenomenon'[7, 44, 81, 121, 221, 317, 318]. A correlation of the 'no-reflow phenomenon' with selective vulnerability has been suggested[130]. However, this concept has been challenged by the work of others and the question of perfusion artifacts has been raised as the basis of the 'no-reflow' observed[248].

CEREBRAL METABOLISM

Normal cerebral metabolism

(See previous chapter.)

Effects of hypoxia

Hypoxia is defined as a decrease in arterial oxygen tension (PaO_2) and results in a reduction in oxygen availability to the brain. As PaO_2 decreases below 65 mmHg, ventilation is stimulated and $PaCO_2$ is reduced, resulting in a reduction of cerebral blood flow which exaggerates the effects of low PaO_2 on the brain. With a reduction of alveolar oxygen tension below 55 mmHg short-term memory is affected[79]. As PaO_2 falls below 50 mmHg progressive impairment of performance and judgment occurs. Unconsciousness occurs at a PaO_2 of approximately 30 mmHg.

Carbohydrate metabolism

During hypoxia an increase in glycolytic rate occurs[69]. There is evidence that the initial activation of this increase in glycolysis occurs at the phosphofructokinase (PFK) step[310]. Although the pyruvate kinase step is also activated[15, 92], this probably occurs after the initial activation at the PFK step. What triggers this activation is not clear.

A significant rise in lactate concentration occurs in the brain when arterial oxygen tension is reduced to 50 mmHg[388]. At a PaO_2 of 35 mmHg, a significant increase in cerebral glucose consumption and lactate production occurs without any change in cerebral metabolic rate for oxygen, which suggests an increase in anaerobic glycolysis under these conditions[69]. A decrease in oxygen consumption at the mitochondrial level does not occur until mitochondrial PO_2 falls below 1 mmHg *in vitro*, although it is not clear if this also occurs in intact tissues[62, 411].

When inspired oxygen is reduced below 7% an increase in γ-aminobutyric acid (GABA) content occurs[460]. It has been hypothesized that GABA may play a role in the control of brain metabolism during hypoxia[459]. Catecholamine and indolamine synthesis is significantly reduced even with mild hypoxia (i.e. 10% inspired O_2) levels of PaO_2 at which tissue lactate and energy charge potential are unaffected but at which functional changes occur. On the basis of such data it has been postulated that the early functional alterations may be related to neurotransmitter abnormalities rather than to energy failure.

Energy metabolism

Phosphocreatine concentration decreases below a PaO_2 of 35 mmHg, while no change in ATP, ADP or AMP occurs even at a PaO_2 as low as 20 mmHg, as long as blood pressure is maintained. One homeostatic mechanism that has been proposed for maintaining the energy state of the brain in spite of low PaO_2 is that brain cells might reduce their energy consumption during hypoxia; however, there is very little experimental evidence to support this concept[25, 92, 191]. Another mechanism is the increase in cerebral blood flow that occurs when PaO_2 is reduced below approximately 50 mmHg[220, 255]. A fall in extracellular pH has been postulated as the factor responsible for this increase in cerebral blood flow during hypoxia. Evidence in favor of this has come from a number of sources. The PaO_2 at which tissue lactate increases coincides with that at which the increase in cerebral blood flow is observed, while direct observations of pial arteries demonstrate that they dilate in response to micro-injections of solutions with reduced pH[224]. However, when the time course of pH change is examined, it is found that it cannot explain the cerebral blood flow changes that occur[9, 308]. Adenosine also has been postulated as a chemical mediator of the CBF response; however, the data available in support of this hypothesis are meager[351, 371, 445].

Effects of ischemia

Carbohydrate metabolism

Tissue glucose declines rapidly following ischemia, such that by 30 s it is at a level of only 15% of normal[261]. This is accompanied by marked changes in the utilization of glucose. In animal studies of focal ischemia, a severe derangement of glucose metabolism within the ischemic area has been observed which consists of a central zone of decreased glucose utilization and a peripheral zone of greatly enhanced glucose metabolism[132]. A general depression of glucose metabolism in the ischemia hemisphere relative to the nonischemic hemisphere is also present. The areas of increased glucose utilization may represent increased anaerobic glycolysis. During cerebral ischemia, a mechanism may exist by which glucose utilization in the brain is inhibited despite the availability of glucose substrate[49]. Thus, cerebral glucose metabolism may be impaired during cerebral ischemia by mechanisms that do not depend upon cerebral blood flow. A similar effect on energy metabolism has been postulated during hypoxia (*see above*).

Similarly brain glycogen declines during ischemia while lactate concentration increases. Lactate increases almost linearly during the first two minutes of ischemia and then levels off with depletion of the supply of glucose[253]. The degree of tissue lactic acidosis produced during complete ischemia depends upon the tissue glucose and glycogen stores, being greater with large stores and lower with small stores[249]. Anoxia leads to higher brain lactate levels than does complete ischemia because of the continued supply of glucose in the former situation. There is a delay in depletion of glycogen until almost all the creatine phosphate and glucose have disappeared. This may be due to changes in levels of inorganic phosphate and other cofactors which modify the activity of phosphorylase in the brain[40, 307].

Pyruvate increases within 10 s of the onset of ischemia[134]. However, during ischemia tissue pyruvate concentration is reduced to very low values due to its metabolism to lactate[249, 315]. Fructose-6-phosphate and glucose-6-phosphate decline to about one-half their normal levels after 30 s of ischemia, while fructose diphosphate almost doubles within the first 4 s of ischemia[259].

The citric acid cycle fails early in ischemia. α-Keto-glutarate declines rapidly. This may be related to a shift of the glutamic dehydrogenase reaction due to an increase in ammonia and NADH. Succinate changes in a triphasic manner: increasing initially, then declining, and then increasing again after 30 s of ischemia. Fumarate and malate increase after the onset of ischemia, while oxalo-acetate declines.

Cerebral energy metabolism

One of the early changes in metabolism following ischemia is a failure of glycolysis to supply high-energy phosphates. This is due to a lack of oxygen which, following occlusion of a vessel, falls to zero in 30–150 s in the cerebral cortex. Based on the Krogh tissue cylinder model[434], metabolic alterations would be predicted to begin when tissue PO_2 reaches a level of 11 mmHg. However, it has been found that the first change in pyridine nucleotide reduction occurs when mitochondrial oxygen tension falls to 0.6 mmHg, a much lower critical oxygen tension than suggested by the Krogh model[61]. Some of the assumptions of the Krogh model have been challenged on the basis of these and other data.

While the aerobic metabolism of 1 molecule of glucose produces 38 molecules of ATP, the anaerobic metabolism of glucose generates only two molecules of ATP. ATP therefore declines rapidly in the first minute after ischemia and then its rate of decline slows. There is still some ATP detectable even after 10 min of ischemia. This may represent compartmentalized ATP which is not available as an energy source to the cell[253, 261]. AMP rises rapidly during the first 2 min of ischemia. Although it declines after this, it is still elevated after 10 min of ischemia. Normally the production of ATP is tightly coupled to the energy needs of the brain[240]. This regulation of energy supply is mediated through the relative amounts of ATP, ADP and Pi in the tissue[273].

During ischemia there is a decrease in the size of the adenine nucleotide pool[253]. No changes in phosphocreatine, ATP, ADP or AMP occur until cerebral perfusion pressure is reduced below 40 mmHg[390, 391]. When cerebral perfusion pressure is lowered to 30–25 mmHg, changes in brain energy metabolism occur[193, 368, 391]. There is an increase in lactate and the lactate/pyruvate ratio, a decrease in phosphocreatine and ATP, and an increase in AMP and ADP. Changes in lactate and lactate/pyruvate ratio occur at higher cerebral perfusion pressures, i.e. between 50 and 100 mmHg. Changes in NADH fluorescence occur at similar levels of cerebral perfusion pressure[144]. CMRO$_2$ is reduced when cerebral perfusion pressure is lowered to 40 mmHg[143]. Cerebral blood flow must be reduced to approximately 45% of normal before changes in energy metabolism occur[96]. Changes in phosphocreatine, ATP and lactate occur when cerebral blood flow is reduced to between 40% and 35% of normal[267].

With complete ischemia phosphocreatine is depleted within about one minute. The energy sources disappear in the following order: phosphocreatine, glucose, ATP and glycogen. Only about 10% of phosphocreatine remains after 2–3 min of ischemia and the adenylate energy charge is reduced to about 25% of normal. However, the adenylate energy charge does not become maximally depleted until after 5–7 min of ischemia[92, 116, 134, 250, 251, 253]. Thus even though brain oxygen rapidly falls to zero during ischemia, the anaerobic utilization of endogeneous glucose and glycogen stores in addition to the utilization of ketone bodies is capable of preventing complete energy depletion for a period of 5–7 min[273].

Ischemia is associated with an increase in cyclic AMP and a decrease in cyclic GMP[52, 215, 254, 414]. The rise in cyclic AMP may be due to release of neuroadrenalin and accumulation of adenosine[33, 323, 410].

There are localized heterogeneous changes in energy metabolism in response to incomplete ischemia. In rats with arterial blood pressure reduced to between 60 and 45 mmHg, signs of moderate energy failure are present even though cerebral venous PO_2 values are as high as 25–30 mmHg[94]. This may be due to hetero-geneous areas of poor perfusion in which energy metabolism is impaired while the well-perfused areas disproportionately contribute to the high venous oxygen tension. This inhomogeneity of perfusion may be exaggerated by hypercapnia[95].

The amount of lactic acid accumulating during complete ischemia is determined by the pre-ischemic substrates stores[249]. Severe incomplete ischemia can yield tissue lactic acid concentrations considerably in excess of those produced in hyperglycemic animals undergoing complete ischemia[97]. It has been shown by Myers *et al.*[301, 302] that fasted animals subjected to periods of ischemia had a significantly better outcome than those that were not in the fasting state. This difference is attributed to the accumulation of lactic acid in excess of 25 µmol/g in the latter group. Similar results were reported by Siemkowicz and Hansen[386], and Welsh *et al.*[452]. A correlation between the degree of lactic acidosis during ischemia and the extent of metabolic recovery was also shown by Rehnacrona *et al.*[352]. Those animals that had a lactic acid level greater than 20–25 µmol/g failed to recover a normal cerebral energy state. If blood glucose level is raised during the recirculation period, recovery is not adversely affected. Thus, cellular acidosis during ischemia appears to be an important factor in the production of cell damage.

Incomplete ischemia may be more harmful than complete ischemia in the following two ways.

(1) The continued supply of glucose allows more lactic acid to be produced.
(2) The small amount of oxygen present may allow certain autolytic processes to occur which require the presence of oxygen (i.e. lipid peroxidation by free radicals).

Free fatty acids

During ischemia there is an accumulation of free fatty acids, a reduction in polyphosphoinsoitides occurs[27], and no significant synthesis of lipids takes place because of the concomitant energy failure[68]. The greatest change in free fatty acids occurs in arachidonic and stearic acids[21, 22, 23, 58, 120, 138, 225, 226, 264]. The free fatty acid content of the brain following ischemia increases about 4-fold after five minutes and 10-fold after thirty minutes of complete ischemia[345]. The accumulation of free fatty acids does not differ between complete and incomplete ischemia[355]. There is a relatively greater increase in polyenoic free fatty acids than in saturated free fatty acids.

It has been postulated that these free fatty acids are produced from the breakdown of polar membrane phospholipids by the activation of phospholipases. Free fatty acids are inhibitors of oxidative phosphorylation by their ability to uncouple ATP formation and oxygen consumption[66, 108]. There is evidence that during ischemia uncoupling of oxidative phosphorylation occurs[338]. The alterations in free fatty acids may have pathological significance in that they may cause brain edema[59], may adversely affect mitochondrial function[458] and can cause an increase in prostaglandin synthesis during recirculation[122].

pH changes

The tissue acidosis that occurs during ischemia is mainly due to the accumulation of lactic acid in the tissues[251]. Extracellular pH changes do not occur until 15–20 s after an intracellular pH decrease occurs following an ischemic event[394]. If the blood supply is not totally occluded, the pH declines more slowly but reaches more acidic levels than with complete ischemia. Recovery from cerebral ischemia is associated with a decline in brain lactate and a more slowly occurring restoration of normal extracellular pH. This recovery process is variable. In some regions the pH returns to normal within 2–3 min of restoration of blood supply while in others the extracellular pH remains low for as long as 50 min. This latter state can be present even where hyperemia occurs.

Tissue acidosis has been demonstrated to be associated with an impairment of cation transport and neuronal excitability[422]. The development of tissue acidosis during ischemia has also been postulated to be of importance in activating certain lysosomal enzymes which may cause tissue autolysis. Recovery following cerebral ischemia may be critically dependent upon the degree of lactic acidosis that develops. In animal studies of ischemia in which cortical lactate concentration reached 15–16 μmol/g considerable recovery of the cortical energy state occurred upon recirculation, as did return of spontaneous electrocortical activity and somatosensory evoked responses, while only slight neuronal changes were detectable by light microscopy[345]. In contrast, in animals in which cortical lactate concentration increased to about 35 μmol/g brain energy state and neurophysiological functions did not recover upon recirculation and extensive neuronal damage was observed by light microscopic examination.

Amino acids

No significant changes occur in a large number of amino acids following a period of ischemia[433]. The exceptions to this are alanine and γ-aminobutyric acid (GABA) which increase. The increase in GABA has been attributed to the continued functioning of glutamic decarboxylase while the GABA shunt pathway is inhibited[460].

Enzymes

In general, no significant changes in enzyme activities occur during ischemia[304, 364, 403]. However, a few specific alterations have been reported in several enzymes, e.g. a decline in phosphofructokinase activity has been observed.

Ion fluxes

During ischemia, changes in ion concentrations occur early. This is not unexpected since the maintenance of electrochemical gradients across cell membranes is dependent on an adequate supply of energy. When cortical PO_2 falls below 8 mmHg a net shift in sodium to the intracellular space occurs, followed within a few seconds by a net shift of potassium to the extracellular space[279, 280]. An increase in potassium and decrease in sodium concentrations of the cerebral venous blood occurs during hypoxia. There is also an immediate increase in CSF potassium and a decrease in CSF sodium. Hypoxia alone produces mild changes in brain extracellular K^+. Superimposed ischemia causes more precipitous and dramatic changes. In hypoxia, there is an initial fall in pericellular K^+ lasting for about 20 s, followed by a progressive slow rise in extracellular K^+ lasting for about 2.5–4 min[393]. However, after about 3 minutes of hypoxia, there occurs a sudden dramatic increase in extracellular K^+ and hydrogen ion and a decrease in sodium ion activity.

It has been reported that very low levels of rCBF (i.e. 6 ml 100 g^{-1}/min^{-1}) are required before K^+ release first occurs in acute ischemia[11]. This is well below the rCBF level of 15 ml 100 g^{-1}/min^{-1} at which the somatosensory evoked response is abolished[37]. With ischemia a massive efflux of potassium ion occurs within one to two minutes of interruption of the cerebral circulation[10, 172]. The increase in K^+ and local osmolarity is due to the release of normally bound intracellular cations. It has been suggested that there may be K^+-activated metabolic mechanism in mammalian brain by which potassium plus chloride are taken up into glial cells, concomitant with a decrease in ATP and consumption of oxygen. The simultaneous uptake of K^+ and Cl^- carries obligatory water and would account for astrocytic swelling induced by potassium. The uptake of potassium ion and chloride ion and swelling of the glia has been noted when extracellular potassium ion activities rise to values above 10 mmol/l[36, 206].

After release of potassium into the extracellular space, clearance apparently occurs via several different mechanisms. Diffusion accounts for some clearance of potassium over short distances. Second, K^+ may exchange across capillaries.

Finally, there is cellular re-uptake of K^+. The latter requires the Na–K ATPase system and may operate particularly for that K^+ released in the course of neuronal activation.

These ion fluxes are associated with EEG alterations. The earliest EEG change occurs within 5 s of the onset of total ischemia[436]. By 10–12 s there is definite slowing of the EEG followed by a decrease in amplitude. The EEG becomes isoelectric within 20–25 s. These changes begin while the overall levels of high energy phosphates are still quite high, suggesting that a significant portion are not readily available for maintaining synaptic ionic gradients[207, 208].

With asphyxia the increase in extracellular K^+ precedes the occurrence of electrical silence[209]. Slowing of the EEG occurs when cortical subarachnoid K^+ rises above 3.5 mEq/l[210]. Threshold levels of PO_2 below which potassium changes occur have been estimated at 29 mmHg for arterial blood and 20 mmHg for jugular venous blood.

During graded hypoxia, electrical silence occurs when inspired O_2 is reduced to 5% despite the absence of dramatic changes in extracellular K^+. At further reductions of O_2, there is a gradually accelerating rise in extracellular K^+ until a critical point is reached (PaO_2 approximately 22 mmHg) at which even the resupplying of oxygen fails to bring about restoration of cell membrane potential. In contrast, acute ischemia results in a more rapid onset of potassium release and pH change, but with time these changes do not accelerate as fast as during hypoxia.

The ion fluxes responsible for the EEG may occur in the dendritic trees of the neuropil. There is some evidence that this is also the location of the most rapid energy changes during ischemia. A high rate of phosphocreatine disappearance has been found in the molecular layer of the cerebellum which is richest in neuroptil compared to the other layers[260].

Release of neurotransmitters in the brain is triggered by an influx of calcium ion into nerve terminals[26]. Restoration of the ionic gradients requires extrusion of calcium ion from the cell. This is achieved in part by a calcium sodium translocase whose energy source is the sodium gradient created by the ATP-ase activity. Cells also contain a calcium ion pump which uses ATP directly[55]. In addition, calcium ion is also sequestered by the smooth endoplasmic reticulum by an ATP dependent uptake mechanism[380] and the mitochondria also contribute to the sequestration of calcium ion[55, 272].

Ischemia is associated with a marked decrease in extracellular calcium ion activity[148, 306]. Intracellular calcium ion probably rises sharply as calcium disappears from extracellular fluid. The increased intracellular calcium ion can trigger lipolysis and futile recycling of ions across mitochondrial membranes.

Histological changes

Two principal cellular alterations have been noted in ischemia: (1) swelling of perineuronal and perivascular glial elements ('Status spongeosis') and (2) 'ischemic cell change' in which the neurones appear shrunken and darkly staining, often with triangular nuclei. The cells have a micro-vaculated appearance. These microvacules represent swollen mitochondria with disintegration of internal structure[41, 43,]. Ischemia also causes clumping of nuclear chromatin and fragmentation of microtubuli[190, 194].

The earliest histological change following hypoxia-ischemia is microvacuolation in the cytoplasm due to ballooning and swelling of mitochondria[44, 46]. This is followed by ischemic cell change which consists of changes in the staining characteristics of neurons, and then by ischemic cell change with incrustations and finally by disruption of the cell.

These changes occur first in the classically vulnerable regions of the brain, that is, layers 3, 5 and 6 of the cortex, layers 1 and 3–5 in the hippocampus, and the Purkinje cell layer of the cerebellum. The cells in these regions that are most susceptible to hypoxia are the smaller cortical neurons, the pyramidal cells of the hippocampus, and the Purkinje cells of the cerebellum. Cortical layer 3, the internal granular layer, appears to be particularly sensitive to hypoxia. This layer has a richer neuropil, lower cell body density, and the same glial concentration as the other cortical layers[154, 180]. It also has a somewhat greater respiratory capacity. However, the laminar pattern of susceptibility has also been attributed to vascular factors[409].

Histopathological lesions following hypotensive episodes in man are usually confined to the arterial boundary zones[3, 42, 470]. Experimental studies in monkeys in which cerebral perfusion pressure was reduced below 25 mmHg for at least 15 min have reproduced these lesions[41, 42]. Usually the lesions were in the arterial boundary zones in the cortex or basal ganglia and less frequently in the hippocampus and cerebellum. The parietal-occipital cortex seems to be the region of the cortex most involved.

These changes do not appear to be due to a failure of reperfusion as once postulated[242]. The primary lesion appears to be neuronal and not vascular. Neurons appear to be more sensitive to hypoxia than are glial cells or vascular endothelium. Histological changes during ischemia affect the various cerebral elements in the following order: neurons, glia, myelinated fibers and mesodermal elements. Purkinje cells and small neurons degenerate before other neurons and oligodendroglia degenerate before astrocytes[188]. This difference in susceptibility to ischemia has been attributed to factors such as differences in metabolic rate, differences in local blood supply, and neuronal stimulation during ischemia[154]. Some evidence suggests that neurons and oligodendroglia have higher rates of oxidative metabolism[336]. Capillary density appears to be greater in areas rich in synaptic terminals rather than those rich in neuronal cell bodies[176].

Immature animals can withstand ischemia better than adult animals. This may be due to:

(1) the lower brain temperature of immature animals under experimental conditions with consequent lower metabolic rates;
(2) the proliferation of synaptic endings with maturation and their higher metabolic requirements; and
(3) the establishment, with maturation, of ionic gradients across cell membranes which require energy[257].

The changes in metabolite concentration during ischemia occur at a significantly lower rate in the immature animal although the pattern of change is similar to the adult[253]. High-energy phosphate levels are maintained almost three times as long in 10 day-old mice as in the adult, and ATP levels are sustained approximately four times longer in newborn mice compared to 10 day-old mice during ischemia[438].

Redox state

A rapid reduction of cortical pyridine nucleotide occurs 30 to 80 seconds after middle cerebral artery occlusion, followed by a slower reoxidation despite the continued presence of vascular occlusion[132]. A significant correlation has been observed between the peak value of pyridine nucleotide fluorescence after vascular occlusion, and the degree of cerebral blood flow decrement.

Complete ischemia results in sustained increases of NADH, whereas incomplete ischemia with the possibility of collateral circulation results in transient increases in NADH with a relatively prompt return to control levels. NADH tissue assays also demonstrate a significant increase when cerebral perfusion pressure is lowered to 40 mmHg.

Mitochondrial respiratory function

The cellular ionic shifts associated with ischemia, that is, influx of sodium ion and loss of potassium ion and accumulation of free fatty acids, favor the loss of calcium ion and potassium ion from mitochondria. Lysophospholipids and free fatty acids inhibit adenine nucleotide translocase[33, 410] and either inhibit state 3 respiration or uncouple oxygen consumption and ATP production[28, 35, 63, 64, 165, 323]. Ischemic periods as short as 3–6 minutes markedly reduce state three respiration and respiratory control ratio (RCR) values. Ten minutes of ischemia lower the ADP/O ratios as well[258, 329]. Other studies of ischemic periods up to 30 minutes, however, showed only reduced state three respiration and RCR values without any increase in state four respiration or decline in ADP/O ratios[128, 350, 378]. Recirculation after 30 min of complete ischemia is associated with a return of mitochondria function toward normal, suggesting that the mitochondria are not irreversibly damaged by these periods of ischemia. A similar recovery was not observed with recirculation after 30 min of incomplete ischemia, suggesting that persistent mitochondrial dysfunction may underlie failure of recovery of the tissue energy state in this situation[349]. However, results of *in vitro* studies of mitochondrial function must be interpreted with caution when making inferences about *in vivo* mitochondrial function.

Free radicals

It has been suggested that ischemia produces cell damage by production of free radicals and subsequent peroxidative degradation of cell membranes[84, 85, 109, 110, 246]. Free radicals can produce fragmentation of fatty acids with the formation of malondialdehyde and fluorescent products[271, 429]. Normally cells have defense mechanisms against free radicals. These consist of enzyme scavengers, chiefly superoxide dismatase, catalase, and peroxidase; there are also endogenous dismutase scavengers of free radicals, mainly α-tocopherol (vitamin E), ascorbic acid (vitamin C) and thiol-containing amino acids and peptides. Additionally, cell membranes provide a physical separation of normally occurring free radicals and sensitive biomolecules.

When recirculation is instituted after an ischemic period, the concentration of arachidonic acid only gradually returns to control values[355, 466].

Therefore, conditions exist for oxidative degradation of fatty acids during this period. The accumulation of arachidonic acid triggers the production of cycloxygenase which in turn produces endoperoxides[112, 228, 294, 376]. Some of the endoperoxides formed have free radical characteristics (endoperoxides include the classical prostaglandins (PG_2, PGE_2 and $PGF_2\alpha$) as well as proxtacycline (PGI_2) and thromboxane A_2). There is evidence that prostaglandins accumulate during the recirculation period[122]. Neurological recovery can be improved if animals are pretreated with indomethacin, a potent blocker of cycloxygenase[111].

Arachidonic acid also produces lipoxygenase[34, 189, 300, 330] which in turn produces leucotrienes. These events constitute another arachidonic acid cascade. Some of the compounds formed are hydroperoxides. There is, as yet, no direct evidence for the accumulation of lipoxygenase products during the recirculation period. There is, however, indirect evidence that the lipoxygenase pathway is involved during the reperfusion period[45]. From studies of cGMT accumulation, guanylate cyclase appears to be activated by hydroperoxide breakdown products of arachidonic acid[133, 155, 299]. The products of the cycloxygenase and lipoxygenase pathways are potentially toxic agents.

In vitro studies have shown that extensive lipid peroxidation can occur in brain tissue homogenates when incubated with agents known to promote free radical formation[354]. However, in studies with glutathione, an endogeneous free radical scavenger, an increase in the oxidized form could not be demonstrated in studies of incomplete or complete ischemia. If increased lipid peroxidation were occurring, this might be expected[71, 348]. Studies of phospholipid concentration or fatty acid composition also failed to indicate the presence of lipid peroxidation[353, 355]. On the basis of malondialdehyde measurements, Yoshida *et al.*[466] concluded that lipid peroxidation did not occur during ischemia. These data, suggesting that free radical formation is not a mechanism of cell damage in ischemia, are contradictory to those of others[84, 89, 109, 110]. The models of ischemia studied by the different groups of investigators were not the same and may account for some of the contradictory data. Thus the evidence for free radical generation and lipid auto-oxidation playing a significant role during ischemia is not clear. The protective effect of barbiturates in ischemia does not appear to be related to their efficacy in scavenging free radicals[404].

Heterogeneity of circulatory and metabolic effects

A widespread spectrum of regional cerebral blood flow alterations may be observed within a focus of cerebral ischemia[29]. Furthermore, there may be a gradation within a zone of ischemia of the degree to which CO_2 reactivity is depressed[427]. CO_2 reactivity has been found to be most reduced in those portions of the ischemic zone which also have the greatest rCBF reduction and least affected in areas with the more nearly normal rCBF. Considerable inhomogeneities of rCBF and vasomotor regulation may exist within a focus of cerebral ischemia.

Small differences in rCBF among brain regions may lead to marked differences in their metabolic behavior when critical or threshold levels of rCBF exist. CBF must be reduced to below 50% of normal before biochemical alterations of ischemia occur[97]. Such levels of CBF compromise oxygen delivery prior to a limitation of glucose supply and result in increased anaerobic glycolysis in association with elevated brain lactate and deficient formation of citric acid cycle intermediates[310, 375]. When CBF is reduced from 50% to 40% of normal, the cerebral metabolic rate for glucose increases but the rate of brain oxygen utilization declines; this suggests a shift to anaerobic glycolysis once a certain critical threshold of oxygen delivery to the tissue has been passed[49]. Similar findings have been demonstrated during normocarbic hypoxia in man[69]. There is a critical level of cerebral blood flow produced by a perfusion pressure between 20 and 40 mmHg below which high-energy phosphates in the brain are reduced[267, 391].

During severe generalized ischemia significant inhomogeneities of rCBF and of energy metabolism may exist in the brain[389]. It is possible that the determinants of suppressed versus enhanced glucose metabolism in ischemic tissue may involve small but critical differences in regional blood flow among the variously affected regions.

Studies of the couple between flow and metabolism during focal ischemia demonstrate that this relationship tends to be preserved even in ischemic brain regions. However, when cerebral blood flow falls below 40% of normal, a dissociation of flow and metabolism occurs with an increase in metabolic rate for glucose above that which would be predicted from the flow rate. This phenomenon occurs in ischemic grey matter and may represent increased anaerobic metabolism of glucose.

DIASCHISIS

The phenomenon of diaschisis was first described in 1914 by Von Monakow[444]. Following a focal injury to the brain, temporary depression of function in remote areas may occur. These remote effects, or diaschisis, can be transhemispheric or propagated by the corticospinal projections.

The first report of bilateral reduction of cerebral blood flow in patients with unilateral cerebral infarction was that of Kempinsky *et al.*[198]. Since then this has been confirmed by several different investigators[160, 397]. It has been hypothesized that a transneuronal depression of metabolism is produced by the unilateral infarct which then results in reduced blood flow in both hemispheres. The bilateral depression of blood flow persists for 2 to 3 weeks, reaching its nadir at about 1 week and then gradually returning toward normal[284, 401]. These data suggest that a neuronal depression secondary to disconnection from afferent stimulation is not the only cause of diaschisis since, if that were the case, the maximum decline in flow would be expected immediately. The time course of flow changes are quite similar in the two hemispheres, suggesting the presence of factors affecting both hemispheres in an almost identical manner.

Metabolic alterations have also been observed in the hemisphere contralateral to a focal ischemic insult. In an animal model in cats a 31% decrease in glucose consumption was found in the contralateral cortex[132]. A corresponding depression of cortical blood flow contralateral to the ischemic hemisphere was demonstrated in the same model[359]. A depression of cerebral oxygen metabolism in the nonischemic hemisphere has also been observed in patients following stroke[284].

In a case reported by Kuhl *et al.*[222] studied within one week after a unilateral stroke there was a 32% reduction in LCMRgl in the contralateral hemisphere which had returned to normal when studied again three months later. Baron *et al.*[16a] have observed a significant decrease in regional cerebral blood flow and oxygen consumption in the cerebellar hemisphere contralateral to a supratentorial infarction. This was present only in patients who were studied less than two months after their stroke. They postulated that these effects were a manifestation of diaschisis. A significant asymmetry of cerebral glucose consumption has been observed in a group of patients with acute unilateral cerebral hemispheric lesions[224a]. Hypometabolism was present in the cerebellar hemisphere contralateral to the cortical lesion. The likelihood of observing this crossed cerebellar hypometabolism seemed to be related to the extent of the hemispheric hypometabolism rather than to the degree of motor impairment.

The norepinephrine and epinephrine content of CSF and plasma in patients with cerebral infarction has been found to be elevated for a period of 2 weeks following the ictus[285]. In addition, a release of vasoactive substances into brain tissue has been observed following a cerebral infarction. After a unilateral ischemic insult, a bilateral depression of norepinephrine content has been reported[219]. The norepinephrine depletion observed has been thought to be due to decreased energy metabolism with interference with the transport of tyrosine across the cell membrane, since this is an ATP-dependent process[65, 461]. It has been hypothesized that a focal vascular occlusion produces a generalized release of norepinephrine from pre-synaptic terminals throughout the brain, constricting cerebral vessels and causing widespread ischemia even in distant areas in the opposite hemisphere. Constriction of cerebral arteries and diffuse cortical pallor have been regularly observed in animal studies. Local vascular occlusion has been shown to produce diffuse cerebral vasoconstriction[80, 289, 449].

Dopamine is significantly elevated bilaterally soon after a unilateral ischemic insult. The time course of the dopamine change parallels that of the fall and recovery of ATP[217]. A defect in conversion of dopamine to norepinephrine by dopamine β oxidase has been postulated. Others have observed a reduction in brain dopamine on the side of carotid occlusion at later times following occlusion[467].

Other biochemical changes have also been observed in the cortex contralateral to an ischemic insult. Glucose and phosphocreatine are increased and pyruvate is unchanged, whereas in the ischemic hemisphere all three of these compounds are depleted[243]. Decreased ATP and increased lactate concentrations have been found in the contralateral hemisphere[217, 219].

Studies of the effects of an ischemic insult in animals where the corpus callosum had been sectioned lend support to the hypothesis of a transcallosal mechanism as the basis of the phenomenon of diaschisis[197]. It is hypothesized that impulses from one hemisphere facilitate the activity of neurons in the opposite hemisphere, and then when a focal injury is produced this source of facilitation is lost. There is consequently reduced neuronal activity following injury of the contralateral hemisphere. Over time after the injury, the contralateral hemisphere assumes greater autonomy and ultimately functions at a level approaching that present prior to the injury.

Recovery following ischemia

Duration of ischemia

Classical clinical teaching has emphasized the susceptibility of the brain to injury from ischemia of even a few minutes' duration, but more recent investigations have provided evidence that under certain circumstances much longer periods of circulatory arrest may be endured without cerebral damage. In the dog, recovery after 25 min of total cerebral ischemia has been reported[305]. In monkeys cerebral circulatory arrest of up to 20 min was well tolerated and in some animals produced only minor clinical deficits[292, 293]. A variety of physiological and metabolic variables reflecting cerebral function have been shown to be capable of partial or complete restitution following 1 hour of complete cerebral ischemia in cats and monkeys[167, 170, 175, 249].

In rats after 1 to 15 min of ischemia phosphocreatine, energy charge potential, lactate and lactate–pyruvate ratio rapidly returned to normal; however, the sum of the adenine nucleotides and the ATP concentration remained below normal even after 3 hours of reperfusion[250, 251]. If the period of ischemia is increased to 30 min, phosphocreatine, ADP, AMP, lactate–pyruvate ratio and energy charge return to normal, but lactate content remains slightly elevated[312, 315]. Metabolic recovery after 90 min of recirculation in rats is present following 30 min of complete ischemia but not following 30 min of incomplete ischemia[314]. Mitochondrial function in the same models was normal following recirculation after complete ischemia but not following incomplete ischemia[350]. Contradictory data, however, have been published by other investigators[265, 412]. In spite of this recovery of energy metabolism, gross functional deficits were present in rats subject to periods of ischemia of 3 min or more. There is evidence, however, that it may take from days to weeks for complete recovery of function to occur following ischemia in these animal models[86, 157, 292].

After 8 min of ischemia in rabbits the alteration in PCr, ATP, AMP, adenylate energy charge and lactate recover within a few minutes and are almost normal after 2 hours[297].

In cats after 1 hour of cerebral ischemia restoration of the energy charge potential to about 93% of control occurs after 3–7 hours of recirculation[168]. Protein synthesis may also be resumed after 30–60 min of ischemia. Even though these animals showed functional recovery, energy metabolism did not return completely to normal, even if the recovery period was extended to 24 hours[167]. This failure of complete restoration of ATP levels during recirculation may be important in influencing the extent of neuronal recovery. In part, this persistently reduced adenylate level may be due to the measurement technique which involves the averaging of normal and variably damaged tissue in the cortex.

In the gerbil biochemical abnormalities lessen with restoration of flow following 1 hour of unilateral ischemia but do not return to control levels even after 24 hours. Total adenylates decline during ischemia and remain low throughout the 24 hour recovery period.

Thus recovery after an ischemic insult is quite variable depending upon the function being measured and depending to a great extent on the animal model used.

Redox state and mitochondrial function

During recovery following ischemia, mitochondrial reoxidation of NADH occurs. In this process pyruvate, which is derived from lactate, is utilized with the subsequent reduction of lactic acidosis. There is a reduced delivery of pyruvate by the glycolytic chain and a fall in cerebral glucose consumption[249]. The redox state of the cerebral cortex has been examined during total and partial ischemia in the cat. In the former circumstance, there is maximal reduction of NAD to NADH during the first minutes of ischemia. Complete reoxidation of NADH appears to be possible when total ischemia is less than 5 min; the recovery of brain redox state following longer periods of total ischemia has not been systematically studied. However, following ischemia for as long as 30–60 min, recovery of mitochondrial function occurs[129, 378]. Thus mitochondria are relatively resistant to complete ischemia as is attested to by the recovery of energy metabolism and normalization of citric acid cycle intermediates in the post-ischemic period.

Neurotransmitters

Neurotransmitter function is disturbed following complete ischemia[47, 462]. There are increases in GABA and alanine, which are amino acids with inhibitory properties; and decreases in glutamate and aspartate, which have excitatory properties[116]. What significance these changes have for the recovery of function following ischemia is unknown at present.

Energy metabolism

Super-normal phosphocreatine levels have been reported in brain during recovery from ischemia[243, 267]. Studies of energy flux reveal that metabolic activity increases by at least 50% in the previously ischemic cortex of clinically affected gerbils after 4 hours of recovery[243]. In an isolated canine brain preparation, a period of increased oxygen consumption following complete ischemia has been reported[229]. Increased oxygen uptake 3 hours after a 1-hour period of complete cerebral ischemia in cats has been found[171]. This additional energy in the recovery phase following ischemia may be utilized for increased cation pumping associated with cerebral edema. It has been estimated that cation transport accounts for about 40% of tissue oxygen consumption in brain slices[453]. Repletion of lost proteins and neurotransmitters during ischemia would also require additional energy.

Recovery of electrical activity

The factors determining recovery of the EEG following cerebral ischemia are poorly understood. One factor, however, appears to be CBF. In cats in which the EEG recovers following ischemia, cerebral blood flow increased by 2 to 4 times during the first hour of the recovery period and then gradually returned to normal levels[168, 169]. Return of the EEG coincided with the termination of hyperemia and the resumption of normal cerebral blood flow. The abnormal intracellular conditions (acidosis, etc.) which develop during ischemia may be responsible for both the hyperemia and the EEG suppression. When the intracellular milieu is restored to normal the hyperemia disappears and EEG recovery occurs. In animals in which the EEG failed to recover, post-ischemic hyperemia did not occur; rather, cerebral blood flow gradually declined. It has been observed that, when ischemia is incomplete, subsequent recovery of EEG and of the pyramidal response during recirculation fails to occur; whereas in animals in which the ischemia has been complete prior to recirculation EEG recovery does occur[169, 170, 328]. As discussed previously, one factor involved in the more deleterious effects of incomplete ischemia may be the greater degree of intracellular acidosis produced[395].

On the other hand, a poor correlation has been observed between metabolic recovery and functional recovery. Following compression ischemia in the rat lasting 5 min or more, the EEG remains abnormal during 3 hours of subsequent recirculation, despite the fact that there is a rapid return to normal of cerebral energy compounds[250]. A return of EEG, evoked potentials, and certain metabolic functions can occur following an insult of as long as 60 min of complete ischemia[166, 167, 213, 214]. The return of these functions, however, has never been shown to be accompanied by recovery of neurological function.

Post-ischemic perfusion pressure

The question has arisen as to whether the irreversible damage produced by ischemia is due to a lack of reperfusion during the recovery phase, i.e. the no reflow phenomenon[7, 8, 54, 107]. This concept has not been substantiated by rCBF studies and other investigations. In fact, studies have shown that there is a reactive hyperemia following periods of ischemia of 15–60 min duration and that a decrease in flow occurs much later[169, 174, 266, 405].

It is known that autoregulation fails during acute cerebral ischemia[425]. Thus it is to be expected that hypotension would be particularly deleterious to the ischemic focus in which blood flow would be expected to fall passively. A normal or even increased post-ischemic perfusion pressure may be necessary for recovery of various parameters following ischemia[372]. Improvement in neurological function in patients following an ischemic brain episode is often associated with a rise in blood pressure[87,384, 455, 456]. Conversely, cerebral infarction is much greater following induced hypotension after major vessel occlusion[435]. The reversibility of cerebral ischemic damage with blood pressure elevation in monkeys has been reported[88]. On the other hand, a deleterious effect of elevation of systemic blood pressure (to 150 mmHg) following unilateral common carotid artery occlusion was found in the gerbil. This occurred in spite of the fact that cerebral blood flow was increased in these animals. One deleterious effect of increased perfusion pressure may be the exacerbation of edema formation.

If cerebral perfusion pressure is restored at the end of an ischemic period, cerebral blood flow initially may increase above normal[387]. Subsequently, cerebral blood flow may fall and may reach markedly low values[127,141, 167, 347, 469]. In the immediate post-ischemic period $CMRO_2$ is reduced[171,312,405]. Subsequently, cerebral metabolic rate increases toward control values and, in some circumstances, may rise above control values[171,216, 243]. If this occurs during the period when CBF is falling tissue oxygenation may undergo a secondary decline. Thus, the post-ischemia period of recirculation may be accompanied by potentially harmful events as recently pointed out by Siesjo[387]. For example, a post-ischemic decline in the activity of some membrane-bound enzymes has been reported[211,379,440,441], there is evidence that abnormal protein metabolism occurs during the recirculation period[72] and there is evidence that the phenomenon of selective vulnerability is a function of the recirculation period, i.e. immediately after an ischemia event the histopathological alterations are homogeneous with no preferential sites of damage[190,194]. Furthermore, barbiturates administered in the recirculation period seem to have a beneficial effect[30,244] although contradictory results have been published[365,413].

Hypothermia

Hypothermia reduces $CMRO_2$ by about 5% per degree centigrade reduction in body temperature. Animals subjected to cerebral ischemia under hypothermic conditions can survive a significantly longer period of ischemia than can normothermic animals[159]. Hypothermia retards the accumulation of lactic acid and the depletion of phosphocreatine and ATP during ischemia. This effect may be due to the reduction in metabolic rate produced and/or its effect on the rate of enzymatic reactions.

Anesthetics

Certain anesthetics, particularly barbiturates, afford protection from ischemia[31,290, 291, 402, 428, 465]. Pentobarbital anesthesia given in experimental animals after middle cerebral artery occlusion diminished both the size and incidence of infarcts and neurological deficits[288,402]. Pentobarbital affords protection in terms of the cerebral energy state in incomplete ischemia[313, 315]. This protective effect is not due to a diminution of acidosis nor does it seem to be due to a reduced metabolic demand. The mechanism of this protection remains obscure[311]. One postulate has been that barbiturates exert their protection effect via their role as efficient free radical scavengers. There is some evidence that free radicals are released during ischemia by peroxidation of membrane lipids[83, 118,196]. Their protective effect has also been attributed to their ability to decrease neuronal activity and consequently the metabolic requirements of the tissue[290, 291, 402, 465]. Additional mechanisms that have been suggested for their protective effect have been their effect on reducing mitochondrial enzymatic auto-oxidation preventing cellular autolysis with secondary endothelial membrane damage and reducing platelet adherence and microcirculatory obstruction[110, 428].

Acknowledgements

Supported in part by U.S.P.H.S. Program Project Grants NS 10939–10 and NS 14867–04.

References

1 ACKERMAN, R. H. Positron imaging in stroke. In *Cerebrovascular Disease, 12th Research (Princeton) Conference*, edited by J. Moossy and O. M. Reinmuth, 67–72. New York: Raven Press (1981)

2 ACKERMAN, R. H., CORREIA, J. A. and ALPERT, N. M. Positron imaging in ischemic stroke disease using compounds labeled with oxygen 15: initial results of clinicophysiologic correlations. *Archives of Neurology*, **38**, 537–542 (1981)

3 ADAMS, J. H., BRIERLEY, J. B., CONNOR, R. C. R. and TREIP, C. S. The effects of systemic hypotension upon the human brain. Clinical and neuropathological observations in 11 cases. *Brain*, **89**, 235–268 (1966)

4 AGNOLI, A., FIESCHI, C., BOZZAO, L., BATTISTINI, N. and PRENCIPE, M. Autoregulation of cerebral blood flow: studies during drug-induced hypertension in normal subjects and in patients with cerebral vascular disease. *Circulation*, **38**, 800 (1968)

5 AGNOLI, A., PRENCIPE, M., PRIORI, A. M., BOZZAO, L. and FIESCHI, C. Measurements of rCBF by intravenous injection of ^{133}Xe. A comparative study with the intra-arterial injection method. In *Cerebral Blood Flow*, edited by M. Brock *et al.* Berlin: Springer-Verlag (1969)

6 ALEXANDER, S. C., WOLLMAN, H., COHEN, P. J., CHASE, P. E., MELMAN, E. and BEHAR, M. Krypton-85 and nitrous oxide uptake of the human brain during anesthesia. *Anesthesia*, **25**, 37 (1964)

7 AMES, A. III. Incidence and significance of vascular occlusion in focal and diffuse ischemia. In *Cerebral Circulation and Metabolism*, edited by T. W. Langfitt, L. C. McHenry, Jr., M. Reivich and H. Wollman, 551–554. New York: Springer-Verlag (1975)

8 AMES, A. III, WRIGHT, R. L., KOWADA, M., THURSTON, J. M. and MAJNO, G. Cerebral ischemia. II. The no-reflow phenomenon, *American Journal of Pathology*, **52**, 437–453 (1968)

9 ASTRUP, J., HEUSER, D., LASSEN, N. A., NILSSON, B., NORBERG, K. and SIESJO, B. K. Evidence against H^+ and K^+ as the main factors in the regulation of cerebral blood flow during epileptic discharges, acute hypoxemia, amphetamine intoxication, and hypoglycemia. A microelectrode study. In *Ionic Actions on Vascular Smooth Muscle*, edited by E. Betz, 110–115. Berlin: Springer-Verlag (1976)

10 ASTRUP, J., REHNCRONA, S. and SIESJO, B. K. The increase in extracellular potassium concentration in the ischemic brain in relation to the preischemic functional activity and cerebral metabolic rate. *Brain Research*, **199**, 161–174 (1980)

11 ASTRUP, J., SYMON, L., BRANSTON, N. M. and LASSEN, N. A. Cortical evoked potential and extracellular K^+ and H^+ at critical levels of brain ischemia. *Stroke*, **8**, 51 (1977)

12 AUBINEAU, P. F., SEYLAZ, J., SERCOMBE, R. and MAMO, H. Evidence for regional differences in the effect of β-adrenergic stimulation on cerebral blood flow. *Brain Research*, **61**, 153–161 (1973)

13 AUE, W. P., BARTHOLD, E. and ERNST, R. R. Two-dimensional spectroscopy: application to nuclear magnetic resonance. *Journal of Clinical Pathology*, **64**, 2229 –2246 (1976)

14 AUSTIN, G., LAFFIN, D., ROUHE, S. R., EDWARDS, M. and HAYWARD, M. A non-invasive i.v. isotope method for measuring cerebral blood flow. *Stroke*, **4**, 362 (1973)

15 BACHELARD, H. S., LEWIS, L. D., PONTEN, U. and SIESJO, B. K. Mechanisms activating glycolysis in the brain in arterial hypoxia. *Journal of Neurochemistry*, **22**, 395–401 (1974)

16a BARON, J. C., BOUSSER, M. G., COMAR, D., DUQUSNAY, N., SASTRE, J. and CASTAIGNE, P. Crossed cerebellar diaschisis: a remote functional depression secondary to supratentorial infarction in man. *Journal of Cerebral Blood Flow and Metabolism*, **1** (Suppl. 1) 500–501 (1981)

16b BARON, J. C., COMAR, D., SUSSALINE, F. *et al.* Continuous ^{15}O inhalation technique: an attempt to quantify CBF, CO_2 and $CMRO_2$. *Acta Neurologica Scandinavica*, **60** (Suppl. 72) 194–195 (1979)

17 BARON, J. C., STEINLING, M., TANAKA, T., CAVALHEIRO, E., SOUSSALINE, F. and COLLARD, P. Quantitative measurement of CBF, oxygen extraction fraction (OEF) and $CMRO_2$ with the ^{15}O continuous inhalation technique and positron emission tomography (PET): experimental evidence and normal values in man. *Journal of Cerebral Blood Flow and Metabolism*, **1** (Suppl. 1) 5–6 (1981)

18 BATTOCLETTI, J. H., HALBACH, R. E., SALLES-CUNHA, S. X. and SANCES, A. Jr. The NMR blood flow meter-theory and history. *Medical Physics*, **8**, 435–443 (1981)

19 BATTOCLETTI, J. H., HALBACH, R. E., SANCES, A. Jr., LARSON, S. J., BOWMAN, R. L. and KUDRAVCEV, V. Flat crossed coil detector for blood flow measurement using nuclear magnetic resonance. *Medical and Biological Engineering and Computing*, **17**, 183–191 (1979)

20 BAYLISS, W. M. On the local reactions of the arterial wall to changes of internal pressure. *Journal of Physiology (London)*, **28**, 220 (1902)

21 BAZAN, N. G. Jr. Effects of ischemia and electroconvulsive shock on free fatty acid pool in the brain. *Biochimica et Biophysica Acta*, **218**, 1–10 (1970)

22 BAZAN, N. G. Jr. Free arachidonic acid and other lipids in the nervous system during early ischemia and after electroshock. In *The Function and Metabolism of Phospholipids in the Central and Peripheral Nervous Systems*, edited by G. Porcellati, L. Amaducci and C. Galli, 317–356. New York: Plenum Press (1976)

23 BAZAN, N. G. Jr., BAZAN, H. E. P., KENNEDY, W. G. and JOEL, C. D. Regional distribution and rate of production of free fatty acids in rat brain. *Journal of Neurochemistry*, **18**, 1387–1393 (1971)

24 BERNSMEIER, A. and SIEMONS, K. Die Messung der Hirndurchblutung mit der Stickoxydulmethode. *Pflügers Archiv für die Gesamte Physiologie (Berlin)*, **258**, 149 (1953)

25 BERNTMAN, L., CARLSSON, C. and SIESJÖ, B. K. Cerebral oxygen utilization and blood flow in hypoxia: influence of sympathoadrenal activation. *Acta Physiologica Scandinavica* (in press)

26 BERRIDGE, M. J. Modulation of nervous activity by cyclic nucleotides and calcium. In *The Neurosciences: Fourth Study Program*, edited by F. O. Schmitt and E. G. Worder, 873–889. Cambridge, Mass.: MIT Press (1979)

27 BIRNBERGER, A. C. and ELIASSON, S. G. Experimental ischemia and polyphosphoinositide metabolism. *Neurology*, **19**, 297 (1969)

28 BJORNTORP, P., EHS, H. A. and BRADFORD, R. H. Albumin antagonism of fatty acid effects on oxidation and phosphorylation reactions in rat liver mitochondria. *Journal of Biological Chemistry*, **239**, 339–344 (1964)

29 BLAIR, R. D. G. and WALTZ, A. G. Regional cerebral blood flow during acute ischemia. *Neurology*, **20**, 802–808 (1970)

30 BLEYAERT, A. L., NEMOTO, E. M., SAFAR, P., STEZOSKI, S. W., MICKELL, J. J., MOOSSY, J. and GUTTI, R. R. Thiopental amelioration of brain damage after global ischemia in monkeys. *Anesthesiology*, **49**, 390–398 (1978)

31 BLEYAERT, A. L., NEMOTO, E., SAFAR, P., STEZOSKI, S. W., MOOSSY, J., RAO, G. R. and MICKELL, J. Thiopental amelioration of postischemic encephalopathy in monkeys. In *Cerebral Function, Metabolism and Circulation*, edited by D. H. Ingvar and N. A. Lassen, 144–145. Copenhagen: Munksgaard (1977)

32 BLOCH, F., HANSEN, W. W. and PACKARD, M. E. The nuclear induction experiment. *Physiological Reviews*, **70**, 474–485 (1946)

33 BLOOM, F. E. The role of cyclic nucleotides in central synaptic function. *Revue Physiologie Biochemie et Pharmacologie*, **74**, 1–103 (1975)

34 BORGEAT, B. and SAMUELSSON, B. Arachidonic acid metabolism in polymorphonuclear leukocytes: effects of ionophore A23187. *Proceedings of the National Academy of Sciences, USA*, **76**, 2148–2152 (1979)

35 BORST, P., LOOS, J. A., CHRIST, E. J. and SLATER, E. C. Uncoupling activity of long-chain fatty acids. *Biochimica et Biophysica Acta*, **62**, 509–518 (1962)

36 BOURKE, R. S., KIMELBERG, H. K., WEST, C. R. and BREMER, A. M. The effect of HCO_3 on the swelling and ion uptake of monkey cerebral cortex under conditions of raised extracellular potassium. *Journal of Neurochemistry*, **25**, 323–328 (1975)

37 BRANSTON, N. M., SYMON, L., CROCKARD, H. A. *et al.* Relationship between the cortical evoked potential and local cortical blood flow acute middle cerebral artery occlusion in the baboon. *Experimental Neurology*, **45**, 195–208 (1974)

38 BRANSTON, N. M., SYMON, L., STRONG, A. J. and HOPE, D. T. Measurements of regional cortical blood flow during changes in extracellular potassium activity evoked by direct cortical stimulation in the primate. *Experimental Neurology*, **59**, 243 (1978)

39 BRAWLEY, B. W., STRANDNESS, D. E. and KELLY, W. A. The physiologic response to therapy in experimental cerebral ischemia. *Archives of Neurology*, **17**, 18 (1967)

40 BRECKENRIDGE, B.M. and NORMAN, J. H. Glycogen phosphorylase in brain. *Journal of Neurochemistry*, **9**, 383–392 (1962)

41 BRIERLEY, J. B. Pathology of cerebral ischemia. In *Cerebral Vascular Diseases*, edited by F. H. McDowell and R. W. Brennan, 59–75. New York: Grune and Stratton (1973)

42 BRIERLEY, J. B., BROWN, A. W., EXCELL, B. J. and MELDRUM, B. S. Brain damage in the rhesus monkey resulting from profound arterial hypotension. I. Its nature, distribution and general physiological correlates. *Brain Research*, **13**, 68–100 (1969)

43 BRIERLEY, J. B., LJUNGGREN, B. and SIESJO, B. K. Neuropathological alterations in rat brain after complete ischemia due to raised intracranial pressure. In *Intracranial Pressure*, Vol. 2, edited by N. Lundberg, U. Ponten and M. Brock, 167–171. Berlin: Springer-Verlag (1975)

44 BRIERLEY, J. B., MELDRUM, B. S. and BROWN, A. W. The threshold and neuropathology of cerebral 'anoxic-ischemic' cell change. *Archives of Neurology*, **29**, 367–374 (1973)

45 BRIGGS, R. G. and DeRUBERTIS, F. R. Calcium-dependent modulation of guanosine 3′, 5′-monophosphate in renal cortex. Possible relationship to calcium-dependent release of fatty acid. *Biochemistry and Pharmacology*, **29**, 717–722 (1980)

46 BROWN, A. W. and BRIERLEY, J. B. The earliest alterations in rat neurones and astrocytes after anoxia-ischaemia. *Acta Neuropathologica*, **23**, 9–22 (1973)

47 BROWN, R. M., CARLSSON, A., LJUNGGREN, B. *et al.* Effect of ischemia on monoamine metabolism in the brain. *Acta Neurologica Scandinavica*, **90**, 789–791 (1974)

48 BROWNELL, G. L., BUDINGER, T. F., LAUTERBUR, P. C. and McGEER, P. L. Positron tomography and nuclear magnetic resonance imaging. *Science*, **215**, 619–626 (1982)

49 BRUCE, D. A., SCHUTZ, H., VALPALAHTI, M. *et al.* Interactions between cerebral blood flow and cerebral metabolism. *Surgical Forum*, **23**, 417–419 (1972)

50 BRUETMAN, M. E. *et al.* Cerebral hemorrhage in carotid artery surgery. *Archives of Neurology*, **9**, 458 (1963)

51 BUONANNO, F. S., VIELMAN, J., PYKETT, I. L. *et al.* Proton NMR imaging of normal and abnormal brain, experimental and clinical observations. In *NMR Imaging*, edited by R. L. Witcofski, N. Karstaedt and C. L. Partain, 147–157. Winston-Salem, North Carolina: Bowman Gray School of Medicine (1982)

52 BURKARD, W. P. Catecholamine induced increase of cyclic adenosine 3′, 5′-monophosphate in rat brain *in vivo*. *Journal of Neurochemistry*, **19**, 2615–2619 (1972)

53 BURROWS, G. On disorders of the cerebral circulation and on the connection between affections of the brain and disease of the heart. London, Longman, Brown, Green and Longmans (1846)

54 CANTU, R. C., AMES, A. III, DIXON, J. and DiGIACINTO, G. Reversibility of experimental cerebrovascular observation induced by complete ischemia. *Journal of Neurosurgery*, **31**, 429–431 (1969)

55 CARAIOLI, E. and CROMPTON, M. The regulation of intracellular calcium. *Current Topics in Membrane Transport*, **10**, 151–216 (1978)

56 CARONNA, J. J. and PLUM, F. Cerebrovascular regulation in preganglionic and postganglionic autonomic insufficiency. *Stroke*, **4**, 12–19 (1973)

57 CARTER, C. C., BICHLING, J. O., DAVIS, D. O. and TER-POGOSSIAN, M. M. Correlation of regional cerebral blood flow with regional oxygen uptake using the ^{15}O method. *Neurology*, **22**, 755–762 (1972)

58 CENEDELLA, R. J., GALLI, C. and PAOLETTE, R. Brain free fatty acid levels in rats sacrificed by decapitation versus focused microwave irradiation. *Lipids*, **10**, 290–293 (1975)

59 CHAN, P. H. and FISHMAN, R. A. Brain edema: induction in cortical slices by polyunsaturated fatty acids. *Science*, **201**, 358–360 (1978)

60 CHANCE, B., NAKASE, Y., BOND, M., LEIGH, J. S. Jr. and McDONALD, G. Detection of ^{31}P nuclear magnetic resonance signals in brain by *in vivo* and freeze-trapped assays. *Proceedings of the National Academy of Sciences of the United States of America*, **75**, 4925–4929 (1978)

61 CHANCE, B., COHEN, P., JOBSIS, F. and SCHOENER, B. Intracellular oxidation-reduction state *in vivo*. *Science*, **137**, 499–508 (1962)

62 CHANCE, B., SCHOENER, B. and SCHINDLER, F. The intracellular oxidation-reduction state. In *Oxygen in the Animal Organism*, edited by F. Dickens and E. Neil, 367–392. Oxford: Pergamon Press (1964)

63 CHEFURKA, W. Oxidative phosphorylation in *in vitro* aged mitochondria. I. Factors controlling the loss of the dinitrophenol-stimulated adenosine triphosphatase activity and respiratory control in mouse liver mitochondria. *Biochemistry*, **5**, 3887–3903 (1966)

64 CHEFURKA, W. and DUMAS, T. Oxidative phosphorylation in *in vitro* aged mitochondria. II. Dinitrophenol stimulated adenosine triphosphatase activity and fatty acid content of mouse liver mitochondria. *Biochemistry*, **5**, 3904–3911 (1966)

65 CHIRGOS, M. A., GREENGARD, P. and UDENFRIEND, S. Uptake of tyrosine by rat brain *in vivo*. *Journal of Biological Chemistry*, **235**, 2075–2079 (1960)

66 CHMOULIOVSKY, M., SHORDERET, M. and STRAUB, R. W. Effect of electrical activity on the concentration of phosphorylated metabolites and inorganic phosphate in mammalian non-myelinated fibres. *Journal of Physiology (London)*, **202**, 90P–92P (1969)

67 CHOROBSKI, J. and PENFIELD, W. Cerebral vasodilator nerves and their pathway from the medulla oblongata. *Archives of Neurology and Psychiatry*, **28**, 1257–1289 (1932)

68 COHEN, M. M. The effect of anoxia on the chemistry and morphology of cerebral cortex slices *in vitro*. *Journal of Neurochemistry*, **9**, 337–344 (1962)

69 COHEN, P. J., ALEXANDER, S. C., SMITH, F. C. *et al.* Effects of hypoxia and normocarbia on cerebral blood flow and metabolism in conscious man. *Journal of Applied Physiology: Respiratory, Environmental and Exercise Physiology*, **23**, 183–189 (1967)

70 COOPER, A. Some experiments and observations on tying the carotid and vertebral arteries, and the pneumogastric, phrenic, and sympathetic nerves. *Guy's Hospital Report*, **1,** 457 (1836)

71 COOPER, A. J. L., PULSINELLI, W. A. and DUFFY, T. E. Glutathione and ascorbate during ischemia and postischemic reperfusion in rat brain. *Journal of Neurochemistry*, **35,** 1242–1245 (1980)

72 COOPER, H. K., ZALEWSKA, T., KAWAKAMI, S., HOSSMAN, K. -A and KLEIHUES, P. The effect of ischaemia and recirculation on protein synthesis in the rat brain. *Journal of Neurochemistry*, **28,** 929–934 (1977)

73 COOPER, R., CROW, H. J., WALTER, W. G. and WINTER, A. L. Regional control of cerebral vascular reactivity and oxygen supply in man. *Brain Research*, **3,** 174 (1966)

74 CRAWLEY, J. S., O'BRIEN, M. D. and VEALL, N. The γ spectrum subtraction technique applied to cerebral blood flow measurement by the inhalation of xenon-133. In *Brain and Blood Flow*, edited by R. W. Ross Russell, 54–56. London: Pitman Publishing Co. (1971)

75 CRONQVIST, S. La circulation de luxe: donnees radiologiques et donnees isotopiques. *VIII Symposium Neuroradiologieum, Paris, September 1967*

76 CRONQVIST, S. Regional cerebral blood flow and angiography in apoplexy. *Acta Radiologica Diagnosis*, **7,** 521 (1968)

77 CRONQVIST, S. and LAROCH, F. Transitory 'hyperemia' in focal cerebral vascular lesions studied by angiography and regional cerebral blood flow measurements. *British Journal of Radiology*, **40,** 270 (1967)

78 CROPP, G. J. A. and BURTON, A. C. Theoretical considerations and model experiments on the validity of indicator dilution methods for measurements of variable flow. *Circulation Research*, **18,** 26–48 (1966)

79 CROW, T. J. and KELMAN, G. R. Effect of mild acute hypoxia on human short-term memory. *British Journal of Anaesthesia*, **43,** 548–552 (1971)

80 CROWELL, R. M. and OLESSON, Y. Impaired microvascular filling after focal cerebral ischemia in the monkey. *Neurology*, **22,** 500–504 (1972)

81 CROWELL, R. M. and OLSSON, Y. Observations on the microvasculature in focal cerebral ischemia and infarction. In *Eighth Princeton Conference: Cerebral Vascular Diseases*, edited by F. H. McDowell and R. W. Brennan. 77–88. New York: Grune & Stratton (1973)

82 D'ALECY, L. G. Sympathetic cerebral vasoconstriction blocked by adrenergic α receptor antagonists. *Stroke*, **4,** 30–37 (1973)

83 DEMOPOULOS, H. B. Control of free radicals in biologic systems. *Federation Proceedings*, **32,** 1903–1908 (1973)

84 DEMOPOULOS, H. B., FLAMM, E. S., SELIGMAN, M. L., JORGENSEN, E. and RANSOHOFF, J. Antioxidant effects of barbiturates in model membranes undergoing free radical damage. *Acta Neurologica Scandinavica*, **56** (Suppl. 64), 152–153 (1977)

85 DEMOPOULOS, H. B., FLAMM, E. S., SELIGMANN, M., POWER, R., PIETRONIGRO, D. and RANSOHOFF, J. Molecular pathology of lipids in CNS membranes. In *Oxygen and Physiological Function*, edited by F. F. Jobsis, 491–508. Dallas, Texas: Professional Information Library (1977)

86 DENNIS, C. and KABAT, H. Behavior of dogs after complete temporary arrest of the cephalic circulation. *Proceedings of the Society for Experimental Biology and Medicine*, **40,** 559–581 (1939)

87 DENNY-BROWN, D. The treatment of recurrent cerebrovascular symptoms and the question of 'vasospasm'. *Medical Clinics of North America*, **35**, 1457–1474 (1951)

88 DENNY-BROWN, D. and MEYER, J. S. The cerebral collateral circulation. II. Production of cerebral infarction by ischemic anoxia and its reversibility in early stages. *Neurology*, **7**, 567 (1957)

89 DONDERS, F. C. Die bewegnung des Gehirns und die Veranderungen der Gefassfullung der Pia mater, auch bei geschlossen, unausdehnbarem Schadel unmittelbar beobachtet. *Nederlands Lancet* (1850)

90 DOYLE, F. H., PENNOCK, J. M. and ORR, J. S. Imaging of the brain by nuclear magnetic resonance. *Lancet*, **2**, 53–57 (1981)

91 DUFFY, T. E., NELSON, S. R. and LOWRY, O. H. Cerebral carbohydrate metabolism during acute hypoxia and recovery. *Journal of Neurochemistry*, **19**, 959–977 (1972)

92 DUFFY, T. E., NELSON, S. R. and LOWRY, O. H. Cerebral carbohydrate metabolism during acute hypoxia and recovery. *Journal of Neurochemistry*, **19**, 959–977 (1972)

93 DYKEN, M. L. Cerebral blood flow and metabolism studies comparing krypton-85 desaturation technique with argon desaturation technique using the mass spectrometer. *Stroke*, **3**, 279–285 (1972)

94 EKLOF, B., MacMILLAN, V. and SIESJO, B. K. Cerebral energy state and cerebral venous Po in experimental hypotension caused by bleeding. *Acta Physiologica Scandinavica*, **86**, 515–527 (1972)

95 EKLOF, B., MacMILLAN, V. and SIESJO, B. K. The effect of hypercapnic acidosis upon the energy metabolism of the brain in arterial hypotension caused by bleeding. *Acta Physiologica Scandinavica*, **87**, 1–14 (1973)

96 EKLOF, B. and SIESJO, B. K. The effect of bilateral carotid artery ligation upon the blood flow and the energy state of the rat brain. *Acta Physiologica Scandinavica*, **86**, 155–165 (1972)

97 EKLOF, B. and SIESJO, B. K. The effect of bilateral carotid artery ligation upon acid-base parameters and substrate levels in the rat brain. *Acta Physiologica Scandinavica*, **86**, 528–538 (1972)

98 EPSTEIN, F.H. Nuclear magnetic resonance, a new tool in clinical medicine. *New England Journal of Medicine*, **304**, 1360–1361 (1981)

99 FAZEKAS, J. R., YUAN, R. H., CALLOW, A. D., PAUL, R. E. Jr. and ALMAN, R. W. Studies of cerebral hemodynamics in aortocranial disease. *New England Journal of Medicine*, **266**, 224 (1964)

100 FICK, A. Uber die Messung des Boutquantums in den Herzventrikeln. *Verhandlungen Physik und Medizinische Gesellschaft Wurzberg*, **2**, 14 (1870)

101 FIESCHI, C. Regional cerebral blood flow in acute apoplexy, including pharmacodynamic studies. *Scandinavian Journal of Clinical and Laboratory Investigation*, **16E** (Suppl. 102) (1968)

102 FIESCHI, C. and AGNOLI, A. Impairment of the regional vasomotor response of cerebral vessels to hypercarbia in vascular disease. *European Neurology*, **2**, 13 (1969)

103 FIESCHI, C., BATTISTINI, N. and NARDINI, M. Experimental cerebral infarction: focal or perifocal reactive hyperemia and its relationship with the red softening. In *Research on the Cerebral Circulation*. Fourth International Salzburg Conference. Springfield: Charles C. Thomas (1970)

104 FIESCHI, C., AGNOLI, A., BATTISTINI, N. and BOZZAO, L. Regional cerebral blood flow in patients with brain infarct. *Archives of Neurology*, **15**, 653 (1966)

105 FIESCHI, C. A., AGNOLI, A., BATTISTINI, N., BOZZAO, L. and PRENCIPE, M. Derangement of regional blood flow and of its regulatory mechanisms in acute cerebrovascular lesions. *Neurology*, **18**, 1166 (1968)

106 FISCHER, C. M. and ADAMS, R. D. Observations on brain embolism with special reference to the mechanism of hemorrhagic infarction. *Journal of Neuropathology and Experimental Neurology*, **1**, , 92 (1951)

107 FISHER, E. G. and AMES, A. III. Studies on mechanisms of impairment of cerebral circulation following ischemia: effect of hemodilution and perfusion pressure. *Stroke*, **3**, 538–542 (1972)

108 FISHMAN, R. A. Carrier transport of glucose between blood and cerebrospinal fluid. *American Journal of Physiology*, **206**(4), 836–844 (1964)

109 FLAMM, E. S., DEMOPOULOS, H. B., SELIGMAN, M. L., POSER R. G. and RANSOHOFF, J. Free radicals in cerebral ischemia. *Stroke*, **9**, 445–447 (1978)

110 FLAMM, E. S., DEMOPOULOS, H. B., SELIGMAN, M. L. and RANSOHOFF, J. Possible molecular mechanisms of barbituate mediated protection in regional cerebral ischemia. *Acta Neurologica Scandinavica*, **56** (Suppl. 64) 150–151, 1977

111 FLOWER, R. J. Drugs which inhibit prostaglandin biosynthesis. *Pharmacological Reviews*, **26**, 33–67 (1974)

112 FLOWER, R. J. Biosynthesis of prostaglandins. In *Oxygen, Free Radicals and Tissue Damage*, Ciba Foundation Symposium 65 (new series), 123–138. Amsterdam: Excerpta Medica (1979)

113 FOG, M. Reaction of the pial arteries to fall in blood pressure. *Archives of Neurology and Psychiatry*, **37**, 351–364 (1937)

114 FOG, M. Relationship between blood pressure and tonic regulation of pial arteries. *Journal of Neurology and Psychiatry*, **1**, 187 (1938)

115 FOG, M. Cerebral circulation. II. Reaction of pial arteries to increase in blood pressure. *Archives of Neurology and Psychiatry*, **41**, 260–268 (1939)

116 FOLBERGROVA, J., LJUNGGREN, B. and SIESJO, B. K. Influence of complete ischemia on glycolytic metabolites, citric acid cycle intermediates and associated amino acids in the rat cerebral cortex. *Brain Research*, **80**, 265–279 (1974)

117 FORBES, H. S. Cerebral circulation. I. Observations and measurement of pial vessels. *Archives of Neurology and Psychiatry*, **1**, 187 (1938)

117a FOX, I. J. History and development aspects of the indicator-dilution technique. *Circulation Research*, **10**, 381–391 (1961)

118 FRIDOVICH, I. Superoxide dismutases. *Annual Review of Biochemistry*, **44**, 147–159 (1975)

119 FUJISHIMA, M., SCHEINBERG, P. and BUSTO, R. Cerebral cortical blood flow: variable effect of hypoxia in the dog. *Archives of Neurology*, **25**, 160–167 (1971)

120 GALLE, C. and SPAGNUOLO, C. The release of brain free fatty acids during ischaemia in essential fatty acid-deficient rats. *Journal of Neurochemistry*, **26**, 401–404 (1976)

121 GARCIA, J. H., KAMIJYO, Y., KALIMO, H., TANAKA, J., VELORIA, J. E. and TRUMP, B. F. Cerebral ischemia: the early structural changes and correlation of these with known metabolic and dynamic abnormalities. In *Ninth Princeton Conference: Cerebrovascular Diseases*, edited by J. P. Whisnant and B. A. Sandok. New York: Grune and Stratton (1975)

122 GAUDET, R. J. and LEVINE, L. Transient cerebral ischemia and brain prostaglandins. *Biochemical and Biophysical Research Communications*, **86**, 893–901 (1979)

123 GIBBS, E. L., LENNOX, W. G., NIMS, L. F. and GIBBS, F. A. Arterial and cerebral venous blood. Arterial-venous differences in man. *Journal of Biological Chemistry*, **144**, 325–332 (1942)

124 GIBBS, F. A., MAXWELL, H. and GIBBS, E. L. Volume flow of blood through the human brain. *Archives of Neurology and Psychiatry*, **57**, 137 (1947)

125 GILBOE, D. D., ANDREWS R. L. and DARDENNE, G. Factors affecting glucose uptake by the isolated dog brain. *American Journal of Physiology*, **219**, 767–773 (1970)

126 GILLINGHAM, F. J., MAWDSLEY, C. and WILLIAMS, A. E. *Stroke: Proceedings of the Ninth Pfizer International Symposium*. Edinburgh: Churchill-Livingstone (1976)

127 GINSBERG, M. D., BUDD, W. W. and WELSH, G. A. Diffuse cerebral ischemia in the cat. 1. Local blood flow during severe ischemia and recirculation. *Annals of Neurology*, **3**, 482–492 (1978)

128 GINSBERG, M. D. MELA, L., WROBEL-KUHL, K. and REIVICH, M. Mitochondrial metabolism following bilateral cerebral ischemia in the gerbil. *Annals of Neurology*, **1**, 519–527 (1977)

129 GINSBERG, M., MELA, L., WROBEL-KUHL, K. and REIVICH, M. Mitochondrial metabolism of normal and ischemic brains from urethane anesthetized gerbils. *Annals of Neurology*, **1**, 519–527 (1977)

130 GINSBERG, M. D. and MYERS, R. E. The topography of impaired microvascular perfusion in the primate brain following total circulatory arrest. *Neurology*, **22**, 988–1011 (1972)

131 GINSBERG, M. D., REIVICH, M., FRINAK, S. and HARBIG, K. Pyridine nucleotide redox state and blood flow of the cerebral cortex following middle cerebral artery occlusion in the cat. *Stroke*, **7**, 125–131 (1976)

132 GINSBERG, M. D., REIVICH, M., GIANDOMENICO, A. and GREENBERG, J. H. Local glucose utilization in acute focal cerebral ischemia: local dysmetabolism and diaschisis. *Neurology*, **27**, 1042–1048 (1977)

133 GOLDBERG, N. D., GRAFF, G., HADDOX, M. K., STEPHENSON, J. K., GLASS, D. B. and MOSER, M. E. Redox modulation of splenic cell soluble guanylate cyclase activity: activation by hydrophilic and hydrophobic oxidants represented by ascorbic and dehydroascorbic acids, fatty acid hydroperoxides and prostaglandin endoperoxides. In *Advances in Cyclic Nucleotide Research*, Vol. 9, edited by W. J. George and I. J. Ignarro, 101–130. New York: Raven Press (1978)

134 GOLDBERG, N. D., PASSONNEAU, J. V. and LOWRY, O. H. Effects of changes in brain metabolism on the levels of citric acid cycle intermediates. *Journal of Biological Chemistry*, **241**, 3997–4003 (1966)

135 GONZALEZ, L. L. and LEWIS C. M. Cerebral hemorrhage following successful endarterectomy of the internal carotid artery. *Surgery, Gynecology and Obstetrics*, **122**, 773 (1966)

136 GOTOH, F., MEYER, J. S. and TOMITA, M. Hydrogen method for determining cerebral blood flow in man. *Archives of Neurology*, **15**, 549–559 (1966)

137 GOTOH, F., TAZAK, Y. and MEYER, J. S. Transport of gases through the brain and their extravascular vasomotor action. *Experimental Neurology*, **4**, 48 (1961)

138 GREENGAARD, P. and STRAUB, R. W. Effect of frequency of electrical stimulation on the concentration of intermediary metabolites in mammalian non-myelinated fibres. *Journal of Physiology (London)*, **148**, 353–361 (1959)

139 GRUBB, R. L., RAICHLE, M. E., HIGGINS, C. S. and EICHLING, J. G. Measurement of regional cerebral blood volume by emission tomography. *Annals of Neurology*, **4**, 322–328 (1978)

140 HAGGENDAL, E. and JOHANSSON, B. Effects of arterial carbon dioxide tension and oxygen saturation on cerebral blood flow autoregulation in dogs. *Acta Physiologica Scandinavica*, **66** (Suppl. 258) 27 (1965)

141 HALLENBECK, J. M. and FURLOW, T. W. Jr. Prostaglandin I$_2$ and in-of its function and evolution. In *The Neurosciences: Fourth Study Program*, edited by F. O. Schmitt and F. G. Worder, 617–622. Cambridge, Mass.: MIT Press (1979)

142 HALSEY, J. H. and CLARK, L. C. Some regional circulatory abnormalities following experimental cerebral infarction. *Neurology*, **20**, 238 (1970)

143 HAMER, J., HOYER, S., STOECKEL, H., ALBERTI, E. and WEINHARDT, F. Cerebral blood flow and cerebral metabolism in acute increase of intracranial pressure. *Acta Neurochirurgica*, **28**, 95–110 (1973)

144 HARBIG, K., REIVICH, M., CHANCE, B. and KOVACH, A. G. B. Changes in pyridine nucleotide florescence in cerebral ischemia. In *Ninth Princeton Conference Cerebral Vascular Disease*, edited by J. B. Whisnant and B. A. Sandok, 251–255. New York: Grune and Stratton (1975)

145 HARPER, A. M., GLASS, H. I., STEVEN, J. L. and GRANAT, A. H. The measurement of local blood flow in the cerebral cortex from the clearance of Xenon^{133}. *Journal of Neurology, Neurosurgery and Psychiatry*, **27**, 255–258 (1964)

146 HARPER, A. M., DESHMUKH, V. D., ROWAN, J. O. and JENNETT, W. B. The influence of sympathetic nervous activity on cerebral blood flow. *Archives of Neurology*, **27**, 1–6 (1972)

147 HARPER, A. M. and GLASS, H. I. Effect of alterations in the arterial carbon dioxide tension on the blood flow through the cerebral cortex at normal and low arterial blood pressures. *Journal of Neurology, Neurosurgery and Psychiatry*, **28**, 449–452 (1965)

148 HARRIS, R. J., SYMON, L., BRANSTON, N. M. and BAYHAN, M. Changes in extracellular calcium activity in cerebral ischaemia. *Journal of Cerebral Blood Flow and Metabolism*, **1**, 203–209 (1981)

149 HASS, W. K., WALD, A., RANSOHOFF, J. and DOROGI, O. Argon and nitorus oxide ceerebral blood flows simultaneously monitored by mass spectrometry in patients with head injury. *European Neurology*, **8**, 164–168 (1972)

150 HAWKES, R. C., HOLLAND, C. N., MOORE, W. S. and WORTHINGTON, B. S. Nuclear magnetic resonance (NMR) tomography of the brain. *Journal of Computed Assisted Tomography*, **4**, 577–586 (1980)

151 HEDLUND, S., LJUNGGRAN, K. and KOBLER, V. Mean cerebral blood transit time obtained by external measurement of an intravenously injected tracer. *Acta Radiologica: Diagnosis*, **4**, 581–591 (1966)

152 HEISS, W. D., PROSENZ, P. and ROSZUCZKY, A. Technical considerations in the use of a γ camera 1600-channel analyzer system for the measurement of regional cerebral blood flow. *Journal of Nuclear Medicine*, **13**, 534–543 (1972)

153 HERNANDEZ-PEREZ, M. J., RAICHLE, M. E. and STONE, H. L. The role of the peripheral sympathetic nervous system in cerebral blood flow autoregulation. *Stroke*, **6**, 284–292 (1975)

154 HESS, H. H. In *Regional Neurochemistry*, edited by S. S. Kety and J. Elkes, 200–212. New York: Pergamon Press (1961)

155 HIDAKA, H. and ASANO, T. Stimulation of human platelet guanylate cyclase by unsaturated fatty acid peroxides. *Proceedings of the National Academy of Science, USA*, **74**, 3657–3661 (1977)

156 HILL, L. E. *The Physiology and Pathology of the Cerebral Circulation*. London: J. and A. Churchill (1896)

157 HILLMAN, H., LOUPEKINE, J. and FULLBROOK, P. The clinical history of cardiac arrest and recovery of anaesthetized hypothermic rats, and their reproduction. *Resuscitation*, **1**, 51–60 (1972)

158 HIMWICH, H. E. and NAHUM, L. H. Respiratory quotient of brain. *American Journal of Physiology*, **90**, 389–390 (1929)

159 HIRSCH, H., BOLTE, A., SCHAUDIG, A. and TONNIS, D. Uber die Wiederbelebung des Gehirns bei Hypothermie. *Pfugers Archiv fur die gesamte Physiologie*, **265**, 328–336 (1957)

160 HOEDT-RASMUSSEN, K. and SKINHOJ, E. Transneural depression of the cerebral hemispheric metabolism in man. *Acta Neurologica Scandinavica*, **40**, 41–46 (1964)

161 HOEDT-RASMUSSEN, K. Regional cerebral blood flow. *Acta Neurologica Scandinavica*, **43** (Suppl. 27), 1–81 (1967)

162 HOEDT-RASMUSSEN, K. and SKINHOJ, E. *In vivo* measurements of the relative weight of gray and white matter in the human brain. *Neurology*, **16**, 515 (1966)

163 HOEDT-RASMUSSEN, K., SKINHOJ, E., PAULSON, O., EWALD, J., BJERRUM, J. K., FAHRENK-RUG, A. and LASSEN, N. A. Regional cerebral blood flow in acute apoplexy, the 'luxury perfusion syndrome' of brain tissue. *Archives of Neurology*, **17**, 271 (1967)

164 HOEDT-RASMUSSEN, K., SVEINSDOTTIR, E. and LASSEN, N. A. Regional cerebral blood flow in man determined by intra-arterial injection of radioactive inert gas. *Circulation Research*, **18**, 237 (1966)

165 HONJO, J. and OZAWA, K. Lysolecithin inhibition of mitochondrial metabolism. *Biochimica et Biophysica Acta*, **162**, 624–627 (1968)

166 HOSSMANN, K. A. Total ischemia of the brain. In *Brain and Heart Infarct*, edited by K. J. Zulch, W. Kaufmann, K. A. Hossmann and V. Hossmann, 107–122. Berlin: Springer-Verlag (1977)

167 HOSSMANN, K. A. and KLEIHUES, P. Reversibility of ischemic brain damage. *Archives of Neurology*, **29**, 375–382 (1973)

168 HOSSMANN, K. A. and LECTAPE-GRUTER, H. Blood flow of the cat brain after complete ischemia for one hour. *European Neurology*, **6**, 318–322 (1971–1972)

169 HOSSMANN, K. A., LECTAPE-GRUTER, H. and HOSSMANN, V. The role of cerebral blood flow for the recovery of the brain after prolonged ischemia. *Zeitschrift fur Neurologie*, **204**, 281–299 (1973)

170 HOSSMANN, K. A. and OLSSON, Y. Suppression and recovery of neuronal function in transient cerebral orchimia. *Brain Research*, **22**, 313–325 (1970)

171 HOSSMANN, K. A., SAKAKI, S. and KIMOTO, K. Cerebral uptake of glucose and oxygen in the cat brain after prolonged ischemia. *Stroke*, **7**, 301–305 (1976)

172 HOSSMANN, K. A., SAKAKI, S. and ZIMMERMAN, V. Cation activities in reversible ischaemia of the cat brain. *Stroke*, **8**, 77–81 (1977)

173 HOSSMANN, K. and SATO, K. Recovery of neuronal function after prolonged cerebral ischemia. *Science*, **168**, 375 (1970)

174 HOSSMANN, K. A. and ZIMMERMAN, V. Resuscitation of the monkey brain after 1 hour's complete ischemia. I. Physiological and morphological observation. *Brain Research*, **81**, 59–74 (1974)

175 HOSSMAN, U. and HOSSMAN, K. Return of neuronal functions after prolonged cardiac arrest. *Brain Research*, **60**, 423 (1973)

176 HOUGH, H. B. and WOLFF, H. G. The relative vascularity of subcortical ganglia of the cat's brain: the putamen, globus pallidus, substantia nigra, red nucleus and geniculate bodies. *Journal of Comparative Neurology*, **71**, 427–436 (1939)

177 HOULT, D. I., BUSBY, S. J. W., GADIAN, G. G., RADDA, G. K., RICHARDS, R. E. and SEELY, P. J. Observation of tissue metabolites using ^{31}P nuclear magnetic resonance. *Nature*, **252**, 285–287 (1974)

178 HUANG, S., PHELPS, M., CARSON, R., HOFFMAN, E., PLUMMER, D., MACDONALD, N. and KUHL, D. Tomographic measurement of local cerebral blood flow in man with O^{15} water. *Journal of Cerebral Blood Flow and Metabolism*, **1** (Suppl. 1) 31–32 (1981)

179 HUTTEN, H. and BROCK, M. The two minute flow index (TMFI). In *Cerebral Blood Flow*, Vol. 19. Berlin: Springer-Verlag (1969)

180 INGVAR, D. H. In *Regional Neurochemistry*, edited by S. S. Kety and J. Elkes, 55–61. New York: Pergamon Press (1961)

181a INGVAR, D. H. The pathophysiology of occlusive cerebrovascular disorders related to neuroradiological findings, EEG, and measurements of regional cerebral blood flow. *Acta Neurologica Scandinavica*, **43** (Suppl. 31) 93 (1967)

181b INGVAR, D. H., CRONQUIST, S., EKBERG, R., RISBERG, J. and HOEDT-RASMUSSEN, K. Normal values of regional cerebral blood flow in man, including flow and weight estimates of gray and white matter. *Acta Neurologica Scandinavica*, **14** (Suppl.) 72–78 (1965)

182 INGVAR, D. H. and LASSEN, N. A. Quantitative determination of regional cerebral blood flow in man. *Lancet*, **2**, 806 (1961)

183 INGVAR, D. H. and LASSEN, N. A. Regional blood flow of the cerebral cortex tetermined by krypton-85. *Acta Physiologica Scandinavica*, **54**, 325–338 (1962)

184 INGVAR, D.H. and LASSEN, N. A. Methods for cerebral blood flow measurement in man. *British Journal of Anesthesia*, **37**, 216 (1965)

185 INGVAR, D. H. and LASSEN, N. A. Cerebral complications following measurements of regional cerebral blood flow (rCBF) with the intra-arterial ^{133}xenon injection method. *Stroke*, **4**, 658–665 (1973)

186 INGVAR, D. H. and RISBERG, J. Increase of regional cerebral blood flow during mental effort in normals and in patients with focal brain disorders. *Experimental Brain Research*, **3**, 195 (1967)

187 IWABUCHI, T., WATAHAVBE, K., KUTSUZAWA, T. *et al.* Lactate in the cerebrospinal fluid and pressure-flow relationships in canine cerebral circulation. *Stroke*, **4**, 207–212 (1973)

188 JACOB, H. In *Selective Vulnerability of Brain in Hypoxaemia*, edited by J. D. Schade and W. H. McMenemey, 153–163. Philadelphia: F. A. Davis & Co. (1963)

189 JAKSCHIK, B. A., FALKENHEIN, S. and PARKER, C. W. Precursor role of arachidonic acid in release of slow reacting substance from rat basophilic leukemia cells. *Proceedings of the National Academy of Science, USA*, **74**, 4577–4581 (1977)

190 JENKINS, L. W., POVLISHOCK, J. T., BECKER, D. P., MILLER, J. D. and SULLIVAN, H. G. Complete cerebral ischemia. An ultrastructural study. *Acta Neuropathologica*, **48**, 113–125 (1979)

191 JOHANNSSON, H. and SIESJO, B. K. Cerebral blood flow and oxygen consumption in the rat in hypoxic hypoxia. *Acta Physiologica Scandinavica*, **93**, 269–276 (1975)

192 JONES, T. Positron emission tomography and measurements of regional tissue function in man. *British Medical Bulletin*, **36**, 231–236 (1980)

193 KAASIK, A., NILSSON, L. and SIESJO, B. K. The effect of arterial hypotension upon the lactate, pyruvate and bicarbonate concentrations of the brain tissue and cisternal CSF, and upon the tissue concentrations of phosphocreatine and adenine nucleotides in anesthetized rats. *Acta Physiologica Scandinavica*, **78**, 448–458 (1970)

194 KALIMO, H., GARCIA, J. H., KAMIJYO, Y., TANAKA, J. and TRUMP, B. F. The ultrastructure of 'brain death'. II. Electron microscopy of feline cortex after complete ischemia. *Virchows Archiv B*, **25**, 207–220 (1977)

195 KAWAMURA, U., MEYER, J. S., HIROMOTO, H. *et al.* Neurogenic control of cerebral blood flow in the baboon: effects of α-adrenergic blockage with phenoxygenzamine on cerebral autoregulation and vasomotor reactivity to changes in $P_{a CO_2}$. *Stroke*, **5**, 747–758 (1974)

196 KELLOGG, E. E. III and FRIDOVICH, I. Superoxide, hydrogen peroxide and singlet oxygen in lipid peroxidation by a xanthine oxidase system. *Journal of Biological Chemistry*, **250**, 8812–8817 (1975)

197 KEMPINSKY, W. H. Experimental study of distant effects of acute focal brain injury: a study of diaschisis. *Archives of Neurology and Psychiatry*, **79**, 376–389 (1958)

198 KEMPINSKY, W. H., BONIFACE, W. R., KEATING, J. B. A. *et al.* Serial hemodynamic study of cerebral infarction in man. *Circulation Research*, **9**, 1051–1058 (1961)

199 KENNEDY, C. and SOKOLOFF, L. An adaptation of the nitrous oxide method to the study of the cerebral circulation in children; normal values for cerebral blood flow and cerebral metabolic rate in children. *Journal of Clinical Investigation*, **36**, 1130 (1957)

200 KETY, S. S. The theory and applications of the exchange of inert gas at the lungs and tissues. *Pharmacological Reviews*, **3**, 1 (1951)

201 KETY, S. S. Blood flow and metabolism in the human brain in health and disease. In *Neurochemistry*, edited by E. Nurnberger. Springfield: Charles C. Thomas (1956)

202 KETY, S. S. Measurement of local blood flow by the exchange of an inert, diffusible substance. *Methods of Medicine and Research*, **8**, 228–236 (1960)

203 KETY, S. W., HARMEL, M. H., BROMELL, H. T. and RHODE, C. B. The solubility of nitrous oxide in blood and brain. *Journal of Biological Chemistry*, **173**, 487 (1948)

204 KETY, S. S. and SCHMIDT, C. F. Determination of cerebral blood flow in man by use of nitrous oxide in low concentrations. *American Journal of Physiology*, **143**, 53 (1945)

205 KETY, S. S. and SCHMIDT, C. F. The nitrous oxide method for the quantitative determination of cerebral blood flow in man: theory, procedure and normal values. *Journal of Clinical Investigation*, **27**, 476 (1948)

206 KIMELBER, H. K., NARUMI, S., BIDDLECOME, S., and BOURKE, R. S. $(Na^4 + K^4)$ ATPase Rb− transport and carbonic anhydrase activity in isolated brain cells and cultured astrocytes. In *Dynamic Properties of Glia Cells*, edited by E.Schoffeniels, G. Franck, L. Hertz and D. B. Tower, 347–357. Oxford: Pergamon Press (1978)

207 KING, L. J., LOWRY, O.H., PASSONNEAU, J. V. and VENSON, F. Effects of convulsants on energy reserves in the cerebral cortex. *Journal of Neurochemistry*, **14**, 599–611 (1967)

208 KING, L .J., SCHOEPFLE, G. M., LOWRY, O. H., PASSONNEAU, J. V. and WILSON, S. Effects of electrical stimulation on metabolites in brain of decapitated mice. *Journal of Neurochemistry*, **14**, 613–618 (1967)

209 KIRSCHNER, H. S., BLANK, W. F. and MYERS, R. E. Brain extracellular potassium activity during hypoxia in the cat. *Neurology*, **25**, 1001–1005 (1975)

210 KIRSCHNER, H. S., BLANK, W. F. and MYERS, R. E. Changes in cortical subarachnoid fluid potassium concentrations during hypoxia. *Archives of Neurology*, **33**, 84–90 (1976)

211 KLATZO, I. Cerebral oedema and ischaemia. In *Recent Advances in Neuropathology*, edited by W. T. Smith and J. B. Cavanagh, 27–39. Edinburgh: Churchill-Livingstone

212 KLEE, A. The relationship between clinical evaluation of mental deterioration, psychological test results, and the cerebral metabolic rate of oxygen. *Acta Neurologica Scandinavica*, **40**, 337–345 (1964)

213 KLEIHUES, P. and HOSSMANN, K. A. Regional incorporation of (L-3-H) tyrosine into cat brain proteins after 1 hour of complete ischemia. *Acta Neuropathologica*, **25**, 313–324 (1973)

214 KLEIHUES, P., HOSSMANN, K. A., PEGG, A. E., KOBAYASHI, K. and ZIMMERMANN, V. Resuscitation of the monkey brain after 1 hour complete ischemia. III. Indications of metabolic recovery. *Brain Research*, **95**, 61–73 (1975)

215 KOBAYASHI, M., LUST, W. D. and PASSONNEAU, J. V. Concentrations of energy metabolites and cyclic nucleotides during and after bilateral ischemia in the gerbil cerebral cortex. *Journal of Neurochemistry*, **29**, 53–59 (1977)

216 KOFKE, W. A., NEMOTO, E. M., HOSSMANN, K. A., TAYLOR, F., KESSLER, P. D. and STEZOSKI, S. W. Brain blood flow and metabolism after global ischemia and post-insult thiopental therapy in monkeys. *Stroke*, **10**, 554–560 (1979)

217 KOGURE, K., BUSTO, R., SCHEINBERG, P. and REINMUTH, A. M. Energy metabolites and water content in rat brain during the early stage of development of cerebral infarction. *Brain*, **97**, 103–114 (1974)

218 KOGURE, K., SCHEINBERG, P., FUJISHIMA, M. *et al.* Effects of hypoxia on cerebral autoregulation. *American Journal of Physiology*, **219**, 1393–1396 (1970)

219 KOGURE, K., SCHEINBERG, P., MATSUMOTO, A., BUSTO, R. and REINMUTH, A. M. Catecholamines in experimental brain ischemia. *Archives of Neurology*, **32**, 21–24 (1975)

220 KOGURE, K., SCHEINBERG, P., REINMUTH, O. M., FUJISHIMA, M. and BUSTO, R. Mechanisms of cerebral vasodilatation in hypoxia. *Journal of Applied Physiology*, **29**, 223–229 (1970)

221 KOWADA, M., AMES, A. III, MAJNO, G. and WRIGHT, R. L. Cerebral ischemia. I. An improved experimental method for study; cardiovascular effects and demonstrations of an early vascular lesion in the rabbit. *Journal of Neurosurgery*, **28**, 150–157 (1968)

222 KUHL, D. E., PHELPS, M. E., KOWELL, A. P., METTER, E. J., SELIN, C. and WINTER, J. Effects of stroke on local cerebral metabolism and perfusion: mapping by emission and computed tomography of ^{18}FDG and ^{13}NH$_3$. *Annals of Neurology*, **8**, 47–66 (1980)

223 KUHL, D. E., REIVICH, M., ALAVI, A. *et al.* Local cerebral blood volume determined by three-dimensional reconstruction of radionuclide scan data. *Circulation Research*, **36**, 610–619 (1975)

224 KUSCHINSKY, W., WAHL, M., BOSSE, O. and THURAU, K. Perivascular potassium and pH as determinants of local pial arterial diameter in cats. *Circulation Research*, **31**, 240–247 (1972)

224a KUSHNER, M., REIVICH, M, ALAVI, A., DANN, R., HURTIG, H. and GREENBERG, J. Contralateral cerebellar hypometabolism following cerebral hemispheric insult: a positron emission tomographic study. *Annals of Neurology*, **12**, 88 (1982)

225 KUWASHIMA, J., FUJIFANI, B., NAKAMURA, K., KADOKAWA, T., YOSHIDA, K. and SHIMIZU, M. Biochemical changes in unilateral brain injury in the rat: a possible role of fatty acid accumulation. *Brain Research*, **110**, 547–557 (1976)

226 KUWASHIMA, J., NAKAMURA, K., FUJIFANI, B., KADOKAWA, T., YOSHIDA,K. and SHIMIZU, M. Relationship between cerebral energy failure and free fatty acid accumulation following prolonged brain ischemia. *Japanese Journal of Pharmacology*, **28**, 277–287 (1978)

227 LAMMERTSMA, A. A., FRACKOWIAK, R. S. J., LENZI, G. L., HEATHER, J. D., POZZILLI, C. and JONES, T. Accuracy of the oxygen-15 steady state technique for measuring rCBF and rCMRO$_2$: tracer modelling, statistics and spatial sampling. *Journal of Cerebral Blood Flow and Metabolism*, **1** (Suppl. 1) 3–4 (1981)

228 LANDS, W. E. M. The biosynthesis and metabolism of prostaglandins. *Annual Review of Physiology*, **41**, 633–652 (1979)

229 LANG, R., ZIMMER, R. and OBERDORSTER, G. Post-ischemic O$_2$ availability and O$_2$ consumption of the isolated perfused brain of the dog. *Pflügers Archiv fur die gesamte Physiologie*, **334**, 103–113 (1972)

230 LASSEN, N. A. Cerebral blood flow and oxygen consumption in man. *Physiological Reviews*, **39**, 183–283 (1959)

231 LASSEN, N. A. The luxury-perfusion syndrome and its possible relation to acute metabolic acidosis localised within the brain. *Lancet*, **2**, 1112–1115 (1966)

232 LASSEN, N. A. Brain extracellular pH; the main factor controlling cerebral blood flow. *Scandinavian Journal of Clinical and Laboratory Investigation*, **22**, 247 (1968)

233 LASSEN, N. A. Control of cerebral circulation in health and disease. *Circulation Research*, **24**, 749–760 (1974)

234 LASSEN, N. A., HOEDT-RASMUSSEN, K., SORGENSE, S. C., SKINHOJ, E., CRONQUIST, S., BODFORSS, B. and INGVAR, D. H. Regional cerebral blood flow in man, determined by krypton-85. *Neurology*, **13**, 719–727 (1963)

235 LASSEN, N. A. and INGVAR, D. H. The blood flow of the cerebral cortex determined by radioactive krypton. *Experientia*, **17**, 42 (1961)

236 LASSEN, N. A., INGVAR, D. H. and SKINHOJ, E. Brain function and blood flow. *Scientific American*, **239**, 62–71 (1978)

237 LASSEN, N. A. and KLEE, A. Cerebral blood flow determination by saturation and desaturation with krypton-85. *Circulation Research*, **16**, 26 (1965)

238 LASSEN, N. A. and LANE, M. H. Validity of internal jugular blood for study of cerebral blood flow and metabolism. *Journal of Applied Physiology: Respiratory, Environmental and Exercise Physiology*, **16**, 313 (1961)

239 LASSEN, N. A. and MUNCK, O. The cerebral blood flow in man determined by the use of radioactive krypton. *Acta Physiologica Scandinavica*, **33**, 30 (1955)

240 LEHNINGER, A. L. *Biochemistry*. New York: Worth Publishers, Inc. (1975)

241 LENNOX, W. G. and GIBBS, E. L. The blood flow in the brain and leg of man and the changes induced by alteration of blood gases. *Journal of Clinical Investigation*, **11**, 1155 (1932)

242 LEVY, D. E., BRIERLEY, J. B., SILVERMAN, D. G. and PLUM, F. Brain hypoxia in initially damaged cerebral neurons. *Archives of Neurology*, **32**, 450–455 (1975)

243 LEVY, D. E. and DUFFY, T. E. Cerebral energy metabolism during transient ischemia and recovery in the gerbil. *Journal of Neurochemistry*, **28**, 63–70 (1977)

244 LEVY, D. E. and BRIERLEY, J. B. Delayed pentobarbital administration limits ischemic brain damage in gerbils. *Annals of Neurology*, **5**, 59–64 (1979)

245 LEWIS, B. M., SOKOLOFF, L., WECHSLER, R. L., WEUTZ, W. B. and KETY, S. S. A method for continuous measurement of cerebral blood flow in man by means of radioactive krypton (Kr-79). *Journal of Clinical Investigation*, **39**, 707 (1960)

246 LEWIS, D. H. and DEL MAESTRO, R. F. (Eds) Free radical in medicine and biology. *Acta Physiologica Scandinavica* (Suppl. 492) (1980)

247 LIN, S. R. and KORMANO, M. Cerebral circulation after cardiac arrest. *Stroke*, **8**, 182 (1977)

248 LITTLE, J. R., KERR, F. W. L. and SUNDT, T. M. Jr. Microcirculatory obstruction in focal cerebral ischemia: an electron microscopic investigation in monkeys. *Stroke*, **7**, 25–30 (1976)

249 LJUNGGREN, B., NORBERG, K. and SIESJO, B. K. Influence of tissue acidosis upon restitution of brain energy metabolism following total ischemia. *Brain Research*, **77**, 173–186 (1974)

250 LJUNGGREN, B., RATCHESON, R. A. and SIESJO, B. K. Cerebral metabolic state following complete compression ischemia. *Brain Research*, **73**, 291–307 (1974)

251 LJUNGGREN, B., SCHUTZ, H. and SIESJO, B. K. Changes in energy state and acid–base parameters of the rat brain during complete compression ischemia. *Brain Research*, **73**, 277–289 (1974)

252 LOWRY, O. H. Metabolite levels as indicators of control mechanisms. *Federation Proceedings*, **25**, 846–849 (1966)

253 LOWRY, O. H., PASSONNEAU, J. V., HASSELBERGER, F. X. and SCHULZ, D. W. Effect of ischemia on known substrates and cofactors of the glycolytic pathway in brain. *Journal of Biological Chemistry*, **239**, 18–30 (1964)

254 LUST, W. D., MRSULJA, B. B., MRSULJA, B. J., PASSONNEAU, J. V. and KLATZO, I. Putative neurotransmitters and cyclic nucleotides in prolonged ischemia of the cerebral cortex. *Brain Research*, **98**, 394–399 (1975)

255 McDOWALL, D. G. Inter-relationships between blood oxygen tensions and cerebral blood flow. In *Oxygen Measurements in Blood and Tissue*, edited by J. P. Payne and D. W. Hill, 205–219. London: Churchill Ltd (1966)

256 McHENRY, L. C. Jr. Quantitative cerebral blood flow determination: application of a krypton^{85} desaturation technique in man. *Neurology*, **14**, 785–793 (1964)

257 McILWAIN, H. *Biochemistry and the Central Nervous System*. Boston: Little, Brown and Co. (1966)

258 MAJEWSKA, M. D., STROSZNAJDER,J. and LAZAREWIEZ, J. Effect of ischemia anoxia and barbiturate anesthesia on free radical oxidation of mitochondrial phospholipids. *Brain Research*, **158**, 423–434 (1978)

259 MAKER, H. S. and LEHRER, G. M. Effect of ischemia. In *Handbook of Neurochemistry*, Vol. 6, edited by A. Lajtha, 267–310. New York: Plenum Press (1971)

260 MAKER, H. S., LEHRER, G. M., SILIDES, D. J. and WEISS, C. Changes in ATP and creatine phosphate (CP) in mouse cerebellar layers during ischemia. *Neurology*, **19**, 297 (1969)

261 MAKER, H. S., LEHRER, G. M., WEISS, C., SILIDES, D. J. and SCHEINBERG, L. C. The quantitative histochemistry of a chemically induced ependymoblastoma. II. The effect of ischaemia on substrates of carbohydrate metabolism. *Journal of Neurochemistry*, **13**, 1207–1212 (1966)

262 MALLETT, B. L. and VEALL, N. Investigation of cerebral blood flow in hypertension using radioactive xenon inhalation and extracranial recording. *Lancet*, **1**, 1081–1082 (1963)

263 MALLETT, B. L. and VEALL, N. The measurement of regional cerebral clearance rates in man using xenon-133 inhalation and extracranial recording. *Clinical Science*, **29**, 179–191 (1965)

264 MARION, J. and WOLFE, L. Origin of the arachidonic acid released post-mortem in rat forebrain. *Biochimica et Biophysica Acta*, **574**, 25–32 (1979)

265 MARSHALL, L. F., GRAHAM, D. I., DURITY, F., LOUNSBURY, R., WELSH, F. and LANGFITT, T. W. Experimental cerebral oligemia and ischemia produced by intracranial hypertension. Part 1. Pathophysiology, electroencephalography, cerebral blood flow, blood-brain barrier and neurological function. *Journal of Neurosurgery*, **43**, 308–317 (1975)

266 MARSHALL, L. G., GRAHAM, D. I., DURITY, F., LOUNSBURY, R., WELSH, F. and LANGFITT, T. W. Experimental cerebral oligemia and ischemia produced by intracranial hypertension. Part 2. Brain morphology. *Journal of Neurosurgery*, **43**, 318–322 (1975)

267 MARSHALL, L. F., WELSH, F., DURITY, F., LOUNSBURY, R., GRAHAM, D. I. and LANGFITT, T. W. Experimental cerebral oligemia and ischemia produced by intracranial hypertension. Part 3. Brain energy metabolism. *Journal Of Neurosurgery*, **43**, 323–328 (1975)

268 MATHEW, N. T., MEYER, J. S., BELL, R. L., JOHNSON, D. C. and NEBLETT, C. R. Regional cerebral blood flow and blood: volume measured with the γ camera. *Journal of Neuroradiology*, **4**, 133 (1972)

269 MCHEDLISHVILI, G. I., MITAGUARIA, N. P. and ORMOTSADZE, L. G. Vascular mechanisms controlling a constant blood supply to the brain ('autoregulation'). *Stroke*, **4**, 742–750 (1973)

270 MCHEDLISHVILI, G. I. Physiological mechanisms controlling cerebral blood flow. *Stroke*, **11**, 240–248 (1980)

271 MEAD, J. F. Free radical mechanisms of lipid damage and consequences for cellular membranes. In *Free Radicals in Biology*, edited by W. A. Pryor, 51–68. New York: Academic Press (1976)

272 MELA, L. Mechanism and physiological significance of calcium transport across mammalian mitochondrial membranes. *Current Topics in Membrane Transport*, **9**, 321–366 (1977)

273 MELA, L. Mitochondrial function in cerebral ischemia and hypoxia: comparison of inhibitory and adaptive responses. *Neurological Research*, **1**, 51 (1979)

274 MEYER, J. S. Circulatory changes following occlusion of the middle cerebral artery and their relation to function. *Journal of Neurosurgery*, **15**, 653–673 (1958)

275 MEYER, J. S. Importance of ischemic damage to small vessels in experimental cerebral infarction. *Journal of Neuropathology and Experimental Neurology*, **17**, 571 (1958)

276 MEYER, J. S. Localized changes in properties of the blood and effects of anticoagulant drugs in experimental cerebral infarction. *New England Journal of Medicine*, **258**, 151 (1958)

277 MEYER, J. S. and DENNY-BROWN, D. The cerebral collateral circulation. I. Factors influencing collateral blood flow. *Neurology*, **7**, 447 (1957)

278 MEYER, J. S., FANG, H. C. and DENNY-BROWN, D. Polarographic study of cerebral collateral circulation. *Archives of Neurology and Psychiatry*, **72**, 296 (1954)

279 MEYER, J. S., GOTOH, F. and TAZAKI, Y. Circulation and metabolism following experimental embolization. *Journal of Neuropathology and Experimental Neurology*, **21**, 4–24 (1962)

280 MEYER, J. S., GOTOH, F., TAZAKI, Y., HAMAGUCHI, K., ISHIKAWA, S., NOVAILHAT, F. and SYMON, L. Regional cerebral blood flow and metabolism *in vivo*. Effects of anoxia, hypoglycemia, ischemia, acidosis, alkalosis and alterations of blood P_{CO_2}. *Archives of Neurology*, **7**, 560–581 (1962)

281 MEYER, J. S., HAYMAN, L. A., YAMAMOTO, M., SAKAI, M. and NAKAJIMA, S. Local cerebral blood flow measured by CT after stable xenon inhalation. *American Journal of Neuroradiology*, **1**, 213–225 (1980)

282 MEYER, J. S., SHIMAZU, K., FUKUUCHI, T. *et al*. Impaired neurogenic cerebrovascular control and dysautoregulation after stroke. *Stroke*, **4**, 169–186 (1973)

283 MEYER, J. S., SHIMAZU, K., OKAMOTU, S. *et al*. Effects of α-adrenergic blockage on autoregulation and chemical vasomotor control of CBF in stroke. *Stroke*, **4**, 187–200 (1973)

284 MEYER, J. S., SHINOHARA, Y., KANDA, T. *et al.* Diaschisis resulting from acute unilateral cerebral infarction. *Archives of Neurology*, **23**, 241–247 (1970)

285 MEYER, J. S., STOICA, E., PASCU, I., SHIMORZU, K., and HARTMAN, A. Catecholamine concentrations in CSF and plasma of patients with cerebral infarction and hemorrhage. *Brain*, **96**, 277–288 (1973)

286 MEYER, J. S., TERAURA, T., SAKAMOTO, K. and KANDO, A. Central neurogenic control of cerebral blood flow. *Neurology*, **21**, 247–262 (1971)

287 MICHENFELDER, J. D., MESSICK, J. M. Jr. and THEYE, R. A. Simultaneous cerebral blood flow measured by direct and indirect methods. *Journal of Surgery and Research*, **8**, 475–481 (1968)

288 MICHENFELDER, J. D., MILDE, J. H. and SUNDT, T. M. Cerebral protection by barbiturate anesthesia. *Archives of Neurology*, **33**, 345–350 (1976)

289 MICHENFELDER, J. D. and SUNDT, T. M. Jr. Cerebral ATP and lactate levels in the squirrel monkey following occlusion of the middle cerebral artery. *Stroke*, **2**, 319–326 (1971)

290 MICHENFELDER, J. D. and THEYE, R. A. Cerebral protection by thiopental during hypoxia. *Anesthesiology*, **39**, 510–517 (1973)

291 MICHENFELDER, J. D. and THEYE, R. A. The influence of anesthesia and ischemia on the cerebral energy state. In *Ninth Princeton Conference: Cerebrovascular Disease*, edited by J. P. Whisnant and B. A. Sandok, 243–250. New York: Grune and Stratton (1975)

292 MILLER, J. R. and MYERS, R. E. Neurological effects of systemic circulatory arrest in the monkey. *Neurology*, **20**, 715–724 (1970)

293 MILLER, J. R. and MYERS, R. E. Neuropathology of systemic circulatory arrest in adult monkeys. *Neurology*, **22**, 888–904 (1972)

294 MONCADA, S. and VANE, J. R. Unstable metabolites of arachidonic acid and their role in haemostasis and thrombosis. *British Medical Bulletin*, **34**, 129–135 (1978)

295 MONRO, A. *Observations on the Structure and Functions of the Nervous System.* Edinburgh: W. Creech (1783)

296 MOSSO, A. *Uber den Kreislauf des Blutes im Menschlichen Gehirn.* Leipzig: Viet (1881)

297 MULLER, U., ISSELHARD, W., HINZEN, D. H. and GEPPERT, E. Electrocorticogramm und regionaler Energiestoffweschel des Kaninchengehirns in der post-ischamischen Erholung. *Pflügers Archiv fur die gesamte Physiologie*, **320**, 181–194 (1970)

298 MUNCK, O. and LASSEN, N. A. Bilateral cerebral blood flow and oxygen consumption in man by use of krypton[85]. *Circulation Research*, **5**, 163–168 (1957)

299 MURAD, F., ARNOLD, W. P., MITTAL, C. K. and BRAUGHLER, J. M. Properties and regulation of guanylate cyclase and some proposed functions for cyclic GMP. *Advances in Cyclic Nucleotide Research*, **11**, 176–204 (1979)

300 MURPHY, R. C., HAMMARSTROM, S. and SAMUELSSON, B. Leukotriene C: a slow-reacting substance from murine mastocytoma cells. *Proceedings of the National Academy of Science, USA*, **9**, 4275–4279 (1979)

301 MYERS, R. E. Lactic acid accumulation as a cause of brain edema and cerebral necrosis resulting from oxygen deprivation. In *Advances in Perinatal Neurology*, edited by R. Korobkin and G. Guilleminault, 85–114. New York: Spectrum Publishers (1979)

302 MYERS, R. E. A unitary theory of causation of anoxic and hypoxic brain pathology. In *Advances in Neurology*, Vol. 26, *Cerebral Hypoxia and its Consequences*, edited by S. Fahn, J. N. Davis and L. P. Rowland, 195–213. New York: Raven Press (1979)

303 MYERSON, A., HALLORAN, R. D. and HIRSCH, H. L. Technic for obtaining blood from the internal jugular vein and internal carotid artery. *Archives of Neurology and Psychiatry*, **17**, 807 (1927)

304 NAIDOO, D. and PRATT, O. E. The validity of histochemical observations post-mortem on phosphatases in brain tissue. *Enzymologia: Acta Biocatalytica*, **17**, 1 (1954)

305 NEELY, W. A. and YOUMANS, J. R. Anoxia of canine brain without damage. *Journal of the American Medical Association*, **183**, 1085–1087 (1963)

306 NICHOLSON, C. Measurement of extracellular ions in the brain. *Trends in Neurology*, **3**, 216–218 (1980)

307 NIGAM, V. N. Studies on glycogen synthesis in pigeon liver homogenates. Glycogen synthesis from glucose monophosphates and UDP glucose. *Biochemical Journal*, **105**, 515–519 (1967)

308 NILSSON, B., NORBERG, K., NORDSTROM, C. H. and SIESJO, B. K. Influence of hypoxia and hypercapnia on CBF in rats. In *Blood Flow and Metabolism in the Brain*, edited by M. Harper, B. Jennett, D. Miller and J. Rowan. *Proceedings of the Seventh International Symposium*, Aviemore, 17–20 June, 1975, 9.19–9.23. Edinburgh: Churchill-Livingstone

309 NILSSON, B., NORBERG, K. and SIESJO, B. K. Biochemical events in cerebral ischemia. *British Journal of Anesthesia*, **47**, 751–760 (1975)

310 NORBERG, K. and SIESJO, B. K. Cerebral metabolism in hypoxia. I. Pattern of activation of glycolysis, a re-evaluation. *Brain Research*, **86**, 31–44 (1975)

311 NORDSTROM, C. H. and REHNCRONA, S. Postischemic cerebral blood flow and oxygen utilization rate in rats anaesthetized with nitrous oxide or phenobarbital. *Acta Physiological Scandinavica*, **101**, 230–240 (1977)

312 NORDSTROM, C. H., REHNCRONA, S. and SIESJO, B. K. Restitution of cerebral energy state after complete and incomplete ischemia of 30 min. duration. *Acta Physiologica Scandinavica*, **97**, 270–272 (1976)

313 NORDSTROM, C. H., REHNCRONA, S. and SIESJO, B. K. Restitution of cerebral energy state, as well as of glycolytic metabolites, citric acid cycle intermediates and associated amino acids after 30 minutes of complete ischemia in rats anesthetized with nitrous oxide or phenobarbital. *Journal of Neurochemistry*, **30**, 479–486 (1978)

314 NORDSTROM, C. H., REHNCRONA, S. and SIESJO, B. K. Effects of phenobarbital in cerebral ischemia. Part II. Restitution of cerebral energy state, as well as of glycolytic metabolites, citric acid cycle intermediates and associated amino acids after pronounced incomplete ischemia. *Stroke*, **9**, 335–343 (1978)

315 NORDSTROM, C. H. and SIESJO, B. K. Influence of phenobarbital on changes in the metabolites of the energy reserve of the cerebral cortex following compelte ischemia. *Acta Physiologica Scandinavica*, **104**, 271–280 (1978)

316 NYLIN, G., SILVERSKIOLD, B. P., LOFSTEDT, S., REGNSTROM, O. and HEDLUND, S. Studies on cerebral blood flow in man using radioactive labelled erythrocytes. *Brain*, **83**, 293 (1960)

317 O'BRIEN, M. D., JORDAN, N. M. and WALTZ, A. G. Ischemia of edema and the blood–brain barrier: distribution of pertecles albumin, sodium and antipyrine in brains of cats after cases of the middle cerebral artery. *Archives of Neurology*, **30**, 461–465 (1974)

318 O'BRIEN, M. D., WALTZ, A. G. and JORDAN, M. Ischemic edema. *Archives of Neurology*, **30**, 461–465 (1974)

319 OBRIST, W. D., RISBERT, J. and UZZELL, B. P. A spectrum subtraction technique for estimating rCBF by xeonon-133 inhalation. *Circulation* (Suppl. 3) 90 (1974)

320 OBRIST, W. D., THOMPSON, H. K. Jr., KING, C. H. and WANG, H. S. Determination of regional cerebral blood flow by inhalation of 133-xenon. *Circulation Research*, **20**, 124–135 (1967)

321 OBRIST, W., THOMPSON, H. K. Jr., WANG, H. and CRONQVIST, S. A simplified procedure for determining fast compartment rCBF's by xeonon-133 inhalation. In *Brain and Blood Flow*, edited by R. W. Ross Russell, 11. London: Pitman Publishing Co. (1971)

322 OBRIST, W. D., THOMPSON, H. K. Jr., WANG, H. S. and WILKINSON, W. E. Regional cerebral blood flow estimated by xenon-133 inhalation. *Stroke*, **6**, 245–256 (1975)

323 OHGA, Y. and DALY, J. W. The accumulation of cyclic AMP and cyclic GMP in guinea pig brain slices. Effect of calcium ions, norepinephrine and adenosine. *Biochimica et Biophysica Acta*, **498**, 46–60 (1977)

324 OLDENDORF, W. H. and FISAKA, Y. Interference of scalp and skull with external measurement of brain isotope content. *Journal of Nuclear Medicine*, **10**, 177–187 (1969)

325 OLESEN, J. Total CO_2 lactate and pyruvate in brain biopsies taken after freezing the tissue *in situ*. *Acta Neurologica Scandinavica*, **46**, 141 (1970)

326 OLESEN, J. Contralateral focal increase of cerebral blood-flow in man during arm work. *Brain*, **94**, 635–646 (1971)

327 OLESEN, J., PAULSON, O. B. and LASSEN, N. A. Regional cerebral blood flow in man determined by the initial slope of the clearance of intra-arterially injected [133]Xe. *Stroke*, **2**, 519–540 (1971)

328 OLSSON, Y., and HOSSMAN, K. Effect of intravascular saline perfusion on the sequelae of transient cerebral ischemia. *Acta Neuropathologica*, **17**, 68 (1971)

329 OZAWAK, K., KITAMURE, O., SOHAWA, T., MURATA, T. and HONJO, I. Mitochondrial vulnerability and lipid metabolism. Brain and pancreatic mitochondria. *Journal of Biochemistry*, **66**, 361–367 (1969)

330 PARKER, C. W., FISCHMAN, C. H. and WEDNER,H. Relationship of biosynthesis of slow reacting substance to intracellular glutathione concentrations. *Proceedings of the National Academy of Science, USA*, **77**, 6870–6873 (1980)

331 PAULSON, O. B. Regional cerebral blood flow in apoplexy due to occlusion of the middle cerebral artery. *Neurology*, **20**, 63 (1970)

332 PAULSON, O. B., LASSEN, N. A. and SKINHOJ, E. Regional cerebral blood flow in apoplexy without arterial occlusion. *Neurology*, **20**, 125 (1970)

333 PAULSON, O. B., OLESEN, J. and CHRISTENSEN, M. S. Restoration of autoregulation of cerebral blood flow by hypocapnia. *Neurology*, **22**, 286–293 (1972)

334 PENFIELD, W. Intracerebral vascular nerves. *Archives of Neurology and Psychiatry*, **27**, 30 (1932)

335 PHELPS, M. E., HUANG, S. C., HOFFMAN, E. J. and KUHL, D. E. Validation of tomographic measurement of cerebral blood volume with C-11-labelled carboxyhemoglobin. *Journal of Nuclear Medicine*, **20**, 328–334 (1979)

335a PLANIOL, T., FLOYRAE, R., ITTI, R., ROUZAUD, M., DEGIOVANNI, F. and GORIES, P. La gamma-angioencephalographic dans l'insuffisance circulatoire cerebrale. *Revue Neurologique*, **125**, 56–62 (1971)

336 POPE, A. In *Biology of Neuroglia*, edited by W. F. Windel, 211–222. Springfield, Ill.: C. C. Thomas (1958)

337 PURCELL, E. M., TORREY, H. C. and POUND, R. V. Resonance absorption by nuclear magnetic movements in a solid. *Physiological Reviews*, **69**, 37–38 (1946)

338 RAFAELSEN, O. J. Action of insulin on glucose uptake of rat brain slices and isolated rat cerebellum. *Journal of Neurochemistry*, **7**, 45–51 (1961)

339 RAICHLE, M. D. Measurement of local cerebral blood flow and metabolism in man with positron emission tomography. In *Twelfth Princeton Conference, Cerebrovascular Disease*, edited by J. Moossy and O. M. Reinmuth, 47–56. New York: Raven Press (1981)

340 RAICHLE, M. E., LARSON, K. B., HIGGINS, C. S. *et al.* Three-dimensional *in vivo* mapping of brain metabolism and acid base status. *Acta Neurologica Scandinavica*, **56** (Suppl. 64), 9.12–9.13 (1977)

341 RAICHLE, M. E., LARSON, K. B., MARKHAM, J., DEPRESSEUX, J. C., GRUBB, R. L. and TER-POGOSSIAN, M. D. Measurement of regional oxygen consumption by positron emission tomography. *Journal of Cerebral Blood Flow and Metabolism*, **1** (Suppl. 1) 7–8 (1981)

342 RAICHLE, M. E., LARSON, K. B., PHELPS, M. E. *et al. In vivo* measurement of brain glucose transport and metabolism employing glucose[11]C. *American Journal of Physiology*, **228**, 1936–1948 (1975)

343 RAICHLE, M. E., MARKHAM, J., LARSON, K., GRUBB, R. L. Jr. and WELCH, M. J. Measurement of local cerebral blood flow in man with positron emission tomography. *Journal of Cerebral Blood Flow and Metabolism*, **1** (Suppl. 1) 19–20 (1981)

344 RAPELA, C. E. and GREEN, H. D. Autoregulation of canine cerebral blood flow. *Circulation Research*, **14 + 15** (Suppl. 1) 205–211 (1964)

345 RECHNCRONA, S., ROSEN, I., SODERFELDT, B. and SIESJO, B. K. The influence of lactate production in the ischemic brain on the capacity for postischemic recovery. *Brain* (in press)

346 REES, J. E., BULL, J. W., RUSSELL, R. W., DU BOULAY, C. H., MARSHALL, J. and SYMON, L. Regional cerebral blood flow in transient ischemic attacks. *Lancet*, **2**, 1210 (1970)

347 REHNCRONA, S., ABDUL-RAHMAN, A. and SIESJO, B. K. Local cerebral blood flow in the post-ischemic period. *Acta Neurologica Scandinavica*, **60** (Suppl. 72) 294–295 (1979)

348 RECHNCRONA, S., FOLBERGROVA, J., SMITH, D. S. and SIESJO, B. K. Influence of complete and pronounced incomplete cerebral ischemia and subsequent recirculation on cortical concentrations of oxidized and reduced glutathione in the rat. *Journal of Neurochemistry*, **34**, 477–486 (1980)

349 REHNCRONA, S., MELA, L. and CHANCE, B. Cerebral energy state, mitochondrial function, and redox state measurements in transient ischemia. *Federation Proceedings*, **38**, 2489–2492 (1979)

350 REHNCRONA, S., MELA, L. and SIESJO, B. K. Recovery of brain mitochondrial function in the rat after complete and incomplete cerebral ischemia. *Stroke*, **10**, 437–446 (1979)

351 REHNCRONA, S., NORDSTROM, C. H., SIESJO, B. K. and WESTERBERG, E. Adenosine in rat cerebral cortex during hypoxia and bicucuoline-induced seizures. In *Cerebral Function Metabolism and Circulation. Cerebral Blood Flow*, edited by D. H. Ingvar and N. A. Lassen, 220–227. Copenhagen: Munksgaard (1977)

352 REHNCRONA, S., ROSEN, I. and SIESJO, B. K. Excessive cellular acidosis: an important mechanism of neuronal damage in the brain? *Acta Physiologica Scandinavica*, **110**, 435–437 (1980)

353 REHNCRONA, S., SIESJO, B. K. and SMITH, D. S. Reversible ischemia of the brain: biochemical factors influencing restitution. *Acta Physiologica Scandinavica* (Suppl. 429) 135–140 (1980)

354 REHNCRONA, S., SMITH, D. S., AKESSON, B., WESTERBERG, E. and SIESJO, B. K. Peroxidative changes in brain cortical fatty acids and phospholipids, as characterized during Fe^{2+} and ascorbic acid-stimulated lipid peroxidation *in vitro*. *Journal of Neurochemistry*, **34**, 1630–1638 (1980)

355 REHNCRONA, S., WESTERBERG, E., AKESSON, B. and SIESJO, B. K. Brain cortical fatty acids and phospholipids during and following complete and severe incomplete ischemia. *Journal of Neurochemistry*, **38**, 84–93 (1982)

356 REINMUTH, O. M., SCHEINBERG, P. and BOURNE, B. Total cerebral blood flow and metabolism. *Archives of Neurology*, **12**, 49–66 (1965)

357 REIVICH, M., GREENBERG, J., ALAVI, A., HAND, P., RENLETMAN, W., ROSENQUIST, A., CHRISTMAN, D., FOWLER, J., MacGREGOR, R. and WOLF, A. Functional imaging of the brain with F-18-fluorodecy-glucose. In *Twelfth Princeton Conference, Cerebro-vascular Disease*, edited by J. Moossy and O. M. Reinmuth, 57–66. New York: Raven Press (1981)

358 REIVICH, M., JEHLE, J., SOKOLOFF, L. and KETY, S. S. Measurement of regional cerebral blood flow with antipyrine-(^{14}C) in awake cats. *Journal of Applied Physiology: Respiratory, Environmental and Exercise Physiology*, **27**, 296–300 (1969)

359 REIVICH, M., JONES, S., GINSBERG, M., SLATER, R. and GREENBERG, J. Regional hemo-dynamic and metabolic alterations in focal cerebral ischemia: studies of diaschisis. In *Oxygen Transport to Tissue*, Vol. 3, edited by A. Silver, M. Erecinska and H. I. Bicher, 617–622. New York: Plenum Press

360 REIVICH, M., KUHL, D., WOLF, A. *et al.* The ^{18}F-fluorodeoxyglucose method for the measurement of local cerebral glucose utilization in man. *Circulation Research*, **44**, 127–137 (1979)

361 REIVICH, M., SLATER, R. and SANO, N. Further studies on exponential models of cerebral clearance curves. In *Cerebral Blood Flow*, p. 8. Berlin: Springer-Verlag (1969)

362 RISBERG, J., ALI, Z. A., WILSON, E. M. *et al.* Regional cerebral blood flow by ^{133}Xe inhalation: preliminary evaluation of an initial slope index in patients with unstable flow compartments. *Stroke*, **6**, 142–198 (1975)

363 RISBERG, J. and INGVAR, D. H. Patterns of activation in the grey matter of the dominant hemisphere during memorizing and reasoning: a study of regional cerebral blood flow changes during psychological testing in a group of neuro-logically normal patients. *Brain*, **96**, 737–756 (1973)

364 ROBINS, E., SMITH, D. E., DAESCH, G. E. and PAYNE, K. E. The validation of the quantitative histochemical method for use on post-mortem material. II. The effects of fever and uraemia. *Journal of Neurochemistry*, **3,** 19–27 (1958)

365 ROCKOFF, M. A. and SHAPIRO, H. M. Barbiturates following cardiac arrest: possible benefit or Pandora's box? *Anesthesiology*, **49,** 385–387 (1978)

366 ROSENBLUM, W. I. Cerebral microcirculation: a review emphasizing the interrelationship of local blood flow and neuronal function. *Angiology*, **16,** 485–507 (1965)

367 ROSENBLUM, W. I. Neurogenic control of cerebral circulation. *Stroke*, **2,** 429–439 (1971)

368 ROTH, E. W., SCHULER, O., SULEDER, and SOBOL, B. Metabolitkonzentrationen in Herz, Gehirn, Niere und Leber des Hundes bei kontrollierter Hypotension. *Zeitschrift für die Gesamte Experimentale Medizin*, **144,** 258–272 (1967)

369 ROWAN, J. O., HAYSER, A. M., MILLER, J. D. *et al*. Relationship between volume flow and velocity in the cerebral circulation. *Journal of Neurology, Neurosurgery and Psychiatry*, **33,** 733–738 (1970)

370 ROY, C. S. and SHERRINGTON, C. S. On the regulation of the blood-supply of the brain. *Journal of Physiology (London)*, **11,** 85 (1890)

371 RUBIO, R., BERNE, R. M., BOCKMAN, E. L. and CURNISH, R. R. Relationship between adenosine concentration and oxygen supply in rat brain. *American Journal of Physiology*, **228,** 1896–1902 (1975)

372 SAFAR, P., STEZOSKE, W. and NEMOTO, E. M. Amelioration of brain damage after 12 minutes' cardiac arrest in dogs. *Archives of Neurology*, **33,** 91–95 (1976)

373 SAKURADA, O., KENNEDY, C., JEHLE, J. *et al*. Measurement of local cerebral blood flow with iodo (^{14}C) antipyrine. *American Journal of Physiology*, **234,** H59–H66 (1978)

374 SALANGA, V. D. and WALTZ, A. G. Regional cerebral blood flow during stimulation of seventh cranial nerve. *Stroke*, **4,** 213–217 (1973)

375 SALFORD, L. G., PLUM, F. and SIESJO, B. K. Graded hypoxia-oligemia in rat brain. I. Biochemical alterations and their implications. *Archives of Neurology*, **29,** 227–233 (1973)

376 SAMUELSSON, B. Prostaglandin endoperoxides and thromboxanes: role as bioregulators. In *The Neurosciences: Fourth Study program*, edited by F. O. Schmitt and F. G. Worden, 1017–1025. Cambridge, Mass.: MIT Press (1979)

377 SCHEINBERG, P. and STEAD, E. A. The cerebral blood flow in male subjects as measured by the nitrous oxide technique. Normal values for blood flow, oxygen utilization, glucose utilization and peripheral resistance, with observations on the effect of tilting and anxiety. *Journal of Clinical Investigation*, **28,** 1163–1171 (1949)

378 SCHUTZ, H., SILVERSTEIN, P. R., VAPALAHTI, M., BRUCE, D. A., MELA, L. and LANGFITT, T. W. Brain mitochondrial function after ischemia and hypoxia. *Archives of Neurology*, **29,** 408–416 (1973)

379 SCHWARTZ, J. P., MRSULJA, B. B., MRSULJA, B. J., PASSONNEAU, J. V. and KLATZO, I. Alterations of cyclic nucleotide-related enzymes and ATPase during unilateral ischemia and recirculation in gerbil cerebral cortex. *Journal of Neurochemistry*, **27,** 101–107 (1976)

380 SCHWEITZER, E. S. and BLAUSTEIN, M. P. Calcium buffering in presynaptic nerve terminals: free calcium levels measured with arsenazo III. *Biochimica et Biophysica Acta*, **600**, 912–921 (1980)

381 SEVERINGHAUS, J. W., CHIODI, H., EGER, E. I. II, *et al*. Cerebral blood flow in man at high altitude. *Circulation Research*, **20**, 272–275 (1967)

382 SHALIT, M. N. Some hemodynamic aspects of regional brain ischemia. In *Pharmakologic der lokalen Gehirndurchblutung. Messmethoden und Ergebnisse*, edited by E. Betz and R. Wullenweber. Munchen-Grafelfing: Werk-Verlag (1969)

383 SHALIT, M. N., REINMUTH, O. M., SHIMOJYO, S. and SCHEINBERG, P. Carbon dioxide and cerebral circulatory control. I. The extravascular effect. II. The intravascular effect. III. The effects of brain stem lesions. *Archives of Neurology*, **17**, 298–303, 337–341, 342–353 (1967)

384 SHANBROM, E. and LEVY, L. The role of systemic blood pressure in cerebral circulation in carotid and basilar artery thromboses: clinical implications and therapeutic implication of vasopressor agents. *American Journal of Medicine*, **23**, 197–204 (1957)

385 SHENKIN, H. A., HARMEL, M. H. and KETY, S. S. Dynamic anatomy of the cerebral circulation. *Archives of Neurology and Psychiatry*, **60**, 240–252 (1948)

386 SIEMKOWICZ, E. and HANSEN, A. J. Clinical restitution following cerebral ischemia in hypo-, normo- and hyperglycemic rats. *Acta Neurologica Scandinavica*, **58**, 1–8 (1978)

387 SIESJO, B. K. Cell damage in the brain: a speculative synthesis. *Journal of Cerebral Blood Flow and Metabolism*, **1**, 155–185 (1981)

388 SIESJO, B. K. and NILSSON, L. The influence of arterial hypoxemia upon labile phosphates and upon extracellular and intracellular lactate and pyruvate concentrations in the rat brain. *Scandinavian Journal of Clinical and Laboratory Investigation*, **27**, 83–96 (1971)

389 SIESJO, B. K. and PLUM, F. Pathophysiology of anoxic brain damage. In *Biology of Brain Dysfunction*, Vol. 1, edited by G. E. Gaull, 319–372. New York: Plenum Press (1973)

390 SIESJO, B. K. and ZWETNOW, N. N. The effect of hypovolemic hypotension on extra- and intracellular acid-base parameters and energy metabolites in the rat brain. *Acta Physiologica Scandinavica*, **79**, 114–124 (1970)

391 SIESJO, B. K. and ZWETNOW, N. N. Effects of increased cerebrospinal fluid pressure upon adenine nucleotides and upon lactate and pyruvate in the rat brain. *Acta Neurologica Scandinavica*, **46**, 187–202 (1970)

392 SILVER, D. J., ROBERTS, M., OWENS, G. and REMBISH, R. Measurement of regional cerebral blood flow: a comparison of the mass spectrographic and intra-arterial xenon 133 techniques. *Neurology*, **24**, 322–324 (1974)

393 SILVER, I. A. Measurement of pH and ionic composition of pericellular sites. *Philosophical Transactions of the Royal Society, Series B*, **271**, 261–272 (1975)

394 SILVER, I. A. pH changes in local cerebral ischemia. *Stroke*, **8**, 131 (1977)

395 SILVER, I. A. Ion fluxes in hypoxic tissues. *Microvascular Research*, **13**, 409–420 (1977)

396 SINGER, J. R. Blood flow measurements by NMR. In *Nuclear Magnetic Resonance Imaging in Medicine*, edited by L. Kaufman, L. E. Crooks and A. R. Margulis. New York/Tokyo: Igaku-Shoin Medical Publishers (1981)

396a SINGER, J. R. Blood flow rates by nuclear magnetic resonance measurements. *Science*, **130**, 1652–1653 (1959)

397 SKINHØJ, E. Bilateral depression of CBF in unilateral cerebral diseases. *Acta Neurologica Scandinavica*, **41** (Suppl. 14) 161–163 (1965)

398 SKINHØJ, E. Regulation of cerebral blood flow as a single function of the interstitial pH in the brain. *Acta Neurologica Scandinavica*, **42** (Suppl.) 604–607 (1966)

399 SKINHØJ, E., HOEDT-RASMUSSEN, K. and PAULSON, O. B. Regional cerebral blood flow and its autoregulation in patients with transient focal cerebral ischemic attacks. *Neurology*, **20**, 485 (1970)

400 SKINHØJ, E. and PAULSON, O. B. Carbon dioxide and cerebral circulatory control. *Archives of Neurology*, **20**, 249–252 (1969)

401 SLATER, R., REIVICH, M., GOLDBERG, H., BANKA, R. and GREENBERG, J. Diaschisis with cerebral infarction. *Stroke*, **8**, 684–690 (1977)

402 SMITH, A. L., HOFF, J. T., NIELSEN, S. L. and LARSON, C. P. Barbiturate protection in acute focal cerebral ischemia. *Stroke*, **5**, 1–7 (1974)

403 SMITH, D. E., ROBBINS, E., EYDT, K. M. and DAESCH, G. E. The validation of the quantitative histochemical method for use on post mortem material. I. The effect of time and temperature. *Journal of Laboratory Investigation*, **6**, 447–457 (1957)

404 SMITH, D. S., REHNCRONA, S. and SIESJO, B. K. Inhibitory effects of different barbiturates on lipid peroxidation in brain tissue *in vitro*: comparison with the effects of promethazine and chlorpromazine. *Anesthesiology*, **53**, 186–194 (1980)

405 SNYDER, J. V., NEMOTO, E. M., CARROLL, R. G. and SAFAR, P. Global ischemia in dogs: intracranial pressures, brain blood flow and metabolism. *Stroke*, **6**, 21–27 (1975)

406 SOKOLOFF, L. The action of drugs on the cerebral circulation. *Pharmacological Reviews*, **11** (1959)

407 SOKOLOFF, L. Local cerebral circulation at rest and during altered cerebral activity induced by anesthesia or visual stimulation. In *Regional Neurochemistry*, edited by S. S. Kety and J. S. Elkes. Oxford: Pergamon Press (1961)

408 SOKOLOFF, L. Localization of functional activity in the central nervous system by measurement of glucose utilization with radioactive de-oxyglucose. *Journal of Cerebral Blood Flow and Metabolism*, **1**, 7–36 (1981)

409 SPECTOR, R. G. Selective changes in dehydrogenase enzymes and pyridine nucleotides in rat brain anoxic-ischaemic encephalopathy. *British Journal of Experimental Pathology*, **44**, 312–316 (1963)

410 SRAGO, E. The effect of long chain fatty acyl CoA esters on the adenine nucleotide tranlocase and myocardial metabolism. *Life Sciences*, **22**, 1–6 (1978)

411 STARLINGER, H. and LUBERS, D. W. Polarographic measurements of the oxygen pressure performed simultaneously with optical measurements of the redox state of the respiratory chain in suspension of mitochondria under steady-state conditions. *Pflüger Archiv fur die gesamte Physiologie*, **341**, 15–22 (1973)

412 STEEN, P. A., MICHENFELDER, J. D. and MILDE, J. H. Incomplete versus complete cerebral ischemia: improved outcome with a minimal blood flow. *Annals of Neurology*, **6**, 389–398 (1979)

413 STEEN, P. A., MILDE, J. H. and MICHENFELDER, J. D. No barbiturate protection in a dog model of complete cerebral ischemia. *Annals of Neurology*, **5**, 343–349 (1979)

414 STEINER, A. L., FERRENDELLI, J. A. and KIPNIS, D. M. Radiommunoassay for cyclic nucleotides. *Journal of Biology and Chemistry*, **247**, 1121–1124 (1972)

415 STRANDGAARD, S. The lower and upper limits for autoregulation of cerebral blood flow. *Stroke*, **4**, 323 (1973)

416 STRANDGAARD, S., OLESEN, J., SKINHØJ, E. and LASSEN, N. A. Autoregulation of brain circulation in severe arterial hypertension. *British Medical Journal*, **2**, 507 (1973)

417 SUBRAMANYAM, R., ALPERT, N. M., HOOP, B. Jr. *et al.* A model for regional cerebral oxygen distribution during continuous inhalation of $^{15}O_2$, $C^{15}O$, and $C^{15}O_2$. *Journal of Nuclear Medicine*, **19**, 48–53 (1978)

418 SUNDT, T. M., GRANT, W. C. and GARCIA, J. H. Restoration of middle cerebral artery flow in experimental infarction. *Journal of Neurosurgery*, **31**, 311 (1969)

419 SUNDT, T. M. and WALTZ, A. G. Experimental cerebral infarction: retro-orbital, extradural approach for occluding the middle cerebral artery. *Mayo Clinic Proceedings*, **41**, 159 (1966)

420 SUNDT, T. M. and WALTZ, A. G. Cerebral ischemia and reactive hypermia. Studies of cortical blood flow and microcirculation before, during and after temporary occlusion of middle cerebral artery of squirrel monkeys. *Circulation Research*, **28**, 426 (1971)

421 SVEINSDOTTIR, E. Clearance curves of krypton-85 and xenon-133 considered as a sum of compartments each having a non-exponential outwash function description of a computer program for the simple case of only two compartments. *Acta Neurologica Scandinavica*, **14** (Suppl.) 69 (1965)

422 SWANSON, P. D. Acidosis and some metabolic properties of isolated cerebral tissues. *Archives of Neurology*, **20**, 653–663 (1969)

423 SYMON, L. Effects of vascular occlusion on middle cerebral arterial pressure in dogs and *Macacus rhesus*. *Journal of Physiology*, **165**, 62 (1963)

424 SYMON, L. Experimental study of cerebral arterial spasm. *3rd European Congress, Neurosurgery, Madrid*, April Excerpta Medica Foundation International Congress Series No. **139**, Excerpta Medica: Amsterdam (1967)

425 SYMON, L., BRANSTON, N. M., STRONG, A. J. Autoregulation in acute focal ischemia: an experimental study. *Stroke*, **7**, 547–554 (1976)

426 SYMON, L., CROCKARD, H. A., DORSCH, N. W. C., BRANSTON, N. M. and JUHASZ, J. Local cerebral blood flow and vascular reactivity in a chronic stable stroke in baboons. *Stroke*, **6**, 482 (1975)

427 SYMON, L., PASZTOR, E. and BRANSTON, N. M. The distribution and density of reduced cerebral blood flow following acute middle cerebral artery occlusion: an experimental study by the technique of hydrogen clearance in baboons. *Stroke*, **5**, 355–364 (1974)

428 TAMURA, A., ASANO, T., SANO, K., TSUMAGARI, T. and NAKAJIMA, A. Protection from cerebral ischemia by a new imidazole derivative (Y-9179) and pentobarbital: a comparative study in chronic middle cerebral artery occlusion in cats. *Stroke*, **10**, 126–134 (1979)

429 TAPPEL, A. L. Lipid peroxidation and fluorescent molecular damage to membranes. In *Pathobiology of Cell Membranes*, Vol. 1, edited by B. F. Trump and A. V. Arstila, 145–170. New York: Academic Press (1975)

430 TER-POGOSSIAN, M. M., EICHLING, J. O., DAVIS, D. O. and WELCH, M. J. The determination of regional cerebral blood flow by means of water labelled with radioactive oxygen-15. *Radiology*, **93**, 31–40 (1969)

431 TER-POGOSSIAN, M. M., EICHLING, J. O., DAVIS, D. O. and WELCH, M. J. The measure *in vivo* of regional cerebral oxygen utilization by means of oxyhemoglobin labelled with radioactive oxygen-15. *Journal of Clinical Investigation*, **49**, 381–391 (1970)

432 TER-POGOSSIAN, M. M., RAICHLE, M. E. and FICKE, D. C. Dynamic positron emission tomography (PET) of the brain. *Journal of Cerebral Blood Flow and Metabolism*, **1** (Suppl. 1) 1–2 (1981)

433 TEWS, J. K., CARTER, S. H., ROA, P. D. and STONE, W. E. Free amino acids and related compounds in dog brain: post-mortem and anoxic changes, effects of annonium chloride infusion, and levels during seizures induced by picrotoxin and by phenylene tetrazol. *Journal of Neurochemistry*, **10**, 641–653 (1963)

434 THEWS, G. In *Selective Vulnerability of the Brain in Hypoxaemia*, edited by J. P. Schade and W. H. McMenemey, 27–35. Philadelphia: F. A. Davis Co. (1963)

435 THOMPSON, R. K. and SMITH, G. W. Experimental occlusion of the middle cerebral artery during arterial hypotension. *Transactions of the American Neurology Association*, **76**, 203 (1951)

436 THORN, W., PFLEIDERER, G., FROWEIN, R. A. and ROSS, I. Stoffwechselvorgange im Gehirn bei akuter Anoxie, akuter Ischamie und in der Erholung. *Pflügers Archiv für die gesamte Physiologie*, **261**, 334–360 (1955)

437 THULBORN, K. R., WATERTON, J. C. and RADDA, G. K. Proton imaging for *in vivo* blood flow and oxygen consumption measurements. *Journal of Magnetic Resonance*, **45**, 188–191 (1981)

438 THURSTON, J. H. and McDOUGAL, D. B. Jr. Effect of ischemia on metabolism of the brain of the newborn mouse. *American Journal of Physiology*, **216**, 348–352 (1969)

439 TRAYSTMAN, R. J. and RAPELA, C. E. Effect of sympathetic nerve stimulation on cerebral and cephalic blood flow in dogs. *Circulation Research*, **36**, 620–630 (1975)

440 U, Go KG, WALKER, J. T. Jr., SPATZ, M. and KLATZO, I. Experimental cerebral ischemia in mongolian gerbils. III. Behavior of the blood–brain barrier. *Acta Neuropathologica*, **34**, 1–6 (1976)

441 U, Go KG, SPATZ M., WALKER, J. T. Jr. and KLATZO, I. Experimental cerebral ischemia in mongolian gerbils. I. Light microscopic observations. *Acta Neuropathologia*, **32**, 299–323 (1975)

442 VEALL, N. and MALLETT, B. L. The partition of trace amounts of xenon between human blood and brain tissues at 37°C. *Physics in Medicine and Biology*, **10**, 375–380 (1965)

443 VEALL, N. and MALLETT, B. L. Regional cerebral blood flow determination by ^{133}Xe inhalation and external recording: the effect of arterial recirculation. *Clinical Science*, **30**, 353–369 (1966)

444 VON MONAKOW, V. *Die Lokalisation im Grosshirn und der Abbau der Funktion durch Kortikale Herde*. Wiesbaden, Germany: J. F. Bergmann (1914)

445 WAHL, M. and KUCHINSKY, W. The dilatatory action of adenosine on pial arteries of cats and its inhibition by theophylline. *Pflügers Archiv fur die gesamte Physiologie*, **362**, 55–59 (1976)

446 WALTZ, A. G. Effect of blood pressure on blood flow in ischemic and in non-ischemic cerebral cortex: the phenomena of autoregulation and luxury perfusion. *Neurology*, **18,** 613–631 (1968)

447 WALTZ, A. G. Red venous blood: occurrence and significance in ischemic and non-ischemic cerebral cortex. *Journal of Neurosurgery*, **31,** 141 (1969)

448 WALTZ, A. G. Effect of $Paco_2$ on blood flow and microvasculature of ischemic and non-ischemic cerebral cortex. *Stroke*, **1,** 27–37 (1970)

449 WALTZ, A. G. and SUNDT, T. M. The microvasculature and microcirculation of the cerebral cortex after arterial occlusion. *Brain*, **90,** 681–686 (1967)

450 WALTZ, A. G., SUNDT, T. M. and OWEN, C. A. Effect of middle cerebral artery occlusion on cortical blood flow in animals. *Neurology*, **16,** 1185 (1966)

451 WELSH, F. A., DURITY, S. and LANGFITT, T. W. The appearance of regional variations in metabolism at a critical level of diffuse cerebral oligemia. *Journal of Neurochemistry*, **28,** 71–79 (1977)

452 WELSH, F. A., GINSBERG, M. D., RIEDER, W. and BUDD, W. W. Deleterious effect of glucose pretreatment on recovery from diffuse cerebral ischemia in the cat. II. Regional metabolite levels. *Stroke*, **11,** 355–363 (1980)

453 WHITTAM, R. The dependence of the respiration of brain cortex on active cation transport. *Biochemical Journal*, **82,** 205–212 (1962)

454 WILLIAMS, D. J. The innervation of the cerebral circulation in man, an histological study (M.D. Thesis). University of Manchester, Manchester, England (1935)

455 WISE, G. Vasopressor-drug therapy for complications of cerebral arteriography. *New England Journal of Medicine*, **282,** 610–612 (1970)

456 WISE, G., SUTTER, R. and BURKHOLDER, J. The treatment of brain ischemia with vasopressor drugs. *Stroke*, **3,** 135 (1972)

457 WITCOFSKI, R. L., KARSTAEDT, N. and PARTAIN, C. L. *NMR Imaging, Proceedings of an International Symposium on Nuclear Magnetic Resonance Imaging.* Bowman Gray School of Medicine of Wake Forest University. Winston-Salem, North Carolina (1982)

458 WOJTCZAK, L. Effect of long-chain fatty acids and acyl-CoA on mitochondrial permeability transport and energy coupling processes. *Journal of Bioenergetics and Biomembranes*, **8,** 293–311 (1976)

459 WOOD, J. D., WATSON, W. J. and DUCKER, A. J. Oxygen poisoning in various mammalian species and the possible role of γ-aminobutyric acid metabolism. *Journal of Neurochemistry*, **14,** 1067–1074 (1967)

460 WOOD, J. D., WATSON, W. J. and DUCKER, A. J. The effect of hypoxia on brain γ-aminobutyric acid levels. *Journal of Neurochemistry*, **15,** 603–608 (1968)

461 WURTMAN, R. J. Catecholamines. *New England Journal of Medicine*, **273,** 637–646 (1965)

462 WURTMAN, R. J., LAVYNE, M. H. and ZERVAS, N. T. Brain catecholamines in relation to cerebral blood vessels. In *Ninth Princeton Conference: Cerebral Vascular Diseases*, edited by J. P. Whisnant and B. A. Sandok, 13–26. New York: Grune and Stratton (1975)

463 WYLIE, E. J., HEIN, M. F. and ADAMS, J. E. Intracranial hemorrhage following surgical revascularization for treatment of acute strokes. *Journal of Neurosurgery*, **21,** 212 (1964)

464 YAMAGUCHI, T., REGLI, F. and WALTZ, A. G. Effect of $Paco_2$ on hyperemia and ischemia in experimental cerebral infarction. In *Brain and Blood Flow*, edited by R. W. Ross Russell. London: Pitman Publishing Co. Ltd. (1971)

465 YATSU, F. M., DIAMOND, I., GRAZIANO, C. and LINDQUIST, P. Experimental brain ischemia: protection for irreversible damage with a rapid acting barbiturate (methohexital). *Stroke*, **3**, 726–732 (1972)

466 YOSHIDA, S., INOH, S., ASANO, T., SANO, K., KUBOTA, M., SHIMAZAKI, H. and UETA, N. Effect of transient ischemia on free fatty acids and phospholipids in the gerbil brain. Lipid peroxidation as possible cause of postischemic injury. *Journal of Neurosurgery*, **53**, 323–331 (1980)

467 ZERVAS, N. T., HORI, H., NEGOLA, M., WURTMAN, R. J., LARIN, F. and LAVYNE, M. H. Reduction in brain dopamine following experimental cerebral ischemia. *Nature*, **247**, 283–284 (1974)

468 ZIERLER, K. L. Equations for measuring blood flow by external monitoring of radioisotopes. *Circulation Research*, **16**, 309–321 (1965)

469 ZIMMER, R., LANG, R. and OBERDORSTER, G. Postischemic reactive hyperemia of the isolated perfused brain of the dog. *Pflügers Archiv fur die gesamte Physiologie*, **328**, 332–343 (1971)

470 ZULCH, K. J. Neue Befunde und Deutungen aus der Gefasspathologie des Hirns und Ruckenmarks. *Zentralbl att fur Allgemeine Pathologie*, **90**, 402 (1953)

Part 2
Clinical applications

6
'Natural' history of ischemic stroke

Mark L. Dyken

The world watches as an ex-general of the armies and former president of the United States stands on the beaches of Normandy and describes vividly and lucidly his recollections of what had occurred there twenty years before. As he talks, the greatest invasion ever mounted by mankind is re-lived.

Millions of television viewers are entranced as a beautiful lady with charm and intelligence describes the thrill of becoming Miss America in 1963, the subsequent tragedy and victory over that tragedy.

In both instances, audiences are spellbound. Among the millions of viewers only a few neurologists note that as the speakers begin to tire, they occasionally block on words and develop a slight flattening of the lower side of the right face.

A grey-haired lady in a wheelchair sits in a corner staring straight ahead. The nursing home attendants and other occupants ignore her. She slumps to the right, held up by straps that keep her in place. She never moves the right arm or leg and does not seem to understand nor does she talk. On rare occasions, when loved ones visit, she will sometimes respond with explosive crying or, rarely, with laughter.

All three have had a stroke in the past. Each had weakness and difficulty with language. Two recovered almost completely and the other will require total care for the rest of her life. To these three people and to their physicians the natural history of their disease process is not important as each is atypical. What is important is what happened to them as individuals. In addition, an emphasis on natural history implies that we are willing to accept the inevitable and wait for the 'natural' results. What the patient, family and the physician want to know is how the outcome may be affected by our present knowledge and the best possible intervention.

Would it be possible to know 'natural' history if we wanted to? The answer is obviously no, as it constantly changes depending on the time, the hospital, the geographical location, the types of treatment selected and a number of other things, not all of which can be identified. Therefore, although the subject of this chapter is the 'natural' history of ischemic stroke, we will really be discussing 'unnatural' history. In addition, some comments will be made concerning cerebral embolism and transient ischemic attacks (TIAs). Attempts will be made to identify changes that are occurring and factors that are known to alter the outcome. Once these are identified, we will try to predict what an individual patient with many different characteristics might expect in general, including the odds of living through the acute illness, returning to independent activity, working again, having another attack and being alive some years later. We want to estimate from our present knowledge what will happen with the most intervention to create a better outcome.

CHANGING 'NATURAL' HISTORY

For some years up until 1975, it has been noted that death rates for heart disease and stroke have decreased in the United States, England, Wales and many other countries (*see* Chapter 2). Although many problems are associated with diagnosing stroke from death certificates[23], these changing rates appear to be real[56, 68, 73, 96, 97]. Epidemiological studies in Rochester, Minnesota, suggest that this may be at least partially due to a decline in incidence in all age groups[51, 52]. As part of ongoing monitoring in the state of Indiana, analyses of mortality have continued through 1980[34, 64, 65]. Between 1975 and 1980, dramatic differences in rate of decline were noted between heart disease and cerebrovascular disease. United States statistics were obtained from publications and from personal communication with Robert Pokras of the National Center for Health Statistics[82, 83, 103]. In addition, the Center performed some special analyses at our request. Rates were age-adjusted for the United States population for 1940 from tables supplied by the National Center for Health Statistics. These statistics from 1968 to 1978 showed trends similar to those in Indiana. Until 1975, a progressive decrease in mortality rates for both heart disease and stroke was noticed. It was presumed that favorable changes were occurring which affected the mortality for both[51]. In 1975, the mortality rates for heart disease began to level off but those for stroke decreased even faster (*Figure 6.1*). Many changes occurred during this time. The Co-operative Study of Hospital Frequency and Character of Transient Ischemic Attacks reported that in 1973 and 1974 antiplatelet aggregating agents were prescribed for 38% of all patients with TIAs[35, 36]. Another identifiable change was an increase in the performance of carotid endarterectomies in civilian non-institutionalized patients[84] (15 000 in 1971, 23 000 in 1974 and 55 000 in 1980) – personal communication with Robert Pokras at the National Center for Health Statistics. Whether or not these have any relationship to the mortality changes is pure conjecture and they were only two of many changes in our society that were occurring during this time. Regardless of this something different is happening that is affecting the 'natural' history. Despite the cause, because of these changes it is not appropriate to compare studies done before 1965 to those done in the 1970s.

Other reasons must be considered. Earlier studies showed rather remarkable differences from hospital to hospital. The mortality in two hospitals staffed by one department in one medical center may differ considerably (8% vs 43)[32]. In addition, within a single institution dramatic changes in mortality can occur[100]. Also, if one reviews the many studies of specific therapy of stroke and of associated factors such

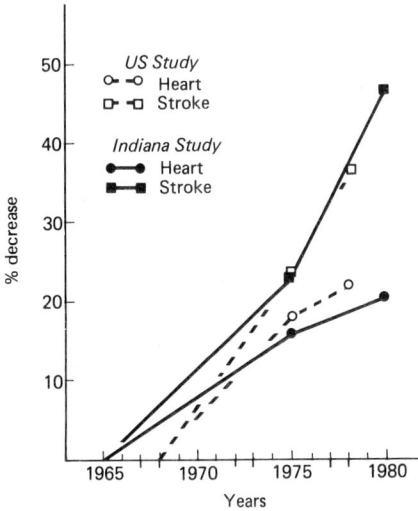

Figure 6.1 Percentage decrease in mortality by age-adjusted mortality rates. Heart disease: (US) ○ – – ○, (Indiana) ● – – ●; Stroke: (US) □ – – □, (Indiana) ■ – – ■. (From Dyken *et al.*[34], courtesy of the Publishers. In *Cerebral Vascular Diseases Thirteenth Research (Princeton) Conference*)

as hypertension and heart disease after stroke, one notes that the 'natural' history is often quite different. Unfortunately, this is frequently ignored by clinicians and the literature is teeming with uncontrolled anecdotal studies concerning a surgical or medical treatment which is concluded to be beneficial because the results were different from some other selected group of patients even though these were not randomly selected, prospectively followed and therapy double-blinded. As the 'natural' history studies are reviewed, we will be particularly attentive to the effect of specific factors as well as to general prognosis.

THE 'NATURAL' HISTORY OF ATHEROTHROMBOTIC INFARCTION

Introduction

Because of the very large number of studies reviewed, it is not possible, nor is it appropriate, to include them all in this communication. In most instances when studies are summarized, those included are selected for quality and comparability of data. In some instances published data were re-calculated so it would be in comparable form. The changing 'natural' history of infarction indicates that those studies reported most recently should be given more weight than earlier studies. Therefore, they are analyzed in much greater detail. However, if information is not available in the recent literature, the most appropriate studies are summarized regardless of when they were reported. Also, many large studies do not attempt to divide stroke into specific diagnostic categories. Although these are not given equal weight to those that specifically address cerebral infarction, large studies will frequently be analyzed for comparison. The rationale for this is that athero-thrombotic infarction is the major contributor to stroke and becomes an even larger contributor to the group of patients that survive the acute illness.

Several studies are given special attention because they are large, well-designed and recent. These include two ongoing community epidemiological studies and two studies of patient populations from multiple hospitals. The two community studies are the Framingham[55, 95], and the Rochester[51, 52, 79, 112]. The two hospital studies are the National Survey of Stroke[109] and the Regional Stroke Survey[116]. The material from the Framingham study is based on a stratified general population sample of the residents of the town of Framingham, Massachusetts, which began in 1949 with an initial cohort of 5209 men and women aged between 30 and 62 at entry. A population of 5184 men and women found to be free of stroke on their first examination was followed prospectively for 26 years for disease occurrence, including stroke and death. This study has resulted in a recent publication concerning survival and recurrence following stroke published in the spring of 1982[95] and an earlier report concerning residual disability in survivors of stroke published in November of 1975[55].

The Rochester study is based on information obtained from medical records on practically all patients of Rochester, Minnesota, who received medical care for stroke in any medical facility in the community. Pertinent publications concern the declining incidence of stroke[51], changing pattern of cerebral infarction[52] and natural history of stroke[79, 112]. The National Survey of Stroke[109] was sponsored by the National Institute of Neurological and Communicative Disorders and Stroke which was designed to provide statistics on the incidence, prevalence and economic impact of the hospitalized stroke and is primarily a chart-review study. The Regional Stroke Survey is an analysis of the demographic, diagnostic features and outcome of all stroke patients admitted to the comprehensive stroke centers of North Carolina, Oregon and Rochester, New York[116]. Two other single hospital studies were looked at closely because of special characteristics. The Mississippi study[58] was included because of the large number of black patients and the Cornell study[72] because of the identification of a number of risk factors. Because almost all studies fail to analyze for some risk factors, many prior to 1965 and some less well-designed and smaller studies are cited in an attempt to get as much information as possible to develop a logical approach to estimating the prognosis for a specific patient.

Average of all patients

The importance of this section is to establish a base upon which variations produced by risk factors can be calculated.

Acute mortality

Table 6.1 summarizes the observed, acute and long-term survival in a number of studies. For those reported in the 1970s to date, the percentage of patients who survived the acute stage ranges from 75% to 89%. For those completed before 1965 this is lower (71% to 80%). In addition, when one looks at 'all stroke', the survival in the earlier studies is much lower (38% to 63%) than in the later (70% to 81%). The differences between 'all stroke' and infarction might be due to a decrease in more lethal cerebral hemorrhage in recent years[49]. The two community epidemiological studies report 82%[52] and 85%[95] survival after acute infarction, and the hospital studies, a range from 75%[9] to 89%[58]. The Rochester Study[52] is unique as survival rates for the same community are known for two different time intervals (1945–1949 and 1970–1974). Despite the observation that as a group the early studies have a lower survival rate than the more recent ones, in Rochester this difference was only 2% over 25 years. As the Rochester survival rate from 1945 to 1949 was higher than any of the other pre-1965 studies, one possible explanation for the minimal change is that the quality of care was relatively higher in the Rochester community at an earlier time. Of course, there are many other possibilities.

If the National Stroke Survey[109] were excluded, the survival rates of the hospital studies become remarkably similar (87%, 88% and 89%) and on the average better than the community studies. The differences in reported survival rates are not surprising as the hospitals represented are totally different. Of the 124 hospitals in the National Stroke Survey, 74 had less than 500 beds with an average of 130. The three other hospital studies represented five hospitals with stroke centers and recognized experts in the diagnosis and treatment of cerebrovascular disease. Therefore, it is quite conceivable that the 12–14% difference in survival rates between these and the National Survey could have been based on expertise and quality of care. Therefore, if these studies are valid one might expect that a hospitalized patient with cerebral infarction to have approximately a 75% chance of surviving the acute period. This likelihood might increase to 87–89% if the patient were hospitalized at a center with special expertise.

Late mortality

The recent studies indicate that the outlook for surviving five years is not nearly as optimistic as that for surviving the acute stage. Although the patients who had anterior circulation infarction in Mississippi[58] were followed only three years, they are included in this analysis because of the high percentage of blacks. Only the Framingham study[95] indicates a greater than 50% chance of living five years and the National Survey of Stroke[9] estimates that only 32% will survive this long (*Table 6.1*). To illustrate these data, *Figure 6.2* has been developed as a composite from the life tables published for Framingham[95], the National Survey of Stroke[9] and for Rochester for 1970 to 1974[52]. Obviously the prognosis for surviving five years is much lower after an infarction than it is for the standard population. Despite this bleak outlook, the prognosis is now more hopeful than it was once. Earlier studies reported a 16–40% survival. The change is particularly impressive in Rochester where, from 1945–1949, only 29% survived five years. By 1970–1974 a further 16% (45%) survived. This gives further support to the basic premise that mortality and morbidity are changing.

Table 6.1 Survival after stroke

	Framingham[95]	National[9] Survey of Stroke	Regional[116] Stroke Survey	Mississippi[58]	Cornell[72]	Rochester[52]	Rochester[52]	Range of Pre-1965 Studies[2,8,13,20,31,40,61,74,76,87,89,90,91,92,107]
Entry	1949–1975	1971, 73, 76	1979	1967–1972	Reported to 1982	1970–1974	1945–1949	1940–1964
Followed to	1975	July, 1977	1982	1972–1977		1970–1974	1945–1949	1962–1965
Type study	Community	Hospital	Hospital	Hospital	Hospital	Community	Community	Community
Country	USA Northern White	USA	USA	USA Southern Black (79%)	USA New York	USA Northern White	USA Northern White	USA England Australia Denmark
Acute	30 Days	30 Days	Hospital	Hospital	30 Days	30 Days	30 Days	Hospital to 3 months
All stroke	78%	70%	81%	ND	ND	ND	ND	38–81%
Infarct	85%	75%	88%	89%	87%	82%	80%	71–77%
5-year survival	*All*	*All* / *Surviving 6 months*		*All* / *Surviving hospital*		*All*	*All*	*All†* / *Survive† acute stage*
All stroke	56%	30% 53%		39% 49%		36%	ND	15–39% 34–66%
Infarct	60%	32% 52%		40%* 47%* (Ant. Circ.)		45%	29%	16–40% 27–62%

* 3-year survival.
† 4–5-year survival.

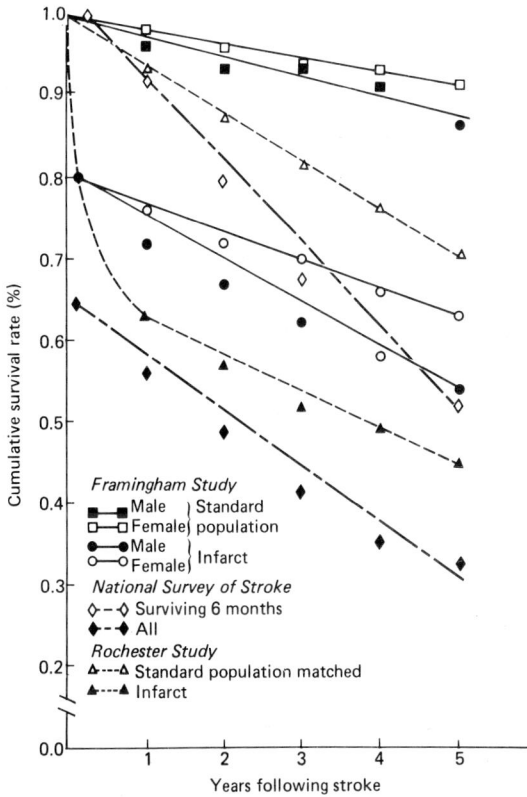

Figure 6.2 Composite of expected survival following cerebral infarct from the Framingham study[95], the Rochester study[9] and the National Survey of Stroke[52] (Modified from Garraway et al.[52], Sacco et al.[95] and Weinfeld et al.[109])

To return to our approach of considering 'natural' history from the viewpoint of the individual patient and the personal physician, we are now in a position to answer several more general questions. The question concerning the chance of surviving the acute illness has been answered in general terms in the previous section. The next question that must be considered when the patient presents with the acute illness concerns the chances for living longer. For five years the answer appears to be an insecure 30–60% survival. Fortunately, we may take each step at a time and delay the answer until survival is assured. Once the patient has survived the acute illness, the long-term prognosis improves to a better than 50% likelihood[9, 95]. To continue in this vein, from *Figure 6.2* it is apparent that the major mortality occurs during the first year and the slope of the life table lines begins to level off. Therefore, one might ask what is the possibility of long-term survival after one has survived one year? Although the danger of playing games with life tables and other investigators' statistics is recognized, the author could not resist manipulating the figures published in the Framingham and Rochester studies. In each case, the data were manipulated by considering those patients who had survived one year to be the total population and the lines were elevated so that this point was 1.0 or 100%. *Figure 6.3* was traced from *Figure 6.2* in the Framingham report[95]. The slope of the line for females who have had cerebral infarction is almost identical to that of males in the standard population and the slope for males

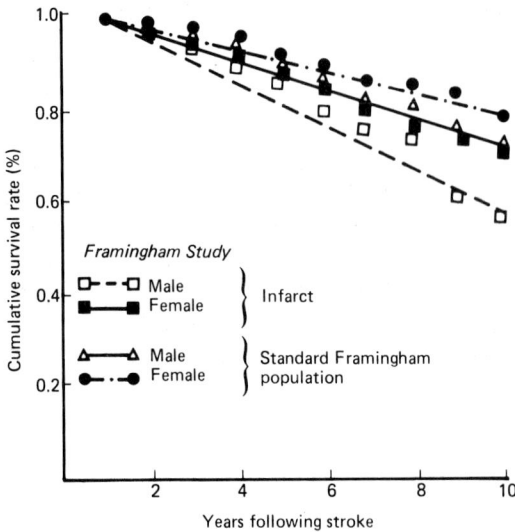

Figure 6.3 Adjustment of *Figure 6.2* of the Framingham study[95] comparing slope of cumulative survival rate for patients after atherothrombotic brain infarction who survived one year to the standard Framingham population (Modified from Sacco *et al.*[95])

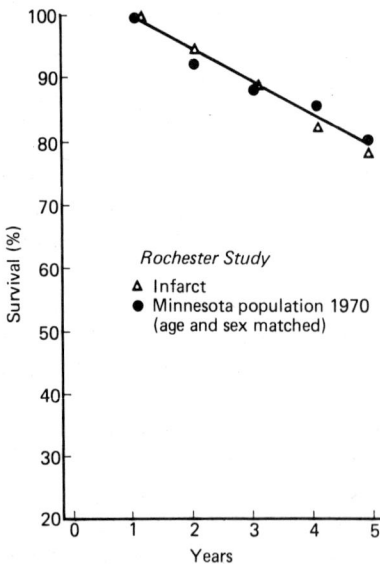

Figure 6.4 Adjustment of *Figure 3* of the Rochester study[52] comparing the probability of survival for patients after cerebral infarct who survived one year to the Minnesota population of same age and sex distribution (Modified from Garraway *et al.*[52])

who have had infarction is not much steeper. *Figure 6.4* is the result of an identical manipulation of the Rochester data[52]. In this instance the slopes of all patients who survived cerebral infarction for one year were identical to those of the age- and sex-matched Minnesota population. One can conclude from these two studies that once a patient has survived a cerebral infarction for a year that the life expectancy is not too greatly different from a standard population.

Functioning level

The ability to function independently is almost as important as survival. Unfortunately, the studies that describe the functioning status of the survivors do not always use easily comparable criteria. For example, in many of the studies reviewed, 'independence in activities of daily living' was not specifically mentioned; however, the functioning level was so described that one could reliably estimate whether the patients were independent or not. Because of these problems, for the purposes of this review, only three clear-cut types of functioning were compared (*Table 6.2*):

(1) ambulation,
(2) activities of daily living, and
(3) residence of the patient.

Three studies describe ambulation. Marquardson, in his pre-1965 study[76], reported that 74% of the survivors could walk unaided. The Rochester study[52] was similar. The Mississippi Study[58] noted that only 48% walked unaided. The exact definition of aided and unaided was not made and, in addition, these patients included a large number of high risk patients, predominantly blacks, with anterior circulation infarction. The two studies that commented on place of residence were identical (84% resided in the home)[55, 76]. Because of the advanced age of many of the survivors, work history was not as reliable as other means of evaluation. However, two studies did estimate ability to work. The Elkhart Study[31] revealed that only 23% of the patients were working or able to work, but later, after examination, it was established that 52% were capable of working. A Rochester report[79] indicated that, in addition to 29% who were normal, 36% of the patients were noted to be working or able to work six months after stroke. These estimates may be rather optimistic as a later Rochester report[52] indicated that at one year only 52% of the patients were capable of independent daily living, and one would assume that the 48% that were dependent would not be able to work.

In all studies where it was possible to estimate the ability to perform activities of daily living, 50% to 74% of the survivors were independent[1, 2, 8, 31, 52, 55, 59, 72, 88, 93] Although there appears to be a rather wide variation in study results the Elkhart data[31] indicates that this might not have been too unexpected. In this study, before the patients were physically examined, a determination was made by history of the patients' ability to perform independent daily-life activities. Later this was checked by actual examination. By history, 52% of the survivors were independent but after each had been examined by the team of neurologists, 78% were assessed as being

Table 6.2 Functioning status of survivors

	Marquard-sen[76]	Missis-sippi[58]	Rochester[52] (Garraway)	Tilberg[59]	Cornell[72]	Framing-ham[55]	Elkhart[31]	VAH[8]	Acheson & Hutchinson[1,2]	Worcester[93]	Pincock[87]
Survival	21 days to discharge	36 months	1 year	21 days	1 month to 2 years	to 25 years	>3 years	Maximum recovery	Average 4.6 years	Discharge	8 years
Type CVD	All	Infarction Ant. Circ.	Infarction	All (84% Infarct)	Infarction	All (76% Infarct)	Infarction	Infarction	All	Infarction	Infarction
Ambulation											
Unaided	74%	48%	75%	50%							
Aided	16%	41%		25%							
No	18%	13%	25%	25%							
ADL*							Hx§ Exam**				
Independent			52%	50%	74%	69%	52% 78%	73%	64%	52%	62%
Part Dependent				25%							
Dependent			48%	25%	26%	31%	46% 19%	27%	36%	48%	38%
Residence											
Home	84%					84%†					
Institution	16%					16%					

* ADL – Activities of daily living. Estimated from description in paper.
† 18% – Live alone.
§ Hx – Functional level determined by history.
** Exam – Functional level determined by actual examination.

capable of independence. This study raises the possibility that the actual ability of the patient to function may be higher than that estimated from either history or chart review. Regardless of this, one can respond a little more optimistically to the question of patients' future independence as at least 50% will function independently and this is very likely to be closer to 70–75%.

Recurrence

The earlier reviews report that the recurrence rate following atherothrombotic infarction ranges from 13–33% over a period of approximately 5 years. The analyses performed in the National Survey of Stroke[91], the Framingham[95] and Rochester[93] studies were reviewed for comparison. The Rochester studies suggest a recurrence rate of 10% in the first year, reaching 20% by the fifth year. The Framingham Study indicates an overall 5-year recurrence rate for men of 42% and women of 24%. These figures are significantly affected by risk factors which will be discussed under that section. Both the Framingham and Rochester studies were of cerebral infarction. The National Survey of Stroke does not give any 5-year recurrence estimates but it did note that in 1975–1976, of the total patients discharged with the diagnosis of cerebral infarction, 297 000 were first episode and 117 000, or 28.3% of the total, were subsequent episodes. Unfortunately, these figures were 'all stroke' and not just cerebral infarction. The response to the general question of what the chances are of having another episode over a 5-year period must be somewhat guarded. In general this does appear to be, on the average, between 13% to 33%, but these figures are significantly affected by risk factors which will be reported in the next section.

The special patient: the effect of risk factors

Introduction

In this section the 'natural' history as estimated in the previous section will be re-evaluated in the light of how it is affected by risk factors. Whenever possible, numerical predictions will be made. Unfortunately, in most instances, because of disagreement or lack of agreed-upon measurable-criteria, this cannot be done and the outcome can only be listed as favorable or unfavorable.

Acute mortality

Risk factors commonly reported in most studies are age, sex and hypertension. As measurements for these are universally agreed upon, they usually can be compared from study to study, and these are summarized in *Table 6.3*. Age appears to be the most single important factor in predicting survival, both from the acute illness and for the long-term. Unfortunately, different investigators summarize their data in

Table 6.3 The effect of age, sex and hypertension on survival after stroke

	Stroke Type	Follow-up	Survival Time to Enter	% Survive	Age				Sex			Hypertension		
					Range (years)	% Survive	Range (years)	% Survive	% Male	% Female	BP (mmHg)	% Survive	BP (mmHg)	% Survive
Acute														
Framingham[95]	Inf.	30 days	0	85	≤60	92	≥70	77						
Elkhart[31]	Inf.	Discharge	0	71					74	67				
Worcester[93]	Inf.	Discharge	0	77	6th Decade	87	9th Decade	65	82	73			NSD	
Carter[20]	Inf.	4 weeks	0	74	<60	91	≥70	63		NSD				
Mississippi[90]	Ant. Inf.	Discharge	0	89	40–59	92	≥60	88	88	90			NSD	
National Survey[9]	All	30 days	0	70	<65	74	≥85	52						
Middlesex[40]	All	30 days	0	43	<65	59	≥75	39	40	47				
Adams[3]	All	2 months	0	81	<60	94	≥75	76	83	79				
Marquardson[76]	All	21 days	0	53	50–59	66	≥80	35	50	55				
Rabkin[90]	All	30 days	0										*See text*	

Chronic

Table 6.4

Study	Onset	Follow-up	Interval	%	Age group				BP / History	
Framingham[95]	Inf.	5 years	0	60			56	64	>140/90 57	≤140/90 68
*VAH[8]	Inf.	44.5 mths.	0	57						
Worcester[93]	Inf.	5 years	Hospital	40			NSD		NSD	
Howard[60]	Inf.	to 3 years			6th Decade 62	9th Decade 14			Systolic ≥140 50	Systolic <140 70
Mississippi[58]	Ant.Inf.	3 years	Hospital	47	40–59 55	≥60 35	43	51	+ History 43	– History 55
National Survey[9]	All	5 years	6 months	53	<65 75	≥85 23				
Marshall and Shaw[77]	All	4–9 years	Hospital	41	<60 53	≥60 28				
Acheson[1]	All	4.6 years	Hospital	66			65	69	Male Diastolic ≥120 51	Male Diastolic <90 82
Middlesex[40]	All	5 years	1 month	34	<65 54	≥75 19	42	26		
Cornell[72]	Inf.	1 month to 2 years	Hospital	60	≤70 74	>70 43				

* Exclude those lost to follow-up.
NSD = No significant data.

different age groups so it is impossible to prepare a table that treats each study the same. In an attempt to draw some useful comparisons, the data were reviewed and divided into younger age groups and older age groups depending upon the method of reporting and the ability to include a significant number of patients in each group. Although most weight is given to the studies of atherothrombotic infarction, studies that included 'all stroke' were added for comparison. All those in the younger groups demonstrated an increased survival rate for the acute episode as compared to the older. The difference in survival ranges between 13% and 28% depending on the series.

No significant difference was noted between males and females for surviving the acute illness.

The Carter Study[20] and the Worcester Study[93] reported that hypertension did not have any significant effect on survival during the acute stage. Rabkin et al.[89, 90] reported that increasing systolic blood pressure before the stroke was a significant predictor of short-term 30-day mortality. The presence of concomitant heart disease unfavorably affects prognosis. In Carter's series[17] only 53% of his patients with congestive heart failure survived four weeks and 12 of 14 who had a concomitant myocardial infarction died within a week.

The clinical findings of depressed sensorium and lowering of consciousness are usually reported to be bad prognostic signs for survival from the acute illness[8, 17, 21, 59, 76, 93, 106]. As many of these studies do not separate infarction from other types of stroke, it is quite possible that patients with cerebral hemorrhage unduly affect these prognostic signs[21, 59, 76]. The National Survey of Stroke[106] determined patient fatality for acute stroke by selected signs and symptoms. Despite the problems with a chart review analysis, 1846 charts were reviewed of which 1519 were considered to be thrombotic infarction. The tables concerning the

Table 6.4 National survey of stroke[107]: patient fatality for acute thrombotic stroke, 1971, 1973, 1975 and 1976 (1519 charts reviewed)

| | Percent of total | % mortality | |
		Present	Absent
Coma	32.0%	59.8	9.5
Abnormal pupils	20.0%	71.3	56.9
Noncomatose			
Stupor	13.0%	28.8	6.6
Nuchal rigidity	3.9%	25.7	8.9
Nausea and vomiting	18.7%	15.4	8.2
Abnormal pupils	6.3%	15.8	9.1
Seizures	6.4%	15.5	9.1
Disoriented	45.6%	12.3	7.1
Vertigo	15.1%	4.4	10.3
Abnormal sensation	26.7%	5.0	11.2
Hemiplegia	61.9%	7.5	15.0
Facial paresis	46.2%	9.6	14.7

fatality rates were reviewed for this communication. A number of symptoms and signs did not appear to be significantly related to survival. In non-comatose patients with 'thrombotic' infarction, these included agitation, hemianopsia, speech difficulties, abnormal eye movements and severe headaches. Those with a high degree of relationship are summarized in *Table 6.4*. Coma was present at one time in 32%. Of these 59.8% died compared with 9.5% of those who were not comatose. When a comatose patient had abnormal pupils, 71.3% died as compared to 56.9% with normal pupils. In the non-comatose patient 45.6% were disoriented and of these, 12.3% died compared with 7.1% of those who were not. Other major risk factors for decreased survival in the non-comatose patient were nuchal rigidity, nausea and vomiting, abnormal pupils, seizures, disorientation and vertigo. The presence of abnormal sensation, hemiplegia or facial paresis seemed to affect the outcome favorably. The authors noted that this could have been an artifact as many of the hospitals did not have neurological expertise and determination of these findings may have been easier in a patient who was not disoriented or stuporous.

Previous cerebral infarction is reported to decrease the likelihood of survival[17, 29, 87]. Carter[17] reported an immediate mortality of 60% of 25 patients who had a previous history of stroke as compared to 26% of his total series of 612 patients.

Late mortality

Once the patient has survived the acute episode, the effect of risk factors upon the likelihood of long-term survival becomes clearer. As one would expect, age becomes an even more significant risk factor. This is expected, as older people who are healthy will be expected to die sooner than young people. The studies reviewed in *Table 6.3* indicate that the prognoses for up to a five year survival are much better for those who are younger than those in the 60 to 65 age bracket. The National Survey[10] reported that 53% of those patients who survived the initial six months lived for five years. This expectancy greatly increased for those under 65, increasing to a maximum of 75%, and fell precipitously for those 85 or older to 23%.

Although all studies are not in agreement, the two most recent ones of atherothrombotic infarction suggest that the outlook for survival is more favorable for women than men. The Framingham study[95] reported that 64% of women lived for five years after stroke compared to 56% of the men.

Because of its prospective nature and excellent design, the Framingham study must be given special weight in an analysis of this sort. Although an in depth review of the literature can identify factors that predict high risk, seldom are analyses reported showing the inter-relationship of these risks. Therefore, a reviewer cannot summarize or perform appropriate statistical analyses. Fortunately, the Framingham study[95] has done this type of analysis for sex, congestive heart failure (CHF) and/or coronary heart disease (CHD) and hypertension. These data are summarized in *Table 6.5*. The combination of hypertension and CHF and/or CHD in males decreases the expectancy to survive 5 years to 35%. If only hypertension is

Table 6.5 The Framingham study[96]. The percentage of patients expected to survive 5 years after cerebral infarction

	Hypertension in males		Hypertension in females	
	Yes	No	Yes	No
Congestive heart failure or coronary heart disease				
Yes	35%	ND	55%	ND
No	51%	85%	70%	70%

present, the expectancy increases to 51% and if none of the three conditions exist the likelihood of surviving increases to 85%. This is similar to the standard Framingham population for males. For females who have CHF and/or CHD and hypertension, the expectancy to survive 5 years drops from 64% to 55%. Hypertension by itself did not seem to have any great effect on females. In fact, females with hypertension but without heart disease had the same expectancy of surviving 5 years as those with none of the three (70%). These are extremely important observations as they enable one to give a fairly precise probability of survival that is much more reliable than simply listing a long list of factors. Other studies also support the unfavorable long-term effect of hypertension[1, 8, 58, 60]. This raises the enticing possibility that proper treatment of hypertension could conceivably increase the likelihood of survival. In the Framingham paper the authors noted that in Framingham, Massachusetts, women with high blood pressure are more likely to get good therapy than males. They suggest that this may account for the difference between males and females. All evidence indicates that the non-hypertensive has a much more favourable outlook for long-term survival. This subject is reviewed in Chapter 3.

The observations concerning heart disease in the Framingham study are supported by a number of other studies. The Rochester study[79, 112] reveals that when the patient died after surviving the acute illness the cause of death was heart disease nearly twice as often as was subsequent stroke. Likewise, the Veterans Administration Study[8] attributed 23% of the deaths to recurrent cerebral infarction and 42% to heart disease.

There is some indication that the prognosis is poorer for Southern Blacks than it is for Whites. Haerer and Woosley[58] reported that the survival for patients with anterior circulation infarction followed for 36 months was only 45% for Blacks as compared to 52% for Whites.

Although there is some controversy as to whether prognosis is related to the quantitative degree of atherosclerosis, some studies indicate that prognosis is good if an internal carotid artery is occluded[11, 36, 37, 41, 70, 108]. Lee *et al.*[70] followed 91 survivors of unilateral cerebral infarction. Of this group, 44 had occlusion and the rest had normal vessels or stenosis to some degree. The five-year survival rates were 52% for patients with normal angiograms, 50% for those with stenosis and 71% for those with occlusion. The ages were not significantly different.

Some early studies[80] suggested that patients with infarction in the distribution of the posterior circulation had a poorer prognosis than those in the anterior. Most of the evidence now suggests the opposite[7, 16, 29, 47, 58, 66, 72, 77]. Marshall and Shaw[77] observed that 53% of their males and 56% of their females with brain stem 'thrombosis' survived compared to 36% of the males and 53% of the females with hemispheric 'thrombosis'. David and Heyman[29] reported that only 60% of their patients with infarction in the carotid artery system were alive at the end of two years as compared to 72% of those with brain stem disease. Haerer and Woosley[58] noted that at the end of five years only 46% of those patients with anterior circulation infarcts who survived the initial hospitalization were still alive as compared to 67% of those with posterior circulation infarcts.

There is some evidence that cerebral blood flow measurements may be a predictor of outcome. Those with impaired blood flow seem to have a definite decrease in expected survival[48].

Functioning level

The age of the patient does not seem to have a clear-cut direct relationship to increased disability on follow-up. Although several studies do indicate that function is worse as the patient ages[4, 58, 76], other studies note no relationship until the patient becomes very old[42]. In fact, Carter[17] states that there is a better prognosis for functional recovery in the older patient. Glynn[53] supported this observation. It was suggested that this apparent better prognosis was related to the increased acute mortality in the older age groups and the possibility that a severe infarction would prove fatal and those who survived had milder, less severe lesions. Nevertheless, the Cornell Study[72], during a short-term follow-up from one month to two years, indicated that 74% of those under 70 years survived without disability as compared to only 43% of those older than 70 (*Table 6.3*). No clear-cut differences in functional recovery are noted between the sexes.

Several studies indicate that degree of functional recovery is related to localization of the infarction[1, 4, 76]. Although Carter was unable to demonstate a major difference[17], Acheson[1] reported 42% of patients with stroke in the right hemisphere had severe disability compared to only 31% of those when it was in the left hemisphere. Adams and Merrett[4] reported that of their patients who survived two months, 52% of those with right hemisphere insults were long-stay patients as compared to only 43% of those with left hemisphere insults.

In addition, to a better long-term prognosis for survival, patients with posterior circulation infarcts also have a better prognosis for function[1, 8, 16, 47, 66, 72, 76, 101]. The studies comparing groups of patients noted impressive differences[1, 8, 72, 76, 101]. In Acheson's series[1] only 13% of patients with posterior circulation insults were disabled versus 31% and 42% for left and right hemisphere infarctions. In Baker's series[8] only 11% of the posterior circulation patients were severely disabled as compared to 30% of those with hemispheric lesions. Similarly, the Cornell Study[72] reported that 47% of the patients with infarctions in the anterior circulation either died or failed to function, compared to only 14% of those with lesions in the posterior circulation. Other factors that are said to have an adverse effect are severity of motor weakness[8, 43, 76], long onset to admission time[4, 43], severe perceptual and cognitive loss[43, 76], homonymous hemianopsia with motor deficit[43, 72] and prior infarction[8].

Recurrence

The Framingham study[95] revealed that the risk for stroke recurrence for men over a 5-year period was 42% as compared to 24% for women. These differences were not related to age. When patients with hypertension were removed from analysis the recurrence rate fell, particularly for men, and a further reduction occurred when those with prior hypertension and CHD and/or CHF were excluded (28% for men). The impact of hypertension and cardiac co-morbidity on recurrence was much less striking for women. The 5-year recurrence rates were reduced from 24% to 19% by excluding hypertension but no additional reduction was obtained by then excluding those with cardiac co-morbidity.

THE 'NATURAL' HISTORY OF EMBOLIC INFARCTION

Introduction

The 'natural' history of embolic infarction is even more difficult to summarize than that of atherothrombotic infarction. First, in addition to the insult to the brain, the prognosis is variably affected by the types of cardiac disease that produced the source for the embolus. Therefore, an in depth understanding would require a knowledge of the 'natural' history of rheumatic heart disease, atrial fibrillation, myocardial infarction and valvular heart disease of all sorts. In addition, the criteria for diagnosing cerebral embolus varies and the condition is diagnosed much less frequently than atherothrombotic infarction. Therefore, an analysis is handicapped by small numbers and the difficulty of comparing the patients in one series to those of another.

Average of all patients

Acute mortality

The hospital series report that the acute mortality from cerebral embolism ranges from 25–30%[19, 27, 45, 110]. The Framingham study[95] reports a lower 30-day fatality rate and a rather marked difference between men and women. For men, the rate was 23% and for women only 9%. The ages were quite similar and the reasons for these differences could not be identified.

Late mortality

As pointed out by Easton and Sherman[38] in their review of the problem of cardiac embolus, very few long-term studies are available. Although it is commonly said that one-half to two-thirds of patients will die within a year, very few good prospective studies are available. A follow-up study by Daley[27] did indicate that half of the patients with rheumatic heart disease ultimately died from cerebral embolism. Carter[19] reported that one-third of his patients died immediately, one-half within one year, two-thirds by 5 years and four-fifths by 10 years. Unfortunately, this was a very small series.

Functioning level

Fisher[45] reported that 41% of survivors had severe deficit and Carter[19] stated that one-third would be so involved. Wells[110] found that nearly half of the patients were incapacitated by severe defects in motility.

Recurrence

The recurrence rate is quite high despite the etiology of the embolus. When embolus is associated with rheumatic heart disease, the recurrence rate is reported to be from 30–75%[10, 19, 28, 46, 84, 95, 99]. About one-third of the recurrences will be within 2 weeks of the initial embolism[28, 99]. Embolization associated with myocardial infarction recurs in 25% of the cases and if atrial fibrillation is excluded, most of these will occur within fourteen days[28]. Patients with atrial fibrillation without myocardial infarction are reported to have as high as 42% recurrence[28]. Of these, about half will occur within 2 weeks.

The effect of risk factors

The risk for death is reported to be closely related to age[109]. In the Framingham study[95] the mortality for males was more than two times that of females of the same age. In Carter's series[17] 12 of 16 patients with signs of congestive heart failure were dead within a week of the embolism.

The National Survey of Stroke[106] attempted to identify signs and symptoms as risk factors for hospital fatality for patients with embolic infarction. Unfortunately, the total number of cases (93) was rather small for this type of analysis. Because of these small numbers only those factors present in more than 25% will be summarized here. Embolic infarction had a total mortality of 29.3% which was close to the 25.8% for 'thrombotic' ischemic infarction. Coma at one time in the illness was present in 25%, and 59.1% of these died compared to 18.6% of the rest. Disorientation was present in 42.4% of the patients at some time but this did not make any significant difference in mortality. Speech difficulties were also common

(71.2%) but did not affect mortality. Other findings present in greater than 25% of the patients were abnormal sensation (27.1%), hemiplegia or hemiparesis (64.4%), and facial paresis (54.2%). Patients with these three findings showed the same paradoxical differences as patients with thrombotic infarction. The possible reasons were discussed in the previous section.

It has been reported[81, 110] that seizures, depression of level of consciousness, and lack of evidence of some recovery from paresis within 48 hours after onset are associated with greater disability.

Although no well-controlled studies have been performed, virtually all anecdotal reports indicate that recurrence is markedly reduced by anticoagulant therapy,[5, 6, 18, 19, 24, 25, 26, 39, 46, 48, 85, 99, 110, 114, 115]. In rheumatic heart disease the recurrence rate may be reduced from 50% to 5–25%[18, 100], and in myocardial infarction to 25% of the 'natural' rate[39].

COMMENTS ON 'NATURAL' HISTORY OF TRANSIENT ISCHEMIC ATTACKS

The place of transient ischemic attacks (TIAs) in cerebral vascular disease varies depending upon individual philosophy. As the event is always completely reversible and its major importance is as a marker for increased risk for ischemic infarction, heart disease and death, it is considered by some to be only a risk factor. As there is actual dysfunction of the nervous system due to ischemia during the attack, others consider it to be cerebral vascular disease and not just a risk factor. Kurtzke in Chapter 2 of this book discussed TIA as a risk factor. A few more comments will be made in this section to emphasize some of the difficulties of predicting outcome from the results of studies that are not prospective or randomized. Kurtzke[69] has reported that in population studies the male/female sex ratio is approximately 1.34. Yet in clinical studies this ratio increases to around 2.0[14, 30, 35, 44, 102, 117]. In addition, in prospective studies two to three times as many males as females develop stroke or die[30, 33]. When the prospective co-operative studies are analyzed by subgroup, it is noted that antiplatelet aggregating agents decrease the risk for stroke and death in men but never to a point lower than would be expected for women treated with placebo[30]. Therefore, we note that for just a single factor, female sex, TIAs occur less frequently, when they occur they are less severe, and when they are severe enough to cause the patient to enter the medical system the prognosis is better. Also, the response to therapy appears to be different. The United States Hospital Frequency of TIA[15, 22, 35, 50, 54, 57, 88, 104], in order to better assess the risk for further TIA, stroke and death, identified a large number of variables and analyzed them in great detail. Methods used were χ^2 regression and factor analysis for risk factors and, if a combination of risk factors was associated with outcome, they were multifactorially analyzed. In addition, the type of treatment was analyzed as a risk factor. History of multiple TIAs was a significant factor for further TIAs and a single TIA placed the patient at greater risk for early infarction. Older age, male sex and unreliability to take medication were found to be risk factors for cerebral infarction. Anticoagulant therapy, older age, male sex, diabetes mellitus, heart disease, abnormal electrocardiogram and poor surgical risk were factors for death. Increased mortality associated with anticoagulants was confined to the older age group. Those White patients treated with antiplatelet aggregating agents had a lower mortality than those treated otherwise; this was not true among Black patients. The type of TIA did not appear to affect the prognosis. Hypertension was not a risk factor in this study. This was assumed to be related to the very good treatment of hypertension once it was recognized at the participating institutions. The results of this study conclusively demonstrate that a large number of risk factors can affect the prognosis of patients with TIAs and, therefore, one cannot seriously consider any study of therapy that is not prospective, randomly selected, controlled and double-blind. For example, although the death rate per year was 6%, if one selected a subgroup with normal electrocardiograms this could be reduced to 2% per year. On the other hand, in groups of patients with diabetes mellitus or who are considered to be poor surgical risks, the death rate would increase to 13% a year. In fact, it was possible to combine two high risk factors and compare these to a combination of two protective factors. In this way the expected mortality would vary from 1% to 30% per year. The various combinations and permutations are endless and we stress the futility of making firm predictions of 'natural' history even if all factors could be identified.

PREDICTION OF OUTCOME FOR THE INDIVIDUAL

A large number of studies and risk factors have been analyzed in attempts to predict the unnatural history of atherothrombotic ischemic infarction, infarction secondary to cardiac embolus and for transient ischemic attacks. In this final section we will attempt to bring this together so that it can be used to help us in predicting what lies in the future for an individual patient. Ideally, one would like to establish a natural history risk profile similar to the stroke risk profile that Kannel[68] calculated from data from the Framingham study. He synthesized all risk factors into a composite risk estimate using multiple logistic equations which describe the conditional probability of a cerebral vascular event for any given set of risk variables from their known coefficients of regression on incidence and constants for the intercept. Unfortunately, even for the Framingham study the numbers were quite small. In the Hospital Frequency Study of Transient Ischemic Attack[22] we performed similar analyses. Even with a total of 954 analyzable patients, the differences in treatment, the large number of potential risk factors, the small number of patients with such factors and, in some instances, lack of information resulted in most of the groups being too small for meaningful analysis. Therefore, potentially potent factors or a combination of factors were not mathematically significant for an adverse event. For a review of natural history the problems become even more overwhelming. Different studies report their data in different ways, they use different measurements, and many have relatively small numbers. Regardless, some fairly reliable generalizations can be made. Unfortunately, they can only be rough estimates and because known and unknown risk factors vary so widely they cannot and must not be used as a basis for evaluating treatment modalities.

Tables 6.6 through to *6.9* are summaries of the material presented in this chapter and were prepared so that one could quickly obtain an estimate of what might be expected for a specific patient. These must be used with caution, except for hypertension and heart disease in the Framingham study, as the inter-relationship of factors has not been reliably determined. Although one can suggest clinically that it appears that the combination of certain factors may have an additive affect, we do not have any good analyses of data to support these impressions. Nevertheless, the tables can be used to obtain a rough approximation of what might be expected on the average and how certain factors might alter this expectancy.

When a patient presents with an ischemic vascular event, the first step is to determine whether this is due to an atherothrombotic infarction, an infarction from a cardiac source embolus or a transient ischemic attack. Once the diagnosis has been made, then the tables can be of some use. As an example, I will use an actual patient who presented at our institution.

A 59-year-old man presented with a gradual onset of right-sided weakness which came on during a period of one hour. History and examination revealed no other risk factors except for mild hypertension with systolic blood pressures ranging in the 150's and the diastolics in the low 90's. A diagnosis of an atherothrombotic infarction was made. The patient was quite fearful that he was going to die and

Table 6.6 Prediction of chances for survival from acute ischemic insult (% survival)

Atherothrombotic infarction (75–89%)
(1) Age in years
       (a) <60–65 (around 90%)
       (b) >70–75 (in 60s to 70s)

(2) National Survey of Stroke[106] (75%)
       (a) Coma (40%)
              (i) Pupils: Abnormal (29%) Normal (43%)
       (b) No coma (90%)

(i) Stupor	Yes (71%)	No (93%)
(ii) Nausea and vomiting	Yes (85%)	No (92%)
(iii) Abnormal pupils	Yes (84%)	No (91%)
(iv) Seizures	Yes (84%)	No (91%)
(v) Disoriented	Yes (88%)	No (93%)

(3) Other factors that decrease survival
       (a) Previous stroke[17]
       (b) Heart disease[17]

Infarction from cardiac source embolus (67–84%)
(1) Adverse factors
       (a) Sex[95]: Male (77%) Female (91%)
       (b) Congestive heart failure[21]
       (c) Coma[106]
              (i) Yes (41%)
              (ii) No (81%)

Table 6.7 Prediction of long-term survival following survival of acute stage (% survival)

Atherothrombotic infarction (45–60% for 5 years)
(1) Age in years
    (a) < 60–65 (53–75%)
    (b) > 75–80 (19–23%)

(2) Sex[95] (60%)
    (a) Male (56%)
        (i)   Hypertension alone (51%)
        (ii) Hypertension plus heart disease: Both (35%) Neither (85%)
    (b) Female (64%)
        (i)   Hypertension alone (70%)
        (ii) Hypertension plus heart disease: Both (55%) Neither (70%)

(3) Adverse factors
    (a) Hypertension
    (b) Heart disease
    (c) Black race
    (d) Severity of motor deficit
    (e) Right hemisphere as compared to left
    (f) Anterior circulation as compared to posterior
    (g) Impaired cerebral blood flow

(4) Favorable factors
    (a) Posterior circulation compared to anterior
    (b) Left hemisphere infarction compared to right
    (c) Occlusion of an internal carotid artery

Infarction from cardiac source embolus[19, 27] (around 50% in one year)

Table 6.8 Prediction of functioning status of survivors (% independent in activities of daily living)

Atherothrombotic infarction (50–74%)
(1) Unfavorable factors for functioning
    (a) Age in years[72]
        (i)   ≤ 70 (74%)
        (ii) ≥ 70 (43%)
    (b) Right hemisphere[1, 3, 76] compared to left
    (c) Anterior compared to posterior circulation infarction
    (d) Severity of motor weakness
    (e) Long onset to admission time
    (f) Severe perceptual and cognitive losses
    (g) Homonymous hemianopsia with motor deficit
    (h) Prior infarction

Infarction from cardiac source embolus[110]
(1) Adverse factors
    (a) Seizures
    (b) Depression of level of consciousness
    (c) Lack of evidence of some recovery for paresis within 48 hours

Table 6.9 Prediction of recurrence in survivors (% recurrence)

Atherothrombotic infarction (13–33% in 5 years)
(1) Factors associated with increased recurrence
    (a) Male sex[95] (42%) vs females (24%)
    (b) Hypertension[95]
        (i) Males more affected than females
(2) Factors associated with decreased recurrence
    (a) No hypertension or heart disease[95]
        (i) Males (42% to 28%)
        (ii) Females (24% to 19%)

Infarction from cardiac source embolus
(1) Rheumatic heart disease (30% to 35%)
    (a) Anticoagulant therapy reduces to 5–25%
(2) Myocardial infarction (25%)
    (a) Anticoagulant therapy reduces fourfold
(3) Atrial fibrillation (42%)

---

asked for reassurance. As summarized in *Table 6.6*, one notes that acute survival varies from 75–89%, but we know from previous analyses on our unit that 91% of our patients have survived. The patient is less than 60 years of age, which is a most favorable prognostic sign. He is alert, without stupor, nausea, vomiting, abnormal pupils, seizures or disorientation. He has had no previous stroke or heart disease. Each of these are favorable; therefore, we can assure the patient that the odds are overwhelming that he will survive this illness. Once reassured, the patient needs to know what the probabilities are of functioning again. From *Table 6.8*, one could predict that the patient's chances are much better than 50% to return to being independent in activities of daily living. In our hospital our previous analyses indicate that over 80% of our patients return to activities of daily living. Therefore, this portion of the table was not of great value to us, but the rest was still of value to help predict whether this patient would have a better or less than average chance of functioning again. As he had only one of the unfavorable factors, we can tell him that his chances of returning to independent activities are extremely good and better than our established average. Our patient did recover to the point where he left the hospital walking with a mild hemiparetic gait and was able to work as a salesman. The questions that he asked at the time of discharge concerned the likelihood of having another stroke in the future and also for long-term survival. From *Table 6.7* he was told that by surviving the acute insult, an average of 45% to 60% of all patients would survive for five years. Our patient is less than 60 which would raise this likelihood to 75%, but he is a male with hypertension which would decrease the likelihood to 51%. As he has few other adverse factors we would probably conclude that he has a much better probability than 51%, particularly as his risk factor is treatable and there is some evidence that good control of the hypertension might increase the probability of surviving to that of a patient with neither hypertension or heart disease, or 85%, which is not significantly different from the standard population.

To estimate the likelihood of a second stroke within five years, *Table 6.9* indicated that on average 13–33% of patients would have a second stroke, but that this patient's sex would increase this risk to 42% and that his hypertension would also unfavorably affect the prognosis. The possibility that good control of hypertension might reduce the risk to that of patients without hypertension is considered. If this were true, this would decrease his risk from greater than 42% to 28%.

SUMMARY

Data has been presented concerning the expected outcome after an ischemic stroke has occurred and how some risk factors affect these expectations. Possibly, of more importance is the identification of the seriousness of potentially treatable risk factors such as hypertension and heart disease. Although the benefit of treatment of hypertension and heart disease after an infarction has not been conclusively determined, in general the evidence suggests that it is quite likely that it is beneficial[12, 62, 63, 67, 71, 96, 104, 105, 111, 113]. Certainly, significant heart disease and hypertension are very potent unfavorable risk factors which might be significantly reduced by adequate therapy[71].

References

1 ACHESON, J. Factors affecting the natural history of 'focal cerebral vascular disease'. *Quarterly Journal of Medicine*, **157**, 25–46 (1971)

2 ACHESON, J. and HUTCHINSON, E. C. The natural history of 'focal cerebral vascular disease'. *Quarterly Journal of Medicine*, **157**, 15–23 (1971)

3 ADAMS, G. F. Prospects for patients with strokes, with special reference to the hypertensive hemiplegic. *British Medical Journal*, **2**, 253–259 (1965)

4 ADAMS, G. F. and MERRETT, J. D. Prognosis and survival in the aftermath of hemiplegia. *British Medical Journal*, **1**, 309–314 (1961)

5 ADAMS, G. F., MERRETT, J. D., HUTCHINSON, W. M. and POLLOCK, A. M. Cerebral embolism and mitral stenosis: survival with and without anticoagulants. *Journal of Neurology, Neurosurgery and Psychiatry*, **37**, 378–383 (1974)

6 ASKEY, J. M. and CHERRY, C. B. Thromboembolism associated with auricular fibrillation. Continuous anticoagulation therapy. *Journal of the American Medical Association*, **144**, 97–100 (1950)

7 ASPLUND, K., WESTER, P. O., FODSTAD, H. and LILIEQUIST, B. Long-term survival after vertebral/basilar occlusion. *Stroke*, **11**, 304 (1980)

8 BAKER, R. N., SCHWARTZ, W. S. and RAMSEYER, J. C. Prognosis among survivors of ischemic stroke. *Neurology*, **18**, 933–941 (1968)

9 BAUM, H. M. and ROBINS, M. Survival and prevalence. In national survey of stroke. *Stroke*, **12** (Suppl. 1), I-59–I-68 (1981)

10 BELCHER, J. R. and SOMERVILLE, W. Systemic embolism and left auricular thrombosis in relation to mitral valvotomy. *British Medical Journal*, **2**, 1000–1003 (1955)

11 BOGOUSSLAVSKY, J., REGLI, F., HUNGERBUHLER, J. and CHRZANOWSKI, R. Transient ischemic attacks and external carotid artery: a retrospective study of 23 patients with an occlusion of the internal carotid artery. *Stroke*, **12**, 627–630 (1981)

12 BRECKENRIDGE, A., DOLLERY, C. T. and PARRY, E. H. O. Prognosis of treated hypertension: changes in life expectancy and causes of death between 1952 and 1967. *Quarterly Journal of Medicine*, **39**, 411–429 (1970)

13 BREWIS, M., POSKANZER, D. C., ROLLAND, C. and MILLER, H. Neurological disease in an English city. *Acta Neurologica Scandinavica*, **42** (Suppl. 24) 1–89 (1966)

14 CANADIAN CO-OPERATIVE STUDY GROUP. Randomized trial of aspirin and sulfinpyrazone in threatened stroke. *New England Journal of Medicine*, **299**, 53–59 (1978)

15 CALANCHINI, P. R., SWANSON, P. D., GOTSHALL, R. A., HAERER, A. F., POSKANZER, D. C., PRICE, T. R., CONNEALLY, P. M., DYKEN, M. L. and FUTTY, D. E. Co-operative study of hospital frequency and character of transient ischemic attacks. IV. The reliability of diagnosis. *Journal of the American Medical Association*, **238**, 2029–2033 (1977)

16 CAPLAN, L. R. Occlusion of the vertebral or basilar artery. Follow-up analysis of some patients with benign outcome. *Stroke*, **10**, 277–282 (1979)

17 CARTER, A. B. *Cerebral Infarction* New York, Macmillan Company (1964)

18 CARTER, A. B. The immediate treatment of cerebral embolism. *Quarterly Journal of Medicine*, **26**, 335–348 (1957)

19 CARTER, A. B. Prognosis of cerebral embolism. *Lancet*, **2**, 514–519 (1965)

20 CARTER, A. B. Strokes. *Proceedings of the Royal Society of Medicine*, **56**, 483–486 (1963)

21 CHRISTIE, D. Stroke in Melbourne, Australia: an epidemiological study. *Stroke*, **12**, 467–469 (1981)

22 CONNEALLY, P. M., DYKEN, M. L., FUTTY, D. E., POSKANZER, D. C., CALANCHINI, P. R., SWANSON, P. D., PRICE, T. R., HAERER, A. F. and GOTSHALL, R. A. Co-operative study of hospital frequency and character of transient ischemic attacks. VIII. Risk factors. *Journal of the American Medical Association*, **240**, 742–746 (1978)

23 CORWIN, L. I., WOLF, P. A., KANNEL, W. B. and McNAMARA, P. M. Accuracy of death certificate assessment of stroke: the Framingham study. *Stroke*, **13**, 125 (1982)

24 COSGRIFF, S. W. Chronic anticoagulant therapy in recurrent embolism of cardiac origin. *Annals of Internal Medicine*, **38**, 278–287 (1953)

25 COSGRIFF, S. W. Prophylaxis of recurrent embolism of intracardiac origin. Protracted anticoagulant therapy on an ambulatory basis. *Journal of the American Medical Association*, **143**, 870–872 (1950)

26 COULSHED, N., EPSTEIN, E. J., McKENDRICK, C. S., GALLOWAY, R. W. and WALKER, E. Systemic embolism in mitral valve disease. *British Heart Journal*, **32**, 26–34 (1970)

27 DALEY, R., MATTINGLY, T. W., HOLT, C. L., BLAND, E. F. and WHITE, P. Systemic arterial embolism in rheumatic heart disease. *American Heart Journal*, **42**, 566–581 (1951)

28 DARLING, R. C., AUSTEN, W. G. and LINTON, R. R. Arterial embolism. *Surgery, Gynecology and Obstetrics*, **124**, 106–114 (1967)

29 DAVID, N. J. and HEYMAN, A. Factors influencing the prognosis of cerebral thrombosis and infarction due to atherosclerosis. *Journal of Chronic Disease*, **11**, 394–404 (1960)

30 DYKEN, M. L. Antiplatelet aggregating agents in transient ischemic attacks and the relationship of risk factors. *Proceedings of the V Colfarit Symposium on Acetylsalicylic Acid in Cerebral Ischemia and Coronary Heart Disease*, November 13–15. Mainz, Germany (1980)

31 DYKEN, M. L. Precipitating factors, prognosis, and demography of cerebrovascular disease in an Indiana community: a review of all patients hospitalized from 1963 to 1965 with neurological examination of survivors. *Stroke*, **1,** 261–269 (1970)

32 DYKEN, M. L. The stroke center. In *Stroke: Diagnosis and Management, Current Procedures and Equipment*, edited by W. S. Fields and John J. Moossy, pp. 151–163. St. Louis, Warren H. Green, Inc. (1973)

33 DYKEN, M. L. Transient ischemic attacks and stroke: aspirin trials. In *Thrombosis and Atherosclerosis*, edited by Nils Bang, John Glover, Robert Holden and Douglas A. Triplett, pp. 393–402. Chicago–London, Year Book Medical Publishers Inc. (1982)

34 DYKEN, M. L. and CALHOUN, R. A. Changes in stroke mortality that have an effect on evaluating and predicting outcome for therapeutic studies. In *Cerebral Vascular Diseases, Thirteenth Research (Princeton) Conference*, edited by M. Reivich. New York, Raven Press (in press)

35 DYKEN, M. L., CONNEALLY, P. M., HAERER, A. F., GOTSHALL, R. N., CALANCHINI, P. R., POSKANZER, D. C., PRICE, T. R. and SWANSON, P. D. Co-operative study of hospital frequency and character of transient ischemic attacks. I. Background organization and clinical survey. *Journal of the American Medical Association*, **237,** 882–886 (1977)

36 DYKEN, M. L., DOEPKER, J. F., KIOVSKY, R. and CAMPBELL, R. L. Asymptomatic occlusion of an internal carotid artery in a hospital population determined by directional doppler ophthalmosonometry. *Stroke*, **5,** 714–718 (1974)

37 DYKEN, M. L., KLATTE, E., KOLAR, O. J. and SPURGEON, C. Complete occlusion of common or internal carotid arteries. Clinical significance. *Archives of Neurology*, **30,** 343–346 (1974)

38 EASTON, J. D. and SHERMAN, D. G. Management of cerebral embolism of cardiac origin. *Stroke*, **11,** 433–442 (1980)

39 EBERT, R. V. Anticoagulants in acute myocardial infarction. Results of a clinical trial. *Journal of the American Medical Association,* **225,** 724–729 (1973)

40 EISENBERG, H., MORRISON, J. T., SULLIVAN, P. and FOOTE, F. M. Cerebrovascular accidents. Incidence and survival rates in a defined population, Middlesex County, Connecticut. *Journal of the American Medical Association*, **189,** 883–888 (1964)

41 FARIS, A. A., POSER, C. M., WILMORE, D. W. and AGNEW, C. H. Radiologic visualization of neck vessels in healthy men. *Neurology*, **13,** 386–396 (1963)

42 FEIGENSON, J. S., McCARTHY, M. L., GREENBERG, S. D. and FEIGENSON, W. D. Factors influencing outcome and length of stay in the stroke rehabilitation unit. Part II. Comparison of 318 screened and 248 unscreened patients. *Stroke*, **8,** 657–662 (1977)

43 FEIGENSON, J. S., McDOWELL, F. H., MEESE, P., McCARTHY, M. L. and GREENBERG, S. D. Factors influencing outcome and length of stay in the stroke rehabilitation unit. Part I. Analysis of 248 unscreened patients – medical and functional prognostic indicators. *Stroke*, **8,** 651–656 (1977)

44 FIELDS, W. S., LEMAK, N. A., FRANKOWSKI, R. F. and HARDY, R. J. Controlled trial of aspirin in cerebral ischemia. *Stroke*, **8**, 301–316 (1977)

45 FISHER, C. M. Reducing risks of cerebral embolism. *Geriatrics*, **34**, 59–66 (1979)

46 FLEMING, H. A. and BAILEY, S. M. Mitral valve disease, systemic embolism and anticoagulants. *Post Graduate Medical Journal*, **47**, 599–604 (1971)

47 FOGELHOLM, R. and AHO, K. Characteristics and survival of patients with brain stem infarction. *Stroke*, **6**, 328–333 (1975)

48 FUJISHIMA, M., NISHIMARU, K. and OMAE, T. Long-term prognosis for cerebral infarction in relation to brain circulation – a seven year follow-up study. *Stroke*, **8**, 680–683 (1977)

49 FURLAN, A. J., WHISNANT, J. P. and ELVEBACK, L. R. The decreasing incidence of primary intracerebral hemorrhage: a population study. *Annals of Neurology*, **5**, 367–373 (1979)

50 FUTTY, D. E., CONNEALLY, P. M., DYKEN, M. L., PRICE, T. R., HAERER, A. F., POSKANZER, D. C., SWANSON, P. D., CALANCHINI, P. R. and GOTSHALL, R. A. Co-operative study of hospital frequency and character of transient ischemic attacks. V. Symptom analysis. *Journal of the American Medical Association*, **238**, 2386–2390 (1977)

51 GARRAWAY, W. M., WHISNANT, J. P., FURLAN, A. J., PHILLIPS, L. H., KURLAND, L. T. and O'FALLON, W. M. The declining incidence of stroke. *New England Journal of Medicine*, **300**, 449–452 (1979)

52 GARRAWAY, W. M., WHISNANT, J. P., KURLAND, L. T. and O'FALLON, W. M. Changing pattern of cerebral infarction: 1945–1974. *Stroke*, **10**, 657–663 (1979)

53 GLYNN, A. A. Vascular diseases of the nervous system. *British Medical Journal*, **1** (Suppl.) 1216–1219 (1978)

54 GOTSHALL, R. A., PRICE, T. R., HAERER, A. F., SWANSON, P. D., CALANCHINI, P. R., CONNE-ALLY, P. M., DYKEN, M. L., FUTTY, D. E. and POSKANZER, D. C. Co-operative study of hospital frequency and character of transient ischemic attacks. VII. Initial diagnostic evaluation. *Journal of the American Medical Association*, **239**, 2001–2003 (1978)

55 GRESHAM, G. E., FITZPATRICK, T. E., WOLF, P. A., McNAMARA, P. M., KANNEL, W. B. and DAWBER, T. R. Residual disability in survivors of stroke – the Framingham study. *New England Journal of Medicine*, **293**, 954–956 (1975)

56 HABERMAN, S., CAPILDEO, R. and ROSE, F. C. The changing mortality of cerebro-vascular disease. *Quarterly Journal of Medicine*, **39**, 71–88 (1978)

57 HAERER, A. F., GOTSHALL, R. A., CONNEALLY, P. M., DYKEN, M. L., POSKANZER, D. C., PRICE, T. R., SWANSON, P. D. and CALANCHINI, P. R. Co-operative study of hospital frequency and character of transient ischemic attacks. III. Variations in treatment. *Journal of the American Medical Association*, **238**, 142–146 (1977)

58 HAERER, A. F. and WOOSLEY, P. C. Prognosis and quality of survival in a hospitalized stroke population from the South. *Stroke*, **6**, 543–548 (1975)

59 HERMAN, B., SCHULTE, B. P. M., VANLUIJK, J. H., LEYTEN, A. C. M. and FRENKEN, C. W. G. M. Epidemiology of stroke in Tilburg, The Netherlands. The population-based stroke incidence register. I. Introduction and preliminary results. *Stroke*, **11**, 162–165 (1980)

60 HOWARD, F. A., COHEN, P., HICKLER, R. B., LOCKE, S., NEWCOMB, T. and TYLER, H. R. Survival following stroke. *Journal of the American Medical Association*, **183**, 921–925 (1963)

61 HUTCHINSON, E. C. and ACHESON, E. J. Natural history of stroke. In *Stroke: Natural History, Pathology and Surgical Treatment*, pp. 138–153. London, Philadelphia, Toronto, W. B. Saunders Company, Ltd. (1975)

62 HYPERTENSION DETECTION AND FOLLOW-UP PROGRAM CO-OPERATIVE GROUP. Five-year findings of the hypertension detection and follow-up program. I. Reduction in mortality of persons with high blood pressure, including mild hypertension. *Journal of the American Medical Association*, **242**, 2562–2571 (1979)

63 HYPERTENSION-STROKE CO-OPERATIVE STUDY GROUP. Effect of antihypertensive treatment on stroke recurrence. *Journal of the American Medical Association*, **229**, 409–418 (1974)

64 INDIANA STATE BOARD OF HEALTH. Indiana population projections prepared by Division of Research/School of Business/Indiana University, Indianapolis, Indiana (1965–1980)

65 INDIANA STATE BOARD OF HEALTH. Indiana vital statistics, yearly summaries. Indianapolis, Indiana (1965–1980)

66 KANAAN, A. and DYKEN, M. Prognosis vertebral/basilar distribution infarction. Indiana University Cerebral Vascular Disease Unit, unpublished data (1973)

67 KANNEL, W. B. Meaning of the downward trend in cardiovascular mortality. *Journal of the American Medical Association*, **247**, 877–880 (1982)

68 KANNEL, W. D. Epidemiology of cerebral vascular disease. In *Cerebral Arterial Disease*, edited by R. W. R. Russell, pp. 1–23. Edinburgh, Churchill-Livingston (1976)

69 KURTZKE, J. F. Epidemiology of cerebrovascular disease. In *Cerebrovascular Survey Report* for Joint Council Subcommittee on Cerebrovascular Disease, National Institute of Neurological and Communicative Disorders and Stroke and National Heart and Lung Institute, pp. 135–176, edited by R. G. Siekert. Bethesda, Maryland, National Institutes of Health (1980)

70 LEE, M. C., LOWENSON, R. B., KLASSEN, A. C., RESCH, J. A. and GOLD, L. H. Effects of clinical severity in angiographic findings on long-term survivorship in unilateral cerebral infarction patients: a prospective study. *Stroke*, **9**, 105 (1978)

71 LEONBERG, S. C. and ELLIOTT, F. A. Prevention of recurrent stroke. *Stroke*, **12**, 731–735 (1981)

72 LEVY, D. E., CARONNA, J. J., LAPINSKI, R. H., SCHERER, P. D., PULSINELLI, W. A. and PLUM, F. Predicting recovery from ischemic stroke (abstract). *Stroke*, **13**, 114 (1982)

73 LEVY, R. I. Declining mortality in coronary heart disease. *Arteriosclerosis*, **1**, 312–325 (1981)

74 MARQUARDSEN, J. The natural history and prognosis of cerebrovascular disease. In *Cerebral Arterial Disease*, edited by R. W. Ross Russell, pp. 24–29. New York, Churchill-Livingstone (1976)

75 MARQUARDSEN, J. The natural history of acute cerebrovascular disease. A retrospective study of 769 patients. *Acta Neurologica Scandinavica*, **45** (Suppl.) 1–198 (1969)

76 MARQUARDSEN, J. *The Natural History of Acute Cerebrovascular Disease* (a retrospective study of 769 patients), pp. 1–192. Copenhagen, Munksgaard (1969)

77 MARSHALL, J. and SHAW, D. A. The natural history of cerebrovascular disease. *British Medical Journal*, **1**, 1614–1617 (1959)

79 MATSUMOTO, N., WHISNANT, J. P., KURLAND, L. T. and OKAZAKI, H. Natural history of stroke in Rochester, Minnesota, 1955 through 1969: an extension of a previous study, 1945 through 1954. *Stroke*, **4**, 20–29 (1973)

80 McDOWELL, F. H., POTES, J. and GROCH, S. The natural history of internal carotid and vertebral-basilar artery occlusion. *Neurology*, **11**, 153–157 (1961)

81 McDOWELL, F. H. Cerebral embolism. In *Handbook of Clinical Neurology, Vascular Diseases of the Nervous System*, Part I, edited by P. J. Vinken and G. W. Bruyn, pp. 386–414. Amsterdam, North-Holland Publishing Company (1972)

82 NATIONAL CENTER FOR HEALTH STATISTICS. Monthly vital statistics, advance report, final mortality statistics, DHHS, Publication No. (PHS) 80-1120, Volume 29, No. 6, Supplement (2), September 17, 1980. Hyattsville, Maryland (1978)

83 NATIONAL CENTER FOR HEALTH STATISTICS. Vital statistics of the United States, Mortality, Parts A and B, published by US Department of Health, Education and Welfare, Public Health Services, Health Resources Administration. Hyattsville, Maryland (1965–1977)

84 OLESON, K. H., HANSEN, J. F. and LAURIDSEN, P. Systemic arterial embolism after mitral valvulotomy. *Scandinavian Journal of Thoracic and Cardiovascular Surgery*, **6**, 52–56 (1972)

85 OWREN, P. A. The results of anticoagulant therapy in Norway. *Archives of Internal Medicine*, **111**, 158–164 (1963)

86 PARRISH, H. M., PAYNE, G. H., ALLEN, W. C., GOLDNER, J. C. and SAUER, H. I. Mid-Missouri stroke survey: a preliminary report. *Missouri Medicine*, **63**, 816–821 (1966)

87 PINCOCK, J. G. The natural history of cerebral thrombosis. *Annals of Internal Medicine*, **46**, 925–930 (1957)

88 PRICE, T. R., GOTSHALL, R. A., POSKANZER, D. C., HAERER, A. F., SWANSON, P. D., CALANCHINI, P. R., CONNEALLY, P. M., DYKEN, M. L. and FUTTY, D. E. Co-operative study of hospital frequency and character of transient ischemic attacks. VI. Patients examined during an attack. *Journal of the American Medical Association*, **238**, 2512–2515 (1977)

89 RABKIN, S. W., MATHEWSON, F. A. L. and TATE, R. B. Long-term changes in blood pressure and risk of cerebrovascular disease. *Stroke*, **9**, 319–327 (1978)

90 RABKIN, S. W., MATHEWSON, F. A. L. and TATE, R. B. The relation of blood pressure to stroke prognosis. *Annals of Internal Medicine*, **89**, 15–20 (1978)

91 ROBINS, M. and BAUM, H. M. Incidence in natural survey of stroke. *Stroke*, **12** (Suppl. 1), I-45–I-57 (1981)

92 ROBINSON, R. W., COHEN, W. D., HIGANO, N., MEYER, R., LUKOWSKY, G. H., McLAUGHLIN, R. B. and MacGILPIN, H. H. Life-table analysis of survival after cerebral thrombosis – ten-year experience. *Journal of the American Medical Association*, **169**, 1149–1152 (1959)

93 ROBINSON, R. W., DEMIREL, M. and LABEAU, R. J. Natural history of cerebral thrombosis, nine to nineteen year follow-up. *Journal of Chronic Diseases*, **21**, 221–230 (1968)

94 ROWE, J. C., BLAND, E. F., SPRAGUE, H. B. and WHITE, P. D. The course of mitral stenosis without surgery: ten- and twenty-year perspectives. *Annals of Internal Medicine*, **52**, 741–749 (1960)

95 SACCO, R. L., WOLF, P. A., KANNEL, W. B. and McNAMARA, P. M. Survival and recurrence following stroke. The Framingham study. *Stroke*, **13**, 290–295 (1982)

96 SOLTERO, I., LIU, K., COOPER, R., STAMLER, J. and GARSIDE, D. Trends in mortality from cerebrovascular diseases in the United States, 1960–1975. *Stroke*, **9**, 549–558 (1978)

97 STAMLER, J. Primary prevention of coronary heart disease. *American Journal of Cardiology*, **47**, 722–735 (1981)

98 SWANSON, P. D., CALANCHINI, P. R., DYKEN, M. L., GOTSHALL, R. A., HAERER, A. F., POSKANZER, D. C., PRICE, T. R. and CONNEALLY, P. M. A co-operative study of hospital frequency and character of transient ischemic attacks. II. Performance of angiography among six centers. *Journal of the American Medical Association*, **237**, 2202–2206 (1977)

99 SZEKELY, P. Systemic embolism and anticoagulant prophylaxis in rheumatic heart disease. *British Medical Journal*, **1**, 1209–1212 (1964)

100 TAYLOR, R. R. Acute stroke demonstration project in a community hospital. *Journal of the South Carolina Medical Association*, **66**, 225–227 (1970)

101 THYGESEN, P., CHRISTIANSEN, E., DYRBYE, M., EIKEN, M., FRANTZEN, J., GORMSEN, J., LADEMANN, A., LENNOX-BUCHTHAL, M., RONNOV-JESSEN, V. and THERKELSEN, J. Cerebral apoplexy: a clinical, radiological, electroencephalographic and pathological study with special reference to the prognosis of cerebral infarction and the result of long-term anticoagulation therapy. *Danish Medical Bulletin*, **11**, 233–257 (1964)

102 TOOLE, J. F., YUSON, C. P., JANEWAY, R., JOHNSTON, F., COURTLAND, D., CORDELL, A. R. and HOWARD, G. Transient ischemic attacks: a prospective study of 225 patients. *Neurology*, **28**, 746–753 (1978)

103 US DEPARTMENT OF COMMERCE. U.S. population by age, sex, rate, Series P-25, report numbers 519, 614, 643 and 870. *Population Estimates and Projections*, Bureau of Census, Washington, D.C.

104 VETERANS ADMINISTRATION CO-OPERATIVE STUDY GROUP ON ANTIHYPERTENSIVE AGENTS. Effects of treatment on morbidity in hypertension. Results in patients with diastolic blood pressures averaging 115 through 129 mmHg. *Journal of the American Medical Association*, **202**, 116–122 (1967)

105 VETERANS ADMINISTRATION CO-OPERATIVE STUDY GROUP ON ANTIHYPERTENSIVE AGENTS. Effects of treatment on morbidity in hypertension. II. Results in patients with diastolic blood pressure averaging 90 through 114 mmHg. *Journal of the American Medical Association*, **213**, 1143–1152 (1970)

106 WALKER, A. E., ROBINS, M. and WEINFELD, F. D. Clinical findings in national survey of stroke. *Stroke*, **12** (Suppl. 1), I-13–I-31 (1981)

107 WALLACE, D. C. A study of the natural history of cerebral vascular disease. *Medical Journal of Australia*, **1**, 90–95 (1967)

108 WALTIMO, O., KASTE, M. and FOGELHOLM, R. Prognosis of patients with unilateral extracranial occlusion of the internal carotid artery. *Stroke*, **7**, 480–482 (1976)

109 WEINFELD, F. D. (ed). The national survey of stroke. (National Institute of Neurological and Communicative Disorders and Stroke). *Stroke*, **12** (Suppl. 1) (1981)

110 WELLS, C. E. Cerebral embolism. *Archives of Neurology and Psychiatry*, **81**, 667–677 (1959)

111 WHISNANT, J. P. Epidemiology of stroke: emphasis on transient cerebral ischemic attacks and hypertension. *Stroke*, **5**, 68–70 (1974)

112 WHISNANT, J. P., FITZGIBBONS, J. P., KURLAND, L. P. and SAYRE, G. P. Natural history of stroke in Rochester, Minnesota, 1945 through 1954. *Stroke*, **2**, 11–22 (1971)

113 WOLF, P. A., KANNEL, W. B., McNAMARA, P. M. and GORDON, T. The role of impaired cardiac function in atherothrombotic brain infarction: the Framingham study. *American Journal of Public Health*, **63**, 52–58 (1973)

114 WOOD, P. An appreciation of mitral stenosis. Part I. Clinical features. *British Medical Journal*, **1**, 1051–1063, 1113–1124 (1954)

115 WOOD, P. An appreciation of mitral stenosis. Part II. Investigations and results. *British Medical Journal*, **1**, 1113–1124 (1954)

116 YATSU, F. M., COULL, B. M., TOOLE, J. F., McELROY, K., FEIBEL, J. H., SPRINGER, C. and WALKER, M. J. Regional stroke survey: demography and outcome (abstract). *Stroke*, **13**, 124 (1982)

117 ZIEGLER, D. K. and HASSANEIN, R. S. Prognosis in patients with transient ischemic attacks. *Stroke*, **4**, 666–673 (1973)

7
Thromboembolism

M. J. G. Harrison

Much of current thinking about the aetiology of transient ischaemic attacks (TIAs) and ischaemic strokes and about their treatment is based on the belief that the pathological process involved is thromboembolism. It is appropriate at this time to review the evidence for this hypothesis and follow through the logic that underlies modern therapy.

EVIDENCE OF THROMBOEMBOLISM

Transient ischaemic attacks

In 1891 Peabody[36] suggested that repeated attacks of transient hemiparesis might be due to recurrent spasm of the middle cerebral artery. This has never been demonstrated angiographically, and spasm of intracerebral vessels seems unlikely to occur unless they are subjected to direct trauma, or in the context of hemiplegic migraine. The association of TIAs with carotid occlusions and basilar artery occlusion suggested that a reduced perfusion pressure might be enough to cause transient focal symptoms. This haemodynamic view of TIAs was championed by Denny-Brown[9] who produced a neurological deficit in the monkey by inducing hypotension after occluding the middle cerebral artery. That this mechanism can operate in patients and cause transient focal neurological deficit is well established. Anecdotal evidence includes reports of cases in whom TIAs were precipitated by iatrogenic hypotension, postural hypotension, the vasodilatation of a hot bath, and exercise induced cardiac decompensation. A haemodynamically significant cardiac arrythmia may cause TIAs. Normally, hypotension or a fall in cardiac output produces the symptoms of a diffuse impairment of cerebral perfusion, the familiar sensations of syncope[40]. Focal symptoms (TIA) are only likely to develop if a local vascular obstruction or tight stenosis (*Figure 7.1*) makes one cerebral territory more vulnerable to a drop in perfusion pressure. This was the case, for example, in the patient described by Eastcott *et al.*[11]. The woman had episodes of amaurosis

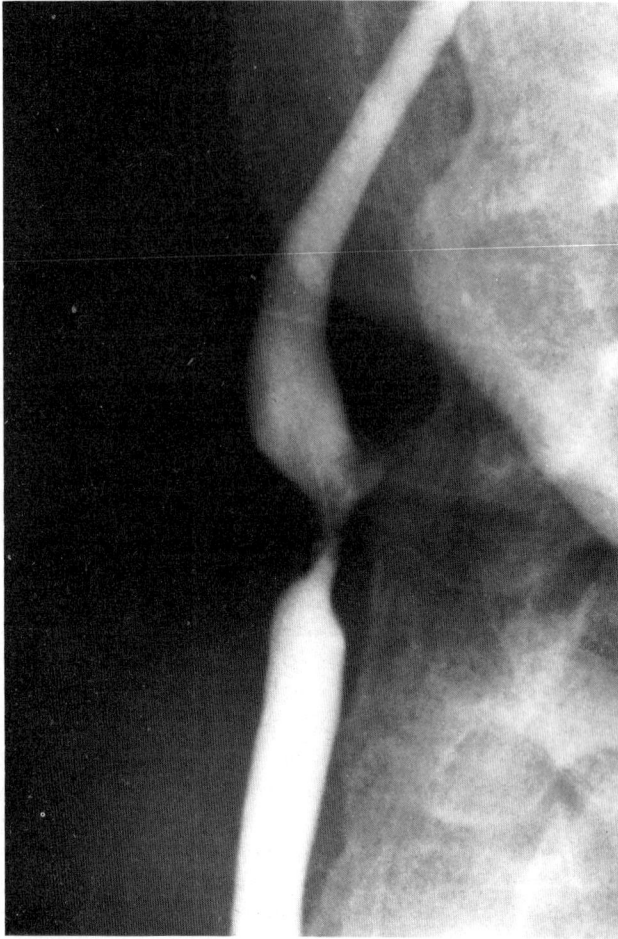

Figure 7.1 Tight stenosis at origin internal carotid artery. (From Harrison[18a], courtesy of the Editor and Publishers, *British Journal of Hospital Medicine*)

fugax and transient hemiparesis (often concurrently) in association with a cardiac tachyarrythmia. The carotid artery ipsilateral to the symptomatic retina and cerebral hemisphere was tightly stenosed. After carotid reconstruction (the first reported in Europe) the patient still had attacks of cardiac arrythmia but these no longer provoked retinal or cerebral symptoms. A similar mechanism must be invoked to explain the TIAs related to the other causes of hypotension when they occur *de novo* in a patient with no previous cerebral lesion.

In the aftermath of cerebral infarction a different haemodynamic mechanism can cause the transient reappearance of a focal deficit. The normal mechanism of autoregulation of cerebral blood flow (CBF) which maintains a level of CBF over a wide range of mean arterial pressure (approximately from 80–180 mmHg) is impaired in the vascular bed of a cerebral infarct. Consequently, blood flow in that area is 'pressure passive' linearly related to the mean arterial pressure. There is evidence that such dysautoregulation may persist after infarction. Hypotension could then provoke a focal reduction of CBF that could be enough to cause symptoms. Riley and Friedman[41] described such a case. Nine months after a hemiplegia producing hemisphere infarct confirmed on a CT scan, a 71 year old developed EEG slow waves and seizures when his blood pressure dropped from 150/100 to 120/70 mmHg.

TIAs after carotid occlusion and in the presence of multiple vessel occlusions may also be due to the fact that the autoregulating reserve is exhausted by compensation for reduced pressure in the Circle of Willis, so that any additional haemodynamic crisis can provoke symptomatic cerebral ischaemia.

Flow problems are, however, documented only rarely and this mechanism can explain only a minority of TIAs. The evidence against the haemodynamic hypothesis rests on a number of clinical observations[2, 19]. Symptoms suggesting a syncopal state are rare in TIA patients and attacks are rarely related to exercise, posture or head position. Although patients with TIAs often have cardiac rhythm disturbances, on 24 hour ECG Holter monitoring arrythmias rarely cause focal symptoms[40]. Although TIAs follow carotid occlusion they are less frequent than after a carotid stenosis not affecting flow. TIAs rarely occur in patients with multiple neck vessel occlusions. Provocative testing of TIA patients, including the induction of tilt table hypotension, rarely causes focal attacks. Finally Price *et al.*[39] managed to collect data on 79 patients examined during a TIA. None had hypotension or a pulse rate below 60 or above 140 mmHg while symptomatic.

In a recent study Ruff *et al.*[42] reported the findings in 132 patients under inpatient investigation for TIAs. Twenty-seven had an episode of documented hypotension. In seven a TIA accompanied the change in blood pressure and four of these had angiographic evidence of a tight stenosis. None of the 20 who had no TIA when they were hypotensive had a tight stenosis. Thulesius noted that occluding collateral flow above a carotid occlusion by manual compression of a superficial temporal artery in eight patients failed to provoke a recurrence of a TIA.

Most of this data has been collected in the context of TIAs in the carotid territory since they are more often studied intensively. There is some evidence that flow problems are more commonly involved in the pathogenesis of TIAs in the vertebrobasilar territory. Thus symptoms suggesting a relationship of attacks to change of posture, head position and exercise are all more common than in the case of carotid TIAs[19]. Dysautoregulation may be more common in patients with vertebrobasilar TIAs, and small ischaemic insults to the brain stem may affect the central neurogenic mechanism of autoregulation, leaving the victim of such a lesion persistently vulnerable to low perfusion pressures[35]. Reduced vertebral artery flow can be caused by head turning and occasionally causes symptoms as a result. Two personal cases developed symptoms, and a local neck bruit, on head turning, presumably due to mechanical stenosis of a dominant vertebral artery.

The evidence for thromboembolism is also largely clinical. Twenty years ago, Fisher and Ross Russell both described the passage of emboli through the retinal circulation in patients during attacks of amaurosis fugax. Subsequent pathological study showed that such white bodies consisted of platelet material. Barnett[2] has recently described a similar white body in a pial vessel on the exposed cerebral

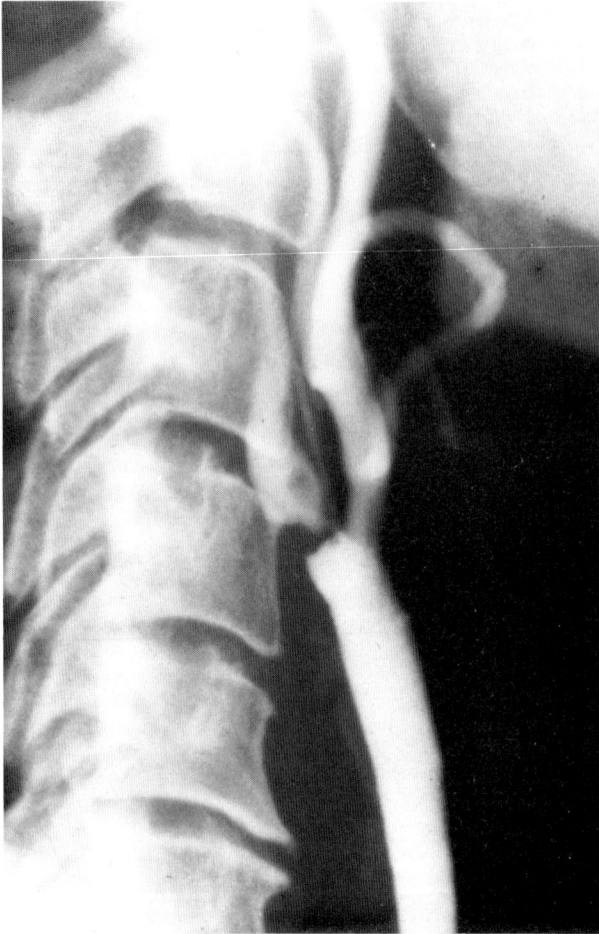

Figure 7.2 Intraluminal mural thrombus visible at site of carotid stenosis (From Harrison[19a], courtesy of the Publishers, *Topical Reviews in Neurology Vol. 1*)

cortex in a patient about to have an extracranial intracranial microvascular anastamosis completed. These direct observations are rare and the presence of a potential *source* for embolism rather than visible embolism constitutes the evidence for this process in most instances.

Carotid angiography reveals a possible source for embolism in the form of a local atheromatous plaque in some 50% of subjects presenting with carotid territory TIAs. Similar abnormalities of the carotid bifurcation are rare in controls[22]. The degree of stenosis is frequently insufficient to affect flow so its association with TIA in its vascular bed can only relate to its potential as a source for thromboembolism. The presence of mural thrombi at the site of carotid stenosis is occasionally demonstrable by angiography (*Figure 7.2*). Operative specimens reveal that embolic material, local mural thrombus or friable atheromatous debris (*Figure 7.3*) is present in 66% of carotid arteries subjected to endarterectomy within one month of a TIA. At longer intervals the chances of finding local embolic material at the

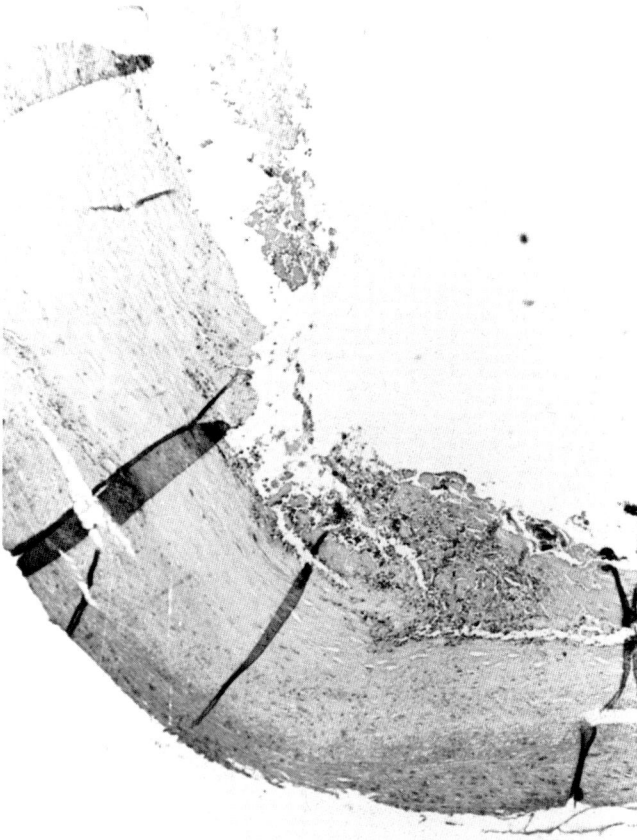

Figure 7.3 Carotid endarterectomy specimen showing friable embolic material on luminal surface

operative site is much less, implying that mural thrombus formation is phasic, and also indicating that such material is very likely to have been present at the time of the TIA[23].

Mural thrombi were found in the study reported by Harrison and Marshall in some 60% of all tightly stenosed lesions, in half of those with stenoses between 25 and 70% and in only 10% in those with less than 25% narrowing of the lumen. The increased prevalence of mural thrombus and the higher potential for embolism of the more severely stenosed lesions may well relate to the frequency with which large plaques show ulceration. The reduced tendency to mural thrombus formation of lesser lesions may explain their reduced stroke risk[4]. Minor lesions show a greater risk of symptom production if ulcerated[34] (*Figure 7.4*).

The circumstances of some patients' attacks support the concept of dislodgement of mural thrombus. Thus cases have been reported of TIAs related to momentary

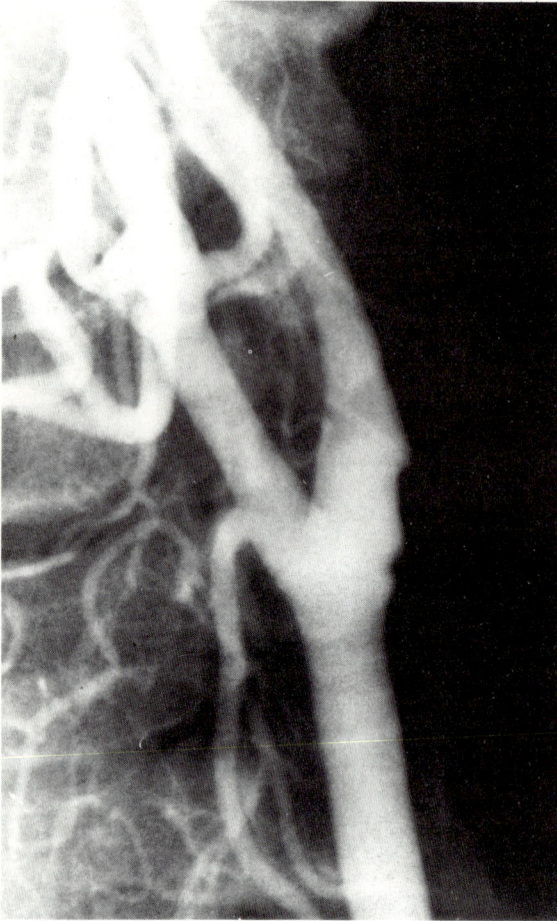

Figure 7.4 Ulcerative atheroma on wall of internal carotid artery at bifurcation

palpation of the carotid, to leaning out of bed, and to sneezing (personal unpublished observations).

The response to treatment also offers some evidence in favour of thromboembolism. Thus carotid endarterectomy may be successful in stopping TIAs even when cerebral blood flow is normal pre-operatively. Similarly, antiplatelet drugs may bring TIAs to a halt in individual patients.

One major criticism of the thromboembolic hypothesis has always been that embolism would not be expected to cause stereotyped attacks. A personal study of the symptoms of patients with multiple carotid territory TIAs revealed that subtle differences, perhaps due to embolism into different middle cerebral artery branches, were present in over 50%. Furthermore, experimental emboli, through streaming of blood flow, follow the same intracranial route repeatedly. Emboli preferentially enter the middle cerebral artery, only entering the anterior cerebral artery when the former is occluded[12]. This is in keeping with the rarity of TIAs attributable to ischaemia restricted to the anterior cerebral artery bed.

Strokes

Cerebral infarction accounts for 90% of major strokes. Haemodynamic crises are rarely responsible though are occasionally documented. As in the case of TIAs focal changes are only likely if there is a local vessel occlusion or tight stenosis to further reduce the local perfusion pressure to a level responsible for infarction. Patients may sustain a hemiplegia under such circumstances in response to haemorrhagic shock, per-operative hypotension or autonomic neuropathy, e.g. diabetes mellitus. In those circumstances watershed territories, those between the major vascular beds of the middle, anterior and posterior cerebral arteries, suffer particularly (*Figure 7.5*). McAuley and Ross Russell[31] (1979) have described the

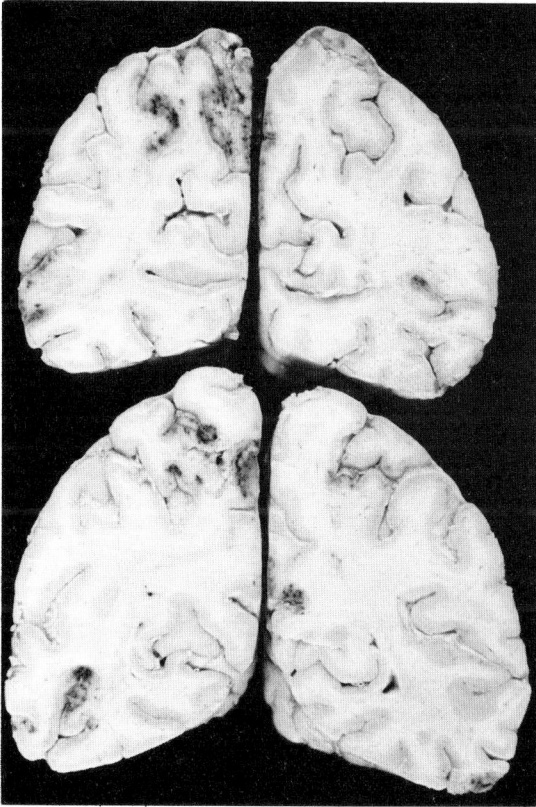

Figure 7.5 Watershed cerebral infarction in patient with severe postural hypotension due to autonomic neuropathy

characteristic visual field defects that distinguish occipital polar watershed infarction after cardiac arrest from the macular sparing hemianopic defect of infarction in the centre of the territory of the calcarine artery due to local vetebral artery occlusion. Clinical experience suggests that haemodynamic crises are most likely to cause infarction when there has already been a previous cerebral infarct, presumably due to poor autoregulatory responses to low perfusion pressures in the damaged area. Thus per-operative strokes occur more commonly during coronary artery and aortoiliac surgery in those with previous symptoms of cerebrovascular disease. The deterioration of patients in the first 2 to 3 weeks after a cerebral infarction may be due to extension of the infarct in relation to cardiac decompensation, whilst autoregulation is still paralyzed in the damaged cerebral hemisphere. A personal case recovering well from a middle cerebral territory infarct extended his infarct when he developed hypotension due to a cardiac dysrrythmia; another suffered the same fate on being sat out of bed for the first time when his mean arterial pressure fell unexpectedly.

Pathological studies suggest that such haemodynamic events are rarely the cause of first cerebral infarcts. Patients who have temporarily survived the effects of a profound hypotension rarely have focal infarcts, even in the presence of cerebral atheroma.

Lhermitte's excellent pathological survey of middle cerebral artery territory infarcts revealed that some 50% were due to carotid occlusion[30]. Those occlusions were embolic from the heart in 20% of instances, but in 80% they were due to thrombus formation on a local arterial stenosis. The stenosis was always severe (75% or more). In another 40% the infarct was attributable to embolic occlusion of the middle cerebral artery itself. Occlusions of the anterior and middle cerebral arteries proved to be due to embolism from the heart in 27%, from neck vessels in 27%, to spread of proximal thrombus in 31% (carotid occlusion) and to local thrombosis in only 10% (*Table 7.1*). It might be argued that fatal cases of cerebral

Table 7.1 Aetiology of intracranial occlusions (from Lhermitte[30])

| | Cerebral arteries | | | | |
	Anterior	Middle	Posterior	Total	(%)
Embolism (proximal vessels)	11	11	15	37	(33)
Embolism (heart)	17	5	1	23	(21)
Spread proximal thrombosis	17*	8	8	30	(31)
Local thrombosis	3	4	3	17	(9)
Undetermined	1	3	3	7	(6)

* Including 4 carotid thrombi that in turn had originated in the heart

infarction might differ significantly from those with survival so it is important to also look at the angiographic data. Studies of strokes of all types reveal carotid occlusion in some 20%. Carotid stenosis that might be the source of embolism occurs more frequently in stroke victims than in controls but the association is much weaker than that of carotid occlusion[20] (*Table 7.2*). Distal, and therefore from the pathological evidence likely embolic occlusions, are common. The timing of angiography is critical. Embolic occlusions disperse and when the interval between the onset of neurological deficit and angiography is more than a few days the number of normal angiograms increases. Ignorance of this effect has led to underestimation of the role of embolic intracranial occlusions in the pathogenesis of cerebral infarction.

Table 7.2 Angiographic appearance of the carotid bifurcation in patients with carotid territory TIAs, completed strokes and supratentorial tumours

| | *n* | *Normal* | *Angiographic appearance (%)* | | *Occlusion* |
			Atheroma	*Stenosis*	
Tumours	211	74	24	2	0
TIA	216	45	23	21	8
Stroke	293	46	15	13	17

Again there are differences between vertebrobasilar territory infarcts and those in the cerebral hemispheres supplied by the carotid artery. Thus, if the middle cerebral artery is the artery of embolism (*Figure 7.6*), the basilar artery is that of thrombosis. *In situ* thrombus formation predominates as a cause of vertebrobasilar occlusion (*Figure 7.7*).

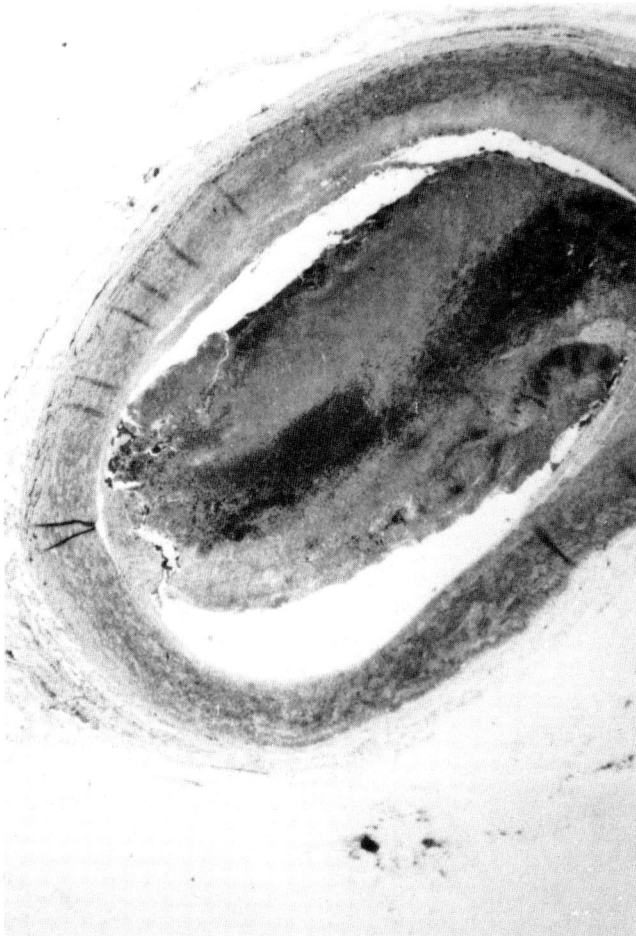

Figure 7.6 Embolus in middle cerebral artery

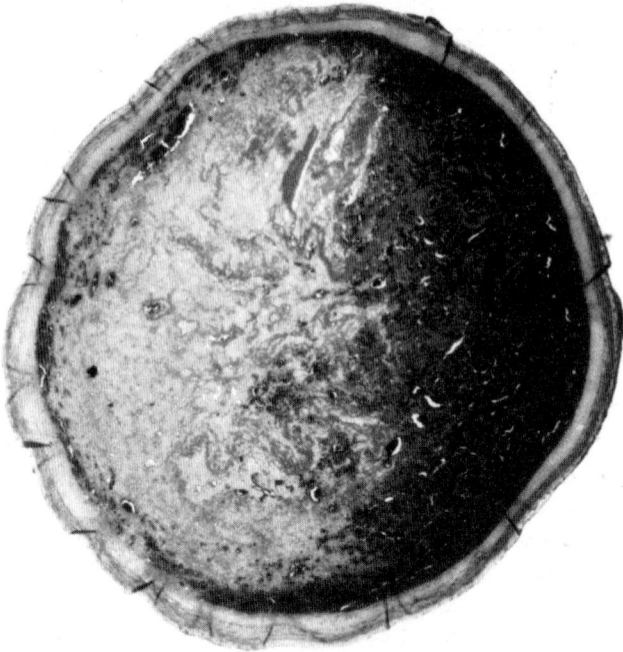

Figure 7.7 Thrombotic occlusion of basilar artery

SOURCE OF EMBOLI

Transient ischaemic attacks

Angiograms suggest that a local abnormality in the parent carotid artery is present in some 60% of cases of carotid TIAs. Endarterectomy in such patients usually reveals that the bifurcation lesion has been the site of mural thrombus formation. Haemorrhage into plaques is commonly encountered or the lesion is ulcerated.

In a further 25% a cardiac source for embolism is detectable[8]. The responsible cardiac lesions are of great interest. Thus they include, as well as rheumatic heart disease with atrial thrombus, mitral valve prolapse, aortic valve stenosis, subacute bacterial endocarditis and marantic endocarditis. These are all situations in which vegetations or small thrombi may develop in association with an abnormal heart valve.

In the remaining 25% no angiographic or cardiac abnormality is found. The aetiology of these patients' TIAs is of great interest and very important in view of their contribution to the number that are included in various therapeutic trials. Are they due to emboli from undetected sites? We know angiography can miss small ulcerated lesions, and the aorta is rarely adequately visualized, though it can be the source of emboli. The development of digital angiography promises to make more extensive angiographic study possible at reduced risk. Some of the cases may have undetected haemodynamic changes, since even repeated Holter monitoring may 'miss' significant arrythmias. Others may have been incorrectly diagnosed as having a TIA. Fisher believes many such events with normal angiography are due to late life migraine. This seems an acceptable hypothesis in those patients who describe a characteristic headache, or march of events, but in many others it is surely better to record a 'don't know' verdict. A very few may prove to be examples of non-convulsive seizure paralysis, a situation that is usually revealed only by electroencephalography or the natural history of the responsible focal cerebral lesion. In vertebrobasilar attacks flow problems may predominate, ulceration of vertebral arteries being infrequent.

Strokes

Autopsy series all suggest that cerebral infarcts can be attributable to embolism from the heart in up to 50%. The clinical experience of most physicians does not match these figures though some careful observers have noted comparable findings. Thus Gautier and Morelot[16] found approximately half of a series of completed stroke victims to have a potentially relevant cardiac lesion. The yield of cardiac abnormalities in stroke patients is increasing with the advent of stroke intensive care units, and the use of sophisticated echocardiography and nuclear scanning. Nuclear scans may detect aneurysms or akinetic segments on which mural thrombus may form. CT scans may reveal the presence of such thrombi in the left ventricle, and echocardiography the presence of atrial thrombi.

The commonest cardiac lesion encountered clinically is atrial fibrillation. Though the risk of cerebral embolism varies with the aetiology of the fibrillation all patients are at risk and in Gautier's neurological series so-called lone fibrillation predominated. Ischaemic heart disease with left ventricular thrombus is perhaps second to cases of atrial thrombus.

The neck vessels seem to be the source of embolism in the causation of cerebral infarction relatively infrequently. Mitchell and Schwartz[33] demonstrated a lack of association between cerebral infarction and carotid stenosis (rather than occlusion). Harrison and Marshall showed only a weak association in a comparable angiographic study[22]. Lhermitte's detailed study of middle cerebral artery territory infarcts found proof of embolism from the carotid artery in only 6 of 122 cases, though persisting occlusions of intracranial vessels were due to artery to artery embolism in some 25%[22].

The difference between TIAs and strokes needs to be noted. The evidence reviewed above points to embolism from the neck vessels predominating in the pathogenesis of TIAs but having a smaller role in completed strokes. Heart lesions causing TIAs are often of the sort that are associated with small embolic masses (vegetations, small thrombi on prolapsing mitral valves, etc.). Stroke victims more frequently have a cardiac source for embolism, and neck vessel disease is relevant because of the development of carotid occlusion by thrombosis of a local stenosis, rather than because of artery to artery embolism. Intracranial atheroma is more common in stroke victims than in those with TIAs[44]. The heart lesions involved may more often be those associated with atrial or ventricular thombus.

Wilson, Warlow and Russell[47] (1979) have recently noted similar differences between the causes of central retinal artery occlusion with retinal infarction, and the aetiology of cases of amaurosis fugax or retinal branch occlusion. Evidence of embolism was detected in most cases of branch occlusion, with visible retinal emboli and a high incidence of cardiac valve disease and carotid stenosis. Cases of central retinal occlusions were older, and had a lower prevalence of valve disease and carotid disease, but were more often hypertensive. Local thrombosis rather than embolism seems responsible for the completed retinal 'stroke'. It is tempting to pursue this speculation to suggest that TIAs are transient because they are produced by small emboli as may develop in a carotid artery or on heart valves, whilst infarction is more often due to blockage of the carotid artery or embolism of larger thrombi that may develop in the chambers of the heart. The nature of emboli might be expected to be highly relevant to such discussions of their behaviour.

NATURE OF EMBOLI

It is likely that some of the differences just discussed relate to the different size and structure of emboli. That there are many pathological types of emboli is clear from accounts of retinal emboli where white bodies, yellow bodies and calcific valve debris have all been described. The white bodies which pass through the retinal circulation have been shown to consist of platelet aggregates. Yellow refractile Hollenhorst bodies consist of cholesterol debris from ulcerated plaques and these have been demonstrated in the brain also. Calcific emboli may arise from aortic valves or rarely from plaques.

The rupture of plaques releasing debris into the circulation is poorly understood. There is considerable evidence that haemorrhage into the base of plaque is frequently the final straw that causes a fracture in the plaque, exposing its base. The moment of haemorrhage may thus precipitate embolism of plaque contents and by exposing subendothelial structures promotes mural thrombus formation[10]. Woodcock (personal communication) has recently shown that the site of a plaque at the carotid bifurcation is liable to abnormal movement patterns during the normal vessel movement at different times in the cardiac cycle. Calcification of advanced plaques may well be a factor in causing excessive mechanical stress on the vessel wall (and hence rupture).

Platelet emboli in the retina are usually associated with reversible ischaemia, presumably due to their friable nature being dispersed by the blood flow. Experimentally such white bodies lodge temporarily at arterial bifurcations provoking little or no response, and moving on in the blood stream. Cholesterol crystals become impacted in retinal vessels and may be seen to stay in place for several weeks. They may not occlude the lumen and so may be asymptomatic. Fields and others have described their passage through the retina after carotid endarterectomy. Calcific emboli in the retina frequently cause a permanent occlusion with retinal infarction[43]. The counterpart to these retinal events in the cerebrum is poorly documented. Patients with amaurosis fugax with no visible retinal emboli often have evidence of asymptomatic hemisphere disturbances (on EEG, CBF studies, etc), and it seems possible that such friable small emboli are often asymptomatic in the cerebral circulation.

The local response to the impaction of an embolus may differ according to its constituents. Platelet emboli may release 5HT and it is possible that local changes are partly related to this. Cholesterol and atheromatous emboli provoke a local histological reaction that may be striking and include giant cell formation. Secondary thrombosis may be provoked. The nature of the lipid material discharged from the plaque may be important in deciding the severity of the local vascular response[27].

Clinical study of patients with pathologically verified embolism of atheromatous material rather than thrombus reveals that fluctuating confusion is more common than a simple completed stroke. Zulch[49] showed that experimental emboli if large tended to enter and occlude the middle cerebral artery, but if small were scattered widely, through the hemisphere. It seems likely that small cholesterol emboli are distributed widely producing diffuse signs. The clinical picture of patients with thrombocytosis and circulating platelet aggregates is similarly one of fluctuating diffuse neurological signs and symptoms rather than of a focal TIA or stroke[38].

The larger emboli derived from heart chambers may well be more stable than those causing TIAs. Fibrin formation stabilizes larger thrombi developing in the left atrium where the composition is more clot-like as in a venous thrombus.

These differences in the site of origin and composition of emboli may well therefore have critical clinical relevance. The rationale for an antithrombotic regime is only logical if thrombosis or embolism of thrombus is involved. Atheromatous embolism would not be expected to respond to antithrombotic measures and perhaps could only be prevented by surgical removal of the ulcerated atheroma. Fibrin stabilized thrombi in heart chambers might be more sensitive to anticoagulation than platelet white bodies developing in the lumen of the open carotid artery.

THROMBOSIS

Thrombus formation in the heart or on the wall of cervical arteries is clearly central to the occurrence of many episodes of cerebral ischaemia. In order to approach its treatment it is necessary to review what is known of the process of thrombus formation, and discuss whether a pre-thrombotic state can be detected in patients at risk.

Histological study of all thrombi shows them to consist of platelet–fibrin masses with entrapped red and white blood cells (*Figure 7.8*). It may, however, be incorrect to assume that the red and white cells are playing a passive role (*see below*). The initial event in mural thrombus formation appears to consist of platelet adherence to the site of endothelial damage, and subsequent platelet aggregation.

Platelets adhere to the subendothelium and to collagen fibres in areas of endothelial damage spreading out to cover, for example, the site of an endarterectomy. Von Willenbrand factor may be involved in the formation of the monolayer. Platelets also adhere one to another in a process which involves calcium

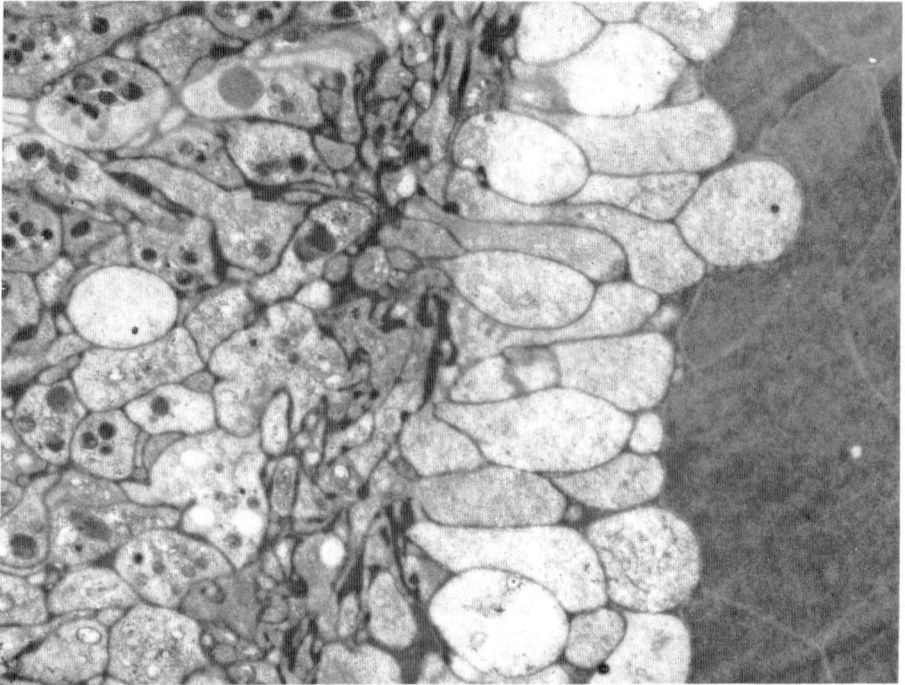

Figure 7.8 Platelet mass with entrapped group of red cells. Note that the platelets adjacent to the red cells are degranulated ($\times$ 8400)

ions, and fibrinogen which probably acts as a molecular bridge between platelets. This process of aggregation is to a degree self propagating since platelets once triggered to aggregate release stores of nucleotides, particularly adenosine diphosphate, which can cause further aggregation (*Figure 7.9*).

The trigger to aggregation *in vivo* may be a combination of the presence of injured endothelium as in an ulcerated plaque with exposure of collagen and subendothelial basement membrane, and of flow characteristics. In whole blood red cells tend to occupy the centre of the flowing column, forcing platelets to the edge. Aggregation tends to occur in vortices so would be anticipated in the area of turbulent flow at the site of a stenosis. However, little is known of the relative roles of thrombotic mechanisms in areas of vessel wall abnormality. When platelets come into contact with collagen or thrombin, phospholipase A_2 and C are stimulated, perhaps through internal calcium ion movement. Platelet membrane phospholipids are hydrolyzed with the production of arachidonic acid. Prostaglandin synthesis then follows (*Figure 7.10*) through the agency of platelet cyclo-oxygenase. Two main endoperoxides, PGG_2 and PGH_2, are formed which have platelet aggregating powers. From endoperoxides a family of prostaglandins are produced, PGD_2 an inhibiting material, PGF_2 and PGE_2 weak inhibitors of platelet aggregation, and TXA_2 (thromboxane A_2) a powerful platelet aggregant. The formation of the latter material is probably responsible for the second wave of aggregation in platelets exposed to collagen. Thromboxane A_2 is very unstable but when it is formed from

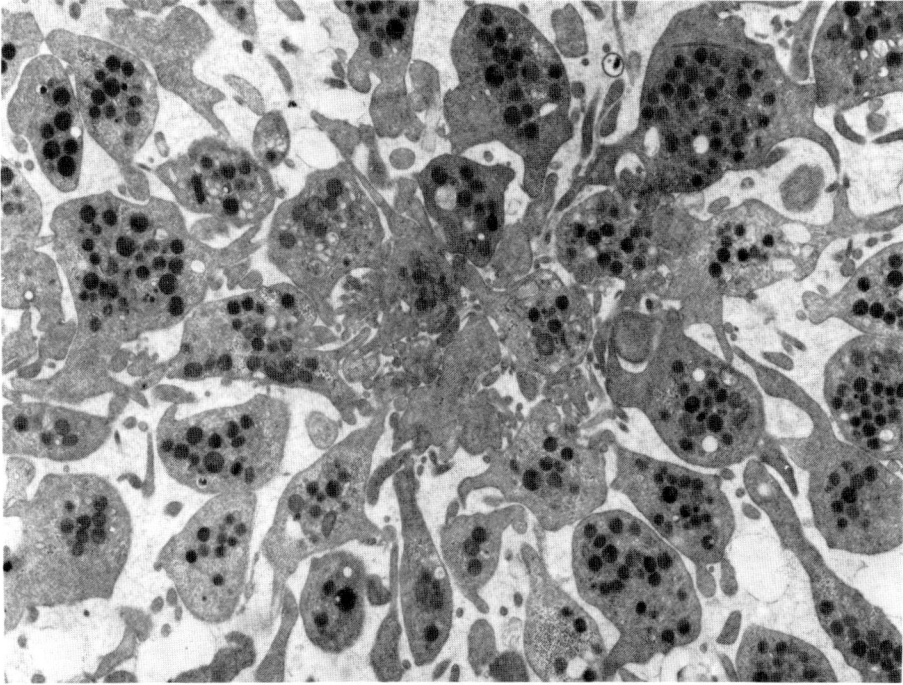

Figure 7.9 Mass of aggregating platelets some showing loss of organelles (release reaction) and pseudopod formation (× 8400)

endoperoxides malondialdehyde is also produced and this stable byproduct can be assayed. Similarly, a stable metabolite of TXA_2, thromboxane B_2, can be assayed. It is thus becoming possible to study the level of prostaglandin activity in platelets which will hopefully reflect the level of pro-aggregating influences affecting platelet adhesive function.

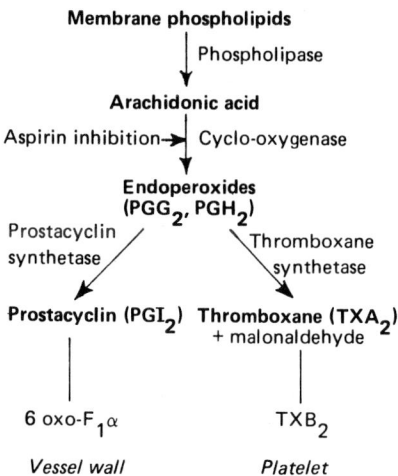

Membrane phospholipids
↓ Phospholipase
Arachidonic acid
Aspirin inhibition→ │ Cyclo-oxygenase
↓
Endoperoxides
(PGG_2, PGH_2)
Prostacyclin ╱ ╲ Thromboxane
synthetase ╱ ╲ synthetase
↓ ↓
Prostacyclin (PGI_2) Thromboxane (TXA_2)
+ malonaldehyde
│ │
│ │
6 oxo-$F_1\alpha$ TXB_2

Vessel wall *Platelet*

Figure 7.10 Pathway of prostaglandin synthesis in platelets and vessel wall

Most cells in the body contain prostaglandins and although vessel walls synthesize TXA_2 they preferentially produce PGI_2 (prostacyclin), a powerful vasodilator and inhibitor of platelet aggregation. It has been suggested that the fact that normal endothelium is antithrombotic is due to its local production of prostacyclin especially in response to local thrombin or the presence of platelet derived endoperoxides. Prostacyclin has been billed as the 'goody' prostaglandin (vasodilator and antiaggregating agent), thromboxane A_2 as the 'baddy' vasoconstricting vessels plugged by platelet masses, and causing further aggregation[32]. Caution is advised before accepting this simple view of affairs, however. It is true that prostacyclin synthesis is impaired in arterial plaques which might favour mural thrombus formation, but congenital deficiency of thromboxane A_2 synthesis has little effect on haemostatic platelet plug formation. Further thrombin can stimulate platelet aggregation by a pathway independent of the arachidonic-prostaglandin pathway. Finally, platelets still do not adhere to vessel walls in which prostacyclin synthesis has been inhibited so that the natural barrier function remains unexplained.

Platelets stimulated to aggregate also release procoagulant phospholipids (platelet factor III), factor V and fibrinogen, and by a variety of means thrombin formation is provoked. This in its own right causes platelet aggregation but by a method partly independent of thromboxane synthesis. The stimulated platelet surface is probably active in promoting many steps in the coagulation cascade and so coagulation and platelet aggregation tend to occur together.

Platelets also release a mitogenic factor that stimulates proliferation of vascular smooth muscle cells. The interaction between endothelial damage, platelet aggregation and a local vessel wall response to the aggregates is thus complex[7].

Do patients with TIAs and strokes show abnormalities of platelet function? Increased platelet aggregation has been demonstrated in patients with major strokes by a variety of methods but the problem has always been that platelet behaviour shows a non-specific response to illness, and such changes may therefore be *post hoc* rather than *propter hoc*. Johnson *et al.*[28] suggest that acute changes in fibrinogen are responsible for the non-specific effect. It is therefore more valuable to look at platelet function in patients with TIAs whose systemic response is minimal and where changes detected weeks after an episode that lasted 20 minutes are unlikely to be a non-specific response to illness. Platelet aggregation measured by the optical density technique in platelet rich plasma using ADP as the stimulus shows an increased tendency to second phase (ADP release; TXA_2 synthesis) aggregation in patients with TIAs. Aggregates are more often detectable in venous samples from patients than from controls. Such aggregates are often assumed to be present in the circulation of such patients, but there is no proof of their existence there and they could be formed in the syringe during sample collection, and their presence needs to be interpreted with caution.

Platelet factor IV and B-thromboglobulin are platelet derived proteins which are released during aggregation. They can all be assayed in venous blood and their levels have been found to be elevated in patients suffering from thrombotic vascular events. Whether the assays are reliable and sensitive enough to detect any evidence of an over-active state of platelets in patients before a major clinical event due to thromboembolism is, however, doubtful. Assays of TXB_2 may in future be more helpful.

Enhanced release reactions may be detected by 5HT release. A subgroup of patients after myocardial infarction have evidence of increased platelet reactivity measured in this way and they have a worse prognosis during follow-up[26].

Thrombin activated platelets can be detected *ex vivo* by differential centrifugation since they are lighter due to release of granules. It may theoretically be possible to detect thrombotic and conceivably pre-thrombotic states by an assessment of the proportions of circulating platelets that go to the light end of such a density gradient.

Platelet survival has been shown to be reduced in a number of situations characterized by thrombosis. The mechanism of consumption of platelets is not fully understood in these techniques[7]. A study of TIA patients revealed a shortened survival in patients with amaurosis fugax in whom an endothelial abnormality was detectable (carotid stenosis, heart valve lesion) but not in a small subgroup with no such lesion[46]. Increased thrombotic events occur in patients with homocystinuria in whom platelet hyperactivity has been found. Endothelial damage is provoked by homocystine infusions, however, So the platelet changes may be secondary.

It is thus possible that shortened platelet survival, high levels of B-TBG and platelet factor IV, increased 5HT release and circulating aggregates all reflect the level of interaction between platelets and diseased vessel wall, rather than demonstrating a primary platelet abnormality.

Using this argument there would be no role for a primary platelet disorder in the genesis of mural thrombosis. Although platelet counts are not elevated in prospective trials of vascular disease, some patients with pathologically elevated platelet counts do present with thromboses. Rare examples of thrombocythaemia produce cerebral and retinal ischaemic events and are controlled by measures that reduce the platelet count or inhibit platelet aggregation. In these rare situations platelet behaviour may be more directly responsible for clinical events.

In patients with prosthetic heart valves, Harker[18] found evidence that the degree of platelet activation was merely a reflection of the size of the area of abnormal material exposed to passing blood. However, a recent study by Walsh *et al.*[45] suggests that the degree of platelet activation, for example by a prolapsing mitral valve may nonetheless be critical to the occurrence of thromboemboli. Thus they tested platelet aggregation and measured platelet coagulant proteins and found evidence of activation in 58% of patients with prolapsing mitral valves, 100% if the patients had cerebral or retinal emboli (6% in controls). Another indirect piece of evidence that platelet behaviour may contribute to pathogenesis comes from a study of patients with hyperlipidaemia. Zahari *et al.*[48] found greater evidence of platelet activation (BTG, pl factor IV and MDA synthesis) in patients with hyperlipidaemia than in patients with established peripheral vascular disease. This suggests that platelet activation may be related to the risk factor rather than just secondary to the presence of atheroma.

Is there any situation where coagulation mechanisms are causative of thromboembolic events? Factor VIII levels, fibrinogen titres and plasma levels of fibrinopeptide A (a small peptide released from fibrinogen by thrombin) are all elevated in clinical circumstances associated with intra-vascular thrombosis. Though these may be secondary events, prospective trials reveal fibrinogen and factor VIII concentrations to be risk factors for cardiovascular deaths. In the case of fibrinogen the mechanism may relate to viscosity factors not just to coagulopathy. Cases of thrombotic tendencies due to abnormalities of individual clotting factors of congenital origin are unfortunately too rare to be of help. Fibrinogen turnover appears to be increased selectively in venous thrombosis, fibrinogen and platelet consumption being increased together in arterial thrombosis[18]. The evidence thus suggests that endothelial damage, platelet reactivity and coagulation factors may all interact in producing the so-called pre-thrombotic state. Arterial disease risk factors may well influence several of these components. For example, smoking and hyperlipidaemia may cause endothelial damage, shorten clotting times and enhance platelet aggregation.

A high haemoglobin or haematocrit proved in the Framingham study to be a weakly active risk factor for stroke, and interest is growing in this aspect of cerebrovascular disease.

Patients with polycythaemia rubra vera have an increased risk of stroke, the level of risk depending on the level of haematocrit rather than on other features of the disease. Although the whole blood viscosity is elevated, the reduced cerebral blood flow in polycythaemia is probably due to a physiological adjustment to the increased oxygen carrying capacity. While such low flow may be of little physiological significance therefore, it may predispose to thrombosis and adversely affect flow in the collaterals distal to a vessel occlusion. Some evidence for this was recently obtained by the finding that the size (on CT scans) of cerebral infarcts due to carotid occlusion was related to the height of the prevailing haematocrit[24] (*Figure 7.11*). We also found haematocrit levels were higher in patients with TIAs[25] especially in those related to carotid occlusion, suggesting *in situ* thrombosis of the carotid might be more prevalent in patients with high haematocrits.

The way red cells might play a role in promoting thrombosis has been receiving attention in the last few years. There are two main possibilities. Firstly, red blood cells contain ADP and haemolysis due to red cell trauma could trigger platelet aggregation by release of ADP. This is the basis of the methods of measuring the glass adhesiveness of platelets[20]. Whole blood rotated in a glass vessel leaks ADP from red cells which activates adhesion and aggregation of the platelets. Red cell ghosts are found in thrombi and Born[3] has suggested that chlorpromazine could have antithrombotic effects by protecting red cell membranes from trauma. Red cells might be damaged by contact with areas of vessel wall abnormality, prosthetic heart valves, etc. causing local elevations of ADP levels. Turbulence might be enough to cause minimal haemolysis. Subclinical haemolysis certainly occurs in patients with prosthetic heart valves but the risk of thromboembolism in such patients does not appear to correlate closely with the presence or absence of haemolysis.

The alternative role for red cells, which may therefore be the more relevant, lies in their effect on flow characteristics. Platelets are forced to travel in the laminar stream in contact with the vessel wall by the presence of larger heavier red cells which occupy the centre of the flowing column of blood. With artificial mixtures of

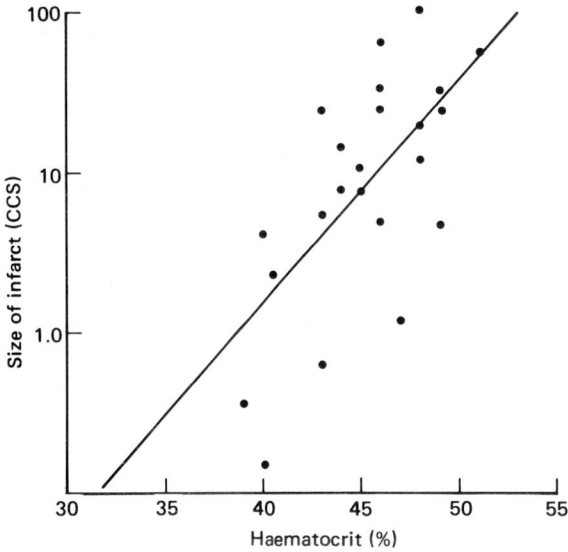

Figure 7.11 Size of cerebral infarcts (on log scale) from CT scan measurements, and prevailing haematocrit in symptomatic patients with angiographically proven carotid occlusion. (From Harrison *et al.*[24], courtesy of the Editor and Publishers, *Lancet*)

platelet rich plasma and red blood cells Baumgartner has demonstrated that platelet adhesion to a preparation of balloon injured rabbit aorta is increased at high haematocrit due to the displacement of platelets on to the intima. This effect of red cells is incidentally enough to override the inhibiting effect of aspirin on platelet adhesion at a haematocrit of only 40%[6]. In the vortex produced by a stenosis platelet aggregation is increased in the presence of red cells, and the number of platelets thrown on to the wall in a model system is also dependent on haematocrit[29]. A model of a bifurcation such as the origin of the internal carotid artery shows that platelets (and red cells) will tend to be thrown against the wall just beyond the point of branching – the usual site of mural thrombus formation in the neck.

It thus seems likely that the mechanical effect of red cells may be enough to give them an important role in influencing flow characteristics and platelet behaviour. In a whole blood aggregometer Pollock *et al.*[37] have shown that platelet aggregation as measured by impedence changes is affected by the relative number of red cells.

White blood cells may also contribute to the pathogenesis of thrombosis and tissue ischaemia. Thus on the one hand leukocytes have a powerful ADP-ase and this may limit the second phase of aggregation *in vivo*, when white cells are incorporated on the edge of growing thrombi. They also contribute to the impaired filterability of whole blood which is detectable in patients with peripheral vascular disease.

ANTI-PLATELET DRUGS

Do the results of trials of anti-platelet drugs add usefully to the information about the role of platelets and thromboembolism in TIA and stroke? Aspirin irreversibly acetylates platelet oxygenase, blocking the breakdown of arachidonic acid in platelets and inhibiting the secondary phase of aggregation to ADP, and blocking that caused by collagen. Theoretically it is therefore a powerful antithrombotic material (if thrombosis is due to pathological activation of this pathway of platelet activation). Aspirin also inhibits prostacyclin formation by the vessel wall and theoretically this could be a prothrombotic effect. However, the effect on the vessel wall is reversible and intermittent aspirin dosages could allow intermittent recovery of prostacyclin synthesis, and maintain a paralysis of TXA_2 production. Also there is a dose response difference. The concentration of aspirin that inhibits platelet cyclo-oxygenase is smaller than that required to block prostacyclin formation by the vessel wall[32]. At high doses aspirin also decreases levels of factors II, VII, IX and X. The net effect is to prolong the bleeding time whether 1.3 G or 0.3 G/day is chosen as the therapeutic regime, suggesting antiplatelet aggregant effects predominate *in vivo*. Neither aspirin, nor sulphinpyrazone which causes reversible inhibition of platelet cyclo-oxygenase, inhibits aggregation induced by high concentrations of collagen or thrombin.

In practice aspirin clearly prevents some patients' TIAs. This is most obvious in cases of frequent episodes of amaurosis fugax[21] and in personal experience in a few patients with cerebral ischaemic attacks lasting 1 to 3 minutes only. These may be the patients in whom pure platelet aggregates form the embolic material. In wider surveys of TIAs, the therapeutic effect of aspirin is less dramatic. Thus the reduction of TIA and stroke frequency in the Canadian Trial was only just significant at the 5% level[5] (*Table 7.3*). Before it is concluded that this represents

Table 7.3 Aspirin treatment of TIAs

Reference	Number in trial	Stroke and/or death	
		Treated	Placebo
Fields *et al.*[15a, 15b]	303	21/153	27/150
Canadian study[5]	585	46/290	68/295

slender evidence that platelets are involved in the pathogenesis of TIAs and strokes it should be remembered that aspirin does not inhibit platelet aggregation under all circumstances, that at doses chosen prostacyclin synthesis is also inhibited, and that many of the patients may have not had thromboembolic attacks.

There is other evidence that aspirin may not *in vivo* live up to its theoretical promise. Thus in a small series of patients Ezekowitz *et al.*[15] (1981) showed that aspirin failed to limit incorporation of indium III labelled platelets into cardiac thrombi. Karino and Goldsmith[29] found no evidence that aspirin could inhibit the formation of platelet aggregates in the vortex below a stenosis. Also Pollock and Harrison[37] found in an impedence platelet aggregometer that aspirin showed much less inhibition of aggregation in whole blood than in platelet rich plasma, and *ex vivo* aggregation in whole blood was little affected (*Table 7.4*). Red blood cells also interfere with the effect of aspirin on platelet adhesion to denuded endothelium[6]. This phenomenon may be due to the way red blood cells cause peripheral

Table 7.4 Mean platelet aggregation following incubation with aspirin or saline ($n = 5$) by impedance and optical density techniques

	Saline	*Aspirin*	*% Change*	
Blood (ohms)	11.7 ± 2.7	15.4 ± 2.7	+ 32	NS
PRP (ohms)	13.0 ± 4.3	9.1 ± 4.7	− 33	$P < 0.02$
PRP (Arbitrary units, OD)	28.0 ± 2.7	21.3 ± 4.4	− 24	$P < 0.05$

movement of platelets on to the vessel wall[29], or to the acceleration of aggregation by red cell haemolysis[3].

Dipyridamole has a weak effect against platelet aggregation *in vitro* but powerfully inhibits the appearance of an intraluminae platelet mass at the site of vascular injury in an experimental model of vessel occlusion[13]. Its effect on platelet behaviour depends on phosphodiesterase inhibition with elevation of platelet cAMP levels. The mechanism of action in the *in vivo* model has not been elucidated, but it has been found that dipyridamole can inhibit the effect of platelet derived mitogenic factor on the proliferation in cell culture of vascular smooth muscle[18]. This potentially anti-atheroma effect of dipyridamole is therefore being pursued (*Table 7.5*). It can be combined with aspirin with synergistic platelet

Table 7.5 Effect of dipyridamole on experimental arteriosclerosis

Baboons	*n*	*Cell loss (%)*	*Platelet survival (loss)*	*Intimal lesion (score)*
Control	8	0	5.4 ± 0.1	4 ± 1
Homocysteinemic	15	9.6 ± 2.2	2.8 ± 0.3	63 ± 5
Dipyridamole treated homocysteinemic	11	7.0 ± 0.9	4.8 ± 0.2	16 ± 2

Proportion of aorta not covered by endothelium after homocysteine infusions (cell loss); platelet survival by Cr method; and degree of smooth muscle cell proliferation and connective tissue formation (intimal lesion score) with or without oral dipyridamole given for 3 months from Harker *et al.*17

aggregation effects. Trials of the combination are under way in North America. In a small study, dipyridamole alone failed to affect the outcome in patients with TIAs[1] (*See* Chapter 10).

Sulphinpyrazone reversibly inhibits platelet cyclo-oxygenase and thereby inhibits platelet aggregation. Unlike aspirin it prolongs the shortened life span of labelled platelets in patients with, for example, prosthetic heart valves. Despite these apparently beneficial antithrombotic properties sulphinpyrazone failed to show a stroke-preventing effect in the Canadian trial[5] though it had apparently, like aspirin, stopped some patients' attacks of amaurosis fugax[14].

These differences in trial success of aspirin, sulphinpyrazone and dipyridamole raise certain important points. Simple platelet aggregation as produced *in vitro* by collagen or ADP cannot be the cause of the majority of strokes or at least two of these three agents would have shown greater efficacy in the preliminary trials.

Tests for abnormal platelet behaviour in patients with vascular disease are again called into question. One drug (ASA) unable to affect the shortened platelet half-life of patients with thromboembolic problems, is more effective in a clinical trial than one able to affect that half life (sulphinpyrazone). Perhaps the tests are assessing the wrong parameters of platelet function – perhaps the platelets are the innocent cars in a traffic jam caused by a fault in the tar macadam – to test their engines and brakes is unlikely to explain why the traffic jam occurred. We need to develop techniques that reveal the dynamic disturbances due to the development of atheroma, the effect of plaque rupture and haemorrhage, the causes for ulceration and the interaction between diseased intima and passing platelets. We need to consider the red and white cells as active, rather than inactive, participants in thrombosis and as determinants of flow characteristics. Finally we need to realize that when we carry out a therapeutic trial we are asking two parallel questions – does the intention to treat TIA and stroke patients with an 'antithrombotic' drug succeed in preventing strokes during follow-up – and does such success help to tell us the mechanism by which such strokes develop? The success of drugs such as aspirin and dipyridamole will not in any simple way reveal the exact mechanism of thrombogenesis and their failure will not necessarily negate a role for thrombosis. However, the explosion of knowledge, particularly of prostaglandin pathways in platelets and vessel walls, promises much in the coming years.

References

1 ACHESON, J., DANTA, G. and HUTCHINSON, E. C. Controlled trial of dipyridamole in cerebrovascular disease. *British Medical Journal*, **1**, 614–615 (1969)

2 BARNETT, H. J. M. Pathogenesis of transient ischaemic attacks. In *Cerebrovascular Disease*, edited by R. Scheinberg, 1–14. New York: Raven Press (1976)

3 BORN, G. V. R. and WEHMEIER, A. Inhibition of platelet thrombosis formation by chlorporamazine acting to diminish haemolysis. *Nature*, **282**, 212–213 (1979)

4 BUSUTTIL, R. W., BAKER, J. D., DAVIDSON, R. K. and MACHLEDER, H. I. Carotid artery stenosis – haemodynamic significance and clinical course. *Journal of the American Medical Association*, **245**, 1438–1441 (1981)

5 CANADIAN CO-OPERATIVE STROKE STUDY GROUP. A randomised trial of aspirin and sulphinpyrazone in threatened stroke. *New England Journal of Medicine*, **299**, 53–59 (1978)

6 DAVIES, J. A., ESSIEN, E., CAZENAVE, J. P., KINLOUGH-RATHBONE, R. L., GENT, M. and MUSTARD, J. F. The influence of aspirin and sulphinpyrazone on platelet adherence to damaged rabbit aorta. *British Journal of Haematology*, **42**, 283–291 (1979)

7 DAVIES, J. A. and McNICOL, G. P. Detection of a prethrombotic state. In *Haemostasis and Thrombosis*, edited by A. L. Bloom and D. P. Thomas, 593–609. Edinburgh: Churchill Livingstone (1981)

8 DE BONO, D. P. and WARLOWE, C. P. Potential sources of emboli in patients with presumed transient cerebral or retinal ischaemia. *Lancet*, **1**, 343–346 (1981)

9 DENNY-BROWN, D. and MEYER, J. S. The cerebral collateral circulation. 2. Production of cerebral infarction by ischaemic anoxia and its reversibility in early stages. *Neurology* (Minneapolis), **7**, 567–579 (1957)

10 DUGUID, J. B. *The Dynamics of Atherosclerosis*. Aberdeen: University Press (1976)

11 EASTCOTT, H. H. G., PICKERING, G. W. and ROB, C. Reconstruction of internal carotid artery in a patient with intermittent attacks of hemiplegia. *Lancet*, **2**, 994–946 (1954)

12 EINSIEDEL-LECHTAPE, H. Secondary emboli: a frequent sequela of complete internal carotid occlusion. *Neuroradiology*, **16**, 96–100 (1978)

13 EMMONS, D. R., HARRISON, M. J. G., HONOUR. A. J. and MITCHELL, J. R. A. Effect of a pyrimido-pyrimidine derivative on thrombus formation in the rabbit. *Nature*, **208**, 255–257 (1965)

14 EVANS, G. Effect of platelet suppressive agents on the incidence of amaurosis fugax and transient ischaemia. In *Cerebral Vascular Diseases, 8th Conference*, edited by F. McDowell and R. Brennan 297–299. New York: Grune and Stratton (1973)

15 EZEKOWITZ, M. D., COX, A. C. and TAYLOR, F. B. Failure of aspirin to prevent incorporation of indium-III labelled platelets into cardiac thrombi in man. *Lancet*, **2**, 440–443 (1981)

15a FIELDS, W. S., LEMAK, N. A., FRANKOWSKI, R. F. and HARDY, R. J. Controlled trial of aspirin in cerebral ischemia. *Stroke*, **8**, 310–315 (1977)

15b FIELDS, W. S., LEMAK, N. A., FRANKOWSKI, R. F. and HARDY, R. J. Controlled trial of aspirin in cerebral ischemia; part II – surgical group. *Stroke*, **9**, 309–318 (1978)

16 GAUTIER, J. C. and MORELOT, D. Infarctus cerebraux. *Nouvelle Presse Medicale*, **4**, 75–80 (1975)

17 HARKER, L. A., ROSS, R., SLICHER, S. J. and SCOTT, C. R. Homocipten induced arteriosclerosis. The role of endothelial cell injury and platelet response in its genesis. *Journal of Clinical Investigation*, **58**, 731–741 (1976)

18 HARKER, I. A. Platelets. In *Recent Advances in Haematology*, Volume 2, edited by A. V. Hoffbrand, M. C. Brain and J. Hirsch, 349–373. Edinburgh: Churchill Livingstone (1977)

18a HARRISON, M. J. G. Surgery for ischaemic stroke. *British Journal of Hospital Medicine*, **24**, 108–112 (1980)

19 HARRISON, M. J. G. Pathogenesis. In *Transient Ischaemic Attacks*, edited by C. Warlowe and P. Morris. New York: Marcel Dekker Ltd (1982)

19a HARRISON, M. J. G. Carotid endarterectomy. In *Topical Reviews in Neurosurgery Vol. I*, edited by J. M. Rice Edwards, Bristol: Wright, P. S. G. (1982)

20 HARRISON, M. J. G. and MITCHELL, J. R. A. The influence of red blood cells on platelet adhesiveness. *Lancet*, **2**, 1163–1164 (1966)

21 HARRISON, M. J. G., MEADOWS, J. C., MARSHALL, J. and ROSS RUSSELL, R. W. Effect of aspirin in amaurosis fugax. *Lancet*, **2**, 743–744 (1971)

22 HARRISON, M. J. G. and MARSHALL, J. Angiographic appearance of carotid bifurcation in patients with completed stroke, transient ischaemic attacks and cerebral tumour. *British Medical Journal*, **1**, 205–207 (1976)

23 HARRISON, M. J. G. and MARSHALL, J. The finding of thrombus at carotid endarterectomy and its relationship to the timing of surgery. *British Journal of Surgery*, **64,** 511–512 (1977)

24 HARRISON, M. J. G., POLLOCK, S., KENDALL, B: E. and MARSHALL, J. Effect of haematocrit on carotid stenosis and cerebral infarction. *Lancet,* **2,** 114–115 (1981)

25 HARRISON, M. J. G., POLLOCK, S., THOMAS, D. and MARSHALL, J. Haematocrit, hypertension, and smoking in patients with transient ischaemic attacks and in age and sex matched controls. *Journal of Neurology, Neurosurgery and Psychiatry*, **45,** 550–551 (1982)

26 HEPTINSTALL, S., MULLEY, G. P., TAYLOR, P. M. and MITCHELL, H. P. A. Platelet release reaction in myocardial infarction. *British Medical Journal*, **1,** 80–81 (1980)

27 JEYNES, B. J. and WARREN, B. A. Thrombogenicity of components of atheromatous material. *Archives of Pathology and Clinical Medicine*, **105,** 353–357 (1981)

28 JOHNSTON, R. V., REAVEY, M. M., LOWE, G. D. O., FORBES, C. D. and PRENTICE, C. R. M. Platelet aggregates in cerebrovascular disease – correlation with fibrinogen. In *Progress in Stroke Research*, Volume 1, edited by R. M. Greehalgh and F. C. Rose, 212–216. London: Pitman Medical (1979)

29 KARINO, T. and GOLDSMITH, H. L. Aggregation of human platelets in an annular vortex distal to a tubular expansion. *Microvascular Research*, **17,** 217–237 (1979)

30 LHERMITTE, F. Sites of cerebral arterial occlusions. In *Modern Trends in Neurology*, **6,** edited by D. Williams, 123–140, London: Butterworths (1975)

31 McAULEY, D. and ROSS RUSSELL, R. W. Correlation of CAT scan and visual field defects in vascular lesions of the posterior visual pathways. *Journal of Neurology, Neurosurgery and Psychiatry*, **42,** 298–311 (1979)

32 MITCHELL, J. R. A. Prostaglandins in vascular disease: a seminal approach. *British Medical Journal*, **282,** 590–594 (1981)

33 MITCHELL, J. R. A. and SCHWARTZ, C. J. *Arterial Disease.* London: Blackwells (1965)

34 MOORE, W. S. and HALL, A. D. Importance of emboli from carotid bifurcation in pathogenesis of cerebral ischaemic attacks. *Archives of Surgery*, **101,** 708–716 (1970)

35 NARITOMI,H., SAKAI, F. and MEYER, J. S. Pathogenesis of transient ischaemic attacks within the vertebrobasilar arterial system. *Archives of Neurology*, **36,** 121–128 (1979)

36 PEABODY, G. L. Relations between arterial disease and visceral changes. *Transactions of the Association of Physicians*, **6,** 154–178 (1891)

37 POLLOCK, S., MOTT, G., STEWART, B. and HARRISON, M. J. G. The effect of aspirin on platelet behaviour in whole blood measured by impedance aggregometry. *British Medical Journal* (in press)

38 PRESTON, F. E., MARTIN, J. F., STEWART, R. M. and DAVIES-JONES, G. A. B. Thrombocytosis circulating platelet aggregates and neurological dysfunction. *British Medical Journal*, **2,** 1561–1563 (1979)

39 PRICE, T. R., GOTSHALL, R. A., POSKANZER, D. C., HAERER, A. F., SWANSON, P. D., CALANCHINI, B. R., CONNEALLY, M., DYKEN, M. L. and FUTTY, D. E. Co-operative study of hospital frequency and character of transient ischaemic attacks. *Journal of the American Medical Association*, **238,** 2512–2515 (1977)

40 REED, R. L., SIEKERT, R. G. and MERIDETH, J. Rarity of transient focal cerebral ischaemia in cardiac dysrythmia. *Journal of the American Medical Association*, **223**, 893–895 (1973)

41 RILEY, T. J. and FRIEDMAN, J. M. Stroke, orthostatic hypotension and focal seizures. *Journal of the American Medical Association*, **245**, 1243–1244 (1981)

42 RUFF, R. L., TALMAN, W. T. and PETITO, F. Transient ischaemic attacks associated with hypotension in patients with carotid artery stenosis. *Stroke*, **12**, 353–355 (1981)

43 RUSSELL, R. W. R. The source of retinal emboli. *Lancet*, **2**, 789–792 (1968)

44 THIELE, B. L., YOUNG, J. V., CHIKOS, P. M., HIRSCH, J. H. and STRANDNESS, D. E. Correlation of arteriographic findings and symptoms in cerebrovascular disease. *Neurology*, **30**, 1041–1046 (1980)

45 WALSH, P. N., KANSU, T. A., CORBETT, J. J., SAVINO, P. J., GOLDBURGH, W. P. and SCHATZ, N. J. Platelets thromboembolism and mitral valve prolapse. *Circulation*, **63**, 552–559 (1981)

46 WILSON, J. A. Platelets in *Amaurosis fugax*. In *Acetylsalicylic Acid in Cerebral Ischaemia and Coronary Heart Disease* edited by K. Breddin, W. Domdorf, D. Loew and R. Marx, 113–117. Stuttgart: Slatteuer Verlag (1978)

47 WILSON, L. A., WARLOW, C. P. and ROSS RUSSELL, R. W. Cardiovascular disease in patients with retinal arterial occlusion. *Lancet*, **1**, 292–294 (1979)

48 ZAHARI, J., BETTERIDGE, J. D., JONES, N. A. G., GALTON, D. U. and KAKKAR, V. V. Enhanced *in vivo* platelet release reaction and malonaldehyde formation in patients with hyperlipidaemia. *American Journal of Medicine*, **70**, 59–64 (1981)

49 ZULCH, K. J. Discussion in *Brain and Heart Infarct*, edited by K. J. Zulch, W. Kaufman, K. A. Hossman and V. Hossmann, 205. Berlin: Springer Verlag (1977)

8
Angiography and computed tomography scanning
Michael J. G. Harrison

The neuroradiological investigation of patients with ischaemic cerebrovascular disease is directed towards two different problems, the analysis of cerebral lesions and the vascular pathology.

(1) Firstly, what is the nature of any cerebral lesion?
(2) Have brief symptoms (transient ischaemic attack – TIA –) nonetheless been produced by a demonstrable infarct?
(3) Have established symptoms been caused by haemorrhage or infarction?
(4) Further, is that infarct lacunar or cortical?
(5) How large is the infarct.?
(6) Is it accompanied by oedema and mass effect?
(7) How old does the infarct look?
(8) Where is it? Is it in the centre of the territory of a major cerebral vessel, or is it in a watershed zone?
(9) Is the infarct haemorrhagic, raising doubts about the safety of anticoagulation, or is it multifocal and bilateral suggesting a cardiac source for embolism?

These questions are now answerable in most patients by computed tomography (CT) scanning. Additional evidence may soon be available on the extent of infarction and ischaemic oedema from nuclear magnetic resonance (NMR) scanning[3].

The second set of questions surround the nature of the vascular lesion.

(1) Is there a source for embolism in major neck vessels or are they occluded?
(2) Are there intracranial stenoses and occlusions, and if so has a collateral circulation developed?
(3) Is there an anomalous Circle of Willis limiting collateral potential?
(4) What do the arterial walls look like?
(5) If there is evidence of plaque formation does it appear ulcerated, and does it seem likely that any stenoses are haemodynamically significant?

(6) Are there signs of an unusual arterial pathology such as an arteritis, fibro-muscular dysplasia, or dissection of a major vessel?

(7) Is the lesion after all venous and not arterial (Chapter 12)?

Most of these questions are to be answered by angiography sometimes sup-plemented by non-invasive techniques (Chapter 9), and by methods of assessment of cerebral blood flow (Chapter 4). To date the use of arterial angiography predominates, providing high resolution imaging of arterial vessels extracranially and intracranially albeit with a small, but definite, mortality and morbidity[19, 23]. The advent of digital subtraction angiography (DSA)[26] promises to provide essentially the same information after intravenous injection at much less risk to the patient, and with the possibility of serial studies rarely ethically acceptable with arterial injections. DSA studies are currently producing films of diagnostic quality in some 85% of cases, but there are problems with movement and swallowing artefact, and in obtaining intracranial views and extracranial views simultaneously.

NATURE OF THE CEREBRAL LESION

Transient ischaemic attack (TIA)

The definition of a TIA implies that only reversible paresis of cerebral metabolism has occurred, flow presumably remaining above the critical threshold for cell death or recovering to such a level before irreversible changes have occurred[13]. The arbitrariness of the definition i.e. symptoms resolving within 24 hours, means that it should have come as no surprise when CT scans revealed evidence of small areas of infarction or atrophy in many such patients. At first it might seem that only those patients whose symptoms have lasted many hours will be found to show infarction but in fact several cases have been described with symptoms lasting only 5 minutes with an appropriately sited small infarct (*Table 8.1*)[21]. EEG studies and measures of regional cerebral blood flow also attest the lasting sequelae of some brief TIAs. Personal experience suggests that brief symptoms with associated irritative phe-nomena e.g. twitching of the mouth combined with transient weakness of the ipsilateral arm and leg are most likely to be accompanied by CT scan evidence of infarction.

Table 8.1. CT scan evidence of infarction in TIA and RINDs, modified from Hum-phrey and Marshall[21]

Infarction (%)	Duration of symptoms
17	5 min
23	5–30 min
14	30 min–24 h
52	1–21 d

Although haemorrhage may produce brief symptoms, TIAs are probably never due to this cause. TIAs are rare in the histories of patients with proven cerebral haemorrhage[12] and I am not aware of a single report of a haemorrhage in any of the surveys of TIAs. The shortest clinical episode associated with a proven haemorrhage in personal experience lasted 5 days.

The value of CT scans in TIA patients includes the detection of infarction, the presence of which may add to the risks of vascular surgery[35] (Chapter 11), and the possibility of finding unsuspected other causes of transient symptoms such as tumours, arterio-venous malformations, and subdural haematomas[13].

Reversible ischaemic neurologic deficit (RIND)

The stroke programme at the National Institutes of Health Bethesda has proposed that patients recovering from ischaemic focal deficits inside 3 weeks should be separately classified. The term reversible ischaemic neurologic deficit (RIND) has been adopted for these cases. Infarction is assumed to have occurred but to have been small or so placed as to have had limited effects on structures like the motor cortex or capsule. Many lacunar lesions are included in this group. Humphrey and Marshall showed that some 50% of such cases have an infarct on CT scanning, a prevalence greater than for TIAs[21] (*Table 8.1*). Perrone also found that the infarcts (on CT scans) in RINDs were larger than those less frequently encountered in TIA[31].

Amongst those with the clinical features of lacunar infarction (pure motor hemiplegia, pure sensory stroke, the dysarthric clumsy hand syndrome, homolateral ataxia and crural paresis) the yield of infarcts on CT scanning is also about 50%. Though many of these lacunar strobes are found to be due to small deep infarcts, some have cortical larger infarcts suggesting that not all are due to hypertensive lipohyalinosis of small vessels.

As mentioned above, an occasional RIND will be found to be due to haemorrhage (*Figure 8.1*), or to tumour.

Completed stroke

Infarction can be reliably distinguished from haemorrhage thanks to the high density lesion accompanying the latter, as long as the scan is obtained within 2 to 3 weeks of the stroke[22]. After this old haematomas may be indistinguishable from old infarcts. The distinction between infarction and tumour may not be as easy since in the early days following infarction oedema may give the latter mass effect (*Figure 8.2*). The use of contrast enhancement may be helpful (*see later*) but in some cases angiography or serial scanning may be necessary. After about 25 days infarcts no longer show mass effect so its presence late after a single clinical ictus would favour a tumour[4]. Chronic subdural haematomas may present with a stroke like sudden hemiplegia (*Figure 8.3*). They are readily detected by CT scanning except when isodense and bilateral. Xenon enhancement of the scan may help delineate the non-enhancing haematoma from the enhancing normal hemisphere. Xenon

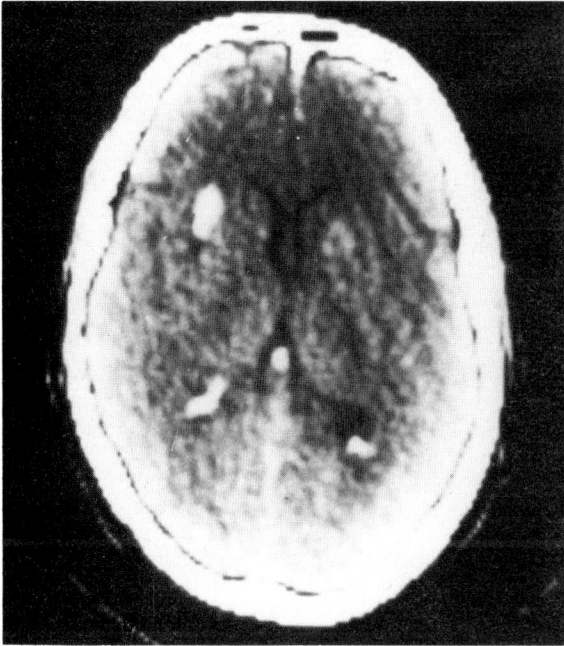

Figure 8.1 CT scan showing small fresh haematoma on left and fading haemorrhage on right. The patient's symptoms lasted 5 days

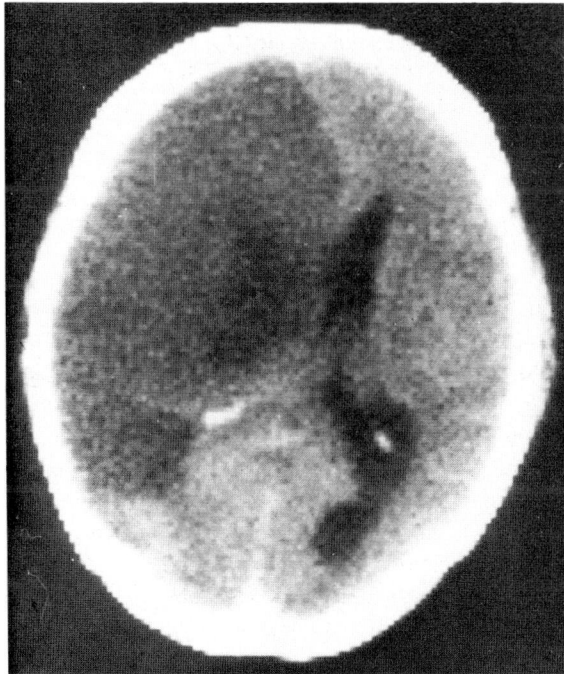

Figure 8.2 CT scan showing homogenous low density lesion due to recent infarction with oedema causing mass effect

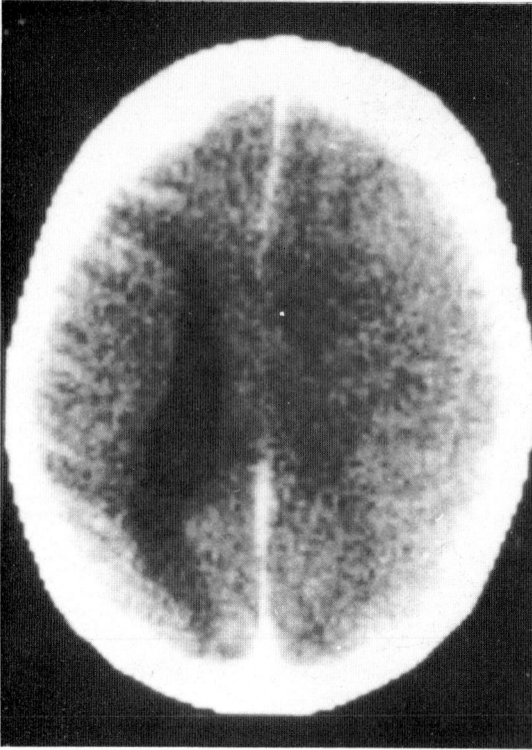

Figure 8.3 CT scan showing midline shift and occlusion of one ventricle due to an isodense sub-dural haematoma

enhancement may also help distinguish tumour and infarction which shows a slow build-up of enhancement[32].

Haematomas produce a focal high density lesion often surrounded by a rim of low density thought to represent the marginal zone of ischaemic necrosis seen pathologically[22]. Enhancement around the periphery may be difficult to interpret when the haematoma has resolved and at this stage the appearance can be of a low density lesion with ring enhancement. The differential diagnosis includes cerebral abscess etc. though the latter usually produces more associated oedema than expected with a mature haematoma. Cerebral haemorrhage is discussed in detail in Chapter 13.

Infarction may be identified as a low density lesion in 50–75% of cases[30]. Normal scans may be attained when the lacunar infarcts are small, especially in the brain stem and pons. Other scans are negative because of their timing. Thus though scans are often positive on day 1, the low density change at this stage is often vague and it's margins are ill defined. The highest yield is at about 8–11 days after the clinical onset. Mature infarcts show an area of density which has a sharp margin 10–20 Houndsfield numbers below that of the surrounding brain (*Figure 8.4*). There is associated atrophy with dilation of the ipsilateral ventricle, and of overlying cortical sulci. As early scans may not reveal an infarct, a normal appearance in the context

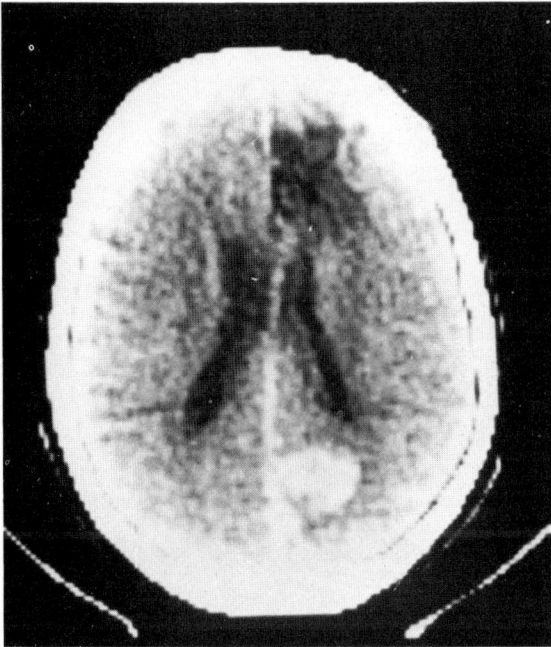

Figure 8.4 CT scan showing a recent enhancing occipital infarct and a mature non-enhancing frontal infarct. (Scan kindly supplied by Dr. A. Valentine)

of a sudden hemiplegia, say, may be considered to be evidence of an ischaemic lesion. When this happens the scan should be repeated in a week or so for confirmation. In some patients the infarct is initially isodense but enhances (*Figure 8.5*). Injections of contrast should therefore be given to increase the rate of detection of infarcts, and to provide more information about any low density lesion. Contrast enhancement is often characteristically of a gyral pattern (*Figure 8.5*) but may be central, peripheral, homogenous (*Figure 8.6*) or heterogenous[30]. In some it is indistinguishable from the enhancement seen in intracerebral tumours. With high volumes of injected contrast material the vast majority of infarcts will show enhancement. Enhancement may be seen in the first 24 hours but is best seen in weeks 1 to 4[7]. Rarely enhancement is still detectable months later. Xenon enhancement may reveal a peripheral zone of enhancement around a non-enhancing centre.

Oedema is common though usually only minor in extent. Initially the low density area is homogenous and the only evidence that part of this oedema is the accompanying mass effect (*Figure 8.2*). The relative extent of necrosis and oedema may be discernible from NMR imaging. Infarct oedema is of mixed aetiology (cytotoxic and vasogenic), and infarcts only rarely show the digital pattern on CT scans characteristic of vasogenic oedema around tumours and abscesses. Swelling of the infarcted area may be detectable on the first day when it is probably a reflection of early vasogenic change associated with necrosis. It is at its greatest however, after 3 to 5 days and this coincides with the peak incidence of death due to

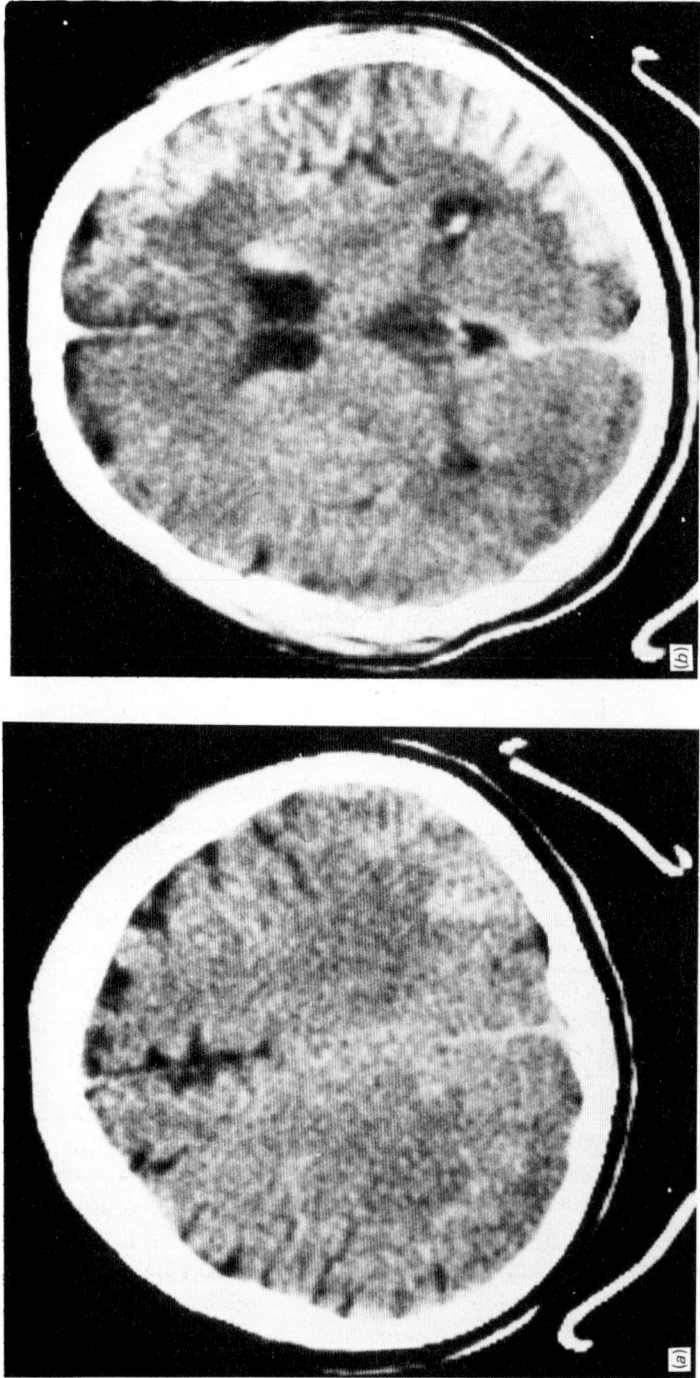

Figure 8.5 CT scans (a) with and (b) without contrast medium in a patient with a recent infarct. There is extensive 'gyral' enhancement (Scans kindly supplied by Dr. A. Valentine)

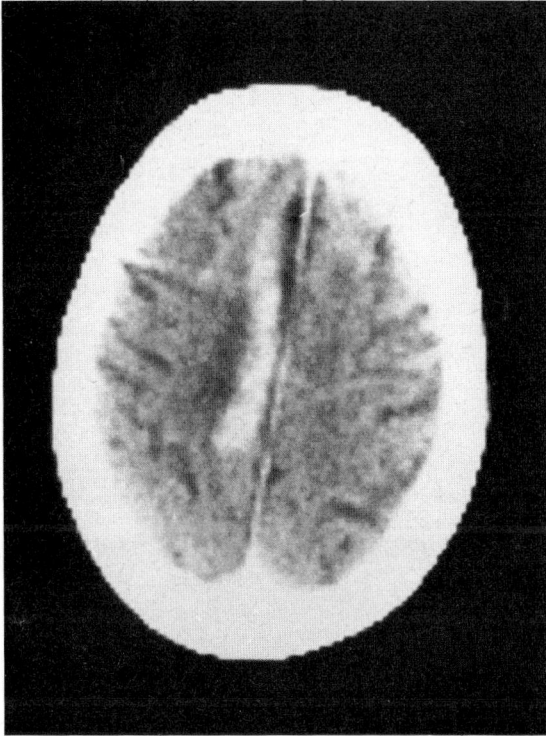

Figure 8.6 CT scan showing homogenous enhancement of a recent infarct in the territory of the anterior cerebral artery. (Scan kindly supplied by Dr. C. J. Earl)

herniation. Oedema resolves by 10–20 days and is rarely detectable in the absence of re-infarction after 25 days.

Haemorrhagic infarction produces an appearance intermediate between that of infarction and frank haemorrhage. The hyper-density is patchy and is seen within an overall area of low density that may be wedge-shaped and occupy the territory of say the middle cerebral artery. There is no low density rim as seen with a primary haematoma. Follow-up scans show the development of a mature infarct.

Watershed infarction occurs in a systemic haemodynamic crisis e.g. cardiac arrest or, occasionally with extracranial carotid artery occlusion. Low density areas appear at the junction of the territories of the posterior and middle, and middle and anterior cerebral arteries. These appearances are thus an indication to consider a haemodynamic mechanism for the clinical picture.

If CT scanning is unavailable radionuclide scans may prove useful and indeed the two techniques can be complementary[4, 9]. Campbell studied 141 infarcts and found that 8% were only detectable by CT scans, and 8% only visible on isotope encephalography. The differential diagnosis of tumour and infarction may be possible tumours tending to give a rounded area of uptake of isotope sparing the cortex, and infarcts a wedge-shaped area including the cortex. Subdural haematomas produce a crescentic area of uptake in 90% of instances. Unfortunately

204

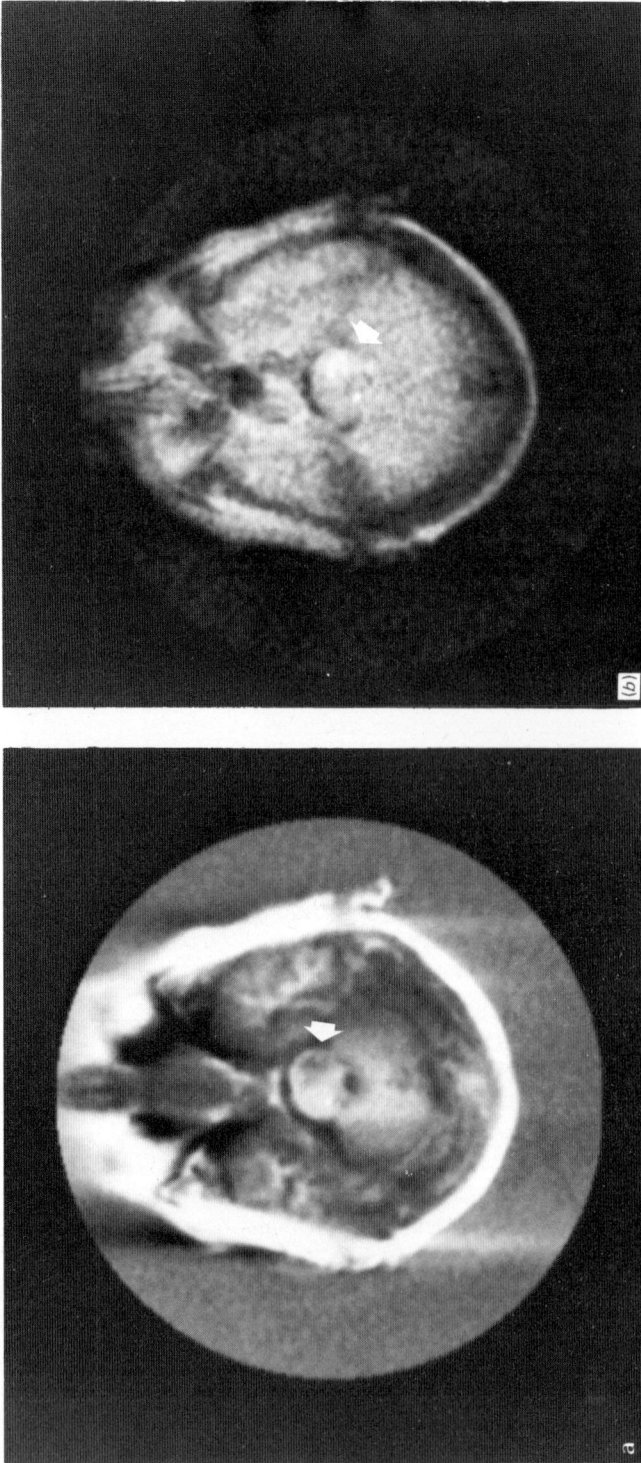

Figure 8.7 NMR scans showing a brain stem infarct, which appears dark on the T1 (a) scan and white on the T2 (b) scan. (Scans kindly supplied by Professor R. Steiner and Dr. N. J. Legg)

haematoma and infarction can not be distinguished reliably and this limits the value of isotope scanning in the investigation of the nature of the cerebral lesion in stroke victims.

The use of new isotopes, e.g. ^{123}I-labelled amphetamine derivatives, promises to provide extra information; uptake reflecting regional blood supply as well as being influenced by metabolic parameters. Infarcts appear as areas of non-perfusion, tumours as areas of high uptake.

NMR scanning also promises to help in the distinction between necrosis and oedema. The loss of grey-white matter contrast on NMR scans may prove to be the most sensitive index of infarction (*Figure 8.7*)[26].

Angiography may be needed to make the distinction between haematoma, infarct and tumour, especially in centres lacking CT scanning facilities. Tumours show mass effect with abnormal tissue vascularity including tumour circulation. Haematomas cause an avascular mass, rarely with extravasation of contrast medium, or visualization of the origin of the bleed if aneurysmal or due to an arteriovenous malformation. Infarcts are revealed as areas of avascularity with loss of capillary blush. Flow abnormalities are commonly present with slow flow, late filling of branches, stasis and delayed venous opacification being more common than high flow with early filling veins in hyperemic areas[34].

The detection of areas of ischaemia and infarction by positron emission tomographic scanning is discussed in Chapters 4 and 5.

NATURE OF THE VASCULAR LESION

Transient ischaemic attack (TIA)

In the discussion on pathogenesis in Chapter 7 it was argued that haemodynamic events rarely cause focal TIAs, and that a cardiac source for embolism may account for up to 25% of cases. Careful cardiac auscultation, chest X-rays, and a 12 lead ECG may well detect most of the relevant cardiac conditions but Holter monitoring and 2D echocardiography may be necessary to exclude vegetations, and to detect mitral valve prolapse and arrythrmias. Radionuclide cardiac scans may also be valuable in detecting akinetic segments due to old myocardial infarction. These may be the site of mural thrombus which may also be detectable by Indium III platelet scanning or CT chest scans. Left venticulography may be possible with DSA as an additional means of detecting intra-cardiac thrombus.

In some 60% of cases however the evidence is that the source of embolism lies in the neck vessels[14]. The role of non-invasive investigation in the detection of plaques of atheroma in neck vessels is discussed in detail in Chapter 9. Whilst angiography is recognised as the gold standard for the detection of such changes, and is currently the only sure way of identifying stenosis of intracranial vessels, arterial injections carry a mortality and morbidity. In the co-operative study[19] (1968) the mortality of angiography was 0.7% and the risk of permanent neurological deficit 0.5%. The risks of neurological deterioration were greater in those with preceding neurological deficit and in the presence of occlusion or tight stenosis

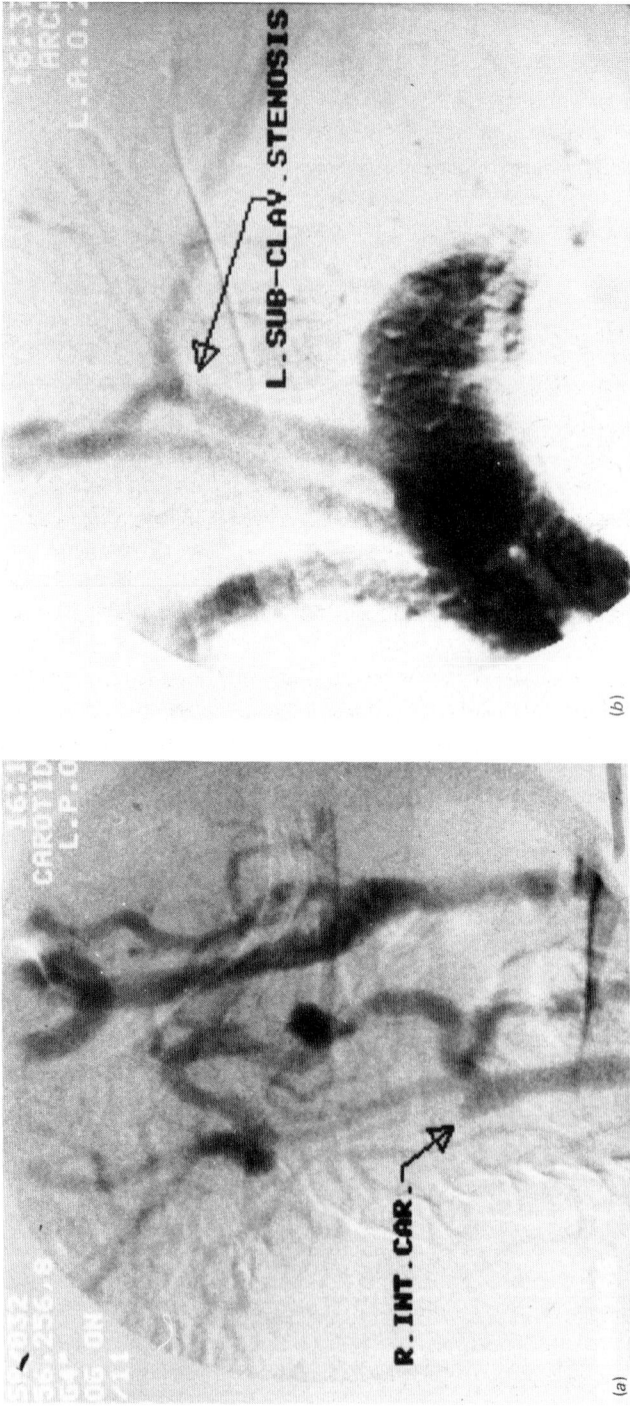

Figure 8.8 Digital subtraction angiograms revealing internal carotid artery occlusion (a) and subclavian artery stenosis (b). (Films kindly supplied by Dr. A. Valentine)

of major vessels. Subintimal tears and intramural injections had caused some of the deterioration. In a recent study of catheter angiography[27] the mortality had fallen to 0.02% and the serious morbidity to 0.04%. Because of this risk, only patients being considered for vascular surgery will be referred for conventional (arterial) angiography.

A larger number of individuals can be considered for intravenous DSA as it carries a much smaller risk (*Figure 8.8*). If DSA is used to screen patients with TIA for surgical lesions, it must be accepted that some will fail to get films of diagnostic quality and arterial injection will then be necessary[26]. Non-invasive techniques may also be used to screen these patients and those with asymptomatic bruits. Selective catheter angiography may then be used to get detailed views of any lesion being considered for endarterectomy. Digital subtraction may be chosen for the selective angiography since it permits use of a smaller volume of contrast medium reducing its hyperosmolar or other effects. The other advantage of intravenous angiography with simultaneous opacification of all neck vessels is that it reveals the state of collateral supply around and above any tight stenosis or occlusion. Hand injection of selected neck vessels only reveals the anatomy of potential collateral. The intravenous technique is capable of showing the route by which blood is actually reaching the territory distal to vascular lesions.

When patients with TIAs in the carotid territory are investigated by angiography 50 to 60% are found to have atheromatous disease at the carotid bifurcation and/or intracranially[14]. Intracranial stenosis, for example of the carotid artery in the carotid siphon, in patients with severe stenosis at the bifurcation (the so-called tandem lesion) must be interpreted with caution since low flow may give an artefactual appearance of a narrow lumen. Such appearances intracranially may return to normal after successful endarterectomy at the bifurcation.

The carotid lesion is classically in the carotid sinus and the plaques are often eccentrically placed and only detectable if biplanar views are obtained after selective injection of the common carotid artery. Otherwise plaques enface are missed. Magnification may help detect small plaques as may the technique of trickle angiography. The degree of abnormality varies enormously from a tight stenosis with slow distal flow (the rat tail sign) to minor irregularity. Comparison with angiograms carried out in patients with cerebral tumours reveals that minor irregularities are also common in such individuals and it is therefore unwise to conclude that such appearances are necessarily causually related to symptoms of cerebral ischaemia[16].

It is believed that ulceration of plaques and intraplaque haemorrhage trigger mural thrombo-embolism in TIA patients (Chapter 7). The angiographic detection of ulceration is however problematical (*Figure 8.9*). A double shadow or obvious filling of a crater is held to be indicative of ulceration. Unless the changes are gross however, the accuracy of prediction of the surgical or pathological findings proves poor. A post mortem study revealed that minor irregularity could be misconstrued as due to ulceration, and smooth looking plaques could prove to be the site of endothelial loss[5].

Although surgical specimens reveal haemorrhage into plaques to be common in TIA patients having a carotid endarterectomy, the radiological identification of

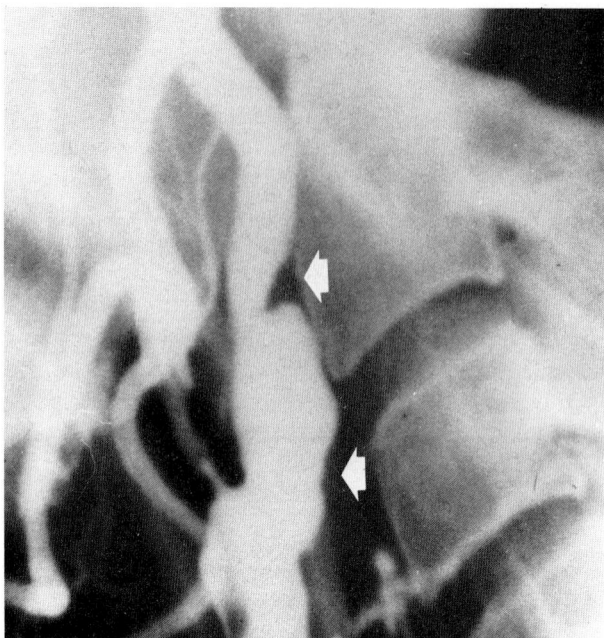

Figure 8.9 Carotid angiogram showing complicated irregular stenotic lesion at the bifurcation.

such a change is probably impossible, though a rounded filling defect has been suggested to be indicative. Surgical studies also reveal the presence of mural thrombus or friable loose material in 66% of those operated upon within a month of their last TIA. Despite this, angiographic identification of intraluminal thrombus is unusual (less than 10% in personal experience). Platelet scanning with Indium III as label may help detect such thrombi.

In some 10% of patients with carotid territory TIAs, angiograms reveal occlusion of the extracranial internal carotid (ECIC) artery. Whilst some of these patients' TIAs are haemodynamic in nature, and may be prevented by a successful ECIC bypass (Chapter 11), there is good evidence that embolism can occur above a carotid occlusion[1]. Emboli may leave the tail of the occluding thrombus. Einsiedel-Lechtape[8] showed by careful study of the intracranial circulation on the side of carotid occlusion (by injection of the contralateral carotid) that small embolic branch occlusions were present in some 60%. Barnett and his group have also drawn attention to the role of the stump of an occluded carotid artery as a source of emboli. The blind stump may harbour ulcerated plaques with fresh thrombus which may be swept into the external carotid artery and cause TIAs on entering the cerebral circulation through collaterals. If TIAs persist after prior demonstration of carotid occlusion, repeat angiography should both examine the bifurcation for evidence of a source of embolism in the stump, common carotid or external carotid artery, and provide the necessary information about the collateral bed and superficial temporal artery in preparation for bypass surgery.

Angiography is less often indicated in the case of TIAs in the vertebrobasilar territory. This is because surgical lesions are less commonly found, and surgery is less well established. Ulceration is unusual in plaques in the vertebral arteries. TIAs in this area may often be haemodynamically produced. Angiograms may reveal that neck turning occludes a dominant vertebral artery, or that there is a local narrowing opposite a prominent cervical osteophyte. Arch angiography may reveal the features of the subclavian steal syndrome with occlusion or stenosis of the proximal subclavian artery, and retrograde filling of the vertebral artery. Although this haemodynamic state of affairs is detected in up to 5% of patients with cerebrovascular disease it is rarely the cause of TIAs and rarely warrants surgery. It may, however, be important in planning surgery of other symptomatic lesions, such as a carotid stenosis.

On rare occasions angiography reveals an unusual non-atheromatous abnormality of neck vessels in patients with TIAs. Coils and kinks may or may not be relevant, their presence being little more frequent than in the control population[13]. Atheroma may develop at the site of a kink however and become a source for emboli. Arteritis or fibromuscular dysplasia may be revealed, the latter affecting the cervical part of the carotid artery often opposite C2, giving a beaded appearance to the vessel[20, 28]. Dissection of the internal carotid artery perhaps due to Marfans syndrome or to fibromuscular disease may produce a tapered appearance to the whole extracranial course of the vessel, a picture also occasionally seen in systemic lupus erythematosus, and after therapeutic irradiation of the neck. Dissection of the middle cerebral artery proved the cause of a TIA in one personal case (*Figure 8.10*).

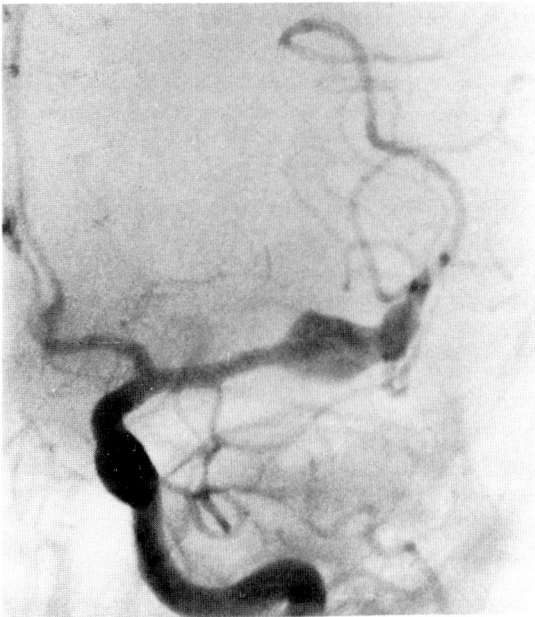

Figure 8.10 Carotid angiogram showing a dissecting aneurysm of the middle cerebral artery. (From Harrison, M. J. G. Dysphasia during sleep due to an unusual vascular lesion. *Journal of Neurology, Neurosurgery and Psychiatry*, **44**, 739 (1981), courtesy of the Editor and Publishers)

Reversible ischaemic neurologic deficits and lacunes

Angiographic study of patients with minor completed strokes recovering in a few weeks produces a mixed yield of carotid stenosis, intracranial embolic occlusions, and intracranial atheromatous disease. Patients presenting with lacunar syndromes commonly have little or no atheromatous change in neck vessels or major intracranial vessels and in these cases hypertensive changes in penetrating arteries are assumed. However Nelson *et al.*[29] showed that some of these patients had carotid stenosis or embolic middle cerebral occlusion so their angiographic investigation can be rewarding. Any suggestion of previous embolic events e.g. amaurosis fugax, bruits over neck vessels or evidence of large vessel disease elsewhere should prompt investigation for a possible source of embolism before attributing the neurological episode to small vessel changes. This is particularly true of the pure motor stroke. Lacunar syndromes such as homolateral ataxia and crural paresis are rarely thought to be due to embolism, and surgery in the vertebro-basilar territory is less likely to be considered in any case, so their angiographic investigation is unlikely to be considered. The yield of angiographic investigation in Humphrey and Marshall's study[21] of patients with stroke syndromes of different durations showed that patients with RINDs commonly (43%) had normal angiograms in keeping with the concept of small vessel disease. Thirteen per cent had a carotid stenosis and 17% occlusion however.

Completed strokes

At autopsy up to 50% of completed strokes are due to occlusion of neck vessels or more commonly intracerebral branches due to cardiac embolism[2]. This may partly reflect the mortality of such strokes since clinical studies suggest that perhaps only 25% have relevant cardiac disease. The yield of abnormalities on 2D echocardiography is small unless there is clinical evidence of heart disease. Atrial fibrillation of any cause is probably the commonest relevant cardiac abnormality.

A series of autopsy studies at the Salpetriere in Paris[25] revealed that infarcts in the middle cerebral territory were often due to extracranial carotid occlusion or to middle cerebral embolism from the heart or neck. Occlusions of the posterior cerebral artery and anterior cerebral artery were usually embolic from neck vessels. Occlusion of the basilar artery by contrast was normally due to *in situ* thrombosis. The rationale for the angiographic study of patients with established strokes due to cerebral infarction is thus to distinguish between occlusion of extracranial and intracerebral vessels and their branches, to search for a source of embolism, and to assess the development of collateral supply to the ischaemic area.

Angiographic surveys of completed hemisphere strokes due to infarction reveal occlusion of the internal carotid artery in some 20% of instances[11, 15, 16]. Embolic occlusions may be detected above such an occlusion in the siphon or in the anterior or middle cerebral arteries[8]. A rather larger number will have demonstrable embolic occlusions intracranially, proximal to carotid stenosis or atheroma or related to cardiac disease. The frequency with which such intracranial occlusions are discovered depends critically on the timing of angiography. This is due to the dissolution of embolic occlusions as first documented by Dalal[6]. In a valuable study Fieschi and Bozzao[10] showed that 49 of 86 patients studied within 3 days of sustaining a hemisphere infarct had vessel occlusions. Sixteen had occlusion of the internal carotid in the neck, six in the siphon (*Figure 8.11*). Twenty-seven had occlusions of the middle or anterior cerebral artery or of their branches. Subsequent angiograms or post mortem study showed dissolution of the occlusion in 10 of

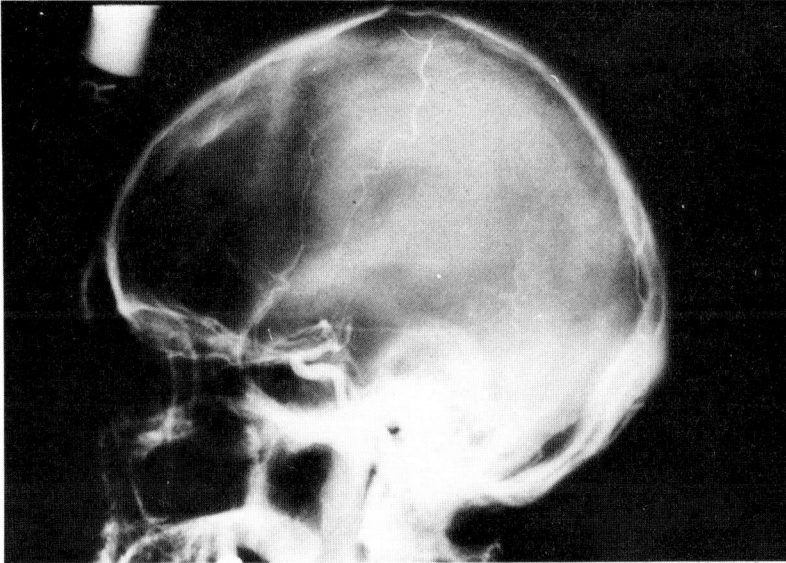

Figure 8.11 Carotid angiogram showing intracranial occlusion due to embolism

the intracranial examples but never of the cervical thrombosis. Normal angiography some days after the onset of an infarct probably therefore reflects the tendency for many intracerebral emboli to break up and move on. Ring[33] also claimed that most patients had evidence of intracranial embolic occlusions if studied early enough and if magnification techniques were used to look at small cortical branches of the middle cerebral arteries.

The difficulty in demonstrating ulceration of carotid atheroma as a source of cerebral emboli has already been noted. Kishore[24] however found angiographic evidence of middle cerebral emboli twice as often above irregular looking carotid plaques than smooth stenoses.

The demonstration of a carotid stenosis in patients with completed strokes may be important to the planning of delayed elective endarterectomy (Chapter 11), or of an ECIC bypass. If such a procedure is planned detailed angiography of the vascular pathology and of collateral channels may be necessary. In addition such patients may need measurement of regional cerebral blood volume and oxygen metabolism by positron emission tomography to define the pathophysiological state of the ischaemic area.

Infarction in the brain stem is not as commonly investigated by angiography. The demonstration of the site of occlusion for example in the basilar artery may

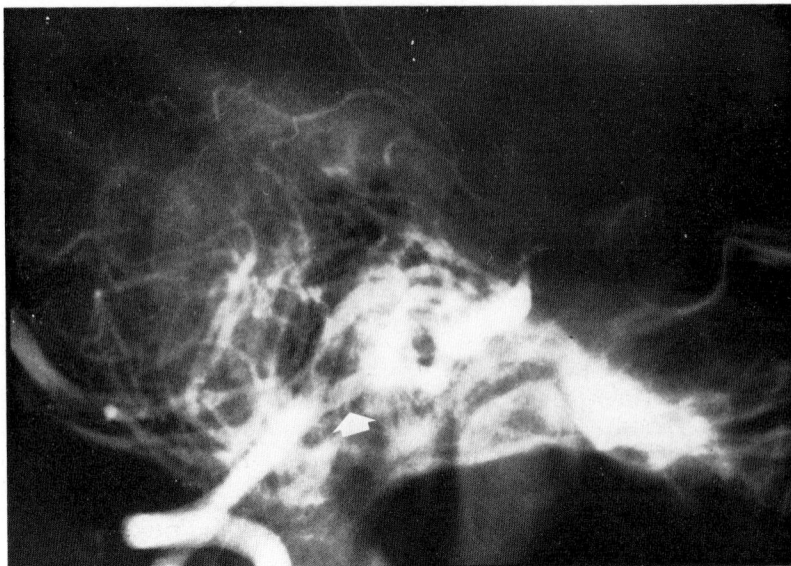

Figure 8.12 Vertebral angiogram showing lack of filling in the basilar artery due to local thrombosis

however have prognostic value (*Figure 8.12*). Surgery is rarely contemplated so the usual indication for angiography concerns the differential diagnosis of the cerebral lesion rather than the vascular cause.

In patients with multi-infarct dementia, angiography reveals intracranial atheromatous changes and in some the features of recent infarction[18].

PROGNOSIS

As already mentioned the site of basilar occlusion may relate to prognosis in patients with brain stem infarction. In the case of carotid disease a recent study has shown some prognostic pointers in the angiographic findings[17]. Subsequent strokes and overall mortality are greatest with carotid occlusion, and least with normal angiograms. The extent and severity of atheroma in patients referred for carotid endarterectomy also correlates with the operative morbidity[35].

References

1 BARNETT, H. J. M., PEERLESS, S. J., and KAUFMAN, J. C. E. Stump of internal carotid artery – a source for further cerebral embolic ischaemia. *Stroke*, **9**, 448–456 (1978)

2 BLACKWOOD, W., HALLPIKE, J. F., KOCEN, R. S. and MAIR, W. G. P. Atheromatous disease of the carotid arterial system and embolism from the heart in cerebral infarction: a morbid anatomical study. *Brain*, **22**, 897–910 (1969)

3 BYDDER G. M., STEINER, R. E., YOUNG, I. R., HALL, A. S., THOMAS, D. J., MARSHALL, J., PALLIS, C. A. and LEGG, N. J. Clinical NMR imaging of the brain: 140 cases. *American Journal of Roentgenology*, **139**, 215–236 (1982)

4 CAMPBELL, J. K., HOUSER, O. W., STEVENS, J. C., WAHNER, H. W., BAKER, H. L. and FOLGER, W. N. Computed tomography and radionuclide imaging in the evaluation of ischaemic stroke. *Radiology*, **126**, 695–702 (1978)

5 CROFT, R. J., ELLAM, L. D. and HARRISON, M. J. G. Accuracy of carotid angiography in the assessment of atheroma of the internal carotid artery. *Lancet*, **1**, 997–1000 (1980)

6 DALAL, P. M., SHAH, P. M., SHETH, S. C. and DESPHANDE, C. K. Cererbral embolism. Angiographic observations on spontaneous clot lysis. *Lancet*, **1**, 61–64 (1965)

7 DAVIS, K. R., ACKERMAN, R. H., KISTLER, J. P. and MOHR, J. P. Computed tomography of cerebral infarction: haemorrhagic, contrast enhancement, and time of appearance. *Computerised Tomography*, **1**, 77–86 (1977)

8 EINSIEDEL-LECHTAPE, H. Secondary emboli: a frequent sequela of complete extracranial internal carotid artery occlusion. *Neuroradiology*, **16**, 96–100 (1978)

9 ELL, P. J., DEACON, J. M. and JARRITT, P. M. *Atlas of Computerised Emission Tomography*. Churchill Livingstone, London. (1980)

10 FIESCHI C. and BOZZAO, L. Transient embolic occlusion of the middle cerebral and internal carotid arteries in cerebral apoplexy. *Journal of Neurology, Neurosurgery and Psychiatry*, **32**, 236–240 (1969)

11 GREITZ, T. Angiography in the investigation of patients with stroke. In *Thule International Symposium on Stroke*, edited by A. Engel and T. Larssen, 159–168 Nordiska: Stockholm (1967)

12 HARRISON, M. J. G. Clinical distinction of cerebral haemorrhage and cerebral infarction. *Postgraduate Medical Journal*, **56**, 629–632 (1980)

13 HARRISON, M. J. G. Pathogenesis In *Transient Ischemic Attacks*, edited by C. P. Warlow and P.J. Morris, 21–46 Dekker: New York (1982)

14 HARRISON, M. J. G. and MARSHALL, J. Indications for angiography and surgery in carotid artery disease. *British Medical Journal*, **1**, 616–618 (1975)

15 HARRISON, M. J. G. and MARSHALL, J. The results of carotid angiography in cerebral infarction in normotensive and hypertensive subjects. *Journal of Neurological Science*, **24**, 243–250 (1975)

16 HARRISON, M. J. G. and MARSHALL, J. Angiographic appearance of carotid bifurcation in patients with completed stroke, transient ischaemic attacks and cerebral tumour. *British Medical Journal*, **1**, 205–207 (1976)

17 HARRISON, M. J. G. and MARSHALL, J. Prognostic significance of severity of carotid atheroma in early manifestations of cerebrovascular disease. *Stroke*, **13**, 567–569 (1982)

18 HARRISON, M. J. G., THOMAS, D. J., DU BOULAY, G. M. and MARSHALL, J. Multi-infarct dementia. *Journal of Neurological Sciences*, **40**, 97–103 (1979)

19 HASS, W. K., FIELDS, W. S., NORTH, R. R., KRICHEFF, I. I., CHASE, N. E. and BAUER, R. B. Joint study of extracranial arterial occlusion. II Angiography, techniques, sites and complications. *Journal of the American Medical Association*, **203**, 961–968 (1968)

20 HOUSER, O. W., BAKER, H. L., SANDOK, B. A. and HOLLEY, K. E. Cephalic arterial fibromuscular dysplasia. *Neuroradiology*, **101**, 605–611 (1971)

21 HUMPHREY, P. R. D. and MARSHALL, J. Transient ischemic attacks and strokes with recovery, prognosis and investigation. *Stroke*, **12**, 765–769 (1981)

22 KENDALL, B. E. and RADUE, E. W. Computed tomography in spontaneous intracerebral haematomas. *British Journal of Radiology*, **51**, 563–573 (1978)

23 KERBER, C. W., CROMWELL, L. D., DRAYER, B. P. and BANK, W. O. Cerebral ischaemia. I Current angiographic techniques, complications and safety. *American Journal of Roentgenology*, **130**, 1097–1103 (1978)

24 KISHORE, P. R. S., CHASE, N. E. and KRICHEFF, I. I. Ulcerated atheroma of carotid artery and cerebral embolism. In *Aspirin Platelets and Stroke*, edited by W. S. Fields and W. K. Hass. 13–27 Warren H. Green: St. Louis (1971)

25 LHEMITTE, F. and GAUTIER, J. C. Sites of cerebral arterial occlusions. In *Modern Trends in Neurology* Vol. 6, edited by D. Williams, 123–140 Butterworths: London (1975)

26 LITTLE, J. R., FURLAN, A. J., MODIC, J. T. and WEINSTEN, M. A. Digital subtraction angiography in cerebrovascular disease. *Stroke*, **13**, 557–566 (1982)

27 MANI, R. L., EISENBERG, R. L., McDONALD, E. J., POLLOCK, J. A. and MANI, J. R. Complications of catheter cerebral angiography: analysis of 5000 procedures. *American Journal of Roentgenology*, **131**, 861–865 (1978)

28 METTINGER, K. L. Fibromuscular dysplasia and the brain. *Stroke*, **13**, 53–58 (1982)

29 NELSON, R. F., PULLICIANO, P., KENDALL, B. E. and MARSHALL, J. Computed tomography in patients presenting with lacunar syndromes. *Stroke*, **11**, 256–260 (1980)

30 NORTON, G. A., KISHORE, P. R. S. and LIN, J. CT contrast enhancement in cerebral infarction. *American Journal of Roentgenology*, **131**, 881–885 (1978)

31 PERRONE, P., CANDELISE, L., SCOTT, G., DE GRANDI, G. and SCIALFA, G. CT evaluation in patients with transient ischaemic attack. *European Neurology*, **18**, 217–221 (1971)

32 RADUE, E. W. and KENDALL, B. E. Xenon enhancement in tumours and infarcts. *Neuroradiology*, **18**, 224–227 (1978)

33 RING, B. A. Diagnosis of embolic occlusions of smaller branches of the intracerebral arteries. *American Journal of Roentgenology*, **97**, 575–582 (1976)

34 SHAH, S., BULL, J. W. D., DU BOULAY, D. H., MARSHALL, J., ROSS RUSSELL, R. W. and SYMON, L. A comparison of rapid serial angiography and isotope clearance measurements in cerebrovascular disease. *British Journal of Radiology*, **45**, 294–298 (1972)

35 SUNDT, T. M., SANDOK, B. A. and WHISNANT, J. P. Carotid endareterectomy: complications and preoperative assessment of risk. *Mayo Clinic Proceedings*, **50**, 301–306 (1975)

9
Non-invasive diagnosis of carotid artery disease
Myron D. Ginsberg and Randall D. Cebul

Occlusive disease of the internal carotid artery is an important cause of stroke, and much of this disease occurs in the form of stenosis-producing atheroma or non-stenotic ulcerative plaques within its extracranial portion, in particular, at or near the bifurcation of the common carotid artery[76]. A number of non-invasive diagnostic methods have been developed over the past three decades to assist the physician in diagnosing extracranial carotid arterial disease and in guiding decisions regarding patient management. In the sections below we discuss general principles pertinent to the evaluation of non-invasive test results; describe the non-invasive methods themselves, giving major emphasis to those methods in wide current use; and examine the clinical indications for non-invasive testing.

NON-INVASIVE TESTING AT THE BEDSIDE

The non-invasive evaluation of the carotid circulation should always begin at the bedside, with cautious palpation of the carotid arteries, auscultation for cervical bruits, and examination of the facial pulses. Cervical palpation itself is of limited reliability inasmuch as the pulsations of the internal carotid artery cannot be readily distinguished from those of the external or common carotid arteries. In contrast, palpation of the internal carotid artery in its pharyngeal segment, when permitted in the co-operative patient, may provide a much more specific impression. Cervical auscultation should be performed with a rubber-rimmed stethoscopic bell, beginning in the supraclavicular fossa and 'inching' progressively toward the angle of the mandible. In this manner, sub-bifurcational bruits and transmitted cardiac murmurs may be distinguished from carotid bifurcational bruits, which are typically heard maximally at the level of the thyroid cartilage and are transmitted rostrally. With increasing degrees of flow-compromising (hemodynamically significant) carotid stenosis, bruit amplitude increases, pitch rises, and the duration of the bruit lengthens. However, when stenosis exceeds 85–90% diameter reduction, bruit amplitude diminishes.

Olivarius[120] has emphasized that pulsations of the external carotid arterial branches of the face and scalp, and in particular the frontal branch of the superficial

215

temporal artery, may become prominent ipsilateral to an occluded or significantly stenotic internal carotid artery, owing to the development of external-to-internal carotid collateral circulation. Fisher[59] has noted that the ipsilateral 'brow pulse' (along the lateral one-half of the eyebrow) and the 'angular pulse' (at the inner canthus), which occur at sites of external-to-internal carotid branch anastomosis about the orbit, may become prominent in the setting of internal carotid occlusion. Caplan[33] has shown that it is occasionally possible to demonstrate reversal of flow in the frontal (supratrochlear) artery, a terminal branch of the ophthalmic artery, with internal carotid occlusive disease. Thus, the systematic examination and bilateral comparison of the facial pulses should be incorporated routinely into the bedside physical examination of the stroke-prone patient.

EVALUATION OF NON-INVASIVE NEUROVASCULAR TESTS

Sensitivity, specificity, predictive value, accuracy and the establishment of reference criteria

Several general principles must be considered when comparing neurovascular tests; these have been sorely ignored in the ever-expanding literature of relatively new technologies. We review below some definitions and concepts of general importance as they relate to non-invasive tests of carotid artery disease.

Test characteristics are most readily understood by referring to a two-by-two table in which the results of a non-invasive test are correlated with corresponding results from a reference test, in this case, arteriography (*Table 9.1*). The diagnostic *sensitivity* of the non-invasive test can be considered its 'positivity-in-disease', that is, the percentage of patients with at least a certain degree of carotid stenosis who have a positive non-invasive test result. Tests with low sensitivity misclassify a considerable proportion of patients with carotid stenosis as normal; that is, they have a high false-negative rate. A test's *specificity* can be considered its 'negativity-in-health', or the percentage of patients with less than a certain degree of carotid stenosis who have negative non-invasive test results. Tests with low specificity misclassify a considerable proportion of patients with normal vessels as having significant carotid stenosis; that is, they have a high false-positive rate. Sensitivity and specificity are generally regarded as being characteristics of the tests themselves and are independent of the prevalence of carotid stenosis in the population being tested.

A test's *accuracy, positive predictive value*, and *negative predictive value*, on the other hand, are related additionally to the prevalence of carotid stenosis, or 'pre-test' probability of disease, in the population being reported. Test accuracy is defined as the proportion of all patients tested who are correctly classified as diseased or non-diseased. The positive and negative predictive values of a test relate, respectively, to the proportion of patients with positive or negative non-invasive test results who are classified correctly by non-invasive tests. These characteristics are a function of the test's sensitivity and specificity as well as the overall prevalance of carotid disease in the population. In populations with an extremely low prevalence of carotid disease (for example, young asymptomatic

Table 9.1 Two-by-two table for interpreting non-invasive test results

| Arteriographic findings | Non-invasive test results | | |
	Negative	Positive	
No stenosis*	TN	FP	TN+FP
Stenosis*	FN	TP	FN+TP
	TN+FN	TP+FP	*Total*

* Arteriographic findings should always explicitly define criteria used for 'stenosis' (e.g. greater than 50%, 60%, etc.).
TN = true negative; TP = true positive; FN = false negative; FP = false positive.

Test characteristics:

Sensitivity (%) = positivity-in-disease $\quad = \dfrac{TP}{TP+FN} \times 100$

Specificity (%) = negativity-in-health $\quad = \dfrac{TN}{TN+FP} \times 100$

Other measures:

Pre-test probability of disease = prevalence $\quad = \dfrac{FN+TP}{Total}$

Test accuracy (%) $\quad = \dfrac{TN+TP}{Total} \times 100$

Positive predictive value (%) $\quad = \dfrac{TP}{TP+FP} \times 100$

Negative predictive value (%) $\quad = \dfrac{TN}{TN+FN} \times 100$

adults with cervical bruits), abnormal results on even highly sensitive and specific non-invasive tests have low positive predictive value. In contrast, in populations with a very high prevalence of carotid disease (for example, patients with anterior circulation transient ischemic symptoms and ipsilateral cervical bruits), even normal results on highly sensitive and specific non-invasive tests have low negative predictive value. Non-invasive tests are only minimally useful in either clinical situation: in the asymptomatic young adult, no testing is warranted, whereas in the symptomatic patient with an ipsilateral bruit, non-invasive studies may be bypassed in favor of proceeding directly to arteriography unless medical contraindications exist.

In principle, all non-invasive tests should be interpreted with reference to criteria concerned with stenosis of a vessel of an explicitly defined degree, as demonstrated by carotid arteriography. Since most non-invasive tests are unable to detect ulcerative non-stenotic carotid lesions, reports that include ulcerative lesions as 'true-positives' in otherwise non-stenotic vessels artificially inflate the actual test sensitivity; these test results are more appropriately considered false-positives, especially when reported for indirect tests, which detect only hemodynamically significant lesions. Arteriography remains the standard of reference against which other tests should be compared. When arteriographic confirmation is unavailable, categories of non-invasive test results thought to represent underlying patho-physiological states should be explicitly defined for different patient groups, and terms such as 'significant', 'compensated' and 'uncompensated' carotid stenosis based solely on non-invasive test results should be abandoned.

In general, studies reporting results of arteriography and non-invasive testing in selected patient populations should be interpreted with caution. Accurate sensitivity and specificity data can be derived only from large, randomly chosen adult populations in which a representative spectrum of underlying carotid pathology is present. From data derived from arteriographic studies performed only in patients with abnormal non-invasive test results, the positive predictive value of the non-invasive tests in that population may be correctly inferred, but one cannot be explicit about test sensitivity or specificity. Knowledge of the positive, predictive value of a test in a specific population is useful for clinical decision-making purposes in that population, but conveys no information about the predictive value of negative test results and very little about the value of positive tests in populations with substantially different underlying disease prevalences.

The literature on non-invasive tests is most useful when the degree of arterio-graphically demonstrable stenosis that is regarded as 'significant' is clearly specified. Tests which are very sensitive for detecting high-grade stenoses may have an appreciable proportion of 'false-negative' results when stenoses in the 40–60% range are considered 'significant'. In the absence of a general consensus as to the degree of cross-sectional diameter reduction that is clinically important, interpretation of non-invasive results according to explicitly stated arteriographic criteria is essential in order to compare different tests and test batteries.

DIRECT NON-INVASIVE METHODS

Direct non-invasive methods are those which directly assess an anatomical or physiological aspect of the common carotid artery bifurcation or its extracranial branches.

Carotid phonoangiography

A simple and widely used form of carotid phonoangiography was developed by Kartchner and McRae[89]. A microphone is used to record vascular sounds from three sites in the neck: immediately below the angle of the mandible; over the carotid bifurcation; and low in the neck. Tracings are displayed on an oscilloscope, and permanent records are made on Polaroid film. The three recording positions may allow differentiation of cardiac murmurs and bruits arising from the great vessels (recorded chiefly in the lowest position), from those arising from the common carotid artery or its branches (*Figure 9.1*). Bruit amplitude is usually graded semiquantitatively (small, moderate, or large). Carotid bruits of moderate

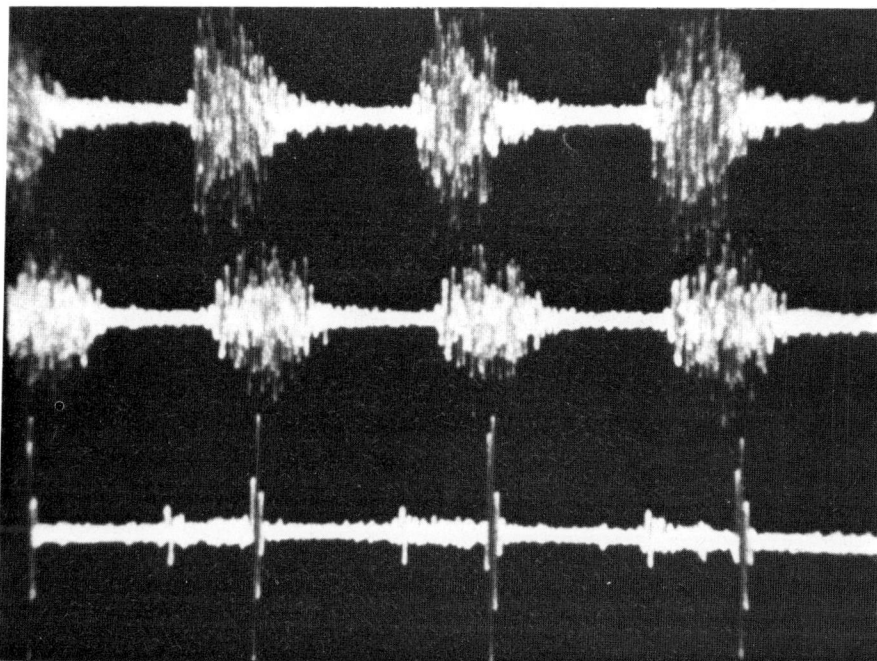

Figure 9.1 Carotid phonoangiogram, showing recordings taken (from top to bottom) just below the angle of the mandible; in the mid-neck; and low in the neck. A typical carotid bifurcational bruit, which extends throughout systole, is present in the top and middle tracings. The normal heart sounds are seen in the bottom tracing. (From Ginsberg *et al.*[66], courtesy of the Editor and Publishers, *Neurology (Minneapolis)*)

and large amplitude characteristically extend throughout the systolic interval and occasionally into diastole.

In their initial evaluation of this method, Kartchner and McRae[89] expressed enthusiasm as to its accuracy in detecting stenosis of 50% or greater, reporting a sensitivity of 91% and a specificity of 82%. Subsequent studies, however, have shown that this type of bruit analysis is an inaccurate predictor of the extent of internal carotid artery stenosis and may be influenced by the presence of contralateral internal carotid stenosis or occlusion[61, 66, 67, 151]. In two angiographically studied series, Ginsberg *et al.*[66, 67] showed that bruits were occasionally recorded even over non-stenotic vessels: 8–11% of vessels with no internal carotid stenosis by arteriography had small bruits, and 3–7% had moderate to large bruits. In addition, bruits of moderate to large amplitude were occasionally heard over completely occluded vessels[67], apparently owing to ipsilateral external or common carotid stenosis.

This type of carotid phonoangiography is useful as an adjunct to other, more definitive non-invasive tests; and for obtaining a permanent record from which sequential comparisons may be made and the progression of extracranial vascular disease may be evaluated[90]. In patients with asymptomatic cervical bruits, phono-angiographic criteria may be of help in differentiating bifurcational bruits from those of sub-bifurcational origin, and in defining a subpopulation of patients more likely to have carotid stenosis[90]. Conversely, the *absence* of a bruit by phono-angiography in the presence of a positive hemodynamic test such as oculo-plethysmography may denote complete occlusion or pre-occlusive stenosis of the internal carotid artery[66, 67, 90].

A more sophisticated, quantitative version of phonoangiography was proposed by Lees and Dewey[99], who applied the theory of turbulent flow in pipes to the analysis of the sound spectrum produced in arteries narrowed by atherosclerosis. In the clinical application of this method[50], recorded bruits are digitized and subjected to spectral analysis by fast Fourier transformation to yield a representation of the intensity or loudness of each frequency present in the bruit (between 10 and 1000 Hz). In turbulent flow, there is a single identifiable 'break frequency' (f), beyond which bruit intensity diminishes with increasing frequency (*Figure 9.2*). The higher the 'break frequency', the greater is the degree of stenosis. The diameter (d) of the residual lumen within the stenotic vessel is given by d = U/f, where U is the peak systolic flow velocity of the unobstructed portion of the artery. In practice, a value for U is assumed (50 cm/sec) on the basis of published data[16]. Duncan *et al.*[50] showed that the predicted diameter of the stenotic vessel agreed to within 1.0 mm of the angiographically demonstrated diameter in 73% of cases, and to within 1.5 mm in 91% of cases. A more recent study using similar methods reported

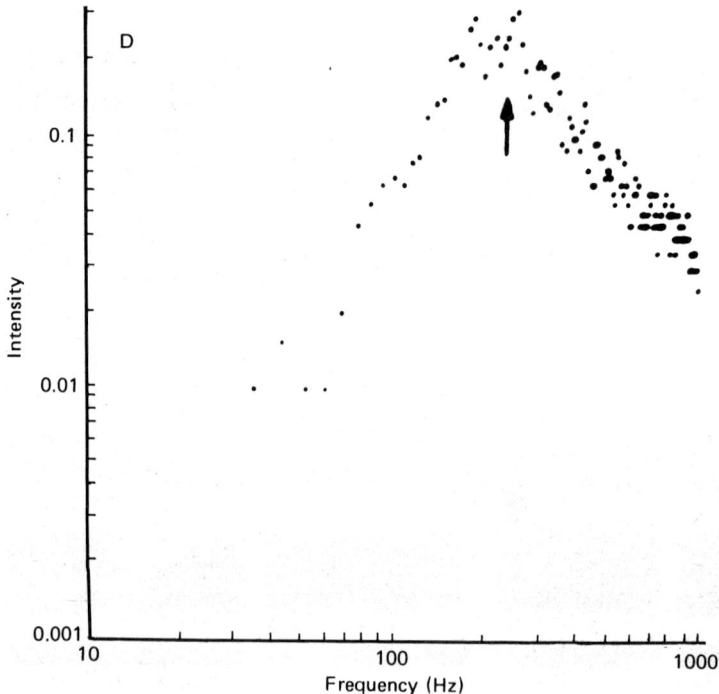

Figure 9.2 Spectral analysis of carotid phonoangiogram in a patient with a carotid bifurcational bruit. The arrow denotes the position of the 'break frequency', beyond which there is a sharp decline in intensity. (From Duncan *et al.*[50], courtesy of the Editor and Publishers, *New England Journal of Medicine*)

agreement to within 1 mm in 85% of cases[95]. Alternatively, when peak flow velocity U is predicted empirically from the peak spectral intensity, it is possible to estimate angiographic stenosis with even greater accuracy[50]. However, approximately 10–15% of bruits have properties such that they cannot be satisfactorily evaluated by this method[50, 95]. Experimental studies employing controlled stenoses and known flow velocities have confirmed that the relationship between 'break frequency', flow velocity and residual lumen holds over a wide range of values[114]. More recent studies have refined the ability of this method to analyze carotid bruits in the presence of superimposed bruits radiating from the great vessels or the heart[94].

Doppler ultrasonic imaging methods

In these methods, a Doppler ultrasonic transducer attached to a position-detecting arm is applied to the neck and passed back and forth over the carotid arterial system in successive transverse sweeps in a progressively cephalad direction. A signal is registered on the screen of a storage oscilloscope at those points at which a moving column of red cells is encountered. In this fashion, a static anatomic image is generated, corresponding to areas of flowing blood within the common, internal and external carotid arteries (*Figure 9.3*). This image itself may reveal zones of stenosis or of complete occlusion (absent flow signal). More importantly, the image

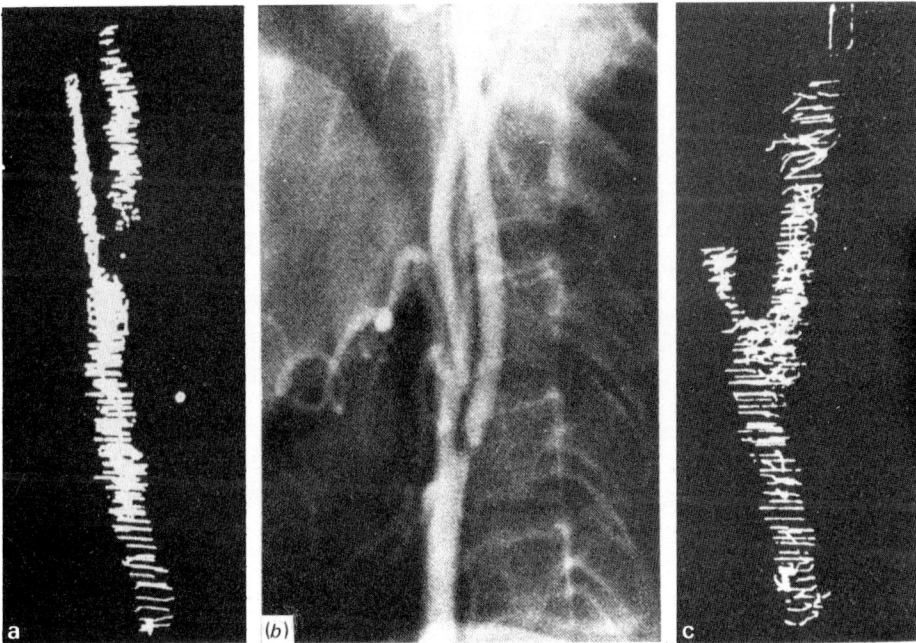

Figure 9.3 Left internal carotid artery stenosis as shown by continuous-wave Doppler imaging (a) and by arteriography (b). Doppler image (c) was performed following carotid endarterectomy. (From Thomas *et al.*, courtesy of the Editor and Publishers, *American Journal of Surgery*, **128**, 168–174 (1974))

serves as a map to permit precise probe placement, from which the local characteristics of the Doppler signal may be assessed, either by listening to the audio signal or by spectral analysis.

Two types of instruments are employed. In continuous-wave instruments, separate transmitting and receiving transducer elements are used, and flow is detected simultaneously from any vessel lying within the path of the sound beam. In contrast, pulsed Doppler imaging systems utilize a single transmitter–receiver crystal, which emits short ultrasonic bursts. Pulsed Doppler circuitry is capable of resolving flow from sample volumes (or 'gates') lying at several different depths along the path of the sound beam. This has the advantage of permitting analysis of the Doppler signal at various points along a vessel's cross-section. Pulsed Doppler information may also be used to reconstruct novel planes of section from the primary data.

In their initial experience with continuous-wave Doppler imaging, Spencer *et al.*[136] reported the most definitive sign of internal carotid artery stenosis to be a narrow visualized segment associated with (1) a large increase in frequency within the segment, and (2) a flow signal of turbulent quality distal to it. Spencer and Reid[137] subsequently stated the theoretical relationships predicted between blood flow, mean velocity, and lumen diameter in an axially symmetric stenosis (*Figure 9.4*). A lumen diameter of approximately 1 mm is associated with a sizeable decrease in blood flow and a peaking of flow velocity (and hence Doppler frequency); whereas with still tighter stenoses, the flow velocity declines precipitously. In asymmetric stenoses, the ratio of the Doppler frequency within the stenosis to that downstream from the stenotic segment was found to be the best quantitative predictor of the degree of stenosis observed angiographically[137]. Subsequent series have confirmed a high degree of accuracy in detecting severe stenoses and occlusions near the carotid bifurcation[24, 25]. Continuous-wave Doppler imaging appears to be best at detecting internal carotid stenoses of 50% or greater. Lesser degrees of stenosis are not as consistently detected, though semi-quantitative schemata for grading percentage stenosis based upon characteristics of the audible Doppler signal have been proposed[148].

A comparable or somewhat greater degree of diagnostic accuracy has been reported with pulsed Doppler imaging systems. Sumner *et al.*[138] found that this method detected 89% of all stenoses greater than 40% and that ultrasonic and arteriographic estimates of percentage stenosis agreed to within 20% in 81% of these studies. Hobson *et al.*[79] noted a sensitivity of 89% and a specificity of 83% in differentiating vessels having less than, from those having greater than, 50% stenosis. Pulsed Doppler is most accurate in confirming normal vessels and in diagnosing completely occluded arteries; in the latter, a sensitivity as high as 93% has been reported[79]. Indeed, this method has been recommended as an effective means of distinguishing high-grade internal carotid artery stenosis from complete occlusion – a distinction of considerable importance in clinical decision-making[79, 80]. However, its ability to make this distinction is not infallible[147]. The addition of spectral analysis to the pulsed Doppler examination enhances its ability to specify the precise degree of stenosis[11]: lesions having less than 50% stenosis produce only spectral broadening, whereas stenosis of greater than 50% is

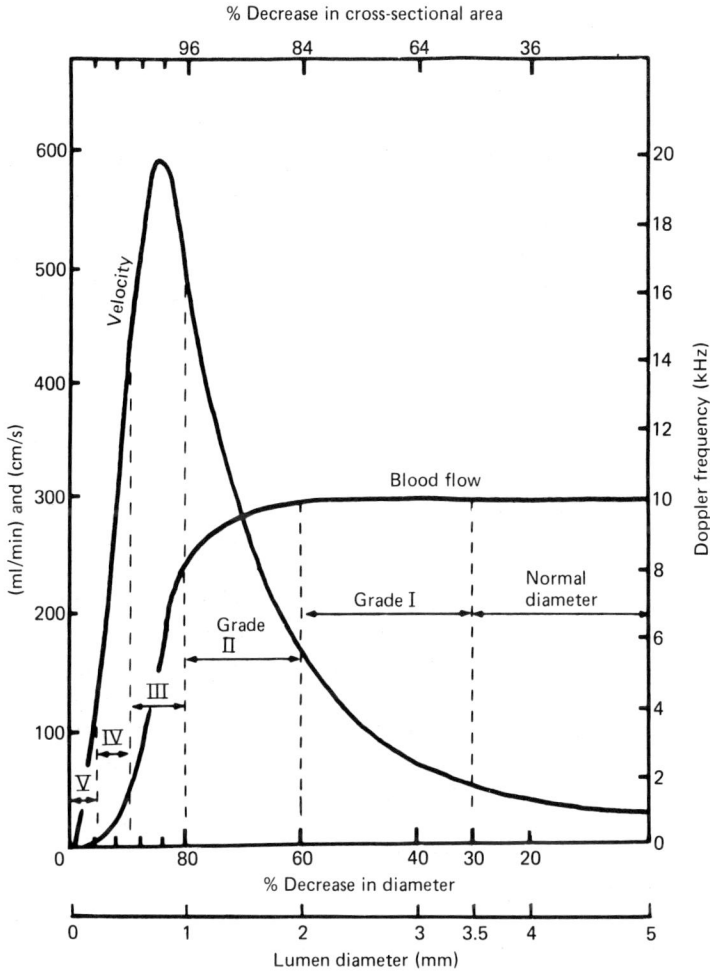

Figure 9.4 Predicted relationships between lumen diameter, blood flow and flow velocity in a graded, axially symmetric arterial stenosis. Blood flow declines abruptly and flow velocity peaks as luminal diameter decreases below 1 mm. (From Spencer *et al.*[137], courtesy of the Editors and Publishers, *Stroke*)

associated in addition with an elevation of peak frequency[22]. A recently devised pulsed Doppler instrument with 30 'gates' appears to have the consistent ability to detect stenosis of greater than 25%[147].

Echo-free areas occur in Doppler ultrasonic images owing to calcification within atherosclerotic plaques. These zones may be found throughout the range of stenosis but are somewhat more common with hemodynamically significant lesions[79, 80]. Imaging of the external carotid artery tends to be far less satisfactory than the internal carotid artery, perhaps owing to its smaller size[25, 147]. When the internal carotid artery is occluded the external carotid artery may be mistaken for the internal carotid, or two external carotid branches may be mistaken for the common carotid artery bifurcation[3].

Real-time (B-mode) ultrasonic imaging

B-mode scanners employ ultrasound to generate a dynamic image of the extra-cranial carotid arterial system in longitudinal or transverse section. Best results are obtained with instruments designed specifically for carotid artery studies, which employ 5–10 MHz ultrasound and are capable of a linear resolution of 0.5–0.8 mm or less. Within the transducer module, which is hand held against the neck and moved along the path of the carotid artery, the ultrasonic beam is deflected in a fan-shaped plane at 15–60 frames/sec by either mechanical or electronic means. Structures are imaged by the reflection of sound waves from tissue interfaces, and the brightness or sonodensity within the image is related to the acoustical impedence of the tissue component. Thus, the normal vessel wall appears bright and the blood column dark; a thin sonodense line, presumably representing the vascular intima, is often apparent within the common carotid artery (*Figure 9.5*).

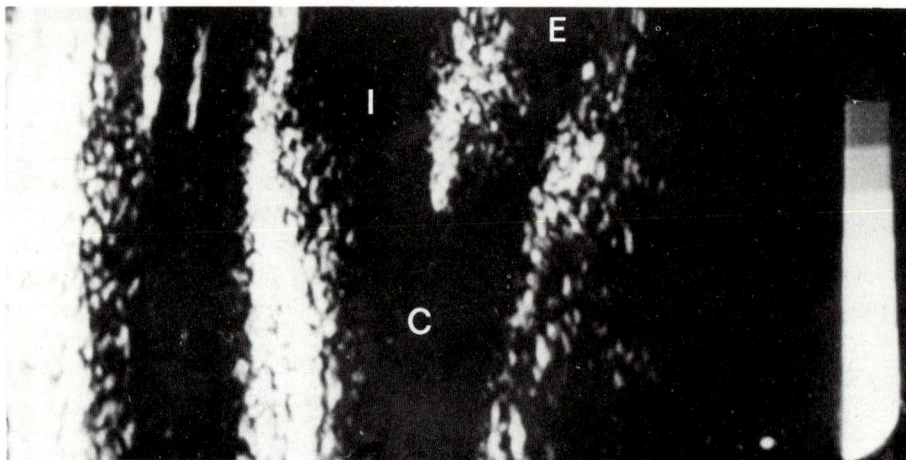

Figure 9.5 Real-time B-mode ultrasonic image of a normal carotid bifurcation in longi-tudinal section, showing the common (C), internal (I) and external (E) carotid arteries

Because the ultrasonic image is generated in real-time on a video monitor, pulsatile motion of the vessel wall and abnormal shear-motion of atherosclerotic plaques may be appreciated.

Ultrasonic examination of human arterial specimens has confirmed that the major factor affecting transmission of ultrasound through diseased vessels is the calcium content of the plaque material, calcified plaque typically having 1000 times the sound absorption of normal artery wall[75]. Calcium-containing atherosclerotic plaques appear as irregular sonodense accumulations (*Figure 9.6*). Plaque of sufficient sonodensity often casts acoustical shadows, rendering visualization of deeper structures impossible. Non-calcific plaque is less consistently visualized, and thrombus is characteristically very difficult to distinguish from blood[22].

Real-time ultrasound has been employed for carotid artery imaging for over a decade[26, 119], yet relatively few thorough clinical assessments of its diagnostic

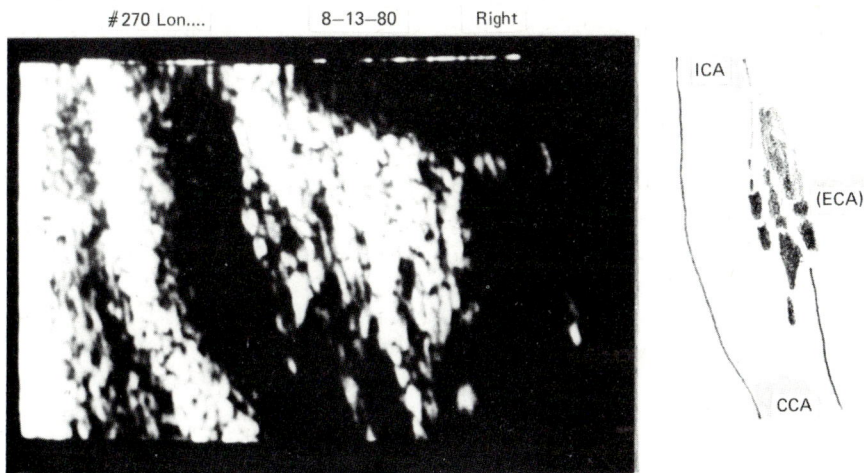

Figure 9.6 Diseased carotid artery bifurcation as shown by B-mode ultrasound. Multifocal sonodense plaque material narrows the common carotid artery lumen and involves the origin of the internal carotid artery as well

capabilities have been published. As with other non-invasive tests, contrast arteriography has been used as the standard reference, yet real-time images and arteriographic images entail fundamentally different principles of visualization. With B-mode scanning, the image is formed only at the points of intersection of the narrow ultrasonic beam-plane with the superficial and deep surfaces of a vascular structure; thus, multiple angles of view are needed to gain a representative impression[41]. Contrast arteriography, however, is most sensitive at revealing indentations of the intravascular dye column by lesions lying in a plane orthogonal to the X-ray beam. Thus, B-mode scans often reveal small focal zones of vessel thickening or plaque which may be obscured by the dye column on contrast studies[68, 69]. When discrepancies of interpretation of plaque arise by good-quality B-mode scanning and arteriography, surgical findings often correlate better with the ultrasonic than with angiographic findings[41, 69]. However, the quality of B-mode scans tends to deteriorate as the degree of atherosclerotic disease increases, in part owing to the obscuring effect of acoustical shadows cast by sonodense lesions, and in part by the uncertainty of identifying vascular structures when their pulsations are diminished. Thus, while the overall diagnostic accuracy of ultrasound in several published reports is in the range of 75–80%[26, 41], this appears to be highly dependent upon the quality of the scan, which in turn is related to the degree of underlying stenosis. Comerata *et al.*[41] found that patients with 0–39% stenosis by arteriography tended to have B-mode scans of good quality, whereas patients with 40–69% stenosis had only fair-to-good-quality scans, and the average scan quality was even lower in patients with stenosis of 70% or greater. B-mode scans could exclude lesions of 40% or greater with a specificity of 86%, but they could accurately identify only 38% of occluded vessels[41]. Hobson *et al.*[80] found B-mode scans to be approximately 80% accurate in vessels with 0–50% stenosis by angiography, but only 58% accurate with lesions producing 50–99% stenosis, and 18% accurate in the setting of total occlusion.

The major strength of B-mode ultrasound is its ability to exhibit structural detail of plaque which produces only mild-to-moderate stenosis. False-negative results are uncommon in B-mode scans of *good quality*. Thus, a normal vessel diagnosed on an ultrasound examination of good quality may be sufficient in some cases to exclude the need for contrast arteriography. However, 13–18% of ultrasound scans are of unsatisfactory quality[5, 26, 80], and, as noted above, this is particularly true with moderate to severe stenotic disease[41]. In particular, it is extremely difficult to distinguish between severe stenosis and total occlusion by B-mode ultrasound[68]. In general, the internal carotid artery image is less intense and of less acceptable quality than that of the common carotid artery or bifurcational zone.

The inaccuracy of B-mode ultrasound in diagnosing high-grade stenotic lesions may be improved by the use of duplex scanners, which combine real-time ultrasonic images with pulsed Doppler devices that provide flow velocity information at selected sample sites[22, 56] or at multiple range points along the profile of a cross-sectional vascular image[53, 71]. The Doppler information may allow the hemodynamics of a vessel to be assessed in a zone from which an ambiguous or poor-quality ultrasound image is obtained. The ability to detect over 90% of flow-reducing lesions has been reported for duplex scanners[22, 56]. However, combining real-time ultrasound with a pulsed Doppler system within a single instrument represents a formidable technological challenge which has not been met in a fully satisfactory manner by the current generation of duplex scanners.

Other direct non-invasive methods

Digital subtraction angiography (DSA)

This is a newly developed technique of remarkable potential which enables the cerebral circulation to be imaged with great clarity following the intravenous administration of iodinated contrast medium. The method utilizes computerized fluoroscopy and image-intensification technology[38, 39, 45]. A 'mask image' formed prior to contrast injection is digitally subtracted from the sequential images formed during passage of iodinated contrast medium through the circulation. The iodine-contrast images are thus isolated and selectively enhanced, so that vessels can be imaged although they contain only one-tenth the concentration of contrast required for visualization by intra-arterial angiography. In a study comparing intravenous DSA with conventional angiography of the common carotid bifurcation[38], vascular images of good to excellent quality were obtained bilaterally in 60% of patients and unilaterally in an additional 23%. In those vessels there was excellent correlation between the two methods, with sensitivity and specificity of 95–99%; ulcerative carotid lesions were well visualized in images of good or excellent quality. DSA requires that 40–50 ml of contrast medium be administered intravenously. Rare allergic reactions and extravasation of contrast constitute the chief risks of the procedure. Although minimally invasive, the potential of this new method is so great that it promises to become the direct 'non-invasive' test of choice for imaging the carotid arterial system. A unique advantage of DSA is its ability to image the intracranial as well as extracranial circulation.

Velocity waveform analysis

This mode of analysis of common carotid artery Doppler signals makes use of a variety of descriptive indices of velocity waveform tracings, including systolic and diastolic velocities and peak widths, heights and slopes. Discriminant analysis is used to optimize the predictive value of this method. High levels of accuracy have been reported, particularly in the identification of hemodynamically significant degrees of carotid stenosis[129]. The ratio of mean peak internal carotid artery flow velocity to mean peak common carotid flow velocity at systole (measured using a duplex scanning system) has been found to be highly reliable in diagnosing stenosis of 60% or greater diameter reduction[21].

INDIRECT NON-INVASIVE METHODS

Indirect non-invasive methods provide information concerning hemodynamic changes occurring in cerebral and orbital circulatory beds as a result of obstructive lesions within the extracranial carotid vasculature.

Oculoplethysmography

In common with plethysmographic procedures used to study peripheral vascular disease, studies in animals and in man have shown that the amplitude and contour of the ocular pulse waveform is altered by ipsilateral carotid stenosis, particularly when greater than 50%[18, 19]. However, in human studies the correlation between internal carotid stenosis and ocular pulse amplitude reduction has been poor. Kartchner, McRae *et al.*[92, 93] devised a practicable instrument to record and compare the relative timing of ocular pulses recorded simultaneously from the two eyes. This method, termed oculoplethysmography (OPG), has become widely popular and has been studied extensively. In this method, topical anesthesia is first applied to the corneas. Small corneal cups, filled with sterile water and connected to pressure transducers, are held against the corneas by 50–55 mmHg of suction. The ocular pulse waveforms resulting from the expansion of the ocular globes during each cardiac systole are recorded simultaneously from each eye on rapidly moving chart paper. The two ocular pulses are subtracted electronically to produce a differential recording, which is superimposed on the ocular pulse tracings. A light opacity sensor simultaneously registers the external carotid artery pulse from the ear lobe. The characteristic finding with unilateral ICA stenosis is a delay of the ipsilateral ocular pulse, most readily detected in the differential tracing (*Figure 9.7*)

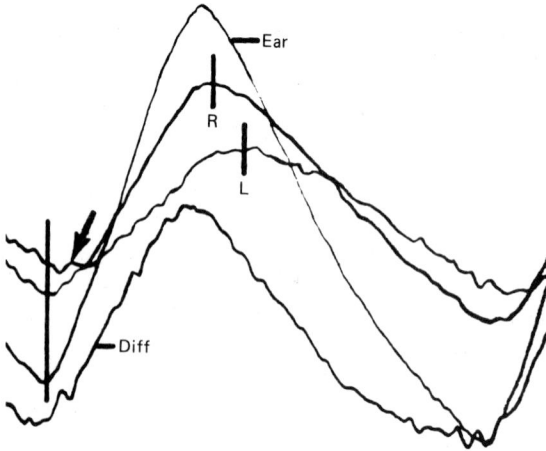

Figure 9.7 Oculoplethysmographic tracings in a patient with hemodynamically significant left internal carotid artery stenosis. A marked left ocular pulse delay is apparent in the pronounced upward bowing of the differential tracing (DIFF), the delayed takeoff of the left ocular pulse (arrow) relative to the ear (external carotid artery) pulse, and the shift of the left ocular pulse peak (L) relative to the right (R). (From Ginsberg *et al.*[66], courtesy of the Editor and Publishers, *Neurology (Minneapolis)*)

but, if moderate in degree, apparent as a visible delay of one ocular pulse peak relative to the other. With bilateral ICA stenosis, the differential tracing may fail to show an inflection, but a delay in the upstroke of each ocular pulse may be apparent when compared to the ear (external carotid artery) pulse.

In the initial studies, an arterial diameter reduction of 40% or more was considered to be hemodynamically significant because it correlated with at least a 20% reduction of ICA blood flow measured intraoperatively[92, 93]. This notion has given rise to a grading scheme from which, it is asserted, the degree of carotid flow reduction may be inferred from a combination of OPG and phonoangiographic findings[1]. The use of such simplistic schemata, however, is to be decried since there appears to be no published detailed experimental substantiation. Kartchner's group initially reported OPG to be abnormal in 76% of internal carotid arteries with stenosis of at least 40%, and to be normal in 97% of arteries with stenosis less than 40%[93]. In a later study[92], these figures were 88% and 92% respectively. Others, however, have found OPG to be relatively insensitive to 40% arterial stenosis[138]. The study of Gross *et al.*[73] suggested that the lowest degree of accuracy with OPG was obtained in the 40–59% range of ICA stenosis. Ginsberg *et al.*[66] found that an ICA stenosis of at least 60% was required to produce a consistent ocular pulse delay, and a variety of other studies have used 50% diameter stenosis as the criterion of hemodynamic significance for OPG[6, 23, 79, 107]. Using the arteriographic standard of 60% diameter reduction as the criterion of hemodynamic significance, Ginsberg *et al.*[66] showed OPG to have a specificity of 95% and a sensitivity of 86% in detecting ICA stenosis. With the criterion of a 50% diameter reduction, Hobson *et al.*[79] noted a specificity of 87% and sensitivity of 81%, whereas Blackshear *et al.*[23] reported a considerably lower sensitivity. A common source of false-positive OPG findings is the presence of a second arterial stenosis in a more proximal vessel[66]. The predominant source of false-negative findings is the presence of bilateral ICA stenosis, resulting in a flat OPG differential tracing.

An OPG refinement of questionable merit was the introduction of an air-filled system that employed digital microprocessor circuitry and permitted direct quantification of eye-to-eye, eye-to-ear, and ear-to-ear pulse delays. In a study undertaken to assess this modification, the optimal criteria for detecting a 60% or greater diameter reduction were found to be a delay of one ocular pulse, relative to the other, of greater than 12 msec; and a delay of an ocular pulse relative to the earlier ear (external carotid) pulse of greater than 36 msec[67]. In that study, the OPG was inconclusive or inaccurate in 26% of vessels studied, so that the test sensitivity was 76% and the specificity was 73%. A similar sensitivity was noted in a second study employing this instrument[107]. At least a third of patients having bilateral hemodynamically significant stenoses remained undetected despite the capability of quantification[67]. A recently reported application of quantitative OPG is in monitoring intraoperative carotid flow and shunt patency during endarterectomy[122]. In summary, OPG of the Kartchner type is an effective though not error-free diagnostic tool. Greater accuracy is achieved by combining OPG with a complementary, direct non-invasive method and using the 'both positive' criterion[79, 138].

The physiological basis of the ocular pulse delay in carotid stenosis has been subjected to experimental scrutiny in a recent study[146]. Increasing stenosis produced only a small ocular pulse delay until a critical areal stenosis of 70–80% was reached, at which point the ocular pulse delay increased abruptly, approaching 30 msec with total occlusion. The OPG pulse delay correlated directly with increasing arterial compliance distal to the stenosis, suggesting that the delay is produced at least in part by a decreased pulse wave velocity resulting from increased poststenotic vascular compliance.

Ophthalmodynamometry

Ophthalmodynamometry (ODM) employs a hand-held, calibrated spring-loaded gauge, used in conjunction with an ophthalmoscope, to measure ophthalmic artery (central retinal artery) blood pressure[17, 102, 130]. The footplate of the instrument is placed on the lateral sclera, and increasing pressure is applied to the globe. Ophthalmic artery diastolic pressure is signalled by an intermittent collapse of the retinal arterioles; when systolic pressure is reached, pulsations cease. The ODM gauge gives values in grams of force, which may be converted to mmHg from a knowledge of intraocular pressure, by means of conversion tables. Normally, ophthalmic arterial pressure is approximately two-thirds to three-quarters of the brachial arterial blood pressure. A side-to-side ODM difference of 15–20% in systolic or diastolic values, or absolute values at or below 40 (systolic) or 10 (diastolic), are observed with hemodynamically significant ICA stenosis[130]. The test is less useful with bilateral ICA stenoses, and ophthalmic artery stenosis is a source of false-positive results.

The accuracy of ODM in detecting carotid artery stenosis of 50% or greater is in the range of 70–75% and is thus comparable to other indirect non-invasive methods such as OPG and periorbital Doppler[83, 130]. The accuracy of the method rises with higher grades of stenosis or with complete ICA occlusion[83, 121], although retinal arterial pressures may tend to equalize in the presence of well-developed ophthalmic collateral circulation. ODM is an old test[8, 102]. The instrument is inexpensive and suitable for use at the bedside. However, ODM requires consistent technique and the co-operation of the patient, and is best performed by an experienced physician.

Oculopneumoplethysmography

Oculopneumoplethysmography (OPPG) adapts the principle of ophthalmodyna-mometry to estimate systolic ophthalmic artery blood pressure in an automated fashion. After topical anesthesia, small suction cups connected to volume transduc-ers are applied to the lateral sclera of each eye. Suction applied to the cups deforms the sclera and elevates the intraocular pressure until it exceeds ophthalmic artery systolic pressure. As the vacuum is then gradually released, a pulsatile waveform becomes apparent in the pressure tracing of each eye at intraocular pressures equal to or below ophthalmic systolic pressure. A third recorder channel registers the degree of applied vacuum itself. A table to convert vacuum pressure to systolic ophthalmic arterial pressure has been derived from a series of OPPG measure-ments made during recording of internal carotid artery stump pressure at carotid surgery[63].

The method of OPPG was first used to assess the adequacy of collateral blood flow in patients undergoing carotid endarterectomy, by employing the test during brief proximal common carotid artery compression. The pressures thus recorded were generally within 5 mmHg of the directly measured internal carotid stump pressure[63]. Early studies with this method suggested 100% reliability in detecting unilateral carotid occlusion or pre-occlusive (greater than 90%) stenosis[65] and an accuracy of 92% in detecting diameter stenosis of 75% or greater[64].

This method has subsequently been employed in many laboratories, usually without carotid compression. Optimal criteria have evolved for identifying hemodynamically significant stenoses. These are:

(1) a side-to-side difference in ophthalmic artery pressure of 5 mmHg or more;
(2) if ophthalmic artery pressure exceeds 110 mmHg, a side-to-side difference in eye pulse amplitude of 2 mm or more at 100 mmHg; and
(3) a ratio of ophthalmic artery pressure to systolic brachial cuff-pressure of 0.66 or less[110, 111].

Early OPPG studies employed a maximal applied vacuum of 300 mmHg, corres-ponding to a systolic stump pressure of 110 mmHg[63]; this relatively low upper limit tended to mask side-to-side differences occurring in hypertensive patients. More recently, the maximal applied vacuum has been extended to 500 mmHg[62], corres-ponding to an intraoperative internal carotid stump pressure of 144 mmHg[63].

Arteriographic correlations from many laboratories indicate that this method is capable of high accuracy. Sensitivity and specificity values of 87–98% and 89–100% respectively have been reported from laboratories using a 50–60% diameter stenosis as the arteriographic criterion of hemodynamic significance[85, 110, 111] with overall accuracy figures of 92–97% in detecting diameter stenosis of 60% or above[9, 106, 111]. In common with other indirect tests, this method is most sensitive in detecting high-grade stenosis (75% or above), and less accurate in the 60–75% range[111]. The addition of carotid compression to this test may reduce the incidence of false-negative results in the 75–100% range of stenosis[111]. In bilateral carotid disease, Gee *et al.*[62] have reported an accuracy of 92%, compared to a much lower success rate using other indirect methods. However, a minority of workers has reported less than satisfactory results with this method[73]. A recent study has suggested that a negative OPPG test result is relatively unreliable in excluding significant anatomic stenosis, as demonstrated by a combination of arteriography plus intraoperative assessment[118]. These false-negative results with tight stenoses may reflect compensation via the development of collateral circulation in at least some patients[118].

OPPG has been applied successfully to monitor ophthalmic artery pressure during carotid endarterectomy and during gradual carotid artery occlusion for inoperable intracranial aneurysms[20]. It has also been used to identify recurrent stenosis in patients post-carotid endarterectomy[96]. OPPG is a highly useful indirect test: it does not require extraordinary technician skills; only a few minutes is required for its execution and a permanent record is provided. Occasional ocular erythema may result. A history of ocular injury or operation within the previous six months or a history of retinal detachment are considered contraindications to this test[65]. The patient must be warned of transient loss of vision during application of the vacuum[65]. Carotid compression is not required in this test, but when employed must be done with great caution, particularly in the presence of atheromatous disease; neurological sequelae have been noted occasionally.

Directional Doppler ultrasonography of periorbital vessels

This indirect test characterizes the external–internal carotid arterial collateral circulation around the orbit by defining the direction of flow in the supratrochlear (or 'frontal') and supraorbital arteries. These are branches of the ophthalmic artery, which in turn arises from the internal carotid artery. The normal direction of collateral flow is from the internal carotid circulation of the orbit into the external carotid circulation of the forehead and face (superficial temporal and facial arteries). Thus, compression of the preauricular segment of the ipsilateral superficial temporal artery characteristically produces an augmentation of normal flow. In contrast, with ICA stenosis the external carotid artery may provide collateral circulation to the internal carotid distribution via the supratrochlear and supraorbital arteries and thus produce a reversal in their direction of flow. External carotid artery branch compression may then lead to a diminution or re-reversal of flow. The directional Doppler examination should be considered abnormal either with reversal of resting flow or in the presence of an abnormal response to external carotid artery branch compression, inasmuch as the latter is occasionally observed without the former[15].

This test makes use of a Doppler ultrasonic velocity detector emitting a 5–10 mHz continuous-wave signal and having the capability of sensing whether the direction of blood flow is toward or away from the Doppler probe. The published literature reveals considerable variation in the application of this method. The most comprehensive approach is to record from both the supraorbital and supratrochlear arteries, which may respond differentially in the presence of disease (see below). Ackerman (R. H. Ackerman, personal communication) and Barnes *et al.*[15] advocate a comprehensive series of external carotid artery branch compression maneuvers, including the preauricular segments of each superficial temporal artery, each facial artery at the angle of the mandible, the infraorbital artery, and the ipsilateral supratrochlear artery (while recording the supraorbital Doppler signal). Barnes, whose group has obtained the most satisfactory published results with this method, in addition recommends brief compression of the ipsilateral and contralateral common carotid arteries low in the neck, which may provide information as to intracranial collateralization in ICA stenosis. Bone *et al.*[28] showed that the distal carotid artery back-pressure measured during endarterectomy exceeded 48 mmHg in all patients having antegrade supratrochlear flow during transient common carotid artery compression, and fell below 41 mmHg in virtually all patients with reversal or obliteration of supratrochlear flow.

Published studies using periorbital Doppler have had widely varying success in detecting hemodynamically significant carotid artery occlusive disease. In two personally studied series[66, 67], the sensitivity of *supraorbital* Doppler in detecting ICA stenosis of 60% or greater varied from 75 to 88%, with a specificity of 70 to 87%. A high proportion of false-positive test results has occurred without hemodynamically significant stenosis in several series[73, 84, 101] but not in all reports[104]. Technically remediable factors may account for some of this variability but cannot explain all false-positive results[66].

Several workers have noted the relative insensitivity of *supraorbital* Doppler to non-occlusive stenosis[73, 101, 103, 106]. In one series, flow reversal occurred in 94% of ICA occlusions but in only 68% of non-occlusive stenoses exceeding 70%[101]. False-negative Doppler findings may result from combined stenoses of the external and internal carotid arteries, or from common carotid artery stenoses since these lesions restrict the amount of external carotid collateralization[84, 104, 105]. *Supratrochlear* Doppler is far more *specific* than supraorbital Doppler in detecting hemodynamically significant ICA stenosis, but in general is far less sensitive. The specificity in excluding 60% diameter stenosis in two personal series[66, 67] was 95 and 99%, but the sensitivity was only 44–48%. Other studies have confirmed the insensitivity of supratrochlear Doppler to stenosis of less than 70–75%[27, 101, 116]. Supratrochlear Doppler abnormalities are most highly correlated with severe ICA stenosis or occlusion[66].

From published series, the following conclusions appear warranted: (1) the method is a technically demanding one, and wide variations in technique and accuracy are evident among investigators; (2) although sensitive to hemodynamically significant stenosis, the method is less sensitive than OPG to lesions producing only 50–74% stenosis[29] and most successful in detecting severe degrees of stenosis or occlusion; this is particularly true of supratrochlear Doppler[4]; (3) neither supratrochlear nor supraorbital Doppler can infallibly distinguish tight ICA stenosis from complete occlusion; and (4) only uncommonly have accuracy figures exceeding 90% been reported with periorbital Doppler[15, 107]. Thus, despite its relatively low cost, periorbital directional Doppler suffers from greater inconsistency and less accuracy than reported for several of the other indirect non-invasive tests. It cannot be recommended for use as a single test of hemodynamically significant occlusive disease.

Other indirect non-invasive methods

Facial thermography

This methodology utilizes a camera sensitive to infrared wavelengths to register the skin temperature of the face. In advanced ICA stenosis or occlusion an abnormally cool patch is observed on the side of the lesion, centered over the medial canthus or medial two-thirds of the supraorbital region, corresponding to those forehead areas supplied by the supratrochlear and supraorbital arteries – branches of the ophthalmic artery[98, 150]. Occluding the superficial temporal artery increases the sensitivity of the method. This test is positive only with hemodynamically significant degrees of carotid narrowing and is most sensitive (80–90%) to complete carotid occlusion[98].

Direct thermometry

Similar information may be gained from direct thermometry of the supraorbital region with a thermistor probe[7, 125, 134]. Normally, the two supraorbital regions differ in temperature by only about 0.2°F (0.1°C). With carotid occlusion, the temperature ipsilaterally may fall by about 1–3°F (0.5–1.6°C)[7]. Confusing findings may arise with bilateral occlusive disease. Thermal detection methods in general are less precise in localizing and characterizing extracranial carotid occlusive disease than are other, more commonly used indirect tests, and they appear to be inconsistently sensitive to milder degrees of hemodynamically significant carotid stenosis[125, 134].

Supraorbital photoplethysmography

This is a technique in which pulsations arising from the circulatory beds of the forehead supplied by the supratrochlear and supraorbital arteries are monitored by a transducer utilizing infrared light-emitting diodes. Recordings are made bilaterally during a series of vascular compression maneuvers. Abnormal degrees of pulse-amplitude attenuation (exceeding 33%) in response to compression of ipsilateral external carotid artery branches or of the contralateral common carotid artery (low in the neck) are observed with occlusive disease of the internal carotid artery and signify the presence of collateral circulation[12]. This method has a reported sensitivity of over 95% and a specificity of 80–90% in detecting stenoses exceeding 50%[10]. Concordant results by supraorbital photoplethysmography and directional Doppler examination have a reported accuracy of 98–99% in predicting or excluding hemodynamically significant carotid stenoses[12,49].

Opacity pulse propagation time

This refers to the time (in milliseconds) from the R-wave of the electrocardiogram to the arrival of the corresponding opacity pulse wave in the vascular bed of interest. An interval exceeding 12 msec for the medial supraorbital area of the forehead is consistent with ipsilateral carotid occlusive disease[126]. This test is not widely used.

Carotid compression tonography

Carotid compression tonography assesses the dynamics of intraocular pressure changes during and following compression of the common carotid artery. Specific indices include the amplitude of ocular pulsations and the slopes of the intraocular pressure curves during and following ipsilateral and contralateral common carotid artery compressions[40]. This test is fairly sensitive to hemodynamically significant carotid stenosis[77] but is not widely employed owing to concern as to the potential risks of carotid compression.

Radionuclide angiography

This refers to the rapid sequential scintillation camera imaging of the cervical and cranial intravascular activity of a radiopharmaceutical such as ^{99m}Tc-pertechnetate immediately following its intravenous bolus administration. Although pictorial information is provided, this test is more properly categorized as an 'indirect' method since it primarily depicts flow velocity within the carotid arterial system. A unilateral diminution of activity may be seen with extracranial carotid occlusion or pre-occlusive stenosis, but false-negative results are common with lesser degrees of stenosis[60]. The limited power of this method renders it unsuitable for routine use as a test for carotid artery occlusive disease, although it is appropriate to request this test as an adjunct to a static technetium brain scan when the latter is otherwise indicated.

USE OF NON-INVASIVE TESTS IN COMBINATION

Because of the inherent limitations of the widely available non-invasive methods, most laboratories perform two or three, and some laboratories as many as six tests in parallel to assess the extracranial arterial circulation[2, 3]. This practice creates complexities of interpretation which have not been fully addressed in the literature. Two issues need to be considered: the first relates to the criteria used for designating a battery of tests as 'positive', and the second concerns the nature of the tests being combined.

When multiple tests are performed in parallel, a test battery may be defined either as one in which *all* test results must be abnormal or one in which *any* of the component test results is abnormal. For a battery of six non-invasive tests, for example, 64 possible combinations of test results are possible. In only two of these, however, are all individual test results either abnormal or normal. The decision as to which of these combinations constitutes a 'positive' or 'negative' battery is a formidable one, probably only possible by sophisticated computer analysis of clinical data.

In the more usual situation, only two tests are performed in parallel, and only four combinations of test results require consideration. The requirement that both tests be abnormal in order to designate the battery as positive enhances the battery's aggregate specificity but decreases its sensitivity. The more liberal criterion that *either* test be abnormal to designate the battery as positive increases the battery's aggregate sensitivity at the expense of decreased specificity. An illustrative battery is the parallel use of fluid-filled oculoplethysmography (OPG) and carotid phonoangiography (CPA) (see reference 37 for an analysis of the relevant literature). With the use of the more stringent 'both-abnormal' criterion of positivity, enhanced specificity (98%) for the detection of significant ICA stenosis[66, 90] is achieved only with a reduced sensitivity (54%) of the battery; this increases the proportion of diseased vessels erroneously classified as normal. Conversely, the 'either-abnormal' criterion of positivity increases the sensitivity (93%) at the expense of decreased specificity (72%), with the result that an increased proportion of normal vessels is erroneously classified as diseased. Unfortunately, many reports in the literature do not reveal the arteriographic findings for the results of each component test of the test battery. Criteria differ among studies, rendering comparison of results impossible in the absence of access to the raw data. The determination of which criterion to apply in a given clinical situation depends upon the decision-maker's desire to minimize false-negative as against false-positive classifications[72, 149]. In general, when a 'positive' battery would be followed by a risky procedure or a therapy of unproven or small benefit, the more severe 'both-tests-abnormal' criterion should be used for decision-making purposes in order to minimize false-positive referrals[35]. However, in clinical situations in which subsequent management would be of relatively low risk and high benefit to the patient, the more liberal 'either-test-abnormal' criterion for positivity may be applied.

The second issue to be considered with parallel testing is the determination of which studies are to be combined. In principle, more diagnostic information is obtained when an additional test is included that provides information not obtainable from the other studies in the battery. A complementary test results in a minimum of overlap in the false-positive and false-negative classifications incurred by each test[37, 149]. In practice, this result is best accomplished by parallel combinations using both indirect and direct tests of the extracranial circulation[3]. Batteries including two or more tests of the same type are more likely to result in concordant results at the dual expense of magnifying errors and confusing the interpreter when conflicting results are obtained. This is especially likely in combinations using two or more indirect non-invasive tests, as convincingly demonstrated by Malone *et al.*[107]. In that study, 202 arteries were evaluated by both fluid-filled OPG and supraorbital directional Doppler ultrasonography with arteriographic correlates. Each test had a comparable overall accuracy (91.6% and 94.2% respectively), and the accuracy of the battery (97%) was not significantly improved over either test, even when the 171 vessels with concordant results on both tests were included. More important, however, is the fact that the individual test results disagreed in 15.4% of vessels. In that situation, the diagnostic accuracy of neither test was acceptable (39% if OPG results were relied upon and 61% if directional Doppler results were used).

In summary, the performance of two or more non-invasive tests in parallel can aid in the information content provided by the neurovascular laboratory, but only with the added complexity of interpretation and additional expense that accompanies such battery-testing. The specific component tests in a battery should be carefully selected, and the criterion for a positive battery should be explicitly defined, based in part upon the relative importance of false-negative and false-positive misclassifications in the specific clinical setting. Reports of non-invasive test batteries should include arteriographic correlates whenever possible, and individual as well as aggregate correlations should be available to the reviewer of these reports.

CLINICAL INDICATIONS FOR NON-INVASIVE TESTING

Introduction

Non-invasive neurovascular tests should be performed when decisions about patient management will be guided by their results. Such decisions may include watchful waiting for the appearance of cerebrovascular symptoms; the initiation of therapy with antiplatelet agents or anticoagulants; and the performance of carotid arteriography with the intention of undertaking surgical correction of carotid arterial lesions, should they be detected. Alternatively, specific therapy may be withheld and serial non-invasive studies performed to detect presumed progression of underlying disease. Management decisions should be based upon the known relative risks and benefits of each therapeutic option.

With the possible exceptions of digital subtraction intravenous angiography and B-mode ultrasonic imaging (when optimal), non-invasive tests cannot unequivocally exclude extracranial carotid artery disease. Similarly, with the possible exception of Doppler imaging, non-invasive tests cannot reliably differentiate high-grade carotid stenosis from complete occlusion. Selective carotid arteriography remains the clinical 'gold standard' for both confirmation and exclusion of disease, yet under even optimal conditions this technique is not entirely risk-free. Death (usually secondary to cardiac causes) and permanent neurological deficits occur in approximately 1% of procedures; much higher prevalences obtain at less experienced centers or when the proportion of high-risk patients being studied is larger[52].

Where the risks of arteriography and endarterectomy appear higher than usual[139] or the benefits of surgical management appear relatively low compared to other forms of therapy, management decisions should be guided by the results of a carefully selected and interpreted non-invasive test battery. In these clinical settings, negative results from a highly sensitive battery may be used to exclude the need for arteriography or the initiation of risky therapy. Patients with positive results on a highly specific battery of non-invasive tests can be chosen for evaluation by arteriography or, if the risks of surgical intervention are high, can be selected for medical management. In low-risk patients likely to benefit from surgical treatment, arteriography may be recommended without prior performance of non-invasive neurovascular tests. In the following sections we use these principles to guide the performance and interpretation of non-invasive tests in several selected clinical situations. *Table 9.2* provides a summary of the clinical indications for non-invasive tests.

Table 9.2 Clinical indications for non-invasive neurovascular tests

Clinical setting	If therapeutic choice is:	Recommendation is:*
Otherwise healthy patients with typical anterior circulation TIAs or transient monocular blindness.	(a) Carotid endarterectomy	(a) Proceed to arteriography. Noninvasive tests not needed.
	(b) Antiplatelet agents	(b) Noninvasive tests optional; may help in patient selection.
	(c) Anticoagulation	(c) Highly specific noninvasive test battery strongly recommended to aid in patient selection.
Patients with probable anterior circulation TIAs or transient monocular blindness who have relative contraindications to arteriography.	(a) Carotid endarterectomy	(a) Highly specific noninvasive test battery is strongly recommended to help select patients for arteriography.
	(b) Antiplatelet agents	(b) Noninvasive tests optional; may help in patient selection.
	(c) Anticoagulation	(c) Highly specific noninvasive test battery is strongly recommended to select patients.

Table 9.2 Clinical indications for non-invasive neurovascular tests (contd)

Clinical setting	If therapeutic choice is:	Recommendation is:*
Patients with completed hemispheral strokes and minor neurological residua.	(a) Eventual carotid endarterectomy	(a) If risk of arteriography is low, proceed directly to arteriography. If risk of arteriography is high, use highly specific noninvasive test battery to select patients.
	(b) Antiplatelet agents	(b) Noninvasive tests optional; may help in patient selection.
Patients with nonhemispheral symptoms or other symptoms suggesting a vascular basis.	(a) Watchful waiting or antiplatelet agents	(a) Noninvasive testing is optional; carotid lesion, if present, may not be responsible for symptoms.
Patients with asymptomatic cervical bruits.	(a) Antiplatelet agents	(a) Noninvasive tests optional; may help in patient selection. Positive results may be followed with serial tests to detect high-risk groups.
	(b) Anticoagulation or carotid endarterectomy	(b) Highly specific noninvasive test battery is strongly recommended to select patients.
Patients with asymptomatic cervical bruits in whom major peripheral or coronary vascular surgery is contemplated.	(a) Carotid endarterectomy (efficacy unproven; see text)	(a) Highly specific noninvasive test battery is strongly recommended as basis of patient selection.
Post-carotid endarterectomy patients.	(a) Carotid endarterectomy (for recurrent stenosis)	(a) If symptoms are present, proceed directly to arteriography.
	(b) Antiplatelet agents	(b) Noninvasive tests are optional.
Patients with central retinal artery occlusion.	(a) Carotid endarterectomy	(a) Highly specific noninvasive test battery is strongly recommended to define patient subgroup with carotid artery pathology.

* The recommendations assume that patients are at low- or normal-risk with respect to the specified diagnostic or therapeutic intervention, unless otherwise indicated.

Patients with definite or probable anterior circulation transient ischemic attacks

Typical anterior circulation transient ischemic attacks are associated with ICA stenosis of at least 50% diameter reduction in approximately one-half of patients[123, 143]. In perhaps as many as an additional 15% of patients, carotid arteriography reveals non-stenotic vessels with irregularities or ulcerations which may be related to the ischemic symptoms. Following a thorough clinical evaluation to exclude potentially remediable cardiac or systemic causes[58], the diagnostic plan should be formulated with the therapeutic direction firmly in mind. In healthy patients with surgically accessible carotid lesions in the arterior circulation, carotid endarterectomy may be recommended when an experienced operating team is available[32, 132]. More comprehensive recommendations regarding the indications for endarterectomy are made elsewhere[58]. In brief, these include operating on vessels with greater than 50% stenosis ipsilateral to the symptoms; stenotic vessels contralateral to a carotid occlusion, regardless of the site of the symptoms; and vessels with rough or ulcerative carotid lesions considered to be non-obstructive, in the absence of specific contraindications. While the relative efficacy of endar- terectomy in these situations has not been adequately compared to medical therapy in controlled trials, the intention to manage patients by surgical means should guide decisions concerning the diagnostic evaluation. In these situations, because of the inherent limitations of most non-invasive methods, these studies may be bypassed in favor of proceeding directly to arteriography[131].

For patients with typical transient ischemic attacks who are not ideal candidates for surgery[32, 58, 132, 139], therapeutic options include daily salicylates indefinitely, or anticoagulation for 3–6 months followed by daily salicylates[32, 58, 132]. In these situations, arteriography should not be performed, and non-invasive evaluation may play a limited clinical role. Abnormal results on a battery of specific non-invasive tests may support the physician's impression of carotid occlusive disease and/or assist in the decision to initiate medical treatment in patients with relative contraindications to aspirin or anticoagulants. In patients without such relative contraindications to medical therapy, however, therapy may be initiated on clinical grounds alone, regardless of non-invasive test results.

Non-invasive tests may be more strongly indicated in patients with atypical anterior circulation symptoms, especially if relative contraindications to arterio- graphy, surgery or medical therapy exist. Selection of individuals for arteriography or relatively risky medical therapy may be guided by abnormal results from a highly specific non-invasive test battery in order to minimize inappropriate initiation of these options. Alternatively, entirely normal results from a sensitive battery of tests in these patients may be used to withhold arteriography or risky medical treatment.

Patients with completed hemispheral strokes and minor neurological residua

In some of these patients non-invasive testing may reveal evidence of a carotid artery stenosis ipsilateral to the cerebral infarction. Such lesions should be confirmed by cerebral arteriography if carotid endarterectomy is contemplated. In the case of surgically accessible lesions, endarterectomy may be recommended at a later date to prevent further strokes in the same vascular distribution[32].

Patients with non-hemispheral transient ischemic symptoms and other possibly vascular symptoms of uncertain significance

In this group of patients, non-invasive procedures may suggest the presence of a carotid artery lesion, but it must be decided on clinical grounds whether such lesions are related to the clinical symptoms. Carotid surgery in this setting is controversial[112], and negative results from a sensitive non-invasive test battery may be used with some confidence as the basis of a decision not to perform arteriographic studies in these patients.

Patients with asymptomatic cervical bruits

Prevalence, natural history, and management strategies

The frequency of asymptomatic cervical bruits decreases with increasing age until the fifth or sixth decades, whereas the prevalence of atherosclerotic disease increases with advancing age[74]. Thus, 'cervical bruit' is not synonymous with 'carotid stenosis' despite the fact that these terms are often used interchangeably. Approximately 4–17% of asymptomatic middle-aged and elderly adults have audible bruits[74, 78, 127, 141]. When only mid-cervical bruits are considered, the prevalence in adults is probably 3–10%[133]. The differential diagnosis of cervical bruits is wide-ranging[133, 142]. Although it has been implied that 70–90% of audible bruits in adults reflect significant ICA disease[31, 141, 142], other reports suggest that as few as 16%, but certainly less than 40–50% of individuals over age 50 with cervical bruits, have ICA lesions of greater than 50% diameter reduction[10, 46, 90].

The implications of disease prevalence, or the pre-test probability of disease, for the predictive value and accuracy of a non-invasive test battery have been reviewed in an earlier section. In the case of the asymptomatic bruit, if one assumes the prevalence of significant ICA disease to be, for example, 20%, positive results on a 'good' test battery with 90% sensitivity and specificity would nevertheless result in false-positive classifications 30.8% of the time. Whether this misclassification rate is acceptable for decision-making depends on the relative risks and costs associated with false-negative versus false-positive designations.

Even with arteriographically documented stenosis, the preferred treatment of asymptomatic individuals is widely debated[32, 36, 57, 140]. Watchful waiting until the occurrence of neurological warning symptoms has been advocated by some[82], while antiplatelet agents[57] or surgical approaches[140, 142] have been recommended by others. Advocates of watchful-waiting strategies cite the very low frequency of sudden, unheralded strokes in asymptomatic patients with suspected or documented ICA stenosis followed without therapy for 3–5 years or more[82, 87, 90,

[100, 124, 135]. Data bearing on the natural history of these patients are mostly inferential, however, being derived primarily from population studies of patients with bruits (stenosis not documented) and from surgical series in which a contralateral, unrepaired stenosis existed in patients undergoing endarterectomy ipsilateral to the site of transient ischemic symptoms.

Advocates of surgical management have generally reported a low incidence of subsequent neurovascular events following uncomplicated arteriography and surgery, although there are no adequately controlled trials to date comparing endarterectomy with other management alternatives. In addition, the summed risks of arteriography and endarterectomy must be considered. The approximately 1% risk of serious arteriographic complications has been mentioned previously[55, 76, 81, 108, 143, 145]. The perioperative risks associated with carotid endarterectomy for asymptomatic ICA stenosis have also been well documented[48, 86, 97, 115, 117, 142]. Among studies reporting a total of 365 patients from university centers with experienced surgical teams, there was only one intraoperative death[86] and one death secondary to cerebrovascular causes within the 30-day postoperative period[115]. In these series, the weighted average mortality rate was thus 0.6% with an additional 1.1% incidence of permanent, and 2.2% incidence of transient cerebral events occurring during the perioperative period. The combined serious operative complication rate is therefore 1.6%. It must be cautioned that complications may be much more prevalent in centers without extensive experience in this procedure[51]. Thus, the combined serious complication rate for arteriography plus surgery is approximately 2.6% in university centers. Of those who survive these procedures without complication, most but not all continue to be asymptomatic over the following 3–4 years. As many as 5% will suffer a stroke, and perhaps an equal number will develop transient neurological symptoms. Between 20 and 33% of patients die of non-cerebrovascular causes[86, 115, 117, 142].

Proponents of therapy with antiplatelet agents for asymptomatic ICA disease cite the beneficial results of such treatment for patients with symptoms of transient cerebral ischemia[57]. However, no systematic effort has been made to evaluate antiplatelet agents in the treatment of asymptomatic ICA disease. Nonetheless, it is possible that the natural history of this condition might be favorably altered by long-term therapy with platelet antiaggregant agents.

In summary, while audible cervical bruits are relatively common in asymptomatic elderly individuals, they reflect significant underlying ICA stenosis in perhaps only 20% of these patients. The management alternatives available to the physician have been recommended on the basis of inferential or inadequately controlled clinical data, and none offers a clear medical benefit without simultaneously conferring increased risk of either short- or long-term morbidity and mortality.

Implications of management strategies for non-invasive diagnosis

Guidelines for the use of non-invasive testing in asymptomatic patients may be developed on the basis of the relative risks and benefits of each of the three management strategies. If the strategy of watchful waiting is preferred, non-invasive testing might be considered optional, although negative results from a sensitive non-invasive test battery would serve to reassure the physician that significant ICA disease is not present. Alternatively, testing could be undertaken at periodic intervals to detect progressive lesions at higher risk of becoming symptomatic. Prospective studies to evaluate the clinical correlates of serial non-invasive testing are needed to assess the utility of this option.

If more aggressive surgical management is contemplated, the possible long-term reduction in symptomatic events is counterbalanced in part by the greater immediate hazards of this strategy. Since far fewer than half of all asymptomatic elderly individuals with audible bruits have significant ICA stenosis, careful selection of patients for arteriography is warranted. If endarterectomy is contemplated, arteriography may be reserved for those patients with abnormal results on a highly specific non-invasive test battery in order to minimize false-positive referrals.

The use of antiplatelet agents in patients with asymptomatic cervical bruits might also be guided by the results of non-invasive neurovascular tests. When the risk of such therapy is negligible, treatment may be initiated empirically, although abnormal non-invasive test results may increase the clinician's confidence in the presence of underlying ICA disease.

Patients with known or suspected carotid artery disease in whom major non-cerebrovascular surgery is contemplated

Patients with the recent onset of *symptomatic* focal cerebrovascular disease concurrent with symptomatic cardiac or other vascular disease may benefit from staged or simultaneous surgical procedures[44, 113]. Although controlled studies are lacking, carotid endarterectomy may be recommended in these situations because of its relatively low risk and the possibility of higher postoperative cerebrovascular morbidity and mortality in unoperated patients[42]. The decision to perform staged or simultaneous operations should probably be based upon the relative clinical urgency of the concurrent disease and upon arteriographic criteria[113]. Non-invasive testing may have a role in the selection of a subpopulation of patients for arteriography who are more likely to have significant carotid lesions[85, 113]. However, owing to the inherent limitations in sensitivity of the most widely available non-invasive methods, these techniques should probably be bypassed in favor of proceeding directly to arteriography[44].

When elective non-cerebrovascular surgery is contemplated in patients with remote histories of cerebrovascular symptoms or with asymptomatic cervical bruits, decisions regarding assessment of the extracranial vasculature and possible surgical treatment are much more problematic[13, 30]. In one case-control study, patients with previous histories of cerebrovascular symptoms were said to be at no greater risk of postoperative neurological complications following coronary bypass grafting than patients without such symptoms[70]; however, the number of patients considered was small.

Studies of patients with asymptomatic cervical bruits or evidence of stenosis by non-invasive testing have been consistent in showing no increased risk of perioperative cerebrovascular events[13, 30]. The results of three series of patients undergoing peripheral vascular surgery without carotid procedures were summarized by Corman[42]. No postoperative neurological deficits occurred among 167 patients with audible cervical bruits, whereas there were 8 postoperative deficits among 791 patients without bruits[34, 54, 144]. A more recent study[14] reported one postoperative deficit in a series of 34 bruits; interestingly, that patient had negative non-invasive tests. In several series, no association was noted between cervical bruits or asymptomatic carotid disease and perioperative neurological events in patients undergoing coronary bypass procedures[13, 14, 30, 70].

While cerebrovascular disease may increase the overall mortality rates of these other major operations[13, 14], and although arteriography and endarterectomy may be performed with relatively low risk in these situations[88, 97], there are no convincing data to support the use of these procedures in neurologically asymptomatic patients. The role of preoperative non-invasive neurovascular testing in these situations would therefore appear to be quite limited and should be confined primarily to aiding in the assessment of overall operative risk.

Post-carotid endarterectomy patients

Recurrent stenosis may occur in as many as 10% of these patients if followed serially[91]. Non-invasive studies may serve to document recurrent carotid lesions post-endarterectomy and may help to select patients for anticoagulation or antiplatelet agents. When reoperation is considered for cerebrovascular symptoms, positive non-invasive test results would require confirmation by cerebral arteriography.

Patients with central retinal artery occlusion

In some patients with central retinal artery occlusion who do not have clinically apparent valvular heart disease, internal carotid artery lesions have been found to coexist[2, 3, 128]. Patients with abnormal results on a highly specific non-invasive test battery may be selected for arteriography when carotid endarterectomy would be the therapy of choice[2, 3].

CONCLUDING COMMENTS

The field of non-invasive neurovascular testing is still in its adolescence. Impressive technological innovations have become commonplace, yet certain limitations in the power of non-invasive methods remain. In general, the hemodynamically sensitive, indirect non-invasive tests are capable of detecting carotid stenoses only when the degree of luminal diameter reduction exceeds 50–60%[43, 47, 109]. The differentiation of preocclusive extracranial carotid stenosis (an operable lesion) from complete (and hence inoperable) vascular occlusion, while possible with Doppler imaging methods, is not infallible. Although the delineation of non-stenotic, ulcerative carotid lesions is possible with B-mode ultrasonic imaging, the correspondence between the appearance of the lesion as shown by ultrasound vs arteriography is not always close. Intravenous digital subtraction angiography, the newest comet in the neurovascular diagnostic firmament, is not 'non-invasive' in the strict sense yet will probably prove to be sufficiently safe to permit its wide general application. This method is unique in that it can visualize the entire spectrum of carotid pathology, from ulcerative lesions to preocclusive stenosis and complete occlusion, with consistency and fidelity. Visualization of the vertebrobasilar system and the intracranial carotid system is also possible, within limits.

Given the availability of these technologically sophisticated modalities, the physician's ability to visualize and characterize extracranial carotid pathology has in general come to exceed his capacity to design and execute definitive studies of either the natural history of such conditions or their proper therapy. The asymptomatic cervical bruit is a particularly apposite example (see above). Non-invasive neurovascular methods are well suited both to the acquisition of natural history data and to the characterization of carotid lesions within the context of controlled, randomized therapeutic trials. It is incumbent upon the concerned physician to direct these impressive diagnostic methods toward the realization of these worthy goals.

Acknowledgements

The support of U.S. Public Health Service Grants NS 05820 and NS 15883 is gratefully acknowledged. Ms Tracey Moffitt assisted with the typing of the manuscript.

References

1 ABU RAHMA, A. F. and DIETHRICH, E. B. Diagnosis of carotid arterial occlusive disease. Reliability of combined carotid phonoangiography and oculoplethys-mography. *Vascular Surgery*, **14**, 23–29 (1980)

2 ACKERMAN, R. H. A perspective on noninvasive diagnosis of carotid disease. *Neurology (Minneapolis)*, **29**, 615–622 (1979)

3 ACKERMAN, R. H. Non-invasive diagnosis of carotid disease. In *Cerebrovascular Survey Report*, edited by R. G. Siekert, 190–210. Bethesda, Maryland: National Institutes of Health (1980)

4 ACKERMAN, R. H. and TAVERAS, J. M. Noninvasive and arteriographic diagnosis of hemodynamically significant carotid lesions. *Stroke*, **7**, 2–3 (1976)

5 ANDERSON, R. D., POWELL, D. F. and VITEK, J. J. B-mode sonography as a screening procedure for asymptomatic carotid bruits. *American Journal of Roentgenology*, **124**, 292–297 (1975)

6 ARCHIE, J. P. Jr., POSEY, P. H. and GOODSON, D. S. Accuracy of digitalized differential pulse timing oculoplethysmography. *Surgery, Gynecology and Obstetrics*, **152**, 259–261 (1981)

7 AUSTIN, J. H. and SAJID, M. H. Direct thermometry in ophthalmic-internal carotid blood flow. *Archives of Neurology*, **15**, 376–392 (1966)

8 BAILLIART, P. La pression arterielle dans les branches de l'artere centrale de la retine; nouvelle technique pour la determiner. *Annales Oculistique*, **154**, 648–666 (1917)

9 BAKER, J. D., BARKER, W. F. and MACHLEDER, H. I. Ocular pneumoplethysmography in the evaluation of carotid stenosis. *Circulation*, **62**, I-1–I-3 (1980)

10 BARNES, R. W. Noninvasive evaluation of the carotid bruit. *Annual Review of Medicine*, **31**, 201–218 (1980)

11 BARNES, R. W., BONE, G. E., REINERTSON, J., SLAYMAKER, E. E., HOKANSON, D. E. and STRANDNESS, D. E. Jr. Noninvasive ultrasonic carotid angiography: prospective validation by contrast arteriography. *Surgery*, **80**, 328–335 (1976)

12 BARNES, R. W., GARRETT, W. V., SLAYMAKER, E. E. and REINERTSON, J. E. Doppler ultrasound and supraorbital photoplethysmography for noninvasive screening of carotid occlusive disease. *American Journal of Surgery*, **134**, 183–186 (1977)

13 BARNES, R. W., LIEBMAN, P. R., MARSZALEK, P. B., KIRK, C. L. and GOLDMAN, M. H. The natural history of asymptomatic carotid disease in patients undergoing cardio-vascular surgery. *Surgery*, **90**, 1075–1083 (1981)

14 BARNES, R. W. and MARSZALEK, P. B. Asymptomatic carotid disease in the cardiovascular surgical patient: is prophylactic endarterectomy necessary? *Stroke*, **12**, 497–500 (1981)

15 BARNES, R. W., RUSSELL, H. E., BONE, G. E. and SLAYMAKER, E. E. Doppler cerebrovascular examination: improved results with refinements in technique. *Stroke*, **8**, 468–471 (1977)

16 BARNETT, G. O., GREENFIELD, J. C. Jr. and FOX, S. M. The technique of estimating the instantaneous aortic blood velocity in man from the pressure gradient. *American Heart Journal*, **62**, 359–366 (1961)

17 BATKO, K. A. and APPEN, R. R. Ophthalmodynamometry: a reappraisal. *Annals of Ophthalmology*, **11**, 1499–1508 (1979)

18 BEST, M. Carotid hemodynamics and the ocular pulse in carotid stenosis. *Neurology (Minneapolis)*, **21**, 982–990 (1971)

19 BEST, M. and ROGERS, R. Techniques of ocular pulse analysis in carotid stenosis. *Archives of Ophthalmology*, **92**, 54–58 (1974)

20 BINGHAM, W. F. Neurosurgical applications of ocular pneumoplethysmography. *Journal of Neurosurgery*, **54**, 588–595 (1981)

21 BLACKSHEAR, W. M. Jr., PHILLIPS, D. J., CHIKOS, P. M., HARLEY, J. D., THIELE, B. L. and STRANDNESS, D. E. Jr. Carotid artery velocity patterns in normal and stenotic vessels. *Stroke*, **11**, 67–71 (1980)

22 BLACKSHEAR, W. M. Jr., PHILLIPS, D. J., THIELE, B. L., HIRSCH, J. H., CHIKOS, P. M., MARINELLI, M. R., WARD, K. J. and STRANDNESS, D. E. Jr. Detection of carotid occlusive disease by ultrasonic imaging and pulsed Doppler spectrum analysis. *Surgery*, **86**, 698–706 (1979)

23 BLACKSHEAR, W. M. Jr., THIELE, B. L., HARLEY, J. D., CHIKOS, P. M. and STRANDNESS, D. E. Jr. A prospective evaluation of oculoplethysmography and carotid phono-angiography. *Surgery, Gynecology and Obstetrics*, **148**, 201–205 (1979)

24 BLACKWELL, E., MERORY, J., TOOLE, J. F. and McKINNEY, W. Doppler ultrasound scanning of the carotid bifurcation. *Archives of Neurology*, **34**, 145–148 (1977)

25 BLOCH, S., BALTAXE, H. A. and SHOUMAKER, R. D. Reliability of Doppler scanning of the carotid bifurcation: angiographic correlation. *Radiology*, **132**, 687–691 (1979)

26 BLUE, S. K., McKINNEY, W. M., BARNES, R. and TOOLE, J. F. Ultrasonic B-mode scanning for study of extracranial vascular disease. *Neurology (Minneapolis)*, **22**, 1079–1085 (1972)

27 BONE, G. E. and BARNES, R. W. Clinical implications of the Doppler cerebrovascular examination: a correlation with angiography. *Stroke*, **7**, 271–273 (1976)

28 BONE, G. E., SLAYMAKER, E. E. and BARNES, R. W. Noninvasive assessment of collateral blood flow of the cerebral hemisphere by Doppler ultrasound. *Surgery, Gynecology and Obstetrics*, **145**, 873–876 (1977)

29 BONE, G. E., DICKENSON, D. and POMAJZL, M. J. A prospective evaluation of indirect methods for detecting carotid atherosclerosis. *Surgery, Gynecology and Obstetrics*, **152**, 587–592 (1981)

30 BRESLAU, P. J., FELL, G., IVEY, T. D., BAILEY, W. W., MILLER, D. W. and STRANDNESS, D. E. Jr. Carotid arterial disease in patients undergoing coronary artery bypass operations. *Journal of Thoracic and Cardiovascular Surgery*, **82**, 765–767 (1981)

31 BREWSTER, D. C., ABBOTT, W. M., DARLING, R. C., REIDY, N. C. and RAINES, J. K. Noninvasive evaluation of asymptomatic carotid bruits. *Circulation*, **58** (Suppl. 1), I-5–I-9 (1978)

32 BYER, J. A. and EASTON, J. D. Therapy of ischemic cerebrovascular disease. *Annals of Internal Medicine*, **93**, 742–756 (1980)

33 CAPLAN, L. R. The frontal-artery sign – a bedside indicator of internal carotid occlusive disease. *New England Journal of Medicine*, **288**, 1008–1009 (1973)

34 CARNEY, W. I. Jr., STEWART, W. B., DePINTO, D. J., MUCHA, S. J. and ROBERTS, B. Carotid bruit as a risk factor in aortoiliac reconstruction. *Surgery*, **81**, 567–570 (1977)

35 CEBUL, R. D. Galactosyltransferase II in detection of pancreatic cancer. *New England Journal of Medicine*, **305**, 766–767 (1981)

36 CEBUL, R. D. Asymptomatic carotid bruit. In *Prognosis: Contemporary Outcomes of Disease*, edited by J. F. Fries and G. E. Ehrlich, 438–441. Bowie, Maryland: Charles Press Publishers (1981)

37 CEBUL, R. D. and GINSBERG, M. D. Noninvasive neurovascular tests for carotid artery disease. *Annals of Internal Medicine*, **97**, 867–872 (1982)

38 CHILCOTE, W. A., MODIC, M. T., PAVLICEK, W. A., LITTLE, J. R., FURLAN, A. J., DUCHESNEAU, P. M. and WEINSTEIN, M. A. Digital subtraction angiography of the carotid arteries: a comparative study in 100 patients. *Radiology*, **139**, 287–295 (1981)

39 CHRISTENSON, P. C., OVITT, T. W., FISHER, H. D. III, FROST, M. M., NUDELMAN, S. and ROEHRIG, H. Intravenous angiography using digital video subtraction: intravenous cervicocerebrovascular angiography. *American Journal of Neuroradiology*, **1**, 379–386 (1980)

40 COHEN, D. N., WANGELIN, R., TROTTA, C., BEVEN, E. G., HUMPHRIES, A. W. and YOUNG, J. R. Carotid compression tonography. *Stroke*, **6**, 257–262 (1975)

41 COMEROTA, A. J., CRANLEY, J. J. and COOK, S. E. Real-time B-mode carotid imaging in diagnosis of cerebrovascular disease. *Surgery*, **89**, 718–729 (1981)

42 CORMAN, L. C. The preoperative patient with an asymptomatic cervical bruit. *Medical Clinics of North America*, **63**, 1335–1340 (1979)

43 CRAWFORD, E. S., DeBAKEY, M. E., BLAISDELL, F. W., MORRIS, G. C. Jr. and FIELDS, W. S. Hemodynamic alterations in patients with cerebral arterial insufficiency before and after operation. *Surgery*, **48**, 76–94 (1960)

44 CRAWFORD, E. S., PALAMARA, A. E. and KASPARIAN, A. S. Carotid and noncoronary operations: simultaneous, staged and delayed. *Surgery*, **87**, 1–8 (1980)

45 CRUMMY, A. B., STROTHER, C. M., SACKETT, J. F., ERGUN, D. L., SHAW, C. G., KRUGER, R. A., MISTRETTA, C. A., TURNIPSEED, W. D., LIEBERMAN, R. P., MYEROWITZ, P. D. and RUZICKA, F. F. Computerized fluoroscopy: digital subtraction for intravenous angio-cardiography and arteriography. *American Journal of Radiology*, **135**, 1131–1140 (1980)

46 DAVID, T. E., HUMPHRIES, A. W., YOUNG, J. R. and BEVEN, E. G. A correlation of neck bruits and arteriosclerotic carotid arteries. *Archives of Surgery*, **107**, 729–731 (1973)

47 DeWEESE, J. A., MAY, A. G., LIPCHIK, E. O. and ROB, C. G. Anatomic and hemodynamic correlations in carotid artery stenosis. *Stroke*, **1**, 149–157 (1970)

48 DUKE, L. J., SLAYMAKER, E. E., LAMBERTH, W. C. and WRIGHT, C. B. Carotid arterial reconstruction: ten-year experience. *American Surgeon*, **45**, 281–288 (1979)

49 DUKE, L. J., SLAYMAKER, E. E., LAMBERTH, W. C. and WRIGHT, C. B. Results of ophthal-mosonometry and supraorbital photoplethysmography in evaluating carotid arterial stenosis. *Circulation*, **60**, (Suppl. 1) I-127–I-131 (1979)

50 DUNCAN, G. W., GRUBER, J. O., DEWEY, C. F. Jr., MYERS, G. S. and LEES, R. S. Evaluation of carotid stenosis by phonoangiography. *New England Journal of Medicine*, **293**, 1124–1128 (1975)

51 EASTON, J. D. and SHERMAN, D. G. Stoke and mortality rate in carotid endarterectomy: 228 consecutive operations. *Stroke*, **8**, 565–568 (1977)

52 EISENBERG, R. L. Cerebral angiography: conflicting testimony. *American Journal of Roentgenology*, **134**, 615–617 (1980)

53 EVANS, T. C. Jr. and TAENZER, J. C. Ultrasound imaging of atherosclerosis in carotid arteries. *Applied Radiology*, March–April, 106–115 (1979)

54 EVANS, W. E. and COOPERMAN, M. The significance of asymptomatic unilateral carotid bruits in preoperative patients. *Surgery*, **83**, 522–527 (1978)

55 FAUGHT, E., TRADER, S. D. and HANNA, G. R. Cerebral complications of angiography for transient ischemia and stroke: prediction of risk. *Neurology (Minneapolis)*, **29**, 4–15 (1979)

56 FELL, G., PHILLIPS, D. J., CHIKOS, P. M., HARLEY, J. D., THIELE, B. L. and STRANDNESS, D. E. Jr. Ultrasonic duplex scanning for disease of the carotid artery. *Circulation*, **64**, 1191–1195 (1981)

57 FIELDS, W. S. The asymptomatic carotid bruit – operate or not? Current Concepts of Cerebrovascular Disease – *Stroke*, **13**, 1–4 (1978)

58 FIELDS, W. S. Selection of patients with ischemic cerebrovascular disease for arterial surgery. *World Journal of Surgery*, **3**, 147–154 (1979)

59 FISHER, C. M. Facial pulses in internal carotid artery occlusion. *Neurology (Minneapolis)*, **20**, 476–478 (1970)

60 FOO, D. and HENRICKSON, L. Radionuclide cerebral blood flow and carotid angiogram. Correlation in internal carotid artery disease. *Stroke*, **8**, 39–43 (1977)

61 GAUTIER, J. C., ROSA, A. and LHERMITTE, F. Auscultation carotidienne. Correlations chez 200 patients avec 332 angiographies. *Revue Neurologique (Paris)*, **131**, 175–184 (1975)

62 GEE, W., McDONALD, K. M., KAUPP, H. A., CELANI, V. J. and BAST, R. G. Carotid stenosis plus occlusion: endarterectomy or bypass? *Archives of Surgery*, **115**, 183–187 (1980)

63 GEE, W., MEHIGAN, J. T. and WYLIE, E. J. Measurement of collateral cerebral hemispheric blood pressure by ocular pneumoplethysmography. *American Journal of Surgery*, **130**, 121–127 (1975)

64 GEE, W., OLLER, D. W., AMUNDSEN, D. J. and GOODREAU, J. J. The asymptomatic carotid bruit and the ocular pneumoplethysmography. *Archives of Surgery*, **112**, 1381–1388 (1977)

65 GEE, W., OLLER, D. W. and WYLIE, E. J. Noninvasive diagnosis of carotid occlusion by ocular pneumoplethysmography. *Stroke*, **7**, 18–21 (1976)

66 GINSBERG, M. D., GREENWOOD, S. A. and GOLDBERG, H. I. Noninvasive diagnosis of extracranial cerebrovascular disease: Oculoplethysmography-phonoangiography and directional Doppler ultrasonography. *Neurology (Minneapolis)*, **29**, 623–631 (1979)

67 GINSBERG, M. D., GREENWOOD, S. A. and GOLDBERG, H. I. Limitations of quantitative oculoplethysmography and of directional Doppler ultrasonography in cerebrovascular diagnosis: assessment of an air-filled OPG system. *Stroke*, **12**, 27–32 (1981)

68 GINSBERG, M. D., NAMON, R., QUENCER, R. M. and DAVID, N. J. Ultrasonic B-scan imaging of carotid artery atherosclerosis: correlations with arteriography. *Neurology (Minneapolis)*, **31**, 55 (1981)

69 GOMPELS, B. M. High definition imaging of carotid arteries using a standard commercial ultrasound 'B' scanner. *British Journal of Radiology*, **52**, 608–619 (1979)

70 GONZALEZ-SCARANO, F. and HURTIG, H. I. Neurological complications of coronary artery bypass grafting: case-control study. *Neurology (New York)*, **31**, 1032–1035 (1981)

71 GREEN, P. S., TAENZER, J. C., RAMSEY, S. D. Jr., HOLZEMER, J. F., SUAREZ, J. R., MARICH, K. W., EVANS, T. C., SANDOK, B. A. and GREENLEAF, J. F. A real-time ultrasonic imaging system for carotid arteriography. *Ultrasound in Medicine and Biology*, **3**, 129–142 (1977)

72 GRINER, P. F., MAYEWSKI, R. J., MUSHLIN, A. I. and GREENLAND, P. Selection and interpretation of diagnostic tests and procedures. *Annals of Internal Medicine*, **94** (2), 553–600 (1981)

73 GROSS, W. S., VERTA, M. J. Jr., van BELLEN, B., BERGAN, J. J. and YAO, J. S. T. Comparison of noninvasive diagnostic techniques in carotid artery occlusive disease. *Surgery*, **82**, 271–278 (1977)

74 HAMMOND, J. H. and EISINGER, R. P. Carotid bruits in 1,000 normal subjects. *Archives of Internal Medicine*, **109**, 109–111 (1962)

75 HARTLEY, C. J. and STRANDNESS, D. E. Jr. The effects of atherosclerosis on the transmission of ultrasound. *Journal of Surgical Research*, **9**, 575–582 (1969)

76 HASS, W. K., FIELDS, W. S., NORTH, R. R., KRICHEFF, I. I., CHASE, N. E. and BAUER, R. B. Joint study of extracranial arterial occlusion. II. Arteriography, techniques, sites and complications. *Journal of the American Medical Association*, **203**, 961–968 (1968)

77 HERTZER, N. R., SANTOSCOY, T. G. and LANGSTON, R. H. S. Accuracy of carotid compression tonography in the diagnosis of carotid artery stenosis. Correlation with arteriography in 300 patients. *Cleveland Clinic Quarterly*, **47**, 79–87 (1980)

78 HEYMAN, A., WILKINSON, W. E., HEYDEN, S., HELMS, M. J., BARTEL, A. G., KARP, H. R., TYROLER, H. A. and HAMES, C. G. Risk of stroke in asymptomatic persons with cervical arterial bruits. A population study in Evans County, Georgia. *New England Journal of Medicine*, **302**, 838–841 (1980)

79 HOBSON, R. W. II, BERRY, S. M., JAMIL, Z., MEHTA, K., HART, L. and SIMPSON, H. Oculoplethysmography and pulsed Doppler ultrasonic imaging in diagnosis of carotid arterial disease. *Surgery, Gynecology and Obstetrics*, **152**, 433–436 (1981)

80 HOBSON, R. W. II, BERRY, S. M., KATOCS, A. S. Jr., O'DONNELL, J. A., JAMIL, Z. and SAVITSKY, J. P. Comparison of pulsed Doppler and real-time B-mode echo arteriography for noninvasive imaging of the extracranial carotid arteries. *Surgery*, **87**, 286–293 (1980)

81 HUCKMAN, M. S., SHENK, G. I., NEEMS, R. L. and TINOR, T. Transfemoral cerebral arteriography versus direct percutaneous and brachial arteriography: a comparison of complication rates. *Radiology*, **132**, 93–97 (1979)

82 HUMPHRIES, A. W., YOUNG, J. R., SANTILLI, P. H., BEVEN, E. G. and deWOLFE, V. G. Unoperated, asymptomatic significant internal carotid artery stenosis: a review of 182 instances. *Surgery*, **80**, 695–698 (1976)

83 HURTIG, H. I., BERKOWITZ, H. D., GINSBERG, M. D., GOLDBERG, H. I. and SILBERBERG, D. H. Comparative study of non-invasive cerebrovascular diagnostic methods. *Stroke*, **10**, 107 (1979)

84 HYMAN, B. N. Doppler sonography: a bedside noninvasive method for assessment of carotid artery disease. *American Journal of Ophthalmology*, **77**, 227–231 (1974)

85 JAIN, K. M., HOBSON, R. W. II, JAMIL, Z., MARSTERS, C. and BERRY, S. M. Clinical screening of pre-operative patients for carotid occlusive disease by oculoplethysmography. *American Surgeon*, **46**, 679–685 (1980)

86 JAVID, H., OSTERMILLER, W. E., HENGESH, J. W., DYE, W. S., HUNTER, J. A., NAJAFI, H. and JULIAN, O. C. Carotid endarterectomy for asymptomatic patients. *Archives of Surgery*, **102**, 389–391 (1971)

87 JOHNSON, N., BURNHAM, S. J., FLANIGAN, D. P., GOODREAU, J. J., YAO, J. S. T. and BERIGAN, J. J. Carotid endarterectomy: a follow-up study of the contralateral non-operated carotid artery. *Annals of Surgery*, **188**, 748–752 (1978)

88 KANALY, P. J., PEYTON, M. D., CANNON, J. P., DILLING, E. W. and ELKINS, R. C. The asymptomatic bruit. *American Journal of Surgery*, **134**, 821–824 (1977)

89 KARTCHNER, M. M. and McRAE, L. P. Auscultation for carotid bruits in cerebrovascular insufficiency. *Journal of the American Medical Association*, **210**, 494–497 (1969)

90 KARTCHNER, M. M. and McRAE, L. P. Noninvasive evaluation and management of the 'asymptomatic' carotid bruit. *Surgery*, **82**, 840–847 (1977)

91 KARTCHNER, M. M. and McRAE, L. P. Noninvasive assessment of the progression of extracranial carotid occlusive disease. In *Noninvasive Cardiovascular Diagnosis. Current Concepts*, edited by E. B. Diethrich, 13–18. Baltimore: University Park Press (1978)

92 KARTCHNER, M. M., McRAE, L. P., CRAIN, B. and WHITAKER, B. Oculoplethysmography: an adjunct to arteriography in the diagnosis of extracranial carotid occlusive disease. *American Journal of Surgery*, **132**, 728–732 (1976)

93 KARTCHNER, M. M., McRAE, L. P. and MORRISON, F. D. Noninvasive detection and evaluation of carotid occlusive disease. *Archives of Surgery*, **106**, 528–535 (1973)

94 KISTLER, J. P., LEES, R. S., FRIEDMAN, J., PRESSIN, M., MOHR, J. P., ROBERSON, G. S. and OJEMANN, R. G. The bruit of carotid stenosis versus radiated basal heart murmurs. Differentiation by phonoangiography. *Circulation*, **57**, 975–981 (1975)

95 KNOX, R., BRESLAU, P. and STRANDNESS, D. E. Jr. Quantitative carotid phonoangiography. *Stroke*, **12**, 798–803 (1981)

96 KREMEN, J. E., GEE, W., KAUPP, H. A. and McDONALD, K. M. Restenosis or occlusion after carotid endarterectomy. A survey with ocular pneumoplethysmography. *Archives of Surgery*, **114**, 608–610 (1979)

97 KREMER, R. M. and AHLQUIST, P. E. The prophylactic carotid thromboendarterectomy. *American Surgeon*, **45**, 703–708 (1979)

98 LANCE, J. W. and SOMERVILLE, B. The detection of stenosis or occlusion of the internal carotid artery by facial thermography. *Medical Journal of Australia*, **1**, 97–100 (1972)

99 LEES, R. S. and DEWEY, C. F. Jr. Phonoangiography: a new noninvasive diagnostic method for studying arterial disease. *Proceedings of the National Academy of Sciences*, **67**, 935–942 (1970)

100 LEVIN, S. M. and SONDHEIMER, F. Stenosis of the contralateral carotid artery – to operate or not? *Vascular Surgery*, **7**, 3–13 (1973)

101 LIEBERMAN, A. Directional Doppler in occlusive cerebrovascular disease. *Stroke*, **8**, 629 (1977)

102 LIVERSEDGE, L. A. and SMITH, V. H. The place of ophthalmodynamometry in the investigation of cerebrovascular disease. *Brain*, **84**, 274–288 (1961)

103 LoGERFO, F. W. and MASON, G. R. Directional Doppler studies of supraorbital artery flow in internal carotid stenosis and occlusion. *Surgery*, **76**, 723–728 (1974)

104 LYE, C. R., SUMNER, D. S. and STRANDNESS, D. E. Jr. The accuracy of the supraorbital Doppler examination in the diagnosis of hemodynamically significant carotid occlusive disease. *Surgery*, **79**, 42–45 (1976)

105 MACHLEDER, H. I. Evaluation of patients with cerebrovascular disease using the Doppler ophthalmic test. *Angiology*, **24**, 374–381 (1973)

106 MACHLEDER, H. I. and BARKER, W. F. Noninvasive methods for evaluation of extracranial cerebrovascular disease. A comparison. *Archives of Surgery*, **112**, 944–946 (1977)

107 MALONE, J. M., BEAN, B., LAGUNA, J., HAMILTON, R., LABADIE, E. and MOORE, W. S. Diagnosis of carotid artery stenosis. Comparison of oculoplethysmography and Doppler supraorbital examination. *Annals of Surgery*, **191**, 347–354 (1980)

108 MANI, R. L., EISENBERG, R. L., McDONALD, E. J. Jr., POLLACK, J. A. and MANI, J. R. Complications of catheter cerebral arteriography: analysis of 5,000 procedures. I. Criteria and incidence. *American Journal of Roentgenology*, **131**, 861–865 (1978)

109 MAY, A. G., DeWEESE, J. A. and ROB, C. G. Hemodynamic effects of arterial stenosis. *Surgery*, **53**, 513–524 (1963)

110 McDONALD, P. T., RICH, N. M., COLLINS, G. J., ANDERSEN, C. A. and KOZLOFF, L. Doppler cerebrovascular examination, oculoplethysmography and ocular pneumoplethysmography. *Archives of Surgery*, **113**, 1341–1349 (1978)

111 McDONALD, P. T., RICH, N. M., COLLINS, J. G. Jr., KOZLOFF, L. and ANDERSEN, C. A. Ocular pneumoplethysmography: detection of carotid occlusive disease. *Annals of Surgery*, **189**, 44–48 (1979)

112 McNAMARA, J. O., HEYMAN, A., SILVER, D. and MANDEL, M. E. The value of carotid endarterectomy in treating transient cerebral ischemia of the posterior circulation. *Neurology (Minneapolis)*, **27**, 682–684 (1977)

113 MEHIGAN, J. T., BUCH, W. S., PIPKIN, R. D. and FOGARTY, T. J. A planned approach to coexistent cerebrovascular disease in coronary artery bypass candidates. *Archives of Surgery*, **112**, 1403–1409 (1977)

114 MILLER, A., LEES, R. S., KISTLER, J. P. and ABBOTT, W. M. Spectral analysis of arterial bruits (phonoangiography): experimental validation. *Circulation*, **61**, 515–520 (1980)

115 MOORE, W. S., BOREN, C., MALONE, J. M. and GOLDSTONE, J. Asymptomatic carotid stenosis. Immediate and long-term results after prophylactic endarterectomy. *American Journal of Surgery*, **138**, 228–233 (1979)

116 MULLER, H. R. The diagnosis of internal carotid artery occlusion by directional Doppler sonography of the ophthalmic artery. *Neurology (Minneapolis)*, **22**, 816–823 (1972)

117 NUNN, D. B. Carotid endarterectomy: an analysis of 234 operative cases. *Annals of Surgery*, **182**, 733–738 (1977)

118 O'HARA, P. J., BREWSTER, D. C., DARLING, C. and HALLETT, J. W. Jr. Oculopneumoplethysmography. Its relationship to intraoperative cerebrovascular hemodynamics. *Archives of Surgery*, **115**, 1156–1158 (1980)

119 OLINGER, C. P. Ultrasonic carotid echoarteriography. *Americal Journal of Roentgenology, Radium Therapy and Nuclear Medicine*, **106**, 282–295 (1969)

120 OLIVARIOUS, B. de F. The external carotid artery sign. *Acta Neurologica Scandinavica*, **41**, 539–550 (1965)

121 PAULSON, O. B. Ophthalmodynamometry in internal carotid artery occlusion. *Stroke*, **7**, 564–566 (1976)

122 PEARCE, H. J., LOWELL, J., TUBB, D. W. and BROWN, H. J. Continuous oculoplethysmographic monitoring during carotid endarterectomy. *American Journal of Surgery*, **138**, 733–735 (1979)

123 PESSIN, M. S., DUNCAN, G. W., MOHR, J. P. and POSKANZER, D. C. Clinical and angiographic features of transient ischemic attacks. *New England Journal of Medicine*, **296**, 358–362 (1977)

124 PODORE, P. C., DeWEESE, J. A., MAY, A. G. and ROB, C. G. Asymptomatic contralateral carotid artery stenosis: a five-year follow-up study following carotid endarterectomy. *Surgery*, **88**, 748–752 (1980)

125 PRICE, T. R. and HECK, A. F. Correlation of thermometry and angiography in carotid arterial disease. *Archives of Neurology*, **26**, 450–455 (1972)

126 PRICE, T. R. and HECK, A. F. Opacity pulse propagation measurement and thermometry in the evaluation of carotid occlusive vascular disease: correlations with angiography. *Stroke*, **3**, 601–603 (1972)

127 RENNIE, L., EJRUP, B. and McDOWELL, F. Arterial bruits in cerebrovascular disease. *Neurology (Minneapolis)*, **14**, 751–756 (1964)

128 ROSS RUSSELL, R. W. The source of retinal emboli. *Lancet*, **2**, 789–792 (1968)

129 RUTHERFORD, R. B., HIATT, W. R. and KREUTZER, E. W. The use of velocity wave form analysis in the diagnosis of carotid artery occlusive disease. *Surgery*, **82**, 695–702 (1977)

130 SANBORN, G. E., MILLER, N. R., McGUIRE, M. and KUMAR, A. J. Clinical-angiographic correlation of ophthalmodynamometry in patients with suspected carotid artery disease: a prospective study. *Stroke*, **12**, 770–774 (1981)

131 SANDOK, B. A. Editorial – noninvasive techniques for diagnosis of carotid artery disease. *Stroke*, **9**, 427–429 (1978)

132 SANDOK, B. A., FURLAN, A. J., WHISNANT, J. P. and SUNDT, T. M. Jr. Guidelines for the management of transient ischemic attacks. *Mayo Clinic Proceedings*, **53**, 665–674 (1978)

133 SANDOK, B. A., WHISNANT, J. P., FURLAN, A. J. and MICKELL, J. L. Carotid artery bruits: prevalence survey and differential diagnosis. *Mayo Clinic Proceedings*, **57**, 227–230 (1982)

134 SHAPIRO, H. M., NG, L., MISHKIN, M. and REIVICH, M. Direct thermometry, ophthalmodynamometry, auscultation and palpation in extracranial cerebrovascular disease: an evaluation of rapid diagnostic methods. *Stroke*, **1**, 205–218 (1970)

135 SONDHEIMER, F. K. and LEVIN, J. M. The contralateral diseased but asymptomatic carotid artery: to operate or not? An update. *American Journal of Surgery*, **140**, 203–205 (1980)

136 SPENCER, M. P., REID, J. M., DAVIS, D. L. and PAULSON, P. S. Cervical carotid imaging with a continuous-wave Doppler flowmeter. *Stroke*, **5**, 145–154 (1974)

137 SPENCER, M. P. and REID, J. M. Quantitation of carotid stenosis with continuous-wave (C-W) Doppler ultrasound. *Stroke*, **10**, 326–330 (1979)

138 SUMNER, D. S., RUSSELL, J. B., RAMSEY, D. E., HAJJAR, W. M. and MILES, R. D. Noninvasive diagnosis of extracranial carotid arterial disease. A prospective evaluation of pulsed-Doppler imaging and oculoplethysmography. *Archives of Surgery*, **114**, 1222–1229 (1979)

139 SUNDT, T. M., SANDOK, B. A. and WHISNANT, J. P. Carotid endarterectomy: complications and preoperative assessment of risk. *Mayo Clinic Proceedings*, **50**, 301–306 (1975)

140 THOMPSON, J. E. and GARRETT, W. V. Peripheral – arterial surgery. *New England Journal of Medicine*, **302**, 491–503 (1980)

141 THOMPSON, J. E., PATMAN, R. D. and PERSSON, A. V. Management of asymptomatic carotid bruits. *American Surgeon*, **42**, 77–80 (1976)

142 THOMPSON, J. E., PATMAN, R. D. and TALKINGTON, C. M. Asymptomatic carotid bruit: long-term outcome of patients having endarterectomy compared with unoperated controls. *Annals of Surgery*, **188**, 308–316 (1978)

143 TOOLE, J. F., JANEWAY, R., CHOI, K., CORDELL, R., DAVIS, C., JOHNSTON, F. and MILLER, H. S. Transient ischemic attacks due to atherosclerosis. A prospective study of 160 patients. *Archives of Neurology*, **32**, 5–12 (1975)

144 TREIMAN, R. L., FORAN, R. F., SHORE, E. H. and LEVIN, P. M. Carotid bruit. Significance in patients undergoing an abdominal aortic operation. *Archives of Surgery*, **106**, 803–805 (1973)

145 VITER, J. J. Femoro-cerebral angiography: analysis of 2,000 consecutive examinations, special emphasis on carotid arteries catheterization in older patients. *American Journal of Roentgenology, Radium Therapy and Nuclear Medicine*, **118**, 633–647 (1973)

146 WALDEN, R., L'ITALIEN, G., MEGERMAN, J., BOUCHIER-HAYES, D., HANEL, K., MALONEY, R. and ABBOTT, W. Complementary methods for evaluating carotid stenosis: a biophysical basis for ocular pulse wave delays. *Surgery*, **88**, 162–167 (1980)

147 WARLOW, C. P. and FISH, P. J. Pulsed Doppler imaging of the carotid artery. *Journal of the Neurological Sciences*, **45**, 135–141 (1980)

148 WEAVER, R. G. Jr., HOWARD, G., McKINNEY, W. M., BALL, M. R., JONES, A. M. and TOOLE, J. F. Comparison of Doppler ultrasonography with arteriography of the carotid artery bifurcation. *Stroke*, **11**, 402–404 (1980)

149 WEINSTEIN, M. C. and FINEBERG, H. V. (Eds.) *Clinical Decision Analysis*. Philadelphia: W. B. Saunders Company (1980)

150 WOOD, E. H. Thermography in the diagnosis of cerebrovascular disease. *Radiology*, **85**, 270–283 (1965)

151 ZIEGLER, D. K., ZILELI, T., DICK, A. and SEBAUGH, J. L. Correlations of bruits over the carotid artery with angiographically demonstrated lesions. *Neurology (Minneapolis)*, **21**, 860–865 (1971)

10
Medical treatment
M. J. G. Harrison and R. W. Ross Russell

The last 15–20 years have seen intensive activity in two areas related to the medical treatment of cerebrovascular disease. Firstly patients with transient ischaemic attacks (TIAs) and minor recovered stroke have been included in trials of antithrombotic regimes aimed at preventing subsequent disabling stroke or death. Secondly the increased understanding of the pathophysiology of cerebral ischaemia has led to a variety of new approaches to the immediate sequelae of cerebral infarction. In this chapter we will review progress in these two areas, attempting, by brief reference to basic mechanisms, to explain the rational basis of treatment as well as to review critically the results of clinical trials.

TRANSIENT ISCHAEMIC ATTACKS

Treatment is aimed at prevention of stroke and other causes of cardiovascular morbidity and mortality (e.g. myocardial infarction). The single most important factor in the long term for TIA patients is the presence of hypertension. Harrison *et al.*[32] noted that a blood pressure of 150/90 or more was to be found in 52% of 154 patients presenting with cerebral transient ischaemic attacks but in only 25% of 191 age sex matched controls ($P<0.001$). The difference remains significant after due allowance is made for the interaction of other risk factors such as smoking and haematocrit. Whisnant's[70] study at the Mayo Clinic showed that the risk of stroke in patients with TIAs was greater in hypertensive patients, and that this increased risk was removed by adequate treatment of hypertension. These points are discussed in detail in Chapter 3.

The effect of treatment of other risk factors in TIA patients has not received systemic study. The effect of stopping smoking, reducing haematocrit or treating hyperlipidaemia in this particular group of patients has not been specifically put to the test. The decision to treat these factors therefore is based on a 'common sense' argument that if a factor is present in TIA patients, and is found to be associated with the risk of stroke in prospective epidemiological studies, then removing it might reduce that risk. The argument, of course, implies that risk factors are causally related to the clinical end points when they might equally be epiphenomena. Only an interventional trial can decide the point. This has been satisfactorily achieved in the case of hypertension, (J. R. A. Mitchell Chapter 3), but the case is unproven with the other risk factors. The beneficial effect of reduced smoking has been shown for cardiac disease but not yet for stroke, for example.

Anticoagulants

The first antithrombotic regime to be widely assessed in the early manifestations of cerebrovascular disease was anticoagulant therapy (*Table 10.1*). Initially large uncontrolled trials were enthusiastic. They were followed by a number of small controlled or randomized trials in which there was no significant difference either individually or collectively between anticoagulated and untreated individuals in stroke incidence. The numbers of patients in these small trials (117 treated, 110 untreated) are still far too few on which to judge the issue. If the risk of stroke in patients with TIAs is about 5% per annum 2000 patients would have to be randomized to stand an 80% chance of detecting a significant ($P < 0.05$) reduction of risk by a modest 25[69]. It seems unlikely that a trial of this size will now be set up but the vogue for anticoagulating patients with TIAs has not completely faded.

Table 10.1 Anticoagulants for TIAs (randomised trials) (from Warlow[69], courtesy of the Publishers, *Recent Advances in Clinical Neurology*, Volume 3)

Reference	Number in trial	Treated group		Control group	
		Mortality (%)	Stroke	Mortality (%)	Stroke
Veterans[68]	37	4.5	4.5	0	0
Baker[6]	44	21	12.5	10	25
Pearce[55]	37	0	6	15	10
Baker[5]	60	30	20	17	13
Bradshaw[8]	49	12.5	8	16	8
Total	227	15	11	13	12

Proponents point to the fact that the stroke rate in two of the randomized trials while on treatment was halved in anticoagulated patients[6, 57]. They also quote the advice from the Mayo Clinic[71] that the stroke risk is greatest in the first two months after TIA and the risks of haemorrhagic complication rare before one year. Those that favour anticoagulation therefore have tended to opt for short term treatment, e.g. 6 months. The Canadian trial of antiplatelet agents does not confirm the excess early stroke risk after presentation with TIAs and anecdotal evidence shows that haemorrhage can complicate anticoagulation at any stage. Further, there is evidence that anticoagulation is rarely fully achieved over the first month or two.

Antiplatelet drugs

The logic of the use of these agents is discussed in Chapter 7. It was also pointed out there that the nature of embolic material probably differs widely amongst patients with TIAs. If anticoagulants are inappropriate for platelet emboli, then antiplatelet drugs are equally unlikely to succeed with emboli of cholesterol crystals, calcific heart valve debris, friable atheroma and bacterial vegetations. Our inability to make a bedside diagnosis of the nature of the embolic material in a particular case clearly hampers judgement of the results of trials. There is also an uncritical assumption that the evidence of platelet artery to artery embolism as a cause of TIAs is directly applicable to the pathogenesis of completed stroke (where in fact different thrombotic material may be more commonly involved). It is possible that antiplatelet drugs, for instance, might prevent TIAs, but not affect the more important completed stroke.

Aspirin

Observations on single patients with amaurosis fugax suggested that both aspirin and sulphinpyrazone might reduce the frequency of attacks. There have been two large trials of aspirin though they still have some of the faults of being too small (*Table 10.2*). Fields *et al*. in 1977[19] and 1978[20] reported a co-operative USA trial of 650 mgm b.d. of aspirin or placebo in patients presenting with carotid territory TIAs. The trial was stratified according to whether or not carotid endarterectomy had been carried out. Too few end points occurred for firm conclusions but combining the operated and un-operated halves of the study there were 11 strokes in aspirin takers and 22 on placebo ($\chi^2 = 3.68 < 0.1$), a difference that is not quite significant. As Warlow[69] pointed out a large number were withdrawn from the trial, and the reasons for their failure to complete the protocol are not set out. This may represent a serious source of error if comparison is made on the strictest criteria.

Table 10.2 Aspirin treatment of TIAs

Reference	Number in trial	Stroke and/or death	
		Treated	Placebo
Fields *et al*.[19, 20]	303	21/153	27/150
Canadian study[10]	585	46/290	68/295

The Canadian trial[10] analyzed 585 patients who in four equal groups had received 1300 mgm of aspirin, 800 mgm of sulphinpyrazone, neither or both drugs for a mean follow-up of 26 months. The results have been claimed to show up to 50% reduction in the risk of stroke or death attributable to aspirin. There being no statistical evidence of interaction it was deemed appropriate to combine the results of patients on aspirin and combined treatment in one subgroup and compare with those on sulphinpyrazone and placebo together, to assess the power of the effects of aspirin. Close inspection of the data shows that the significant difference that emerges is compounded of a small benefit of combined treatment, and an adverse effect of those receiving sulphinpyrazone alone. It is strange to see the net conclusion made that aspirin is effective in the prevention of stroke. The oddities of these subgroup data, of course, merely highlight the fact that although some 600 patients were studied, the trial is still too small to be conclusive.

A new UK trial in which some 2000 patients will be randomized to aspirin or placebo will, it is hoped, answer this question more decisively[67].

The Canadian trial which had not separately randomized males and females nevertheless showed a 48% reduction in stroke and/or death in men ($P < 0.005$) while in females there were more end points on aspirin. The UK trial will address itself to this point specifically by randomizing men and women separately.

It is perhaps ironic that the Canadian trial which is by far the best in TIA came in for so much criticism. This probably reflects the belated realization of the criteria by which to judge the adequacy of trial design[56].

Sulphinpyrazone

The 'failure' of the Canadian trial[10] to demonstrate a positive effect of sulphin-pyrazone requires some comment. Evans' small pilot study had suggested a reduction in the frequency of TIAs including amaurosis fugax[18]. A bigger trial in amaurosis fugax could not confirm this effect however (Wilson and Ross Russell, personal communication). Despite the ability of sulphinpyrazone to normalize shortened platelet survival in patients with vascular prostheses it has not had beneficial effects on clinical end points. This raises the intriguing possibility that simple effects on platelet aggregation are not sufficiently close to the pathogenesis of stroke.

An alternative approach is to influence prostaglandin metabolism by dietary means. The prostaglandins synthesized from arachidonic acid have two double bonds in the side chain. Those synthesized in platelets and vessel walls from eicosapentaenoic acid have three double bonds. The thromboxane formed (TXA_3) is not nearly as active as TXA_2 as an aggregating agent, but the prostacyclin formed is an antiaggregant. Increasing the dietary levels of eicosapentaenoic acid, e.g. by a mackerel diet, has been shown to inhibit *ex vivo* platelet aggregation[62]. Eskimoes have a diet rich in eicosapentaenoic acid and have longer bleeding times than Danish controls. The reduced vascular disease morbidity in Eskimoes might partly relate to these differences in prostaglandin metabolism.

Dipyridamole

This vasodilator has little effect on platelet aggregation *in vitro* but it inhibits platelet plug formation in damaged small arteries in animal models[17]. It also

Table 10.3 Cardiac-valve replacement. Treatment with warfarin and dipyridamole (from Sullivan *et al.*[63], courtesy of the Editor and Publishers, *New England Journal of Medicine*)

Warfarin plus:	No. in trial	Patients with emboli	No. of emboli
Placebo	36	6	11
Dipyridamole	27	0	0
Dipyridamole discontinued	7	2	2

increases platelet half life and inhibits the smooth muscle proliferating influence of platelet extracts[27] (*Table 10.3*).

In practice the only situation in which dipyridamole appears to have clinically useful antithrombotic effects is in the presence of prosthetic heart valves[63]. Used in an unselected group of patients with TIAs it failed to demonstrate a protective effect against stroke in the follow-up period though the study was small[1].

Trials are now in progress in France and North America of combinations of dipyridamole and aspirin vs aspirin alone. Until these are completed and reported there is no more than theoretical justification for the use of the combination rather than aspirin alone. Preliminary data from the French study suggests that the combination is no more effective than aspirin alone.

Policy

In patients with TIAs who have no operable stenosis of the appropriate cervical artery (Chapter 7) the present evidence supports the use of aspirin, especially in males. As many patients as possible should be encouraged to enter one of the multicentre trials of antiplatelet agents to obtain a clearer view of the benefit or lack of benefit of such treatment. Patients with gastrointestinal intolerance of aspirin may be tried on enteric coated aspirin though absorption is less predictable. The dose if aspirin should be used is under intensive study experimentally and the use of 1 × 300 mgm a day is being tested in the UK TIA trial. For patients not entering a double blind trial, the 'best bet' regime after consideration of material discussed in Chapter 7 is perhaps no more than 150 mg. For patients with aspirin intolerance there is currently no antithrombotic regime of demonstrable benefit, let alone of proven use.

CEREBRAL INFARCTION

Oedema

Much of the early mortality after cerebral infarction is believed to be due to the development of oedema in the affected hemisphere. It can be severe enough to cause intracranial shifts and tentorial herniation with compression of the upper brain stem. Clinical signs of brain stem lesions consequent upon hemisphere

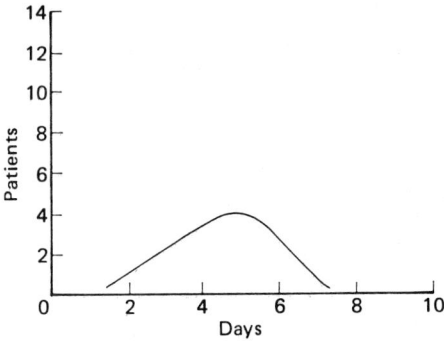

Figure 10.1 Time of death after cerebral infarction due to coning (Modified from White[72])

swelling and of elevated CSF pressures were noted by Plum[57] in 20% of acute hemiplegic stroke victims. The neuropathological sequelae of coning with microhaemorrhages in the brain stem were noted in cases of cerebral infarction dying within 4.5 days. Death from coning occurs between 2 and 10 days (*Figure 10.1*) and is the commonest cause of early death[72]. Less severe degrees of hemisphere swelling are common and mass effect is obvious on CT scans for up to 25 days, and is perhaps seen at some stage in as many as 60% of acute infarcts.

Theory

It is important to consider the nature of the oedema accompanying infarction before going on to discuss attempts to treat it. Klatzo[36] suggested that broadly speaking there were two types of cerebral oedema – cytotoxic oedema which is cellular in origin and due to the inability of damaged cells to maintain normal ion homeostasis, and vasogenic oedema in which plasma constituents flood the extracellular space due to damage to the blood brain barrier (BBB). This useful scheme has successfully been applied, for example, to the oedema of triethyl tin poisoning in which the histological appearances are clearly those of cellular swelling, and to the oedema provoked in the underlying white matter by cold injury to the cortex which fits nicely the vasogenic model with a damaged BBB. In the latter case plasma protein markers are carried through the white matter at a distance from the site of BBB damage, at rates dependent on the perfusion pressure. Induced hypertension increases the extent and amount of extracellular fluid accumulation[37]. There is also evidence that the protein content of the added fluid in vasogenic oedema has deleterious effects itself[65].

The CT scan appearance of white matter swelling in patients with cerebral tumours (*Figure 10.2*) suggests that tumour oedema is largely of this vasogenic type. Biopsy specimens obtained from peritumour oedematous brain by Reulen[58], showed increased water content and concentrations of Na^+ and Cl^- compatible with the concept of plasma leak. Corticosteroids prove very effective in reducing this kind of oedema experimentally. Clinically the response in tumour patients is dramatic and very rapid. It is possible that steroids have effects other than on the BBB and on clearance of vasogenic oedema. Thus they may improve neuronal function even in the presence of oedema. In the case of cold injury oedema in the cat, Pappius showed that the EEG might improve on steroids with only a modest reduction in white matter water content. This contrasted with the lack of EEG improvement despite more complete elimination of water when the diuretic furosemide was used[52].

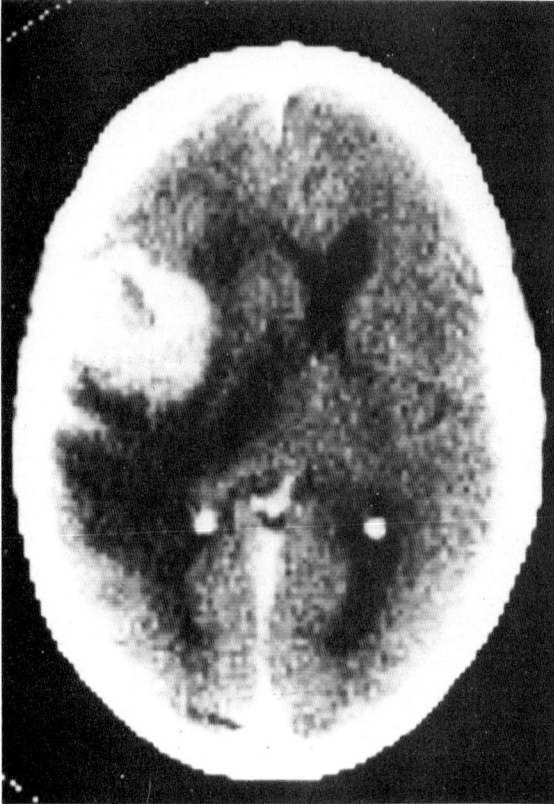

Figure 10.2 CT scan showing digital pattern of white matter oedema associated with a tumour (vasogenic oedema). (From Harrison[29], courtesy of the Publishers, *Geriatrics for the Practitioner*)

CT scans suggest that the oedema of cerebral infarction may not be vasogenic or at least that it differs in important ways from tumour oedema. Thus the swelling is more diffuse, the low attenuation homogenous, and both grey and white matter are affected (*Figure 10.3*). It has been assumed that ischaemic oedema is cytotoxic in nature and that this explains all the differences. Both experimental and clinical data suggest this is too simple a view. In some experimental models of ischaemia, oedema develops in a biphasic fashion and it has been customary to suggest that the early oedema is cytotoxic and that after, say, 24 hours the BBB breaks down, leading to a second more severe phase of vasogenic oedema[50]. The delayed appearance of positive radionucleid brain scans in patients with infarcts (after the

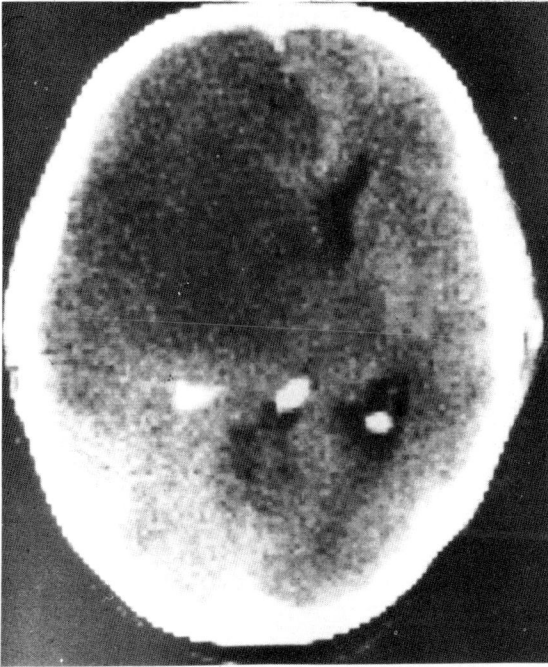

Figure 10.3 CT scan showing hemogenous low density area due to oedema associated with infarction. (From Harrison[29], courtesy of the publishers, *Geriatics for the Practitioner*)

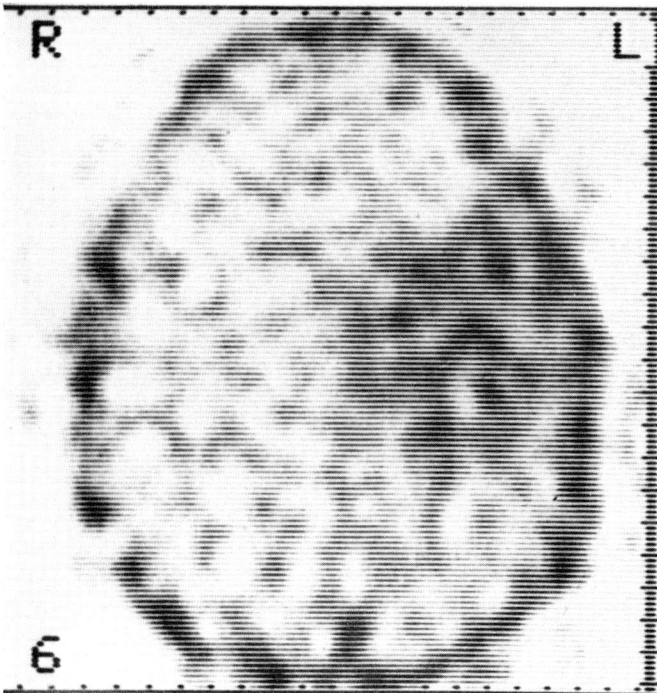

Figure 10.4 ECAT scan after an injection of TC[99m] showing wedge shaped uptake of isotope at site of recent infarct. (From Harrison[29], courtesy of the Publishers, *Geriatrics for the Practitioner*)

peak of oedema has passed) has been thought an analogous situation in man (*Figure 10.4*).

Recent experiments suggest an even more complex picture. Thus Hossman[33, 60] has shown that during complete circulatory arrest tissue water levels do not rise (there is no inflow of water) but water shifts from extracellular to intracellular compartments. This shift, a true example of cytotoxic oedema, appears to parallel failure of membrane ATPases, suggesting that it is due to cell pump failure. On restoration of blood flow the water content of the tissue rises rapidly but tends to fall again after a few hours. The severity of the earlier ischaemia seems to predetermine whether oedema will develop. Symon *et al.*[64] have shown that oedema can develop at levels of flow (20 ml/100 g/min) at which EEG and evoked potentials are affected, but at which indices of cell damage are as yet unaffected. Thus it is not until levels of about 10 ml/100 g/min that potassium and calcium movement occurs and histological change is prominent (*Figure 10.5*). Some of the oedema occurring may be due to increased micropinocytosis therefore rather than to pump failure. Even at this stage of early oedema formation some animals show leak of plasma markers.

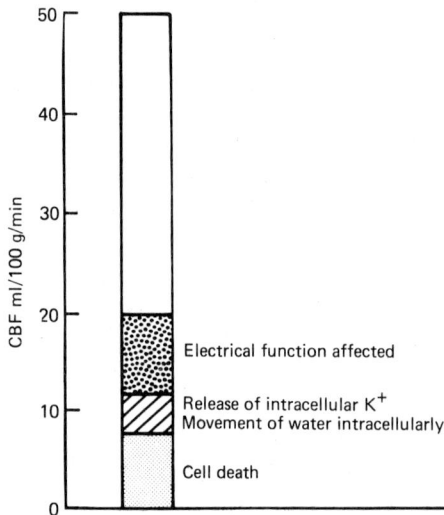

Figure 10.5 Threshold of cerebral ischaemia. (Modified from Symon[64])

In the clinical sphere, Harrison and Ell[30] found evidence of radionucleid leak within 24 hours in patients whose infarcts were showing mass effect on CT scans.

The mixed nature of oedema in cerebral infarction with the possibility of cytotoxic and vasogenic factors coexisting must be recalled when considering the various therapeutic regimes that have been used. It is important to note that raising the hydrostatic pressure increases this mixed oedema.

Practice

In view of the response of experimental vasogenic (cold injury) oedema to steroids and the dramatic clinical response of patients with brain tumours to their use, several attempts have been made to assess their efficacy in the acute stroke victim (*Table 10.4*). Early pilot studies appeared encouraging but were uncontrolled.

Table 10.4 Steroids in acute stroke (trials with at least 50 patients)

Reference	*Number in trial*	*Treated group* Mortality (%)	*Treated group* Improved (%)	*Control group* Mortality (%)	*Control group* Improved (%)
Tellez and Bauer[66]	54	18	57	35	50
Candelise[11]	111	43	ND	35	ND
Norris[49]	53	27	ND	18.5	ND
Santambrogio[59]	89	ND*	31	ND	34
Mulley[46]	118	41	ND	47	ND

* ND – no date.

Patten[53] gave 16 mgm of dexamethasone a day for 10 days to 14 patients and followed 17 controls. Neurological clinical scores suggested a small (12%) improvement in the treated patients and a small (12%) deterioration in the controls. Although this was shown to be a significant trend, the matching of the cases was inadequate. Haemorrhages and infarcts were both included and were not randomly distributed. Nor were brain stem and carotid territory infarcts equally split between treatment and control. Finally the study was too small to be reliable.

Tellez and Bauer[66] (1978) reported an essentially negative double blind study of 50 patients with cerebral infarction. The best single study has come from Mulley *et al.* (1978)[46]. One hundred and eighteen patients with acute strokes (onset less than 48 hours prior to entry into the trial) received 6 hourly injections of sterile water or of 4.2 mgm of dexamethasone for 10 days. Over days 11–14 the injections were tailed off. There was no significant difference in mortality between the two groups (40% at 10 days, 60% at 3 months, 75% at 1 year). Clinical scores revealed no evidence of any significant difference in the quality of life between the two groups. The mean time from onset of stroke to entry to hospital (5½ hours) probably explains the high early mortality. It leaves little doubt that there is no indication for the routine administration of dexamethasone to acute stroke victims. Higher doses of dexamethasone are being assessed currently. None of these trials has had CT scan control, so it remains true that steroids have not been assessed specifically in the subgroup of stroke victims with the greatest degree of delayed hemisphere swelling. There is a risk, however, that members of this subgroup would be rescued from coning, only to survive in a severely damaged state since they have massive hemisphere necrosis.

Oedema has also been treated by the use of hyperosmolar agents which theoretically would have the advantage of having an effect on cellular swelling

Table 10.5 Mannitol in acute stroke

Reference	Number in trial	Treated group Mortality (%)	Improved (%)	Control group Mortality (%)	Improved (%)
Candelise[11]	106	43	ND	35	ND
Santambrogio[59]	77	ND	33	ND	34

* ND – no date.

Table 10.6 Glycerol in acute stroke (randomized trials)

Reference	Number in trial	Treated group Mortality (%)	Improved (%)	Control group Mortality (%)	Improved (%)
Mathew[39]	54	7	76	8	56
Larson[39]	27	33	25	33	27

(*Table 10.5*). Mannitol has been shown to limit the size of the cerebral infarct produced by a middle cerebral clip in the cat but the rebound effect on oedema seen in patients with tumours argues against its routine use in stroke victims. Glycerol has the advantage of low toxicity though hyperosmolar diabetic coma has been provoked (*Table 10.6*). Meyer et al.[41] (1971) reported its use in a dose of 1.2 g/kg/day in 36 patients treated within 3 days of the onset of acute cerebral infarction. Falls in CSF pressure supported the belief that the glycerol had successfully reduced intracranial pressure. In a further study EEG parameters and cerebral blood flow (CBF) improved, suggesting that glycerol, by reducing oedema, had improved microvascular perfusion and thereby local metabolism. As glycerol is metabolized, it is free of the rebound oedema after the use of other hyperosmolar agents like mannitol. In 1972[39] the same group reported a controlled trial of 50 g of glycerol given in 500 ml of 5% dextrose saline daily for 6 days in patients with acute cerebral infarction. There were 2 deaths in 29 treated patients and 2 in 25 untreated. Neurological recovery as judged by a clinical score was better in the treated group. This small study needs confirmation from a larger tightly controlled trial, especially as it was not supported by the results of another small study by Larson et al.[38] (1976).

A controlled trial should also be considered in which hypertonic human albumin infusions are used to produce a reduction in oedema. They too would be free from rebound and could be combined with normovolaemic haemodilution (*v. infra*).

Anticoagulants

Although extension of infarction and reinfarction are causes of deterioration in recent stroke victims they are not common events (*Table 10.7*). The logic of

Table 10.7 Deteriorating stroke

Phase of stroke	Symptoms
Early 3–5 days	Oedema Re-infarction Re-bleed
Late	Cardiac Respiratory Renal Inappropriate ADH, etc.

treating all patients who present with the effects of acute cerebral infarction with anticoagulants is thus suspect. In practice, trials of anticoagulants in acute stroke failed to reveal any benefit. Hill, Marshall and Shaw[34] further showed by comparison of 65 anticoagulated and 64 control cases that anticoagulants did not prevent recurrent stroke.

There are two special circumstances, however, in which anticoagulants must be considered.

Cardiac embolism

Patients who sustain embolic cerebral infarction from a cardiac source probably benefit from anticoagulation[15]. The thrombus that forms in the left atrium of patients with atrial fibrillation, and in the left ventricle of those with myocardial infarction or cardiomyopathy, is thought to be more clot-like than artery to artery emboli, and therefore theoretically more responsive to anticoagulation.

In fatal myocardial infarction mural thrombi are found in 45%[7]. Clinically it is difficult to detect such thrombi but their presence can be suspected if ECG or radiographic evidence shows a ventricular aneurysm, or radionucleid scans show an akinetic segment. CT scans can detect some thrombi in the left ventricular cavity as can images built up by the incorporation of indium labelled platelets into existing thrombi. Two dimensional echocardiography can detect some such thrombi. Digital angiography may enable ventriculograms to be produced noninvasively in the near future, and further improve the diagnostic accuracy.

Davies and Pomerance[14] reported the autopsy findings in patients with chronic atrial fibrillation. Sixty-two per cent had thrombi in the left atrial appendage. Only a minority of the cases had rheumatic heart disease. It is now accepted that atrial thromboembolism occurs in the presence of atrial fibrillation of all aetiological categories. Though the risk of atrial thrombus and embolism is greatest with mitral valve disease and ischaemic heart disease, it is also detectable with atrial fibrillation due to thyrotoxicosis or with 'lone fibrillation'.

In planning preventive therapy it is clearly important to know when recurrences are liable to occur. In the case of rheumatic heart disease Darling[13] noted a recurrence rate of 56% over 10 years with a third of the recurrence occurring in the first 2 weeks after the first embolic episode. The risk of embolism after myocardial infarction is less (2% in Bean's series)[7]. Recurrences were also less likely (one in four according to Darling) although the greatest risk was again in the first 14 days after embolism. Atrial fibrillation doubled the recurrence rate in the ischaemic group and increased it seven-fold in the rheumatic, the recurrence again being most likely to occur in the first month after the initial embolus.

These data clearly suggest that if anticoagulants are to be used in an attempt to prevent recurrent cerebral embolism, then they should be prescribed immediately after the presenting cerebral embolus brings the patient to medical notice. There is a theoretical risk, however, that an infarct might be made haemorrhagic with an increased mortality and morbidity due to anticoagulation during the acute phase when the blood vessels in the infarct are abnormal (showing a damaged blood –brain barrier (BBB) for example). In fact vessel disruption is rarely encountered histologically. However, animal studies have demonstrated more haemorrhagic infarcts after experimental carotid occlusion or embolism if the animals were anticoagulated.

In practice this risk has probably been exaggerated and the fact that up to half the recurrent emboli occur in the first 2 to 3 weeks after the first embolus argues strongly for early anticoagulation. Patients with evidence of haemorrhagic infarction on CT scans or blood stained CSF should not be anticoagulated however. Patients with atrial fibrillation, recent myocardial infarction, rheumatic valve disease, cardiomyopathy and sino atrial disease should all be considered for anticoagulation. In the case of myocardial infarction without atrial fibrillation the risk period is probably encompassed by short term treatment, e.g. 6 months. In chronic atrial fibrillation and rheumatic heart valve disease not amenable to surgery, long term treatment is indicated. Several studies have suggested that dipyridamole should be added to warfarin in the case of prosthetic heart valves of the Starr Edwards type which have a high risk of embolism unless so treated[63]. The combination of aspirin and warfarin was similarly successful in a trial carried out in the Netherlands. The risk of gastric haemorrhage did not prove prohibitive, contrary to one's expectations.

The choice of therapy is more difficult with mitral valve prolapse and with bacterial endocarditis. The association of cerebral infarction with prolapse of a mitral valve leaflet, detectable clinically by a systolic murmur and midsystolic click, and by echocardiography, has recently been debated. The frequency of this abnormality in healthy individuals makes it difficult to be sure of its pathological significance. Geyer and Franzini[22] have described the finding of thrombus on a prolapsing leaflet and this is strong evidence that this valvular abnormality can be a source of cerebral embolism. The emboli are often small, causing rather minor episodes and it may be adequate to treat these patients with antiplatelet agents though there is yet no clear evidence on this point.

In the case of bacterial endocarditis, some early trials showed an increased mortality with the addition of heparin or anticoagulants to the antibiotics. It was generally concluded that anticoagulants were contraindicated in the case of cerebral embolism due to subacute bacterial endocarditis (SBE) though this established policy has been challenged more recently.

In practice the trials of anticoagulants for recurrent cardiac embolism have been inadequate by modern standards. No randomized study has been carried out. Wright and McDevitt[73] compared 1515 patient months on treatment with 1747 patient months off treatment. There were 10 episodes of cerebral embolism on treatment, and 70 off. Adams *et al.*[2] described a retrospective study of 84 patients with mitral valve disease and atrial fibrillation, half of whom had been anticoagulated. Forty-one of the 42 untreated (from earlier years) had died, in 13 cases from a cerebral embolus. Only 26 anticoagulated patients died and in only four cases was this due to cerebral embolism. The authors suggested that the benefit of anticoagulation was only evident for 12 months and that treatment might be unnecessary thereafter.

It seems unlikely that major trials will now be started, so the current recommendation from many sources[15] must remain unsupported by formal proof. Anticoagulants appear to be indicated in the case of cardiac embolism when there is proof of structural cardiac disease or atrial fibrillation. Antiplatelet drugs may suffice in the case of mitral valve prolapse.

Progressing stroke

The second situation in which anticoagulants should be considered is in the case of the so-called progressing stroke[45]. Patients whose deficit continues to increase while under observation form this important group.

Five per cent of patients with carotid occlusion show this temporal pattern failing to stabilize in the first 18–24 hours and this situation may be even more common with basilar occlusion. The cause of deterioration varies. In some, systemic factors such as hypotension, congestive cardiac failure or hypoxia are clearly responsible. If these are absent and if CT scans or CSF examination show no evidence of a haemorrhagic lesion (or other nonvascular lesion) anticoagulants can be considered. The rationale in this case is that thrombus formation may be progressing, for example above a carotid occlusion, threatening collateral flow at the first branching point (ophthalmic artery) or at the siphon.

Short term anticoagulation has been assessed in a number of studies[5, 12]. Unfortunately they fail to satisfy stringent requirements for randomized trials but in each case less treated patients showed further progression after entry than did controls. Untreated series showed further progression occurred in 30 to 40% whilst on anticoagulation 15 to 25% deteriorated (*Table 10.8*).

Table 10.8 Anticoagulants for progressing strokes: (randomized trials)

Reference	Number in trial	Treated group		Control group	
		Mortality (%)	Progression	Mortality (%)	Progression
*Carter[12]	42	5	18	20	30
Baker[5]	128	8	13	15	31

* Report of 76 randomized patients. Only 42 still progressing at time of institution of treatment

The consensus view is thus that anticoagulants should be used in patients with no CT scan evidence of haemorrhage who are showing increasing focal disability while under observation. As the period during which deterioration is seen is commonly only a few days and anticoagulation needs to be achieved promptly, intravenous heparin is preferred.

Blood pressure

Hypertension is the single most important risk factor for ischaemic stroke and clinical experience suggests that 40–50% of acute ischaemic stroke patients are hypertensive on presentation. There immediately arises the problem of how soon and how aggressively such elevated pressures should be treated in the acute stroke victim. The benefit of long term control in the prevention of stroke is discussed in detail in Chapter 3.

Theory

Several problems surround the safety of blood pressure treatment in this context. Firstly, the normal autoregulation of cerebral blood flow in the brain is impaired in the aftermath of cerebral infarction. The area of brain in which autoregulation fails may be extensive or may remain restricted to the infarcted zone. Some evidence suggests that autoregulation is restored in a few weeks but Symon found in an animal model that the centre of a middle cerebral artery infarct might fail to show normal autoregulation even 3 years later. In the area of lost autoregulation blood flow is pressure passive and so any reduction of blood pressure will cause reduced cerebral blood flow and potentially may aggravate local ischaemia. The tissue around an infarct may have a level of ischaemia that is sufficient to paralyze its metabolic activity but that is not severe enough to cause cell death. A fall in blood pressure when autoregulation is lost could convert this vulnerable penumbra, as it is called, from a potentially reversible state of oligaemia to one in which further cell death (infarction) is going to occur[4].

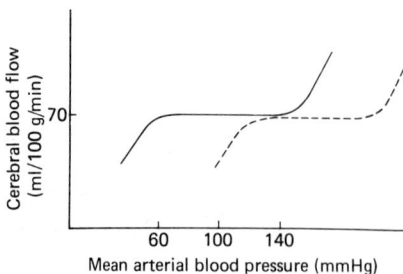

Figure 10.6 Autoregulation of cerebral blood flow in normotensive (—) and hypertensive (– – –) subjects diagram. (From Humphrey[35], courtesy of the Editor and Publishers, *British Journal of Hospital Medicine*)

It must also be noted that the autoregulatory curve is moved to the right in hypertensive patients (*Figure 10.6*) so even in areas where autoregulation is preserved flow may fall at a mean arterial blood pressure which would not be

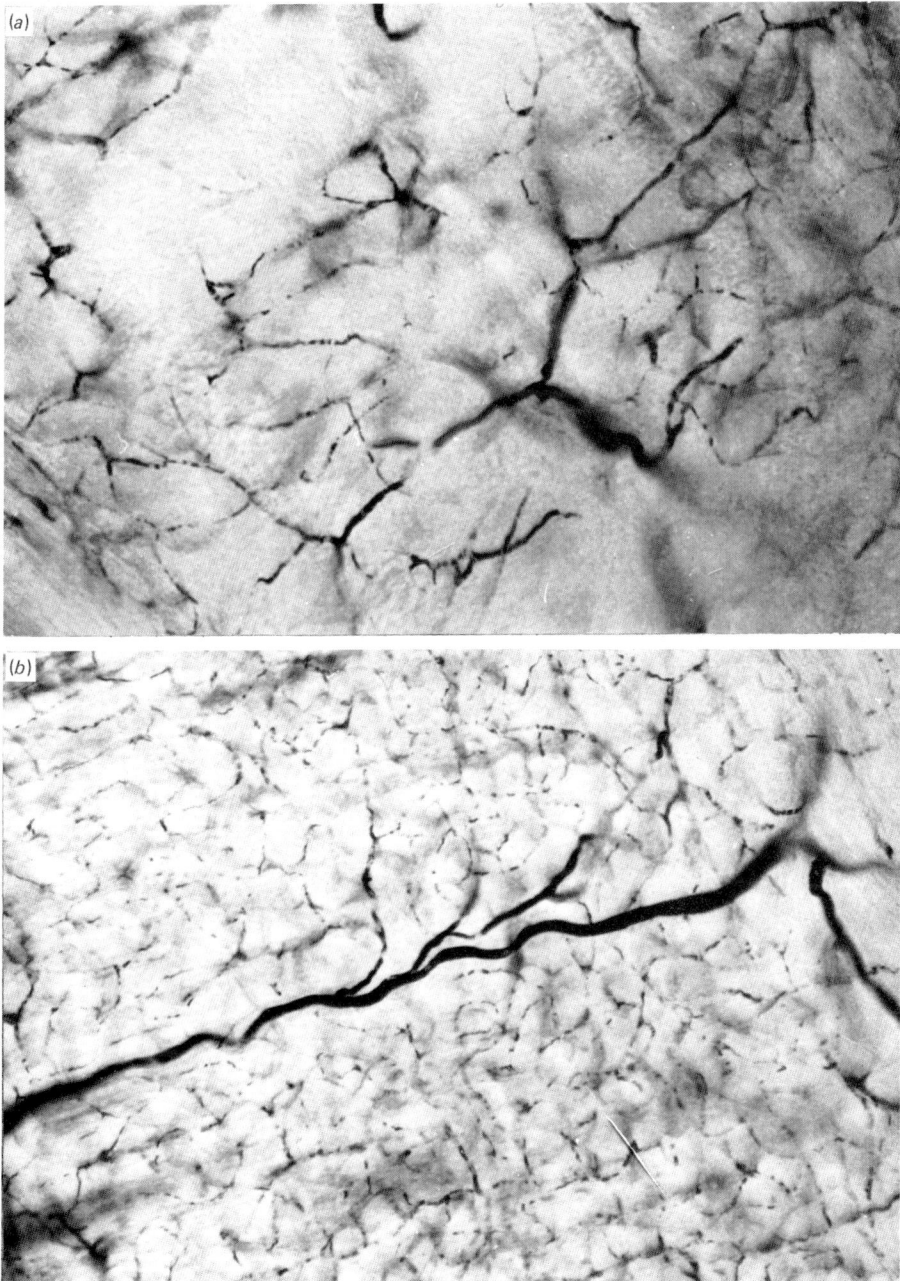

Figure 10.7 (*a*) Patchy refilling of the cerebral microvasculature with a carbon suspension after severe ischaemia – the no reflow phenomenon. (*b*) Normal control

associated with such a fall in a normotensive patient. A blood pressure of 120/80, for example, could well be below the intact autoregulatory limit for a chronically hypertensive patient.

Some years ago Ames showed that after total cerebral ischaemia in the experimental animal, the immediate recirculation of the capillary bed on restoration of blood flow was patchy (the no reflow phenomenon) (*Figure 10.7*). Though many factors may contribute to the production of this problem stagnation of flow is clearly the most important. If some flow persists during ischaemia the no flow phenomenon does not develop. A brief period of hypertension or of haemodilution may be sufficient to prevent no reflow. There is, however, little evidence that the no reflow phenomenon is pathologically very important. Thus its prevention did not affect post ischaemic survival in the gerbil nor does its presence or absence explain the selective vulnerability of some neurones to ischaemia. There are no direct indications of its occurrence of relevance in man however, but it remains possible that it could be a further reason to avoid hypotension in the victim of cerebral infarction.

Thirdly, there is the influence of the level of blood pressure on oedema formation. As discussed, the mixed cytotoxic and vasogenic oedema of cerebral infarcts, especially when collateral flow is possible, is greatly affected by hypertension. In the animal models a rise in blood pressure causes a breakdown of the BBB in the ischaemic bed and greatly increases the influx of water. To leave the blood pressure at a high level therefore, or to increase it in the hope of increasing blood flow in an area of lost autoregulation, could possibly increase the severity of oedema.

Practice

The only solution at present is to avoid sudden or severe falls of arterial pressure lest infarction be extended in an ischaemic 'penumbra'. Other considerations may override this caution, of course. Left ventricular failure, for example, would be a compelling indication for acute blood pressure reduction. Some slight reduction of pressure (acutely) may well be advisable to limit oedema formation. After 2 to 3 weeks when it is believed some recovery of the autoregulatory capacity is likely, long term blood pressure management should commence (Chapter 3).

Blood flow

Superficially it appears obvious that attempts should be made to increase blood flow to ischaemic tissue. If there is any chance that some cells are viable even though electrically inactive it is clear that their survival and return to a functional state could theoretically be achieved by even small changes in flow. The areas around an infarct studied in the baboon after middle cerebral occlusion by Symon's group[64] show levels of flow reduction, e.g. to 15 ml/100 g/min, at which evoked potentials fail but there is no sign of loss of cellular integrity – no loss of K^+ or ingress of Ca^{++} (*Figure 10.5*). Induced hypertension can cause sufficient increase in the blood flow in these border zone areas for an evoked potential to return. We have already discussed the theoretical risk of employing hypertension as a means of achieving this increase in flow because of the risks of oedema formation. What of other means of increasing flow?

Hypercarbia from CO_2 inhalation produces profound vasodilatation in the cerebral vascular bed and CBF rises in normal subjects. The vascular bed of an infarcted area, however, shows a vasoparalysis with maximal vasodilatation probably in response to lactacidosis. CO_2 inhalation in such a situation would cause no further increase in vessel diameter in the ischaemic area but distant normal areas would dilate widely. Blood flow under these circumstances thus increases in the normal areas and may even as a result fall in the ischaemic territory. Millikan[44] reported a comparison of 50 patients treated with 5% CO_2 (which probably

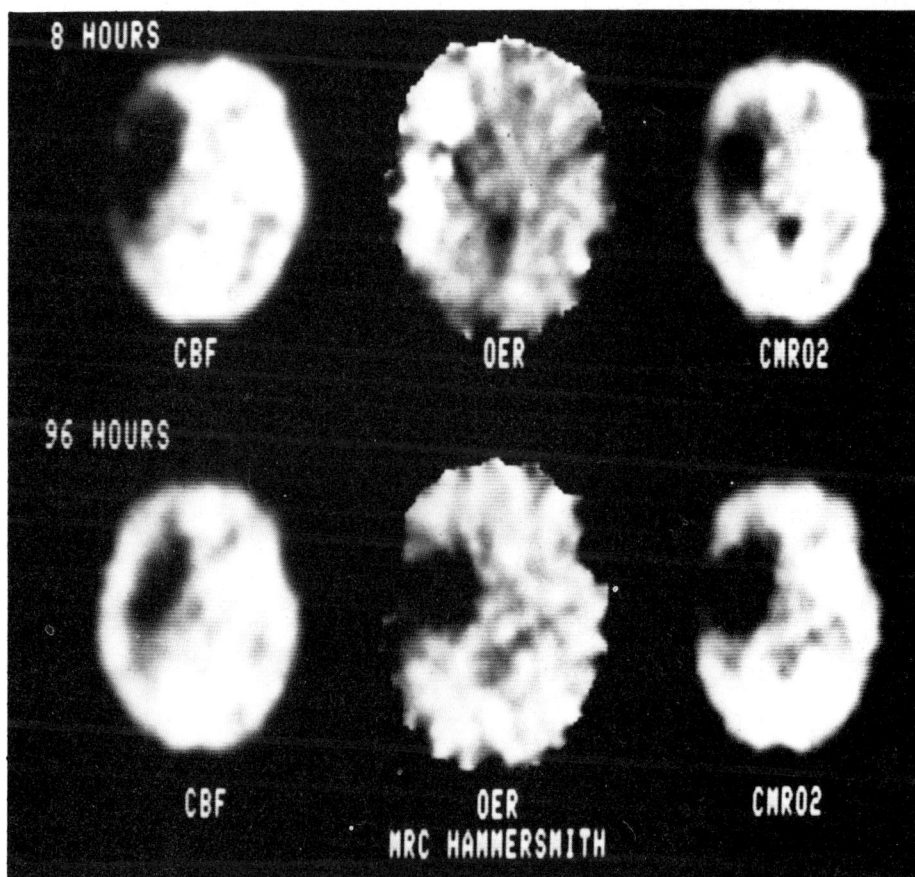

Figure 10.8 PET scan images after inhalation of O_2^{15} and CO_2^{15} reflecting regional O_2 utilization and CBF. Upper frames show white area of high oxygen extraction in an ischaemic area at 8 hours (misery perfusion), and same patient with reduced oxygen extraction in the same infarct at 96 hours. OER = oxygen extraction ratio. (Scans kindly supplied by Drs Frakowiak and Wise and Mr T. Jones)

increased blood flow by 50–75%) and 225 unmatched 'control' stroke cases. He could detect no improvement.

Vasodilator drugs (e.g. papaverine) have the same theoretical problem of potentially stealing further blood supply from ischaemic regions. They may also cause dangerous hypotension. Meyer and Gilroy[43] treated 70 patients with a progressive stroke deficit, 34 with intravenous papaverine. Clinical scoring suggested that those receiving papaverine had benefited. Harper[28] has pointed out that an ideal vasodilator should be more active on cerebral than systemic vessels (so limiting hypotension), should affect vessels in the ischaemic area more than elsewhere (to limit steal) and should have no effect or an inhibiting effect on metabolism (to avoid hypermetabolism). This ideal is most closely approximated by calcium antagonists which are most active on vessels in areas with impaired BBB in the territory of ischaemic damage.

The discovery of the phenomenon of steal of blood from the ischaemic area by measures that increase flow elsewhere led logically to the proposal that hypocarbia might be beneficial. Vasoconstriction in normal areas produced by hyperventilation might lead to an increase in blood supply in vasoparalyzed ischaemic areas. Paulson treated 50 patients in this way, hyperventilating the patients for 72 hours under sedation. There was no evidence of clinical benefit.

PET scanning reveals that few patients show evidence of an area in which high oxygen extraction implies the presence of viable tissue receiving an inadequate blood supply (*Figure 10.8*). Regimes dependent on attempts to improve flow may therefore only be relevant in a small subgroup (?10%). Further, in this group some may show an increase and others a decrease in flow in response to CO_2 or vasodilator drugs depending on the presence or absence of steal phenomena. Theoretically PET scans and CBF studies could identify individual patients in whom a particular strategy would increase flow in an area showing 'misery' perfusion. Frakowiak, Wise and Jones (personal communication) have recently described a case in which such a state of affairs proved transient only. The difficulties in identifying the right patient for a particular protocol are thus enormous. It is perhaps not surprising that indiscriminate use of vasodilator materials has not had clear cut success.

Viscosity

The role of elevated haematocrit in increasing whole blood viscosity has been discussed in Chapter 7. In normal subjects cerebral blood flow is reduced at high haematocrit and increases after venesection. The apparent dependence of CBF on haematocrit probably reflects a homeostatic response to the altered oxygen carrying capacity. High flow rates when the oxygen carrying capacity is low in anaemic blood maintains the same oxygen delivery to the brain that is achieved by a much lower CBF when the haematocrit is high. In the situation where blood flow has stopped, however, the presence of a high haematocrit will tend to increase the perfusion pressure needed to restart flow. In the acute stroke victim a high haematocrit might well adversely affect flow in maximally dilated collateral vessels, and the re-establishment of flow in capillaries in which flow has stopped. Some evidence that such a pathological progress does operate comes from a study of the size of cerebral infarcts produced by carotid occlusion. CT scan measurements suggested that patients with a high haematocrit had larger infarcts[31] (*Figure 10.9*).

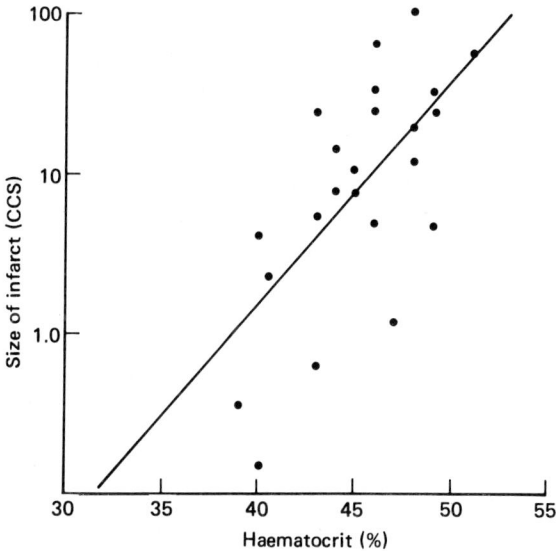

Figure 10.9 Size of cerebral infarcts (on log scale) from CT scan measurements, and prevailing haematocrit in symptomatic patients with angiographically proven carotid occlusion. (From Harrison *et al.*[31], courtesy of the Editor and Publishers, *Lancet*)

In theory, therefore, ischaemic haemodilution would increase blood flow, and this has been demonstrated both in normals and in stroke victims. What, however, has not been proven is whether such a change in bulk flow is of benefit to stroke victims. Reducing the oxygen carrying capacity of the blood may counterbalance some of the rheological benefit produced by haemodilution. Haemodilution does however prevent the 'no reflow' phenomenon after global ischaemia and it is reasonable to consider further the potential therapeutic effect in the case of focal cerebral infarction.

Gilroy[23] described a trial in which 50 patients received dextran 40 for 3 days in the presence of an established deficit of at least 24 hours' duration. Fifty controls received a similar volume of intravenous fluid but no dextran. The treated group had a better mortality and neurological score. Two other trials revealed no benefit under similar circumstances. Mathews[40] randomized 100 patients within 48 hours of an acute stroke. Mortality and initial levels of recovery showed a trend in favour of dextran 40 in the 52 treated subjects, but by 6 months there was no residual benefit. This study also raised the general problem that a marginal benefit might 'move' a patient with massive infarction from the fatal into the severely disabled group (*Table 10.9*).

Table 10.9 Dextran in acute stroke

Reference	Number in trial	Dextran Improved (%)	Dextran Mortality	Control Improved (%)	Control Mortality
Gilroy[23] (10 days)	100	83	4	57	15
Mathews[40]	100	32†	16*	44†	19*

* At 3 weeks
† Independent at 6 months

Oxygen supply

Normally the oxygen content of blood is defined by the equation:
$$O_2 \text{ content} = 1.39\,Hb \times O_2 \text{ saturation } (\%) + 0.002\,pl\ O_2.$$
The oxygen saturation is normally 100% in the absence of severe cardiopulmonary disease and so the oxygen content depends on haemoglobin levels, the plasma dissolved oxygen contributing little. There is evidence that oxygen delivery is homeostatically controlled. Patients with anaemia have a high cerebral blood flow whether their viscosity is low or high (anaemic paraproteinemic patients). In a stroke patient O_2 extraction is rarely limited by the oxygen content of the blood but theoretically more oxygen could be delivered by increasing oxygen saturation. There have been several studies showing clinical or EEG improvement in stroke victims while in hyperbaric oxygen chambers but lasting benefit has not been proven. A study of 122 patients was unfortunately not randomized or adequately controlled, so the authors' cautious optimism about the improved outcome after 10–20 exposures to 1.5 to 2.5 atmospheres O_2 cannot be more than anecdotal evidence[48]. There is a possible risk of inducing epileptic seizures in a hyperbaric oxygen chamber which could have adverse effects on clinical outcome.

There is a clear indication for the use of oxygen if oxygen saturation of the blood is below normal values (*see below*).

Prostaglandins and fatty acids

Theory

There is growing interest in a possible role for altered prostaglandins and fatty acids in ischaemic brain. Siesjo[61] has discussed the breakdown of endogenous phospholipids to prostaglandins and free fatty acids in ischaemic tissue. The free fatty acids have adverse effects on mitochondrial function, and can cause oedema in brain tissue slices.

In an animal model blocking prostaglandin synthesis with indomethacin reduces the oedema that developed in severely ischaemic brain areas.

That endoperoxides and thromboxanes produced in ischaemic brain affect the capillary bed is also suggested by an experimental study by Hallenbeck and Furlow[26] in which indomethacin improved the level of cerebral perfusion after a period of total ischaemia.

It is thus possible to argue that prostaglandins and thromboxanes formed in ischaemic brain both enhance local oedema formation and cause vasoconstriction. Theoretically, cyclo-oxygenase blockers such as indomethacin might therefore have some protective effect.

Practice

There has so far been no report of a controlled trial of the use of agents such as indomethacin in the context of acute cerebral infarction. The strokes that occurred in the patients in the Canadian trial who were receiving aspirin tended to be less severe but the changes were not dramatic and no measurements of infarct size or degree of associated swelling on CT scans have been forthcoming.

Inhibition of cerebral metabolism and hypermetabolism

It has been suggested that a logical stratagem for the protection of cerebral tissue affected by ischaemia in the penumbra of a cerebral infarct is to suppress its metabolic requirement. In this way anerobic metabolism with damaging lactacidosis, prostaglandin synthesis and free fatty acid formation might all be reduced, and oedema formation limited. This idea has been encouraged further by experimental evidence that there is often an overswing to hypermetabolic conditions after ischaemia, further increasing the demand for oxygen.

Both hypothermia and anaesthesia would theoretically produce the desired reduction in metabolism.

Hypothermia

Experimental evidence suggests that hypothermia is protective against severe cerebral ischaemia but its effect on resuscitation, i.e. when instituted after the event, needs to be studied further. In practice, hypothermia has not been pursued clinically in the context of cerebral infarction for a number of reasons. The practical management of patients under hypothermia is very difficult with the risks of cardiac dysrhythmias and hyperviscosity being particularly worrying.

Barbiturate anaesthesia

There have been many experimental studies in recent years demonstrating the protective effect of barbiturate anaesthesia.

Survival, infarct size and neurological deficit have all been claimed to be improved, for example, after middle cerebral and carotid clipping in the dog and middle cerebral occlusion in the baboon. Symon's[9] group also showed that barbiturates produced a small but significant rise in cerebral blood flow in an area of low flow. This effect was assumed to be due to an inverse steal phenomenon with blood being 'diverted' away from the normally perfused areas, when their metabolic demands were suppressed.

Despite these theoretical attractions and experimental support there are grave practical difficulties in transferring the regime to stroke victims. Thus anaesthetic doses are involved with all the attendant difficulties of pulmonary complications and hypotension (the dangers of which have already been stressed). However, Paulson[54] in 1973 described a study of hyperventilation which also involved heavy sedation and could report no significant benefit. Agnoli et al.[3] reported that four patients on barbiturates survived despite an adverse prognostic clinical score from which no untreated patient recovered. There were, however, two deaths due to pneumonia in their barbiturate group, and the authors stressed the problems of cardiac complications and respiratory care. They also noted that assessment of the patients was difficult because of the long acting bariturate preparation employed. Hypothermia may develop with increase in blood viscosity potentially harmful to the microcirculation. Orgogozo[51] has pointed out that logically one should consider drugs like Althesin which suppress cerebral metabolism but do not cause respiratory depression so do not require ventilatory support. The fall in blood pressure is less marked and severe hypothermia is not a problem. Recovery is rapid which aids assessment. Orgogozo found using Althesin in a small group of patients a similar global reduction in CBF to that described by Symon, with an inverse steal increasing flow in the infarcted hemisphere.

The nutritional state of experimental animals influences their recovery from transient ischaemia. Starved animals show a better recovery due to reduced lactic acid production in the face of energy failure[24]. Glucose loading impairs recovery by increasing lactacidosis. It is therefore theoretically arguable that intravenous therapy with glucose may not be ideal in the immediate aftermath of cerebral ischaemia, though this does not appear to have been considered.

Fibrinolysis

Since fibrin stabilizes major thrombi and is a constituent of many emboli especially those originating in cardiac chambers it is logical to consider the possibility of using fibrinolytic agents to disobliterate a recent occlusion. There are two immediate theoretical risks. Firstly, fragmentation of a carotid thrombus might aggravate and increase the intracranial embolism that we know occurs above such an occlusion[16]. Secondly, the haemostasis in an infarct might be tipped in favour of spontaneous haemorrhage by powerful stimuli to fibrinolysis. Extension of infarction or haemorrhage into the ischaemic bed might therefore prove disastrous complications of attempts of thrombolysis. Both Meyer[42] and Fletcher[21] reported trials in which the increased risk of haemorrhage proved unacceptable.

Now CT scans can identify those patients with haemorrhagic infarction, and digital angiography those with carotid or intracranial occlusion it is theoretically possible that fibrinolytic treatment could be reconsidered. The systemic problems may be limited by the strategy of regional fibrinolysis in which the territory of an obstruction is perfused via a catheter.

GENERAL MEASURES

The discussion so far has concentrated on the possibilities for prevention and treatment of the cerebral infarct. Though these are clearly the central issues stroke victims are also affected by a large number of associated conditions, and are subject to complications which threaten their survival and the quality of their recovery.

Associated problems

The experience from stroke intensive care units has shown how frequent general medical conditions are in patients who are admitted with an acute stroke. The associated problems are[25]:

(1) hypertension in 62%;
(2) hypertension and heart disease in 36%;
(3) ischaemic heart disease in 27%;
(4) diabetes in 20%; and
(5) rheumatic heart disease in 2%.

Correction of subnormal cardiac output and oxygenation is clearly important to the victim of a cerebral infarct. This may involve blood gas monitoring if there is any clinical suspicion of arterial desaturation. Twenty-four hour ECG monitoring reveals cardiac arrhythmias in many patients with acute stroke, and some of these may warrant treatment though they are rarely fatal. Similarly poor diabetic control may aggravate neurological deficit and in this context blood monitoring is often needed. A switch to soluble insulin may be required.

The danger of hyperviscosity has been discussed, so dehydration needs to be corrected. Nasogastric tubes may be required to ensure an adequate fluid intake in drowsy patients or those with impaired swallowing due to brain stem infarcts.

Rarely patients develop inappropriate ADH secretion with hyponatremia and increased drowsiness and the risk of seizures. Treatment in this context depends on fluid restriction and monitoring of serum and urine osomolarity.

Epilepsy develops in about 5% of acute stroke victims, sometimes reflected in the appearance of paroxysmal laterilizing epileptic discharges (PLEDS) on the EEG. Focal or generalized seizures may be seen, and should be treated aggressively.

Complications

Bronchopneumonia is a major cause of death in acute stroke patients, accounting for up to a third of fatalities. Predisposing factors include impaired consciousness, reduced mobility of the chest and diaphram in the hemiplegic, impaired respiration and swallowing in brain stem strokes, and the general immobility of the patient. Early recognition of chest infection is important and may be signalled by only a rise in temperature and respiratory rate. Mulley (personal communication) has noted that temperatures if taken in the axilla should be measured on the non-hemiplegic side since the temperature on the immobile side may be up to 1°C lower. Physiotherapy to the chest should be instituted if it looks as though immobility will last more than a day or two, and antibiotics may be necessary.

Deep vein thrombosis defined by non-invasive techniques develops in about 50% of cases of acute hemiplegia, often within the first few days. The paralysed leg is usually affected and severe weakness is probably a predisposing factor, with slow venous blood flow in the hemiplegic leg. The use of anti-embolism stockings is probably helpful though there is little data on this despite the importance and frequency of the problem. Prophylaxis, for example with ultra low dose heparin treatment[47], may therefore be appropriate in patients in whom hemiplegia and attendant immobility is more than transient.

Clinically overt deep vein thrombosis is much less frequent. The decision to use anticoagulants needs to take into account the severity of the stroke and the overall prognosis. Half the patients dying in the aftermath of an acute stroke have autopsy evidence of pulmonary embolism, and these are occasionally the cause of death.

Particular risks apply to the hemiplegic limbs. There is evidence of cortical thinning in the bones of the hemiplegic leg, for example, increasing the risk of fractures during the falls that are likely to occur. Subluxation of the hemiplegic shoulder is common due to loss of tone in the surrounding muscles. Careless lifting of the patient, or over enthusiastic amateur physiotherapy, may aggravate this problem and cause dislocation of the shoulder and increase shoulder pain. Care of the limbs is also essential to prevent contractures, and the role of appropriate positioning during rest is as important as active physiotherapy to that goal.

CONCLUSION: PRINCIPLES OF THERAPY

In a difficult field, it is helpful to have an overall clinical approach to stroke problems. In the case of transient ischaemic attacks the problem is firstly to identify the few cases in which a TIA is mimicked by sensory epilepsy, non-convulsive seizure paralysis, migraine, tumours, sub-dural haematoma, etc. CT scans and EEGs should be performed to achieve a precise diagnosis. The second problem discussed in other chapters is to identify a possible source of embolism in the heart or neck vessels often entailing echocardiography and angiography. Finally a choice has to be made between vascular surgery, anticoagulants and antiplatelet agents.

In the case of completed strokes there are a number of additional problems. Alternate diagnosis for the cause of an acute hemiplegia must be considered, especially tumours which account for as many as 5% of such cases. Rare causes of vessel occlusion, e.g. meningo-vascular syphilis, aortitis, collagen disease and trauma must be sought because of the possibility of specific therapy. Similarly there may be particular risk factors that may be treated to reduce the risk of recurrence, e.g. polycythaemia, anaemia, thrombocytosis, embolic heart disease, hyperlipidaemia. Associated general medical conditions such as cardiac failure and hypertension require treatment, and prophylaxis against certain complications may be clearly indicated by the severity of neurological disability.

The possibility for specific treatment has been considered in detail in this chapter, including antioedema regimes, anticoagulants, vasodilators, etc. In view of the possible hazards it is perhaps prudent to be guided by the principle of not initiating a treatment regime until it has been substantiated by a well designed study of sufficient size to satisfy recognized statistical criteria.

References

1 ACHESON, J., DANTA, G. and HUTCHINSON, E. C. Controlled trial of dipyridamole in cerebral vascular disease. *British Medical Journal*, **1**, 614–615 (1969)
2 ADAMS, G. F., MERRETT, J. D., HUTCHINSON, W. M. and POLLOCK, A. M. Cerebral embolism and mitral stenosis: survival with and without anticoagulants. *Journal of Neurology, Neurosurgery and Psychiatry*, **37**, 378–383 (1974)
3 AGNOLI, A., PALESSE, N., RUGGIERI, S., LEONARDIS, G. and BENZI, G. Barbiturate treatment of acute stroke. In *Advances in Neurology*, Volume 25, edited by M. Goldstein, L. Bolis, G. Fieschi, S. Garini and C. M. Millikan. 269–274. New York: Raven Press (1979)
4 ASTRUP, J., SIESJO, B. K. and SYMON, L. Thresholds in cerebral ischaemia – the ischaemic penumbra. *Stroke*, **12**, 723–725 (1981)
5 BAKER, R. N., BROWARD, J. A., FANG, M. C., FISHER, C. M., GROCH, S. N., HEYMAN, A., KEMP, H. R. and McDEVITT, E. Anticoagulant therapy in cerebral infarction. Report on co-operative study. *Neurology*, **12**, 823–835 (1962)
6 BAKER, R. N., SCHWARTZ, W. S. and ROSE, A. S. Transient ischemic strokes. A report of a study of anticoagulant therapy. *Neurology*, **16**, 841–847 (1966)
7 BEAN, W. B. Infarction of the heart. III. Clinical course and morphological findings. *Annals of Internal Medicine*, **12**, 71–94 (1936)
8 BRADSHAW, P. and BRENNAN, S. Trial of long-term anticoagulant therapy in the treatment of small stroke associated with a normal carotid angiogram. *Journal of Neurology, Neurosurgery, and Psychiatry*, **38**, 642–647 (1975)
9 BRANSTON, N. M., HOPE, J. and SYMON, L. Barbiturates in focal ischaemia of primate cortex: effects on blood flow distribution, evoked potential and extracellular potassium. *Stroke*, **10**, 647–652 (1979)
10 CANADIAN CO-OPERATIVE STUDY GROUP. A randomised trial of aspirin and sulfinpyrazone in threatened stroke. *New England Journal of Medicine*, **299**, 53–59 (1978)
11 CANDELISE, L., COLOMBO, A. and SPINNLER, M. Therapy against brain swelling in stroke patients – a retrospective clinical study on 227 patients. *Stroke*, **6**, 353–356 (1975)
12 CARTER, A. B. Anticoagulant treatment in progressing stroke. *British Medical Journal*, **2**, 70–73 (1961)
13 DARLING, R. C., AUSTEN, W. G. and LINTON, R. R. Arterial embolism surgery. *Gynaecology and Obstetrics*, **124**, 106–114 (1967)

14 DAVIES, M. J. and POMERANCE, A. Pathology of atrial fibrillation in man. *British Heart Journal*, **34**, 520–525 (1972)

15 EASTON, J. D. and SHERMAN, D. G. Management of cerebral embolism of cardiac origin. *Stroke*, **2**, 433–441 (1980)

16 EINSEIDAL-LECHTAPE, M. Secondary emboli: a frequent sequela of complete internal carotid occlusion. *Neuroradiology*, **16**, 96–100 (1978)

17 EMMONS, P. R., HARRISON, M. J. G., HONOUR, A. J. and MITCHELL, J. R. A. Effect of pyridimopyrimidine derivative on thrombus formation in the rabbit. *Nature*, **208**, 255–257 (1965)

18 EVANS, G. Effect of platelet suppressive agents on the incidence of amaurosis fugax and transient ischaemia. In *Cerebral Vascular Diseases, 8th Conference*, edited by F. McDowell and R. Brennan, 297–299. New York: Grune and Stratton (1973)

19 FIELDS, W. S., LEMAK, N. A., FRANKOWSKI, R. F. and HARDY, R. J. Controlled trial of aspirin in cerebral ischemia. *Stroke*, **8**, 310–315 (1977)

20 FIELDS, W. S., LEMAK, N. A., FRANKOWSKI, R. F. and HARDY, R. J. Controlled trial of aspirin in cerebral ischaemia; part II – surgical group. *Stroke*, **9**, 309–318 (1978)

21 FLETCHER, A. P., ALKJAERSIG, N., LEWIS, M., TULENSKI, V., DAVIES, A., BROOKS, J. E., HARDIN, W. B., LANDAU, W. M. and RAICHLE, M. E. A pilot study of urokinase therapy in cerebral infarction. *Stroke*, **7**, 135–142 (1976)

22 GEYER, S. J. and FRANZINE, D. A. Myxomatous degeneration of the mitral valve complicated by nonbacterial endocarditis with systemic embolisation. *American Journal of Clinical Pathology*, **72**, 489–492 (1979)

23 GILROY, J., BARNHART, M. and MEYER, J. S. Treatment of the acute stroke with dextran 40. *Journal of the American Medical Association*, **210**, 2193–2198 (1969)

24 GINSBERG, M. D., WELSH, F. A. and BUDD, W. W. Deleterious effect of glucose pretreatment on recovery from diffuse cerebral ischaemia in the cat. 1. Local cerebral flow and glucose utilization. *Stroke*, **2**, 374–354 (1980)

25 HACHINSKI, V. and NORRIS, J. W. Intensive care of stroke. In *Proceedings of the International Symposium on Experimental Clinical Methodologies for Study of Acute and Chronic Cerebrovascular Diseases*, 375–381. Oxford: Pergamon (1980)

26 HALLENBECK, J. M. and FURLOW, T. W. Prostaglandin I_2 and indomethacin prevent impairment of post-ischaemic brain reperfusion in the dog. *Stroke*, **10**, 629–637 (1979)

27 HARKER, L. A., RUSSELL, R., SLICHTER, S. and SCOTT, C. R. Homocystine-induced arteriosclerosis. *Journal of Clinical Investigation*, **58**, 731–741 (1976)

28 HARPER, A. M., GRAIGEN, L. and KAZDA, S. Effect of the calcium analogonist, nimodipine on cerebral blood flow and metabolism in the primate. *Journal of Cerebral Blood Flow and Metabolism*, **1**, 349–356 (1981)

29 HARRISON, M. J. G. Cerebrovascular disease. Modern methods of investigation applicable in the elderly. In *Geriatrics for the Practitioner*, edited by A. N. J. Reinders-Folmer and J. Schouten, 33–42. Amsterdam: Excerpta Medica (1981)

30 HARRISON, M. J. G. and ELL, P. Ischaemic edema in stroke. *Stroke*, **12**, 888 (1981)

31 HARRISON, M. J. G., POLLOCK, S., KENDALL, B. E. and MARSHALL, J. Effect of haematocrit on carotid stenosis and cerebral infarction. *Lancet*, **2**, 114–115 (1981)

32 HARRISON, M. J. G., POLLOCK, S., THOMAS, D. and MARSHALL, J. Haematocrit, hypertension and smoking in patients with transient ischaemic attacks and in age and sex matched controls. *Stroke* (in press)

33 HOSSMAN, K-A. and SCHUIER, F. J. Experimental brain infarcts in cats. 1. Pathophysiological observations. *Stroke*, **2**, 583–592 (1980)

34 HILL, A. B., MARSHALL, J. and SHAW, D. A. Cerebrovascular disease: trial of long-term anticoagulant therapy. *British Medical Journal*, **2**, 1003–1006 (1962)

35 HUMPHREY, P. R. D. Clinical relevance of measurements of cerebral blood flow. *British Journal of Hospital Medicine*, **26**, 233–241 (1981)

36 KLATZO, I. Neuropathological aspects of brain edema. *Journal of Neuropathology and Experimental Neurology*, **26**, 1–14 (1967)

37 KOGURE, K., BUSTRO, R. and SCHEINBERG, P. The role of hydrostatic pressure in ischemic brain edema. *Annals of Neurology*, **9**, 273–282 (1981)

38 LARSON, O., MARINOVICH, N. and BARBER, K. Double-blind trial of glycerol therapy in early stroke. *Lancet*, **1**, 832–834 (1976)

39 MATHEW, N. T., MEYER, J. S., RIVERA, V. M., CHARNEY, J. Z. and HARTMANN, A. Double-blind evaluation of glycerol therapy. *Lancet*, **2**, 1327–1329 (1972)

40 MATTHEWS, W. B., OXBURY, J. M., GRAINGER, K. M. R. and GREENHALL, R. C. D. A blind controlled trial of dextran-40 in the treatment of ischaemic stroke. *Brain*, **99**, 193–206 (1976)

41 MEYER, J. S., CHARNEY, J. Z., RIVERA, V. M. and MATHEW, N. T. Treatment with glycerol of cerebral oedema due to acute cerebral infarction. *Lancet*, **2**, 993–997 (1972)

42 MEYER, J. S., GILROY, J. and BARNHART, M. Therapeutic thrombolysis in cerebral thromboembolism. In *Cerebral Vascular Disease, Fourth Princeton Conference*, edited by C. M. Millikan, R. G. Siekert and J. P. Whisnant, 211–220. New York: Grune and Stratton (1965)

43 MEYER, J. S., GOTOH, F., GILROY, S. and NARA, N. Improvement in brain oxygenation and clinical improvements in patients with strokes treated with papaverine hydrochoride. *Journal of the American Medical Association*, **194**, 957–961 (1965)

44 MILLIKAN, C. M. Evaluation of carbon dioxide (CO_2) inhalation for acute focal cerebral infarction. *Archives of Neurology and Psychiatry*, **73**, 324–328 (1955)

45 MILLIKAN, C. H. and McDOWELL, F. H. Treatment of progressing stroke. *Stroke*, **12**, 397–409 (1981)

46 MULLEY, G., WILCOX, R. G. and MITCHELL, J. R. A. Dexamethasone in acute stroke. *British Medical Journal*, **2**, 994–996 (1978)

47 NEGUS, D., FRIEDGOOD, A., COX, S. J., PEEL, A. L. G. and WELLS, B. W. Ultra-low dose intravenous heparin in prevention of post-operative deep vein thrombosis. *Lancet*, **1**, 891–894 (1980)

48 NEUBAUER, R. A. and END, E. Hyperbaric oxygenation as an adjoint therapy in strokes due to thrombosis. *Stroke*, **2**, 297–300 (1980)

49 NORRIS, J. W. Steroid therapy in acute cerebral infarction. *Archives of Neurology*, **33**, 69–71 (1976)

50 O'BRIEN, M. D. Ischaemic cerebral edema. A review. *Stroke*, **10**, 623–628 (1979)

51 ORGOGOZO, J. M. Barbiturate treatment of acute stroke (discussion). In *Advances in Neurology*, Volume 25, edited by M. Goldstein, L. Bolis, C. Fieschi, S. Garini and C. M. Millikan, 275–276. New York: Raven Press (1979)

52 PAPPIUS, H. M. Effect of steroids on cold injury edema. In *Steroids and Brain Edema*, edited by H. J. Reulen and K. Schurmann, 57–63. Berlin: Springer Verlag (1972)

53 PATTEN, B. M., MENDELL, J., BRUUN, B., CURTIN, W. and CARTER, S. Double-blind study of the effects of dexamethasone on acute stroke. *Neurology*, **22**, 377–383 (1972)

54 PAULSON, O. B. Discussion. In *Cerebral Vascular Diseases, Eighth Princeton Conference*, edited by F. M. McDowell and R. W. Brennan, 204–205. New York: Grune and Stratton (1973)

55 PEARCE, J. M. S., GUBBAY, S. S. and WALTON, J. N. Long-term anticoagulant therapy in transient cerebral ischaemic attacks. *Lancet*, **1**, 6–9 (1965)

56 PETO, R., PIKE, M. C., ARMITAGE, P., BRESLOW, N. E., COX, D. R., HOWARD, S. V., MANTEL, N., McPHERSON, K., PETO, J. and SMITH, P. G. Design and analysis of randomised clinical trial requiring prolonged observation of each patient. 1. Introduction and design. *British Journal of Cancer*, **34**, 585–612 (1976)

57 PLUM, F. Brain swelling and edema in cerebrovascular disease. *Research Publications Association of Research in Nervous and Mental Diseases*, **41**, 318–348 (1968)

58 REULEN, H. J. Vasogenic brain edema. *British Journal of Anaesthesia*, **48**, 721–752 (1976)

59 SANTANBROGIO, S., MARTINOTTI, R., SARDELLA, J., PORRO, F. and RANDAZZO, A. Is there a real treatment for stroke: clinical and statistical comparison of different treatments in 300 patients. *Stroke*, **9**, 130–132 (1978)

60 SHUIER, F. J. and HOSSMANN, K-A. Experimental brain infarcts in cats. 2. Ischemic brain edema. *Stroke*, **2**, 593–601 (1980)

61 SIESJO, B. K. Cell damage in the brain. A speculative synthesis. *Journal of Cerebral Blood Flow and Metabolism*, **1**, 155–186 (1981)

62 SIESS, W., ROTH, P., SCHERER, B., KURZMAN, I., BOHLIG, B. and WEBER, P. C. Platelet membrane fatty acids, platelet aggregation and thromboxane formation during a mackerel diet. *Lancet*, **1**, 441–444 (1980)

63 SULLIVAN, J. M., HARKEN, O. E. and GORLIN, R. Pharmacologic control of thromboembolic complications of cardiac valve replacement. *New England Journal of Medicine*, **279**, 576–580 (1968)

64 SYMON, L., BRANSTON, N. M. and CHIKOVANI, O. Ischaemic brain edema following middle cerebral artery occlusion in baboons. Relationship between regional cerebral water content and blood flow at 1 to 2 hours. *Stroke*, **10**, 184–191 (1979)

65 TANAKA, K., MARMAROU, A. and SHULMAN, K. Regional cerebral blood flow changes associated with direct infusion edema. *Journal of Cerebral Blood Flow*, **1** (Suppl. 1) 156–157 (1981)

66 TELLEZ, H. and BAUER, R. Dexamethasone as treatment in cerebrovascular diseases. 2. A controlled study in acute cerebral infarction. *Stroke*, **4**, 547–558 (1973)

67 UK-TIA STUDY GROUP. Design and protocol of the UK-TIA aspirin study. In *Drug Treatment and Prevention in Cerebrovascular Disorders*, edited by G. Togroni and S. Garattine. Amsterdam: Elsevier (1979)

68 VETERANS ADMINISTRATION. An evaluation of anticoagulant therapy in the treatment of cerebro-vascular disease. *Neurology*, **2**, 132–138 (1961)

69 WARLOW, C. Transient ischaemic attacks. In *Recent Advances in Clinical Neurology*, Volume 3, edited by W. B. Mathews and G. M. Glaser. London: Churchill Livingstone (1982)

70 WHISNANT, J. P., CARTLIDGE, N. E. F. and ELVEBACK, L. R. Carotid and vertebrobasilar transient ischaemic attacks; effect of anticoagulants, hypertension and cardiac disorders on survival and stroke occurrence. A population study. *Annals of Neurology*, **3**, 107–115 (1978)

71 WHISNANT, J. P., MATSUMATO, N. and ELVEBACK, L. R. The effect of anticoagulant therapy on the prognosis of patients with transient cerebral ischaemic attack in a community Rochester Minnesota – 1955 through 1969. *Proceedings of the Mayo Clinic*, **48**, 844–848 (1973)

72 WHITE, O. B., NORRIS, J. W., HACHINSKI, V. C. and LEWIS, A. Death in early stroke, causes and mechanisms. *Stroke*, **10**, 743 (1979)

73 WRIGHT, I. S. and McDEVITT, E. Cerebrovascular diseases: their significance, diagnosis and present treatment, including the selective use of anticoagulant substances. *Annals of Internal Medicine*, **41**, 682–698 (1964)

11
Surgical treatment for ischemic vascular disease

Thoralf M. Sundt, Jr and Mark L. Dyken, Jr

The complexities of the cerebral circulation and the multiple causes for cerebral infarction and transient ischemic attacks from occlusive vascular disease – coupled with conflicting reports in the literature regarding the etiology and treatment for various stroke syndromes – have produced a state of confusion among physicians and surgeons treating stroke patients. The prevalence and magnitude of the problem has been established in the epidemiology section but beyond this there is no consensus of opinion concerning the ideal type of therapy, either medical or surgical. As with other types of specific medical therapy there has been a long history of anecdotal reports, but only one prospective controlled study has been reported concerning endarterectomy as a potential therapy for transient ischemic attacks[8]. A prospective controlled co-operative study is now in process concerning extracranial and intracranial microsurgical bypass, but this study has not been completed[2]. The endarterectomy study has been variably reported depending upon whether the analyses of events began at the time of hospital discharge or at the time of random assignment. It is not conclusive. In addition, this study was performed in the sixties and could not be expected to reflect the advances in surgical technique, anesthesiology, anesthesia and methods of evaluating blood flow and electro-encephalographic changes.

Despite this inability to specifically identify the exact place and value for surgical procedures, most clinicians, whether they be surgically or medically based, believe that the procedure must be of value in at least some subgroups. The purpose of this chapter will be to present the data as reviewed by the authors and summarize the experience of the senior author. The results will be analyzed as objectively as possible in an attempt to determine where surgical procedures might be of value. The following factors must be considered by the surgeon when selecting those patients who might benefit from an operation: the presenting symptoms; the natural course of the untreated disease; alternate forms of therapies; the risk of preoperative angiography; the presumed long-term benefits of the treatment and the risk of the procedure itself.

BACKGROUND

Anatomical considerations

The cerebral circulation can be divided into a conducting system and a penetrating system. The conducting vessels are the carotid, middle cerebral, anterior cerebral, vertebral, basilar and posterior cerebral arteries, plus their major (named) and minor (unnamed) branches. The branches of these systems form a vast network of interconnecting and anastomosing vessels on the surface of the brain. The conducting vessels may be regarded as non-resistance-type vessels because there is only a 10–15% drop in perfusion pressure from the common carotid artery to major branches of the middle cerebral artery and a similar gradient from these large branches to the level of the penetrating arterioles[1,32]. The penetrating vessels enter the brain parenchyma at right angles to the surface vessels from which they are derived[22]. The system of conducting vessels, modulated by the sympathetic nervous system[11], serves as a pressure head or pressure equalization reservoir to provide an adequate perfusion pressure to the penetrating or nutrient arterioles where primary autoregulation probably resides. The conducting vessels, the recipients of emboli and the site of primary atherosclerosis, form a low-resistance bed ideal for bypass grafting[30]. The penetrating vessels, when involved with anteriolar sclerosis, cause lacunar infarcts.

Cerebral blood flow

Normal blood flow to the human brain is approximately 55 ml/100 g/min (about 800 ml min^{-1} for the whole brain). The brain can, however, accommodate to a substantial reduction in flow and continue to function. Laboratory and clinical studies agree on the minimal amount of blood flow required to sustain normal electrical activity in the brain. This type of activity cannot be equated with normal function, but the electroencephalogram has proved to be a sensitive monitor of cerebral ischemia during carotid endarterectomy. This critical level of flow, which can be defined as that flow at which patients can no longer maintain normal electrical activity, has been found to be about 15 ml/100 g/min[28].

Patterns of large vessel occlusive disease

Fisher *et al.* reported that, in contrast to the carotid arteries where symptomatic occlusions were often extracranial in location, in the vertebral arteries symptomatic occlusions were usually intracranial[10]. This observation, later confirmed by other workers[6], is of considerable importance because the most common site for stenosis or occlusion of the veterbral artery originates from the subclavian artery[25]. Stenotic lesions at this location, however, are usually protected by a collateral system of vessels arising from deep muscular branches of the thyrocervical and costocervical arteries, and cerebral infarction from this source is uncommon. Atherosclerotic plaques are diffusely distributed throughout the vertebral arteries, and ulceration of these plaques is rare[10]. Again, this is in contrast with the carotid system where plaques are often near the bifurcation of the common carotid artery. Ulceration with secondary embolization is common.

Emboli (from the heart or carotid bifurcation) are thought to be the chief cause of occlusion of the major branches of the internal carotid artery. This does not seem to be the case in the vertebral basilar system where Castaigne *et al.* found thrombosis on pre-existing stenosis to be the cause of 90% of basilar artery occlusions and 70% of the intracranial vertebral artery occlusions (the correlation of infarction with basilar artery occlusion was 100% and with vertebral artery occlusion, 50%)[6]. These workers thought that occlusion on pre-existing stenosis was uncommon in the extracranial vertebral artery but common in the intracranial portion of that vessel. In that study, occlusions of the posterior cerebral artery were thought to be embolic in origin in 94% of their cases. This finding indicated that these vessels, the terminal branches of the basilar artery, were the likeliest recipients for emboli and, in this respect, were similar to the major branches of the internal carotid artery.

Although the cause of infarction in the carotid and vertebral basilar systems can be evaluated pathologically, the cause of TIAs is more difficult to assess[9,33]. Various causes have been proposed, but the following two are most often considered: (1) emboli from ulcerated plaques of large vessels to more distal arteries, and (2) hemodynamic changes distal to the site of stenosis of occlusion of an artery. The hemodynamic changes might result from variations in systemic perfusion pressure or from failure of collateral flow. The former seems to occur more often in the carotid circulation, the latter (in Dr. Sundt's judgement), in the vertebro–basilar circulation.

ISCHEMIC SYNDROMES: PATHOGENESIS AND ANGIOGRAPHIC FINDINGS

Transient ischemic attacks (TIAs)

The correlation of clinical symptoms, angiograms, and cerebral blood flow studies have indicated that flows between 20 and 30 ml/100 g/min are borderline. Patients with flow rates this low are often neurologically unstable and particularly vulnerable to the effects of emboli. The development of infarction is related to both the degree and duration of ischemia. It occurs within minutes in areas of zero flow, but it may take hours in regions of marginal flow. Blood flow values in zones of incomplete focal ischemia are non-homogeneous and characterized by areas of reactive hyperemia, as well as zones of decreased perfusion adjacent to infarcted tissue. It is necessary now to consider the pathogenesis of ischemic symptomatology.

Two theories regarding the etiology of TIAs have been proposed: microembolic phenomena and hemodynamic changes. It is quite likely that both mechanisms may produce TIAs. It has been found from cerebral blood flow measurements that cerebral blood flow does not usually become reduced, in terms of static measurements, unless carotid stenosis exceeds 80 to 90%. Although this cannot necessarily be extrapolated to the dynamic state of an active individual in whom autoregulation is impaired, it is probable that perfusion distal to a point of high-grade stenosis or vascular occlusion is vulnerable to alterations in cardiac output and perfusion pressure.

The occurrence of typical TIAs in patients with large dural arteriovenous malformations illustrates the complexity of the problem. In these patients who have increased venous pressure, the transient ischemic event is probably related to alterations in the venous outflow.

Not infrequently, angiograms are found to be normal in patients with typical TIAs and the cause of the events is never determined. This is analogous to the so-called benign amaurosis fugax seen in patients with normal carotid and ophthalmic arteries. In the posterior circulation a rather severe form of TIA can possibly be related to flow alterations through a very small artery. This is also possible in the anterior circulation, particularly in patients with hypertensive disease and arteriolar changes in the striate system.

Amaurosis fugax is transient monocular blindness lasting less than one hour – most commonly, only three to five minutes. The onset is rapid, often described as a shade coming down slowly over one eye.

The presence in the retina of emboli indicates that amaurosis fugax is often embolic in origin. When a carotid artery is occluded or nearly occluded in the presence of retrograde ophthalmic flow (on angiography) and a markedly lowered retinal artery pressure, the possibility exists that transient non-embolic flow alterations can occur and produce retinal ischemia. Nevertheless, amaurosis fugax has been a relatively uncommon finding in our patients with known chronic internal carotid occlusion, in contrast to the high frequency of this symptom in patients with carotid stenosis.

A transient focal neurological deficit of less than 24 hours' duration is considered to represent a TIA.

Carotid system TIAs are most commonly manifested by transient weakness or numbness in the hand area and, when the dominant hemisphere is involved, by dysphasia. Severe TIAs produce transient hemiparesis. Localization of a focal deficit to the foot alone is in general an uncommon form of TIA, but it is not an uncommon form of TIA in patients with occluded carotid artery.

TIAs in the vertebral basilar system are less stereotyped than those in the carotid system. Vertigo is a common component of TIA in the vertebral basilar system; however, vertigo alone is most commonly a manifestation of labyrinthine disorder and, therefore, unless associated with some other manifestations of brain stem ischemia, should not be considered a TIA. Vertigo from the carotid system is rare and occurs only when compensatory collaterals are present. The reports of vertigo from carotid kinking, and relief from resection of loops and kinks, should be considered cautiously.

Transient hemiparesis, hemisensory deficit, or homonymous hemianopia can arise from ischemia in either the anterior or posterior circulatory system, but these are usually considered to represent carotid TIAs unless symptoms are alternating from side to side or associated with cranial nerve palsies. Transient quadriparesis is most commonly of brain stem origin. Dysarthria and dysphagia, which are symptoms of bulbar ischemia, may be seen in patients with pseudobulbar palsy from supratentorial lesions, but they are most commonly brain stem in origin. Transient impairment of function of the extraocular muscles may be of definite localizing value, but if diplopia is due to TIA it will usually be associated with other symptoms. Nausea, vomiting and vertigo may occur with brain stem TIA, but this combination is not useful for distinguishing brain stem from labyrinthine dysfunction.

Data from several centers indicate that, among patients with TIAs, an average of 5–8% will have cerebral infarction in each year of follow-up[16]. Untreated patients who have been observed after onset of the first TIA appeared to have an even higher risk of cerebral infarction in the first few months of observation[34]. However, not all patients with carotid ulcerative stenosis have a TIA before suffering a major stroke, and not all episodes of TIA are due to carotid artery disease. Complicating the problem further for the clinician, no statistically valid reports on large groups of untreated patients are available to establish how the relationship between TIA and subsequent stroke is affected by the presence of a carotid bruit, altered retinal artery pressure (RAP) and angiographically determined degree of ulceration and stenosis. However, there is some recent evidence that patients with a high degree of carotid stenosis (greater than 70%) have a greater risk of subsequent stroke than do those with minimal stenosis[37].

Cerebral infarction

A neurological deficit persisting longer than 24 hours is considered to result from a cerebral infarction. An infarction usually produces a permanent deficit, but small infarctions can result in a reversible deficit, which has been referred to by some as a reversible ischemic neurological deficit (RIND). Localization of an infarction to the anterior or posterior circulation follows the criteria indicated above for TIA.

Cerebral infarction, in contrast to cerebral ischemia, denotes anatomical death of tissue. Analysis of the intracranial and extracranial angiograms of patients considered for carotid endarterectomy has revealed evidence of obstruction of flow in either the intracranial or extracranial circulation in most patients with a known cerebral infarction. Furthermore, about 50% of patients with infarction have angiographic evidence of a focal internal carotid artery or middle cerebral artery slow-flow alteration indicating marginal cerebral blood flow. The cause for cerebral infarction in this group was occlusion or near obstruction of a major intracranial or extracranial conducting vessel with a reduction in the critical perfusion pressure head reservoir.

SURGERY FOR CAROTID ARTERY OCCLUSIVE DISEASE

Endarterectomy

General and review

In patients with high-grade stenotic lesions, carotid endarterectomy restores a normal perfusion pressure to the internal carotid system, and in patients with ulcerative lesions it removes a source of emboli. Deep areas of ulceration are more common in those plaques which are quite thick so that stenosis and ulceration often coexist. A deep ulcerative plaque is much more dangerous than a shallow ulcer crater. For this reason, we have preferred conservative management for shallow ulcer craters in the belief that these craters will heal spontaneously. Examination of plaques removed at surgery for deep ulcer craters commonly reveals coexistence of smaller ulcer craters which have re-endothelialized and apparently are no longer thrombogenic. Until the natural history of individual plaques can be predicted and determined, there will be no unanimity of opinion regarding the proper management of the shallow ulcer crater.

The decision for the clinician is not an easy one. Obviously, those patients with minimal preoperative risk factors should be good surgical candidates whereas those with risks such as complicating medical illness or widespread atherosclerosis should be poor surgical candidates. Unfortunately, most of the patients who present with cerebral vascular disease lie between these two extremes. An analysis of the risk factors could help the clinician determine which patients should be considered for angiography and surgical treatment. Most surgeons would agree that an estimated operative risk in excess of 10% is a contraindication for operation[7]. Many feel that it must be much lower. Doctors Hass and Jonas reviewed the results of the extracranial occlusion joint study which evaluated surgical treatment of extracranial arteries to prevent stroke. They performed calculations which were not to determine whether surgery was better than the best medical therapy but rather what was the highest permissible complication rate and concluded that in TIA patients in stroke complication greater than 2.9% was unacceptable and less than 1.5% was preferable[12, 14].

The major factors that determine the surgical risk for a given patient appear to be:

(1) experience of the operating team;
(2) condition of the patient at the time of operation; and
(3) postoperative care[4].

These factors seemed to be valid in a joint study of extracranial disease[5] in which there was a steady decrease in surgical mortality and morbidity over the ten years of study.

The surgical approach to TIA is confined to approaches to surgically accessible lesions or bypass procedures. The new surgical techniques concerned with microsurgical anastomosis between branches of the external carotid artery to branches of an intracranial artery have been perfected and are being studied but their application has not yet been established. More established procedures include removal of an accessible lesion by endarterectomy with or without patch grafting. At the present time major areas of controversy concern the value of removing surgically accessible lesions in patients who have asymptomatic bruit and whether these lesions should be approached or not in patients who have had completed infarction. Most clinicians would agree that some types of lesions in patients who have TIAs should be approached surgically but there is no general agreement on the types of lesions that would best be handled in this manner. The authors hope that the development of techniques which will visualize the arterial system with minimal risk such as digital subtraction venous angiography, better clarification of structural integrity of the brain and function of the brain such as refinements of computerized tomography, nuclear magnetic resonance techniques and positron emission tomography, will result in a future clear understanding of exactly which kind of patients will benefit most by a surgical procedure and where it is contraindicated.

In terms of symptomatology, an endarterectomy is considered for patients with amaurosis fugax, TIAs, small infarcts with a minimal residual deficit and selected cases of progressing strokes. It is not indicated for a large completed infarct because a neurological deficit at this point is probably irreversible, and the risk of hemorrhage is great. It is not indicated for the non-specific symptom of vertigo and only rarely in selected patients with other forms of symptomatology likely to originate in the posterior circulation.

The management of an acute occlusion of the internal carotid artery is more controversial. On occasion, gratifying results can be achieved from emergency endarterectomy in patients with acute internal carotid artery occlusions if the symptoms have been present for only a few hours. (This does not necessarily correlate with the time of anatomical occlusion as patients can develop ischemic symptomatology one or two days following the point of anatomical occlusion and at the time collateral flow, for one reason or another, fails.) The chance of avoiding a permanent hemiplegia from surgery must be balanced against the risk of hemorrhage and death. This is a decision which must be made by the family. We have achieved normal neurological function in a dramatic fashion from the operative procedure in three of fifteen such hemiplegic patients, but we have also lost three patients from hemorrhage.

Mayo Clinic experience

The primary indiction for surgery in Dr. Sundt's series (1352 operations) has been a recent TIA. Minor degrees of carotid ulceration were treated conservatively (anticoagulants or aspirin). Virtually all patients, with only a rare exception, had greater than 70% stenosis of the involved carotid artery. All patients were monitored with intraoperative xenon cerebral blood flow (CBF) measurements and continuous electroencephalograms, plus postoperative retinal artery pressure measurements.

It is extraordinarily difficult to analyze the results of any operative procedure or to compare the results of surgery form one institution to another without some means of grouping patients according to preoperative risk factors. Therefore, we have grouped our patients according to medical, neurological and angiographically determined risk factors. Medical risk factors included coronary artery disease (angina pectoris) or a myocardial infarction of less than six months' duration, severe hypertension (blood pressure greater than 180/110 systolic), chronic obstructive pulmonary disease, physiological age of more than 70 years and severe obesity.

Neurological risk factors included a progressing neurological deficit, a deficit less than 24 hours old, frequent daily TIAs, or multiple neurological deficits secondary to multiple cerebral infarctions. Angiographically determined risk factors included a coexisting stenosis of the internal carotid artery in the siphon area; extensive involvement of the vessel, with the plaque extending more than 3 cm distally in the internal carotid at the level of the second cervical vetebra, in conjunction with a short, thick neck; occlusion of the opposite internal carotid artery; and evidence of a soft thrombus extending from the ulcerative lesion.

Using the above criteria, it has been possible to classify patients according to preoperative risk factors, the results of surgery, and the operative complications as follows:

Grade 1 neurologically stable patients with no major medical or angiographically determined risks, with unilateral or bilateral ulcerative–stenotic disease – combined major morbidity and mortality 0%, minor morbidity (normal employment but with deficits such as decreased alternate motion rate in one hand) 2%;

Grade 2 neurologically stable patients with no major medical risks but with significant angiographically determined risks – major morbidity and mortality 1%, minor morbidity 2%;

Grade 3 neurologically stable patients with major medical risks with or without significant angiographically determined risks – major morbidity and mortality 4.5% (primarily myocardial infarction), minor morbidity 2%; and

Grade 4 patients with major neurological risks (i.e. neurologically unstable patients) with or without associated major medical or angiographically determined risks – major morbidity and mortality 4% (intracerebral hemorrhage primary complicating factor), minor morbidity 3%.

Complications that resulted in no morbidity (TIA, wound hematoma, paroxysmal lateralizing epileptiform discharges, etc.) are not included in the above figures as these problems did not produce a permanent morbidity. However, immediate attention to complications is imperative to prevent a permanent morbidity. There were postoperative occlusions identified by a reduction in retinal artery pressures with or without TIAs. Flow was restored in each case with emergency surgery. Most of these complications occurred early in the series before venous patch grafting and intraoperative heparinization (without reversal) were standard measures. One of these patients retained a mild hemiparesis and is in the major morbidity column. Two of these patients retained a minor deficit in the hand and are reported in the minor morbidity group. However, the remaining patients left the hospital after a normal period of hospitalization morbidity. This illustrates the major importance of early identification of an occlusion following endarterectomy by retinal artery pressure measurements.

The patency of the vessels following surgery can be accurately determined only through retinal artery pressure measurements by an experienced neuro-ophthalmologist on the day following the operation, or by oculoplysmography or digital subtraction angiography. This is analogous to the presence of a pulse in the foot following peripheral vascular surgery. A reduction in the retinal artery or oculoplethysmometric pressure is an immediate indication for evaluation of the vessel by angiography or re-exploration. It is only through these techniques that the true incidence of postoperative occlusion can be identified. In institutions where these measures are not routinely performed, the incidence of postoperative occlusion may be higher than generally accepted. We have had more inquiries for possible extracranial to intracranial bypass for an internal carotid occlusion that followed endarterectomy than for any other single entity. Unfortunately, most of these patients have already had a large infarction from the carotid occlusion and are not candidates for bypass surgery. The history in these patients reveals that they have seldom been evaluated for possible carotid occlusion at the time of the infarction (usually within 72 hours of the endarterectomy).

Adequate monitoring techniques are advisable for the reduction of morbidity and mortality during carotid surgery. This choice is safer than routine shunting, which increases the risk of embolization. Nevertheless, there is little question that some patients have practically no cross-fill from the opposite circulation, and these individuals can have a cerebral infarction within three to four minutes of carotid occlusion. In fact, we have seen blood flows fall to virtually zero levels at the time of carotid occlusion.

It is imperative that the plaque be removed in its entirety from the internal carotid artery and that no intimal ledge be left to serve as a source of emboli. In our experience, venous patch grafting has proved superior to simple closure of the arteriotomy, except in cases where an unusually large vessel is present. In some cases, it is necessary to remove the plaque from the internal carotid artery prior to

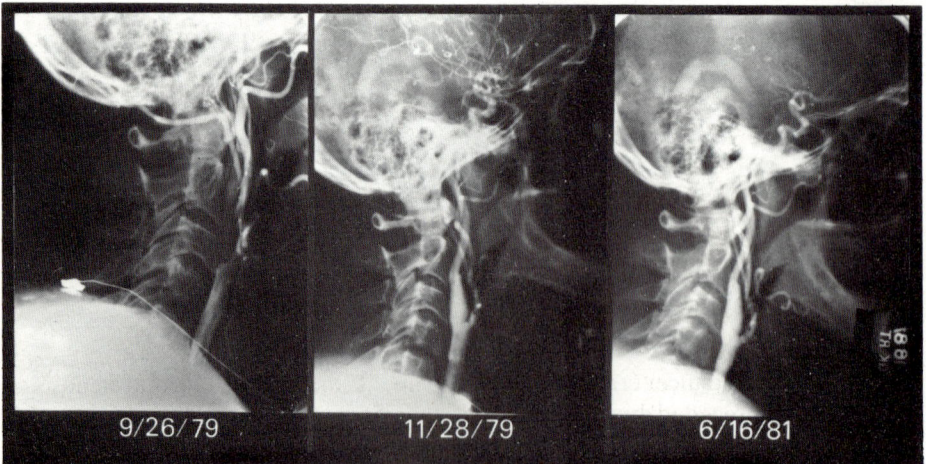

9/26/79   11/28/79   6/16/81

Figure 11.1 Pre- and post-operative angiograms in a patient undergoing endarterectomy for an occlusion of the right internal carotid artery. It will be noted that this vessel remains essentially unchanged during the period between the first angiogram performed approximately eight weeks following the operation and the second angiogram performed 21 months following the operation. The patch graft has extended the bulb of the internal carotid artery distally and rotated the vessel so that the internal carotid artery is more the primary extension of the common carotid artery than is the external carotid artery

placement of a shunt. This is particularly true in patients in whom the plaque extends more than 3 cm past the carotid bifurcation. *Figure 11.1* is an example of the results of endarterectomy.

Effects of endarterectomy

True cerebral autoregulation probably resides in the penetrating arterioles discussed previously. These are apparently modulated by an intrinsic nervous system that has origin in the brain stem[3, 15, 21, 23]. These arterioles must be supplied with an adequate perfusion pressure if they are to function normally. The normalization of retinal artery pressures after endarterectomy indicates the restoration of a normal perfusion pressure in the conducting vessels. This increase in the distal perfusion pressure permits the parenchymal arterioles to return to a more normal tone – from one of maximal dilatation – and thus the autoregulatory ability of the brain is restored.

The microembolic[24, 35] and hemodynamic theories[20] for transient ischemic attacks and infarcts are not mutually exclusive. Areas of brain functioning on a marginal flow of 40 to 50% of the normal flow are particularly vulnerable to the effects of emboli. Furthermore, plaques that have a severe degree of stenosis and that, therefore, represent a significant hemodynamic lesion are more likely to form deep ulcer craters than are plaques of lesser severity.

Thus, endarterectomy in a patient with a high-grade stenosis and ulceration confers the following benefits:

(1) Removes a source of emboli[24];
(2) Restores a normal distal perfusion pressure and the capability for normal autoregulation;
(3) Increases flow through the artery and, depending on collateral flow, increases cerebral blood flow; and
(4) Prevents progression of the stenosis to occlusion.

We believe that patients with the so-called mini-ulcer should not be operated on but rather should be treated conservatively. We have not infrequently noted that in plaques removed at surgery because of high-grade stenosis or a deep ulcer crater, there will be proximal small pits covered with endothelium which probably at one time represented minor ulcerations. Carotid atherosclerosis is not the only cause of TIAs[18, 19], and one should be very cautious about recommending surgery on the basis of a presumed ulcer crater. Conversely, not all strokes from carotid stenosis of occlusion are preceded by a TIA[19] and, therefore, asymptomatic patients with pronounced stenosis and reduced retinal artery pressure may be candidates for surgery[13, 17, 19].

Results of endarterectomy

The operative or surgical results of carotid endarterectomy are summarized in *Table 11.1* according to the grade risk of the patient prior to surgery. The results of

Table 11.1 Results of carotid endarterectomy* between 1 January 1972 and 1 January 1982

Grade of Risk	Procedures	Neurological function			Mortality		
		Normal, unchanged, or improved†	New deficit		From intracerebral hemorrhage	From myocardial infarction	From other complications
			Major	Minor			
1	472	468 (4)	0	4	0	0	0
2	282	278 (4)	2	2	0	0	0
3	357	342 (4)	5	3	0	6	1
4	241	222 (7)	5	5	5	2	2
Total	1352	1310 (19)	12	14	5	8	3

* Overall, mortality was 1.2%, major morbidity was 1%, and minor morbidity was 1%.
† Numbers in parentheses are patients with transient neurological dysfunction (transient ischemic attacks, seizures, migraine variants)

Table 11.2 Cerebral blood flow according to anesthetic used and grade of risk (mean ± SD)

	Halothane											
Time of measurement	Grade 1			Grade 2			Grade 3			Grade 4		
	n	$\bar{x}$	SD	n	$\bar{x}$	SD	n	$\bar{x}$	SD	n	$\bar{x}$	SD
Baseline	149	63±26		85	59±27		135	52±21		80	48±20	
Occlusion	149	35±18		85	31±18		137	27±15		78	24±14*	
Shunt	40	45±15		40	53±18		62	44±17		46	41±12	
Post-occlusion	150	70±27†		86	69±25†		137	62±23†		82	61±21†	

	Ethrane											
Time of measurement	Grade 1			Grade 2			Grade 3			Grade 4		
	n	$\bar{x}$	SD	n	$\bar{x}$	SD	n	$\bar{x}$	SD	n	$\bar{x}$	SD
Baseline	278	49±18		168	45±20		180	42±18		127	38±21	
Occlusion	276	27±12		167	24±14		176	21±11		127	18±11*	
Shunt	97	38±14		86	36±12		97	36±12		78	36±15	
Post-occlusion	280	51±18		170	51±20†		187	49±19†		133	51±22†	

* Two-sample t test applied to differences between grade 1 and grade 4 values at occlusion was significant at $P < 0.001$
† Paired t test applied to differences between baseline and post-occlusion values was significant at $P < 0.001$

Table 11.3 Cerebral blood flow versus electroencephalogram from carotid occlusion

	Number of patients with change in electroencephalogram from occlusion		Number of patients without change in electroencephalogram from occlusion	
Flow*	Halothane	Ethrane	Halothane	Ethrane
0–4	6	27	0	0
5–9	18	73	1	0
10–14	46	84	6	36
15–19	41	64	19	73
20–24	7	8	41	101
25–29	0	0	54	101
≥30	0	0	222	253
Total	118	256	343	564

* In ml/100 g per minute

cerebral blood flow measurements are summarized in *Table 11.2* according to the grade of the patient and the anesthetic agent employed. It is important in this group to note that the occlusion flow was significantly lower in the grade 4 patients than it was in the other groups. This underscores the marginal collateral flow present in these patients and helps to explain their unstable preoperative neurological picture. *Table 11.3* correlates the occlusion blood flow measurements with changes noted in the electroencephalogram[29]. Thus, 2% of the patients had occlusion blood flows below 4 ml/100 g/min and had a shunt not been employed one can be confident that this group of individuals would have suffered an infarction from the occlusion time required for endarterectomy. In another group, 92 patients had occlusion flows that varied between 5 and 9 ml/100 g/min and it is probable that a number of patients in this group (7% of the total) might very well have also suffered an infarction from the period of occlusion. Added to this are the large number of patients having occlusion flows between 10 and 14 ml/100 g/min. Some of these patients (13% of the total) might have also sustained an ischemic deficit from the period of occlusion.

Dr. Whisnant has analyzed data from the Mayo Clinic concerning all patients (151) seen from 1970 through 1974 with transient focal ischemia in whom carotid endarterectomy was performed ipsilateral to the ischemia. Each patient was evaluated by a neurologist and surgery was performed by a single surgeon. It should be noted that this series comprises a slightly different group from the group summarized in *Table 11.1* which includes only patients operated upon after routine monitoring was adopted. Thus there are two years' worth of patients in the chronic group not included in the group summarized in *Table 11.1* and these patients with TIAs fell into various risk categories.

Nevertheless, ischemic stroke in this group occurred in 3% (2% major, 1% minor), either during or within 30 days after surgery. Mortality after endarterectomy was 1% at one month.

After one month, ischemic strokes occurred at a rate of 2% per year (two-thirds were ipsilateral to endarterectomy) vs an expected rate of 6% per year. Mortality was 3% per year and 71% of deaths were due to cardiac cause. It was concluded that stroke morbidity was less than expected in the operative group and that cardiac disease was greater than expected because of the prolongation of life from the endarterectomy.

A multivariant analysis, using 18 variables, detected none related to mortality. Only low cerebral blood flow during carotid clamping was found to be related to stroke morbidity. This coincides with the results of the cerebral blood flow measurements referred to above[36].

Extracranial–intracranial bypass

General and review

It seems possible that a patent bypass graft can be maintained in the vast majority of properly selected patients. Postoperative angiograms have revealed an amazing amount of flow through these grafts and it is not at all uncommon to visualize not only the middle cerebral complex but also part of the anterior cerebral complex from blood derived through the bypass graft (*Figure 11.2*). These dramatic changes in vascular perfusion following bypass procedures lead one to wonder how some particular patients could have functioned prior to revascularization. A brief review of some physiology and pathogenesis of ischemic symptoms will help us understand this question and place this operative procedure in perspective.

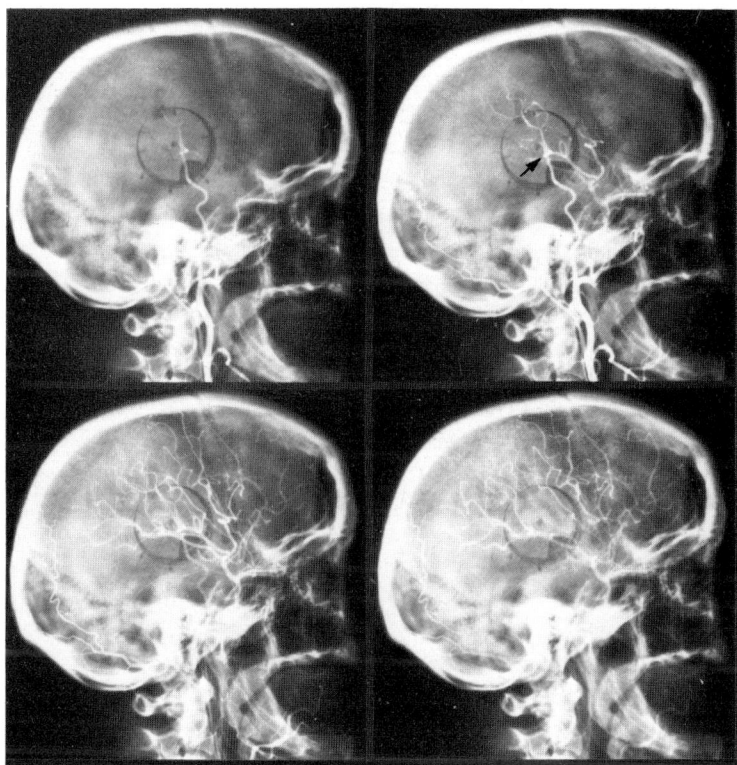

Figure 11.2 Post-operative angiogram in a patient undergoing a temporal artery to middle cerebral artery bypass procedure for occlusion of the ipsilateral internal carotid artery. The bypass graft fills not only the middle cerebral group but also the anterior cerebral artery and its branches. This angiogram was performed three months following the bypass procedure

It is known that normal electrical activity in the brain is commonly preserved with blood flow reduction to 40% of normal. However, the brain is exquisitely sensitive to further reductions of flow and alteration in electrical activity often develops when flow is reduced to between 15 and 20 ml/100 g/min and virtually always develops when flow is reduced below 15 ml/100 g/min. Normal electrical activity cannot be equated to normal neurological function but it does indicate the preservation of physiological function.

It is quite possible that patients with a chronic internal carotid artery occlusion or high grade stenosis of the siphon or middle cerebral artery complex have adequate flow for physiological activity while at rest or during most modern activities. Superimposed alterations in cardiac output or peripheral perfusion pressure result in transient ischemic attacks and in some instances frank infarction. Careful analysis of the case history in many patients with a chronic major vessel occlusion will reveal alterations in sensorium with posture (generalized cerebral ischemia) which must be differentiated from the common lightheadedness or mild vertigo related to a labyrinthine disorder common in the elderly. These individuals have often had a rather major change in cerebral function and mental capacity.

A rare form of chronic ischemia has been referred to as the 'slow stroke'. Patients with this syndrome report to the physician with a chronic progressing neurological deficit localized to the watershed area of cerebral perfusion (the foot and leg area). Less commonly the proximal upper extremity is involved. Computerized tomography in these patients is normal. A coexisting venous stasis retinopathy may be identified on funduscopic examination. The hallmark and identifying feature of this syndrome is the relentless progression of a mild deficit which is most noticeable in the foot and which is accentuated by activity. Quite frequently the individual has a relatively normal neurological examination when initially tested but if observed to walk for as long as 100 yards a definite foot drop develops and in some instances the patient is unable to walk further and must sit down and rest before continuing. This is a classic example of chronic crebral ischemia and is the cerebral analog of chronic retinal ischemia, the well known entity clearly described as venous stasis retinopathy.

Major indications for temporal artery to middle cerebral artery bypass procedures are continued transient ischemic attacks in patients with known internal carotid artery occlusions, or high grade stenotic lesions of the distal internal carotid artery or proximal middle cerebral artery who have continued to have ischemic events while taking anticoagulants or antiplatelet agents. The less common chronic syndromes referred to above often coexist with transient ischemic attacks. Bypass procedures are not indicated for patients with asymptomatic occlusion nor are they indicated for individuals who have sustained a large infarction with irreversible neurological deficits.

Quite recently two separate teams of investigators have documented the vast difference between cortical perfusion pressures in patients with a patent internal carotid artery and those with an internal carotid artery occlusion. In the former group, individuals in whom the cortical perfusion pressure was measured prior to internal carotid artery ligation and supplementary bypass for giant aneurysms, the cortical perfusion pressure in the pressure head reservoir was equal to the mean arterial blood pressure measured at the wrist. However, in patients with a chronic internal carotid artery occlusion both groups of investigators found that the cortical perfusion pressure was approximately 50% of the peripheral perfusion pressure. Following bypass surgery there was an immediate increase in the perfusion pressure and, of course, with delayed dilatation of the graft and increased flow through the graft, the probability is that the perfusion pressure would increase further thereafter.

In spite of the above compelling arguments for the rationale of a bypass procedure, it is a fact that a controlled study has not yet been completed verifying the role of this operation. A co-operative study is currently in progress and results of that study should be available in the near future. It should be recognized, however, that the variability of underlying vascular pathology, differences in patient evaluation from institution to institution, the participation of centers from all over the world with different patient populations, and the major problems related to the control process of true randomization within the reporting institutions and the degree of enthusiasm for the study within each participating institution makes a study of this nature most difficult to evaluate.

Recently a prominent team of investigators have raised questions on the relevance of a stump of the internal carotid artery to continued ischemic events in the territory of an occluded internal carotid artery. Certainly the stump of an external carotid artery in patients with a patent internal carotid artery is a recognized risk for continued ischemic events on an embolic basis. The true contribution of the internal carotid artery stump in these cases can only be determined by evaluating individual cases which have been carefully reported.

In this regard, however, it should be noted that a 'stumpectomy' of the internal carotid artery is not an innocuous procedure. In fact, this can develop into a rather major undertaking. The stump of the internal carotid artery in these cases is contained in a hardened and thick vessel which is involved with atherosclerosis. The stump cannot merely be ligated with a single suture. In order to close the stump an endarterectomy in the internal carotid artery is necessary. *It is not possible to do an internal carotid artery* in most cases without continuing the endarterectomy into the external carotid artery. Quite commonly atherosclerosis is diffuse in the external carotid artery, and does not terminate and feather out smoothly as it does in the internal carotid artery 2–3 cm above the bifurcation. In the external carotid artery atherosclerosis often extends into branches of the external carotid artery and a distal break point in the endarterectomized segment cannot be achieved without leaving a ledge. Thus it is often necessary to tack the wall of the intima to the endarterectomized surface in the external carotid artery and in some instances its branches. In these cases the vessel is best repaired with a saphenous vein patch graft.

The problems related to atherosclerosis in the external carotid artery have led us to recommend the 'on-lay' patch for patients with a coexisting stenosis of the external carotid artery in whom external carotid artery surgery is planned in order to increase collateral flow through the ophthalmic artery, or as a preliminary for temporal artery to middle cerebral artery bypass surgery. In these cases occasional attempts have been made to close the stump of an internal carotid artery if out-pouching is significant, but where it is minor it has been merely ignored. To date we have had no strokes which we could attribute to a residual stump in these patients. The rete mirabile which has developed behind the eye and which is the source of collateral flow through branches of the internal maxillary artery would seemingly serve as a filter system for major emboli.

Mayo Clinic experience

In order to maintain a patent bypass graft, it is necessary to have a perfusion gradient across the site of anastomosis. In this series to date (438 operations), patency approaches 98%. Occlusions in this series have been primarily related to situations in which an adequate perfusion gradient across the site of anastomosis could not be maintained. Postoperative angiograms in such patients have revealed patency of the recipient vessel at the point of anastomosis but no evidence of flow through the bypass graft. We have had graft failure in patients suffering from idiopathic regressing arteriopathy; mild stenotic lesions which, although symptomatic, did not reduce the gradients in the pressure head reservoir; embolic events; and carotid cavernous fistula. *Figure 11.2* is an example of a typical bypass graft in a patient with adequate donor and recipient vessels.

SURGERY FOR VERTEBRAL BASILAR OCCLUSIVE DISEASE

Endarterectomy

General and review

Although there are a few series of vertebral endarterectomies reported, general experience with this procedure has been poor. This is because of the excellent collateral circulation present in most patients distal to the site of the most common area for stenosis in the vertebral artery, the origin of the vertebral from the subclavian artery, and the non-ulcerative character of these stenotic lesions. Furthermore, there is no large series in which postoperative angiograms have been evaluated for patients undergoing this type of operation. Enthusiasm for endarterectomy in this area is not great, and there are few institutions currently recommending this type of procedure.

Carotid–subclavian bypass

Angiographically identifiable subclavian steal syndromes are not rare; however, many patients will have this angiographic picture without symptomatology and, therefore, patients must be evaluated carefully prior to recommending surgery merely because of the angiographic demonstration of this problem. A bypass graft from the proximal carotid artery to the subclavian artery distal to the origin of the vertebral artery is the procedure of choice for patients with a symptomatic subclavian steal syndrome.

Vertebral artery transpositions

The role for this procedure is, as yet, undetermined because no hard data are available for analysis.

Extracranial–intracranial bypass

For intracranial vertebral artery stenosis

An extracranial to intracranial bypass for occlusive disease involving the proximal intracranial vertebral artery can be achieved from an anastomosis between the occipital artery and the posterior inferior cerebral artery (*Figure 11.3*)[30]. As our experience with these procedures to date is still limited (38 procedures), it is premature to predict a role for this operation. Nevertheless, our results have been modestly encouraging, and it is our belief that the operation will have a very definite but limited role in the management of patients with ischemic symptomatology in this system.

It should be emphasized that the patients we have operated on to date have been individuals who have been disabled by the frequency or severity of their ischemic events. These are not individuals who have sustained only one or two TIAs. Patients who have been accepted for surgery have had either bilateral intracranial vertebral artery occlusions proximal to the origins of the posterior inferior cerebral arteries, or unilateral vertebral artery occlusion in combination with a high-grade intracranial stenosis of the opposite vertebral artery. These patients often present with a clinical picture of ataxia, visual disturbances, altered mentation, and changes in sensorium with erect posture. Some patients have been suffering from a progressing stroke in the brain stem or cerebellum. Others have had multiple TIAs not altered by anticoagulant therapy. No patients have been evaluated who have had only one or two TIAs involving the posterior circulation. In our experience, angiograms in such patients are often normal or show only minimal large vessel disease.

To achieve' a high flow and materially alter the hemodynamics of the posterior circulation, it is necessary to perform the anastomosis between relatively large vessels and not resort to using a surface vessel over the cerebellum. Thus, in occlusive disease involving the vertebral arteries, one should perform the anastomosis, if possible, between the occipital artery and the medullary loop of the posterior inferior cerebral artery as that vessel courses around the medulla (*Figure 11.3*).

Grafts have been patent in 90% of the patients in this group. Complications related to the operative procedure have been greater than those in the anterior circulation and in large measure have been related to marginal neurological status of these patients prior to operation. Respiratory complications have been frequent and have usually resulted from previous cranial nerve dysfunction that has made swallowing and handling of secretions difficult. We now often leave a nasotracheal tube in place until the patients are fully awake from surgery and are able to handle their secretions with reasonable facility.

Patients are operated on in the sitting position for occipital to posterior inferior cerebral artery bypass grafts. Thus, risks related to air emboli, hypotension and convexity subdural collections of fluid or air are present in this group; however, it is our judgement that these risks are far outweighed by the exposure achieved from the position. All patients should receive adequate blood volume replacement on a unit for unit basis which helps to prevent air emboli. These patients have areas in

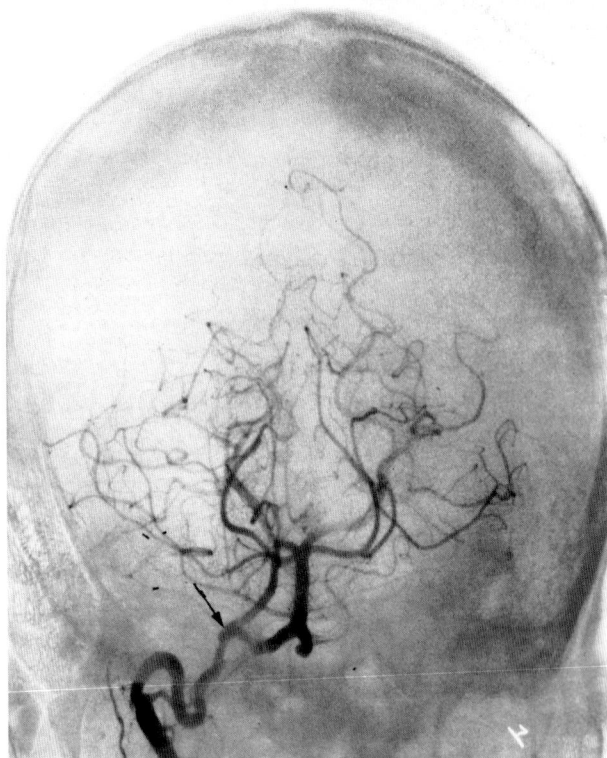

Figure 11.3 Post-operative angiogram in a patient undergoing an anastomosis between the occipital artery and the posterior inferior cerebellar artery. At the time of the bypass procedure both vertebral arteries were patent but stenotic. During the period of follow-up a stenotic lesion progressed to produce total occlusion of both vertebral arteries. However, these occlusions occurred without symptoms. Post-operative angiography demonstrated filling of entire posterior circulation through the bypass graft

the brain in which autoregulation is no longer preserved, and they are extraordinarily vulnerable to fluctuations in perfusion pressure and cardiac output. Accordingly, it is imperative to maintain an adequate perfusion pressure throughout the operation. Complications such as epidural hematoma and aseptic meningitis related to blood in the subarachnoid space are not unique to this type of operation and can be prevented with appropriate measures.

For basilar artery stenosis or occlusion

We have used basically five procedures in the management of occlusive vascular disease in the posterior circulation. The first of these procedures was discussed above and has been used to bypass stenotic lesions of the vertebral artery. It is still the procedure of choice for patients with intracranial vertebral artery occlusions or stenotic lesions proximal to the origin of the posterior inferior cerebellar artery.

The problem relates to the fact that most patients – or at least many patients – have their lesions distal to the posterior inferior cerebellar artery.

Our experience with the second procedure we attempted – that being a superficial temporal artery to proximal superior cerebellar artery bypass procedure – was less rewarding in that high flows were not achieved. Thus far we have only one patient out of seven achieve what we would consider to be a high flow from this operative procedure. However, other workers have had better experience with this operation and perhaps we abandoned it too soon. Nevertheless, at least in our limited experience, the superior cerebellar artery, in contrast to the posterior cerebral artery, tolerates temporary occlusion poorly for a bypass procedure. Infarcts in the area of the cerebellum were not uncommon in patients undergoing this operation in our hands.

The third approach attempted for occlusive disease in this system at our institution was transluminal angioplasty. We believe it is an acceptable approach for patients with very focal lesions but is hazardous for individuals with diffuse disease and probably in light of our current experience (five cases) should be reserved for individuals in whom one form of bypass procedure or another cannot be employed[31].

The fourth procedure or approach for occlusive disease is a side-to-side anastomosis between the posterior cerebral artery and the superior cerebellar

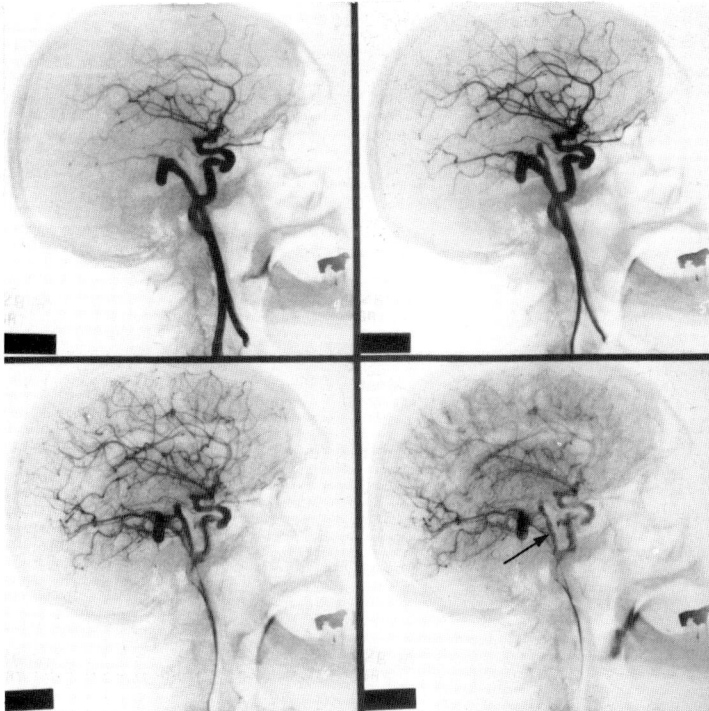

Figure 11.4a Lateral series in a patient undergoing an interposition saphenous vein graft between the external carotid artery and the proximal posterior cerebral artery for basilar artery occlusion. Note retrograde filling of the basilar artery (arrow)

artery in patients with a fetal circulation[26]. A variation of this operation has been used in a patient with a giant aneurysm of the posterior cerebral artery – previously reported – in which the aneurysm was excised and the distal posterior cerebral artery anastomosed to the superior cerebellar artery. High flows are achieved but there are few patients who are candidates for this operation (only five cases to date). Nevertheless, in the individual in whom this anatomical variation is present, it is our judgement that this is the most reliable and lowest risk operative approach for patients with these types of problems.

There remains a large group of patients with either occlusions or diffuse stenotic lesions of the basilar artery who are not candidates for one of the above procedures. An interposition saphenous vein graft between the external carotid artery and the proximal posterior cerebral artery can be lifesaving and dramatic in relief of neurological symptomatology in some of these cases (*Figure 11.4b*)[27]. Flows are very substantial with these types of grafts and the results in patients who have had a patent graft are most rewarding.

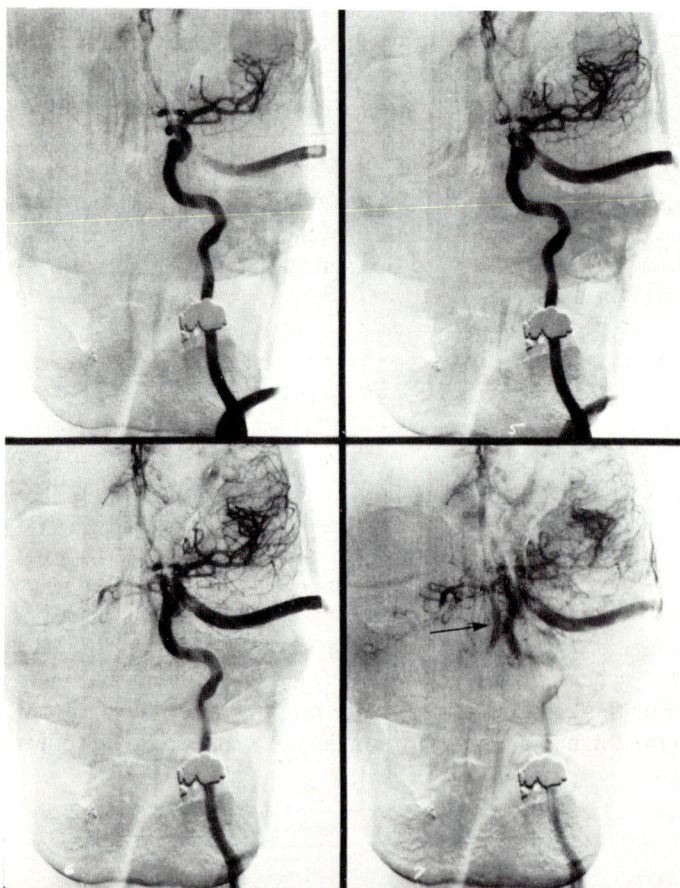

Figure 11.4b Anterior-posterior projection of same case illustrated in *Figure 11.4a*. Saphenous vein graft has been brought across the floor of the middle fossa to be anastomosed to the proximal posterior cerebral artery

So far 27 patients have undergone interposition saphenous vein grafts between the external carotid artery and the proximal posterior cerebral artery at the Mayo Clinic. One patient with a large aneurysm in the posterior circulation had a proximal clipping of her only vertebral artery along with a simultaneous bypass graft. This patient is now normal. All other patients have had major ischemic symptomatology while on adequate medical therapy and were at high risk for a posterior circulation infarct. Twenty-two of these 27 patients were confined to bed or were disabled from the severity of their ischemic events prior to surgery and three of these patients had a progressing stroke in the posterior circulation. Thus, they were all very high risk candidates for surgery.

In the 21 patients with patent grafts, there were 15 excellent results, four good results, and two deaths (both in patients with progressing strokes in whom surgery was a desperation effort). There were three early graft occlusions and three late graft occlusions in the group. In these six patients there were three minor strokes, two major strokes and one death.

Our laboratory data relating to the thrombogenicity of vein grafts is difficult to acquire because of a lack of adequate laboratory models with vein grafts of the length used in these cases. We do know from the work of Kaye *et al.* at the Mayo Clinic that most of the original endothelium of the vein graft is sloughed away some time between the second and tenth day following the time of graft placement. Obviously during this period the graft is relatively thrombogenic. Graft patency can be improved in these cases both clinically and in the laboratory by treatment with combined aspirin and Persantine (dipyridamole). Also, the higher the flow, the less likely the graft is to thrombose. Our measured flows at surgery varied between 35 and 300 ml/min with most flows ranging somewhere between 80 and 100 ml/100 g/min. Grafts with these types of flows have remained patent. Grafts with flows as low as 30 to 40 are marginal and most of our occlusions have occurred in patients with low flows at surgery. The sources for occlusions have included the following problems: atherosclerosis in the recipient vessel at the site of the anastomosis, twisting or angulation of the graft as it is pulled through the previously prepared tunnel which follows a track over the zygoma through the parotid gland and then into the cervical area just superficial to the digastric muscle, possible technical errors at either the distal or proximal suture line, and over-distension of the vein in its preparation. However, we have not been able to correlate graft flows with known technical complications in either suture line.

Late graft occlusions in most instances were related to a mismatch in the size between the donor and recipient vessels and occurred in patients with unusually large saphenous veins. For this reason we have more recently used the vein from the leg rather than from the thigh in patients in whom an obviously adequate vein is present in the leg.

References

1 BAKAY, L. and SWEET, W. H. Cervical and intracranial intra-arterial pressures with and without vascular occlusion. *Surgery, Gynecology and Obstetrics*, **95**, 67–75 (1952)

2 BARNETT, H. J. M. and PEERLESS, S. J. Collaborative EC/IC bypass study: the rationale and a progress report. In *Cerebrovascular Diseases, Twelfth Research (Princeton) Conference*, edited by John Moossy and Oscar M. Reinmuth, 271–288. New York: Raven Press (1981)

3 BATES, D., WEINSHILBOUM, R. M., CAMPBELL, R. J. and SUNDT, T. M. Jr. The effect of lesions in the locus coeruleus on the physiological responses of the cerebral blood vessels in cats. *Brain Research*, **136**, 431–443 (1977)

4 BLAISDELL, W. Extracranial artery surgery in the treatment of stroke. In *Cerebral Vascular Diseases (Transactions of the Eighth Conference)*, edited by F. H. McDowell and R. W. Breenan, 3–15. New York: Grune and Stratton (1973)

5 BLAISDELL, W. F., CLAUSS, R. H., GALBRAITH, J. G. *et al*. Joint study of extracranial arterial occlusion. IV. A review of surgical considerations. *Journal of the American Medical Association*, **209**, 1889–1895 (1969)

6 CASTAIGNE, P., LHERMITTE, F., GAUTIER, J. C. *et al*. Arterial occlusions in the vertebro-basilar system: a study of 44 patients with postmortem data. *Brain*, **96**, 133–154 (1973)

7 CLAUSS, R. H., SANOUDOS, R. M., RAY, J. F. III *et al*. Carotid endarterectomy for cerebrovascular ischemia. *Surgery, Gynecology and Obstetrics*, **136**, 993–1000 (1973)

8 FIELDS, W. S., MASLENIKOV, V., MEYER, J. S. *et al*. Joint study of extracranial arterial occlusion. V. Progress report of prognosis following surgery or nonsurgical treatment for transient cerebral ischemic attacks and cervical carotid artery lesions. *Journal of the American Medical Association*, **211**, 1993–2003 (1970)

9 FISHER, C. M. Occlusion of the vertebral arteries causing transient basilar syndrome. *Archives of Neurology*, **22**, 13–19 (1970)

10 FISHER, C. M., GORE, I., OKABE, N. *et al*. Atherosclerosis of the carotid and vertebral arteries – extracranial and intracranial. *Journal of Neuropathology and Experimental Neurology*, **20**, 82–88 (1970)

11 HARPER, A. M., DESHMUKH, V. D., ROWAN, J. O. and JENNETT, W. B. The influence of sympathetic nervous activity on cerebral blood flow. *Archives of Neurology*, **27**, 1–6 (1972)

12 HASS, W. K. and JONAS, S. Caution falling rock zone: an analysis of medical and surgical management of threatened stroke. *Proceedings of the Institute of Medicine, Chicago*, **33**, 80–84 (1980)

13 JAVID, H. Development of carotid plaque. *American Journal of Surgery*, **138**, 224–227 (1979)

14 JONAS, S. and HASS, W. K. An approach to maximal acceptable stroke complication rate after surgery for transient cerebral ischemia. *Stroke*, **18**, 104 (1979)

15 LANGFITT, T. W. and KASSELL, N. F. Cerebral vasodilatation produced by brain-stem stimulation: neurogenic control vs autoregulation. *American Journal of Physiology*, **215**, 90–97 (1968)

16 MILLIKAN, C. H. Reassessment of anticoagulant therapy in various types of occlusive cerebrovascular disease. *Stroke*, **2**, 201–208 (1971)

17 MOORE, W. S., BOREN, C., MALONE, J. M. and GOLDSTONE, J. Asymptomatic carotid stenosis: immediate and long-term results after prophylactic endarterectomy. *American Journal of Surgery*, **138**, 228–233 (1979)

18 MOHR, J. P., CAPLAN, L. R., MELSKI, J. W., GOLDSTEIN, R. J., DUNCAN, G. W., KISTLER, J. P., PESSIN, M. S. and BLEICH, H. L. The Harvard co-operative stroke registry: a prospective registry. *Neurology (Minneapolis)*, **28**, 754–762 (1978)

19 PESSIN, M. S., DUNCAN, G. W., MOHR, J. P. and POSKANZER, D. C. Clinical and angiographic features of carotid transient ischemic attacks. *New England Journal of Medicine*, **296**, 358–362 (1977)

20 PESSIN, M. S., HINTON, R. C., DAVIS, K. R., DUNCAN, G. W., ROBERSON, G. H., ACKERMAN, R. H. and MOHR, J. P. Mechanisms of acute carotid stroke. *Annals of Neurology*, **6**, 245–252 (1979)

21 RAICHLE, M. E., HARTMAN, B. K., EICHLING, J. O. and SHARPE, L. G. Central noradrenergic regulation of cerebral blood flow and vascular permeability. *Proceedings of the National Academy of Science, USA*, **72**, 3726–3730 (1975)

22 SAUNDERS, R. L. and BELL, M. A. X-ray microscopy and histochemistry of the human cerebral blood vessels. *Journal of Neurosurgery*, **35**, 128–140 (1971)

23 SHALIT, M. N., REINMUTH, O. M., SHIMOJYO, S. and SCHEINBERG, P. Carbon dioxide and cerebral circulatory control. III. The effects of brain stem lesion. *Archives of Neurology*, **17**, 342–353 (1967)

24 SIEKERT, R. G., WHISNANT, J. P. and MILLIKAN, C. H. Surgical and anticoagulant therapy of occlusive cerebrovascular disease. *Annals of Internal Medicine*, **58**, 637–641 (1963)

25 STEIN, B. M., McCORMICK, W., RODRIGUEZ, J. N. *et al*. Incidence and significance of occlusive vascular disease of the extracranial arteries as demonstrated by postmortem angiography. *Transactions of the American Neurological Association*, **86**, 60–66 (1961)

26 SUNDT, T. M. Jr., CAMPBELL, J. K. and HOUSER, O. W. Transpositions and anastomoses between the posterior cerebral and superior cerebellar arteries. Report of two cases. *Journal of Neurosurgery*, **55**, 967–970 (1981)

27 SUNDT, T. M. Jr., PIEPGRAS, D. G., HOUSER, O. W. and CAMPBELL, J. K. Interposition saphenous vein grafts for advanced occlusive disease and large aneurysms in the posterior circulation. *Journal of Neurosurgery*, **56**, 205–215 (1982)

28 SUNDT, T. M. Jr., SHARBROUGH, F. W., ANDERSON, R. E. *et al*. Cerebral blood flow measurements and electroencephalograms during carotid endarterectomy. *Journal of Neurosurgery*, **41**, 310–320 (1974)

29 SUNDT, T. M. Jr., SHARBROUGH, F. W., PIEPGRAS, D. G., KEARNS, T. P., MESSICK, J. M. Jr. and O'FALLON, W. M. Correlation of cerebral blood flow and electroencephalographic changes during carotid endarterectomy. *Mayo Clinic Proceedings*, **56**, 533–543 (1981)

30 SUNDT, T. M. Jr., SIEKERT, R. G., PIEPGRAS, D. G. *et al*. Bypass surgery for vascular disease of the carotid system. *Mayo Clinic Proceedings*, **51**, 644–692 (1976)

31 SUNDT, T. M. Jr., SMITH, H. C., CAMPBELL, J. K., VLIETSTRA, R. E., CUCCHIARA, R. G. and STANSON, A. W. Transluminal angioplasty for basilar artery stenosis. *Mayo Clinic Proceedings*, **55**, 673–680 (1980)

32 SYMON, L. A comparative study of middle cerebral pressure in dogs and macaques. *Journal of Physiology (London)*, **191**, 449–465 (1967)

33 WHISNANT, J. P., FITZGIBBONS, J. P., KURLAND, L. T. *et al*. Natural history of stroke in Rochester, Minnesota, 1945 through 1954. *Stroke*, **2**, 11–22 (1971)

34 WHISNANT, J. P., MATSUMOTO, N. and ELVEBACK, L. R. The effect of anticoagulant therapy on the prognosis of patients with transient ischemic attacks in a community: Rochester, Minnesota, 1955 through 1969. *Mayo Clinic Proceedings*, **48**, 844–848 (1973)

35 WHISNANT, J. P., MILLIKAN, C. H., SAYRE, G. P. and WAKIM, K. G. Effect of anticoagulants on experimental cerebral infarction: clinical implications. *Circulation*, **20**, 56–65 (1959)

36 WHISNANT, J. P., SANDOK, B. A. and SUNDT, T. M. Jr. Endarterectomy for transient cerebral ischemic-long term survival and stroke probability (abstract). *Stroke*, **13**, 113 (1982)

37 ZIEGLER, D. K. and HASSANEIN, R. S. Prognosis in patients with transient ischemic attacks. *Stroke*, **4**, 666–673 (1973)

12
Cerebral venous thrombosis

P. R. D. Humphrey, C. R. A. Clarke and
R. J. Greenwood

Cerebral venous thrombosis was first recorded in the early part of the nineteenth century. Kalbag and Woolf, in their detailed monograph, refer to Ribes, a French physician who in 1825 described a 45-year-old man who developed epilepsy and headaches[15]. At post mortem, six months later, the superior sagittal sinus and lateral sinuses were thrombosed; carcinomatous metastases were present in the brain. Later in the nineteenth century several further reports became available, the majority based on post mortem studies. In many cases, there was a preceding infection. This resulted in the widely held belief that sinus thrombosis tended to occur in severely ill patients with septicaemia and had a grave prognosis. In 1888, Gowers in his textbook pointed out that sinus thrombosis was common in the puerperium[11]. He also stressed the importance of the venous system as an anastomotic network. As the condition became more widely recognized, it became apparent that the outlook was not so gloomy. The true incidence, however, has never been established. Barnett and Hyland reported 39 noninfective cases at autopsy from Toronto General Hospital over a twenty year period[4]. In a study of 182 consecutive autopsies in a chronic institution, there was a 9% incidence of dural sinus thrombosis[31]. Many authors have emphasized that the condition is often not suspected or the appropriate investigations not performed[3, 15, 25]. This review will highlight the varied presentation of cerebral venous thrombosis.

FUNCTIONAL ANATOMY

In clinical practice, although it may not be possible to differentiate between superior sagittal sinus thrombosis, transverse (lateral) sinus thrombosis, and superficial cerebral venous thrombosis, a knowledge of the venous anatomy is important to understand the genesis and spread of these conditions and recovery from them.

The dural venous sinuses (*Figure 12.1*), save for those lying in the free edge of the falx and tentorium cerebelli (the inferior sagittal and straight sinuses), are rigid

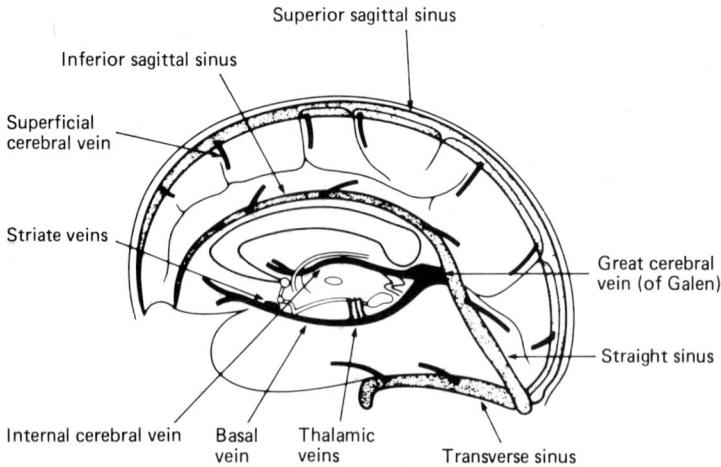

Figure 12.1 Main venous drainage of the brain

tubes, often trabeculated, formed between fibrous dura and endosteum. They drain all the blood from the brain into the internal jugular veins through the following three venous systems:

(1) The superficial cerebral veins, a dozen or so in number, which drain the superficial surfaces of the hemispheres into the superior sagittal sinus.
(2) The superficial middle cerebral veins which drain the cortex adjacent to the lateral sulcus, emptying into the cavernous sinus (*Figure 12.2*).
(3) The deep venous system comprises the basal veins (formed by the deep middle cerebral, anterior cerebral and striate veins) and the internal cerebral veins which meet to form the great cerebral vein of Galen draining into the junction of the inferior sagittal sinus and straight sinus. All the cerebral veins have thin walls lacking muscle fibres and have no valves. The veins on the convexity of the hemispheres lie adherent to the deep surface of the arachnoid. Blood flow within them is frequently in the same direction as in the neighbouring arteries and is reversible.

Numerous and rather variable anastomotic channels interconnect the superficial cerebral veins and the sinuses. The most important are shown in *Figure 12.2*, the great anastomotic vein of Trolard connecting the superior sagittal sinus to the superficial middle cerebral vein and the inferior anastomotic vein of Labbé which connects the transverse sinus to the superficial middle cerebral vein. In addition the diploic veins (which have valves) occupying the cranial bones communicate with the meningeal veins, the dural sinuses and the scalp veins.

The multiple connections between veins and sinuses are clinically important in: (1) facilitating the spread of infections, for example, from the nasopharynx to cavernous sinus or from the scalp via diploic veins to superior sagittal sinus; (2) forming the routes of propagation of established thromboses; and (3) providing

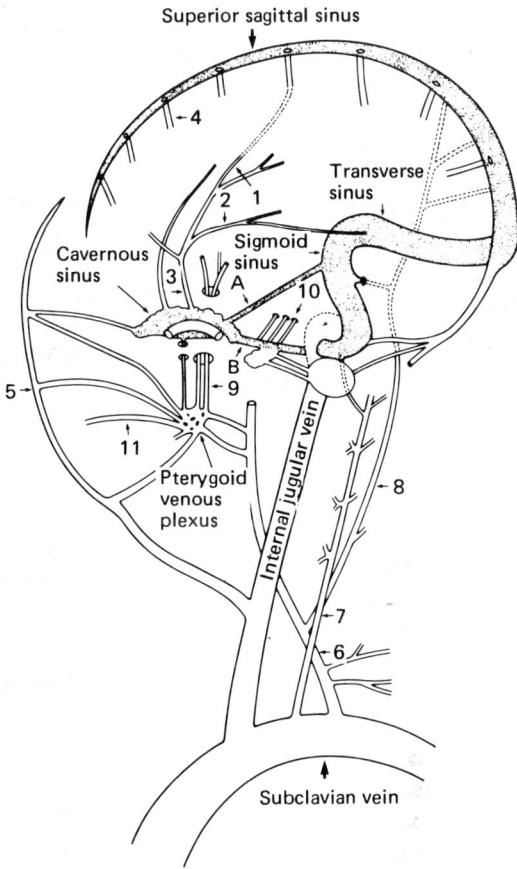

Figure 12.2 Schematic diagram showing some of the major anastomotic channels between the cerebral veins and sinuses and between the extra- and intracerebral systems. A = superior petrosal sinus; B = inferior petrosal sinus; 1 = great anastomotic vein (of Trolard); 2 = inferior anastomotic vein (of Labbé); 3 = superficial middle cerebral vein; 4 = superficial cerebral vein; 5 = facial vein; 6 = external jugular vein; 7 = vertebral vein; 8 = occipital vein; 9 = meningeal veins; 10 = labyrinthine veins; 11 = nasal vein. (Modified from MacEwen[18])

alternative routes whereby blood in the dural sinuses may reach the exterior of the skull when the normal drainage routes are blocked.

PATHOLOGY

A number of interesting points emerge from pathological studies. Haemorrhagic infarction is the prominent intracerebral lesion in intracranial venous thrombosis after early infancy. Perivenous petechial 'ring' haemorrhages involve both grey and white matter with subarachnoid leakage of blood and sometimes asymmetrical confluent white matter haemorrhage. This pathology is invariably associated with cerebral vein thrombosis and there may be involvement of the dural sinuses. Symmetrical thalamic infarction following occlusion of the straight sinus or vein of Galen is an interesting though rare phenomenon. Less florid changes comprise swelling of cerebral white matter.

The scanty pathological material in cases presenting with isolated raised intra-cranial pressure ('otitic hydrocephalus') has confirmed lateral and posterior sagittal sinus thrombosis as the cause and demonstrated few, if any, microscopic or macroscopic changes in the brain (cases 22 and 28[15]).

In neonates and young infants, acute changes in the brain following intracranial venous thrombosis consist of confluent myelin breakdown, which may progress to liquefaction, in the deep white matter of the centrum semiovale with sparing of the cortex and basal ganglia. With prolonged survival, gliosis and cystic encephalo-malacia supervene; the relevance of these changes to cerebral palsy is emphasized by Kalbag and Woolf[15].

CLINICAL FEATURES

Predisposing factors

Recent studies suggest that in many cases no predisposing cause is found[3, 10]. A wide variety of conditions have now been reported to be associated with cortical vein and sinus thrombosis, as follows:

(1) pregnancy[6, 17], puerperium[6, 22] and the contraceptive pill[2, 17];
(2) local factors such as trauma[13], surgery, sepsis[29] and tuberculous meningitis and neurosyphilis or neoplasm[3];
(3) systemic illness including malignancy[26], and metabolic disorders such as dehydration[15], diabetes mellitus[1], ulcerative colitis[12], Behçet's syndrome[20], Budd-Chiari syndrome[15] and congestive cardiac failure[31]; and
(4) haematological disorders such as leukaemia[26], polycythaemia rubra vera[4], thrombocytopenia[3], paroxysmal noctural haemoglobinuria[14], sickle cell trait[24] and haemolytic anaemia[17].

Cortical vein thrombosis

Thrombosis of the cortical veins may occur in isolation but there is often associated thrombosis of the dural sinuses[15, 17, 27]. The clinical features largely result from intracerebral or subarachnoid bleeding.

Headache is generally the initial symptom. It is usually severe and sometimes associated with nausea and vomiting. Neck stiffness may be present and the picture resemble subarachnoid haemorrhage or meningoencephalitis. Epilepsy often occurs early in the presentation and may be focal or generalized. Status epilepticus and coma occur in some cases. The fits are frequently followed by prolonged hemiparesis, with aphasia if the dominant hemisphere is involved. It is unusual for the hemiplegia to precede the fits. Epilepsy, however, is not invariable, in which case the presentation may be difficult to distinguish from cerebral arterial occlusion, haemorrhage or abscess. In rapidly fatal cases, neck rigidity, Cheyne Stokes respiration and hyperpyrexia followed by death may occur within a few hours of presentation.

Many patients are severely ill with raised intracranial pressure and papilloedema. Sometimes mental changes such as confusion and psychotic symptoms are the predominant features[4, 27]; these may be followed by progressive loss of consciousness without the development of focal neurological signs.

Cerebral vein thrombosis is common in the first year of life and may follow many of the common childhood infections[5, 15, 25]. Failure to thrive, refusal to feed, vomiting, weight loss and irritability, sometimes proceeding to coma, may dominate the presentation in these infants.

Dural sinus thrombosis in isolation

Symptoms due to thrombosis limited to the dural sinuses are usually less dramatic than those due to cerebral vein thrombosis and are generally limited to the signs and symptoms of raised intracranial pressure. Recovery is often spontaneous. In 1931 this syndrome, which was noted to follow otitis media, mastoiditis or nasopharyngitis, was termed 'otitic hydrocephalus' by Sir Charles Symonds[28]. It was suggested that the condition was due to excessive secretion from the choroid plexus or defective absorption from the arachnoid villi. Symonds was aware that thrombosis of the transverse (lateral) sinus, which lies close to the middle ear, was often present and did not feel initially that this could explain the whole picture. Unfortunately, the term otitic hydrocephalus has remained: it is now appreciated that this syndrome does, indeed, follow unilateral transverse sinus thrombosis and that ventricular enlargement does not occur unless secondary to other pathology[8, 9]. Thrombus usually extends into the posterior part of the superior sagittal sinus to occlude the contralateral transverse sinus and the straight sinus.

Isolated thrombosis of the sagittal sinus may also produce symptoms and signs of raised intracranial pressure presenting with a picture identical to benign intracranial hypertension[23]. However, sagittal sinus thrombosis is usually accompanied by cortical vein thrombosis with the appropriate signs and symptoms. Proptosis has been reported in sagittal sinus thrombosis although it is much more common in cavernous sinus thrombosis. Oedema of the scalp is sometimes present.

Spread of thrombosis to the inferior petrosal sinus may produce a sixth nerve palsy. Extension of the thrombosis into the jugular veins results in paralysis of the ninth, tenth and eleventh cranial nerves with swelling and tenderness of the neck. Paralysis may sometimes spread to the twelfth nerve and rarely the fifth nerve is involved from thrombosis in the superior petrosal sinus[30].

Thrombosis of the sigmoid sinus may produce oedema and tenderness at the point of exit of the mastoid emissary vein along the posterior border of the mastoid. Scotti *et al.* reported a four-year-old boy who presented with a soft lump behind the ear, over which a bruit was heard[25]. This was an enlarging emissary vein and was the only sign of lateral sinus thrombosis.

Thrombosis of the whole of the straight sinus usually results in extensive fatal haemorrhagic infarctions, particularly in the thalamus.

Cavernous sinus thrombosis

Thrombosis of the cavernous sinus frequently follows infections of the face and paranasal air sinuses. It is usually bilateral since there is a free venous communication between the two cavernous sinuses. The patients are often gravely ill with high fever, headaches, ocular pain and tenderness. There is often paresis of the third, fourth, sixth and ophthalmic division of the fifth cranial nerves. This results in a complete ophthalmoplegia with a fixed mid-position pupil due to involvement of both sympathetic and parasympathetic fibres. Painful proptosis, chemosis and oedema of the periorbital structures follows obstruction of the ophthalmic veins. Lacrimation is often marked. Papilloedema may be seen. Spread of thrombosis to the pterygoid plexus may cause oedema of the pharynx. Recently thrombosis has been recognized to follow fungal infections. Mucormycosis invades blood vessels and causes gangrene with grey-black appearance of infected tissue[19]. This may be apparent on examination of the nasopharynx and is particularly likely to occur in diabetic or immunocompromised patients.

INVESTIGATIONS

Although cerebral venous thrombosis may be suspected, a definite diagnosis is usually impossible on clinical grounds alone.

Fever, leucocytosis and a high erythrocyte sedimentation rate (often over 50 mm) are frequently present, even in the absence of infection. Plain skull films are normal unless there is evidence of local infection. The cerebro-spinal fluid pressure is usually raised. Its constituents vary from being normal to suggestive of a previous (and usually minor) subarachnoid bleed. A mixed mononuclear and polymorph pleocytosis of 10–200 cells per mm^3 may occur with raised protein.

In superior sagittal sinus thrombosis, the EEG usually shows a bilateral diffuse slow wave disturbance, although we have seen a normal record in a patient whose clinical picture suggested benign intracranial hypertension. Focal hemisphere slow waves are common in cortical thrombophlebitis. The periodic discharges seen in herpes simplex encephalitis have not been recorded following cortical thrombosis, so the EEG may be helpful with differential diagnosis.

The computed tomography (CT) scan appearances are variable. Diffuse low attenuation suggestive of widespread oedema is common although this may sometimes be focal, making differentiation from a tumour or arterial infarct difficult[16]. More characteristic are bilateral, multiple, high attenuation areas which are indicative of haemorrhagic infarction. This is particularly suggestive of cortical thrombophlebitis (*Figure 12.3*). Patronas *et al*. suggested that a triangular area of increased density, before contrast, along the course of the superior sagittal sinus was a useful finding[21]. This high attenuation area is thought to be due to

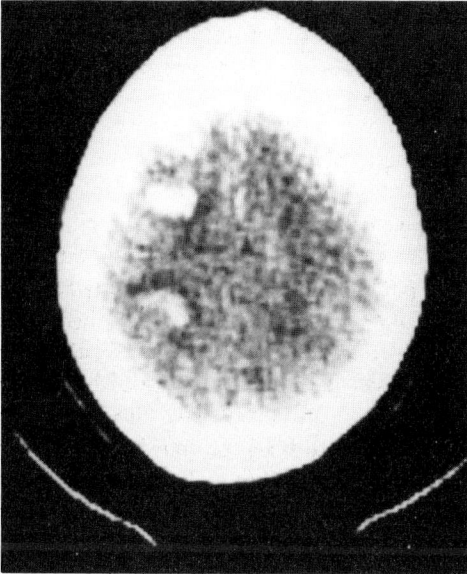

Figure 12.3 CT scan (without contrast) showing several discrete areas of haemorrhagic infarction consistent with cortical thrombophlebitis

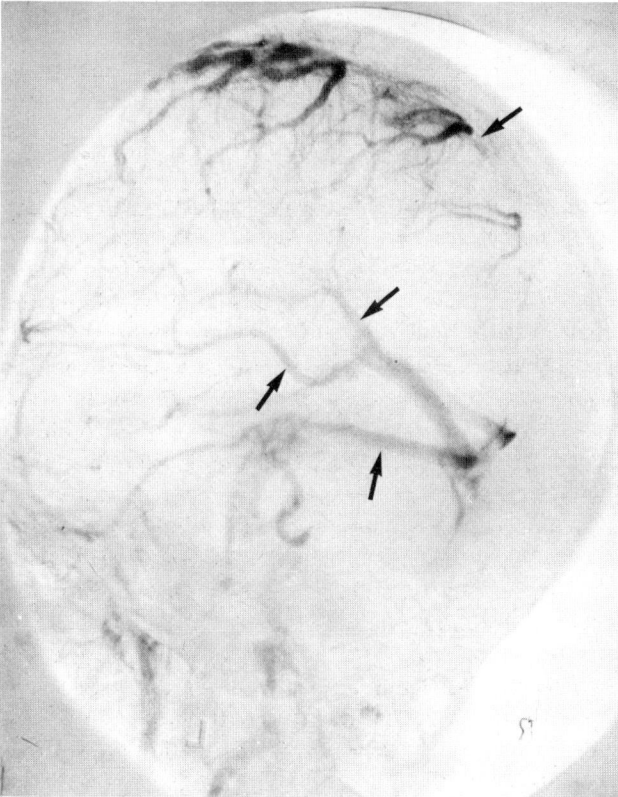

Figure 12.4 Occlusion of the superior sagittal sinus demonstrated on angiography (top arrow) with a patent inferior sagittal sinus, internal cerebral vein and transverse sinus (lower arrows)

unorganized thrombus. It lasts for only a few days and is replaced by a low or normal attenuation area as the clot becomes organized. This low attenuation may be highlighted by giving contrast, following which a triangular area of enhancement appears around the sinus. Normal CT scans have been seen in post mortem verified cases of sagittal sinus and cortical thrombosis. This is frequently the case, however, in lateral sinus occlusion. Ventricular enlargement is not a feature of these conditions and in cases with diffuse hemisphere swelling the ventricles may be small.

Carotid angiography remains the only investigation which can, with certainty, confirm the diagnosis (*Figure 12.4*),[10, 17, 25]. High quality venous-phase films, with lateral and oblique views, are usually sufficient to confirm superior sagittal sinus thrombosis, lateral sinus thrombosis and cortical venous thrombosis. Unless clinical attention is focused upon the venous circulation the possibility remains that these conditions may be missed. Delayed films may be necessary to allow for slow venous filling resulting from raised intracranial pressure. More detailed procedures such as simultaneous, bilateral internal carotid injection with delayed films have been described, but these are not in common use. Local injection of contrast into the sagittal sinus was practised in the 1940s but is now regarded as hazardous.

TREATMENT

First, treatment of cerebral venous thrombosis may be directed towards the primary cause, if any, is identifiable.

Secondly, epilepsy, which may be relatively resistant to treatment, and raised intracranial pressure may threaten life. The rise in intracranial pressure results from blockage of normal CSF absorption due to damaged arachnoid villi and venous stasis. Diuretics and steroids are often administered. Recurrent lumbar puncture, which is not without risk, sometimes provides a temporary and effective means of reducing intracranial pressure until collateral venous drainage becomes established. Lumboperitoneal shunting and optic nerve or subtemporal decompression may help to save vision and lower intracranial pressure.

Thirdly, treatment of the thrombosis itself must be considered. Oral and intravenous anticoagulants and fibrinolytics have been advocated to prevent progression. Unfortunately from CSF, CT scan and pathological data it is clear that haemorrhagic venous infarction, which may only be microscopic, has often occurred at presentation in cortical vein thrombosis. This has led to completely contradicting views regarding the use of anticoagulants. Krayenbuhl advocated anticoagulants; he felt that cerebral haemorrhage was no more frequent in a treated group of 17 patients[17]. The group without treatment had a considerably higher mortality, although the most severely ill seemed to be in this group. Gettelfinger and Kokmen, however, reported that two of their three patients taking anticoagulants died of haemorrhagic intracranial complications[10]. Several other small studies have come to opposing conclusions[2, 4, 15]. Recently Di Rocco *et al.* have reported five patients with aseptic dural sinus thrombosis who were treated with a combination of sodium heparin and urokinase[7]. All made a complete recovery; post operative cerebral angiography showed patency of the involved sinuses in all.

There are no controlled trials on which to base conclusions. There can thus be no definite guidelines. Furthermore it is unlikely that enough cases could be gathered for a controlled clinical trial unless the frequency of this condition has been markedly underestimated.

We suggest that it is only in cases presenting with symptoms of isolated dural sinus thrombosis that anticoagulants be considered. In cases where fits and haemorrhagic infarction occur, their use is hazardous.

CONCLUSIONS

In this review we hope to have emphasized some of the difficulties in the diagnosis and management of cerebral venous thrombosis. The clinical picture may resemble benign intracranial hypertension, cerebral abscess or tumour, subarachnoid haemorrhage, encephalitis or a cerebrovascular arterial event. Frequently the classical predisposing factors such as sepsis and the puerperium are absent. While noninvasive investigations may sometimes suggest the correct diagnosis, they may frequently not provide any clue to the underlying venous thrombosis. This is particularly likely to occur in those who present as an 'encephalitis' with headache, epilepsy and a deteriorating neurological deficit. In such cases the CT scan may merely show low attenuation areas and it is unlikely that angiography would be considered. A similar situation occurs in those who present with the clinical picture of benign intracranial hypertension and have a normal CT scan. Again the diagnosis will be missed as angiography will not usually be carried out.

It is clear that the frequency of this condition is underestimated. The diagnosis is missed for several reasons. First, in many patients the diagnosis is not even considered and angiography is not performed. Secondly, in cases where angiography is carried out, not necessarily with venous thrombosis in mind, insufficient attention may be paid to the venous phase. It is particularly important to take oblique views, with delayed films if necessary.

The use of anticoagulant drugs and fibrinolytic agents remains controversial but may have a role in selected cases.

References

1 ASKENASY, H. K., KOSARY, I. Z. and BRAHAM, J. Thrombosis of the longitudinal sinus. *Neurology*, **12**, 288–292 (1962)

2 ATKINSON, E. A., FAIRBURN, B. and HEATHFIELD, K. W. G. Intracranial venous thrombosis as complication of oral contraceptives. *Lancet*, **1**, 914–918 (1970)

3 AVERBACK, P. Primary cerebral venous thrombosis in young adults: the diverse manifestations of an under-recognized disease. *Annals of Neurology*, **3**, 81–86 (1978)

4 BARNETT, H. J. M. and HYLAND, H. H. Non-infective intracranial venous thrombosis. *Brain*, **76**, 36–49 (1953)

5 BYERS, R. K. and HASS, G. M. Thrombosis of the dural venous sinuses in infancy and in childhood. *American Journal of Diseases of Children*, **45**, 1161–1183 (1933)

6 CARROLL, J. D., LEAK, D. and LEE, H. A. Cerebral thrombophlebitis in pregnancy and the puerperium. *Quarterly Journal of Medicine*, **35**, 347–368 (1966)

7 DI ROCCO, C., IANNELLI, A., LEONE, G., MOSCHINI, M. and VALORI, V. M. Heparin–urokinase treatment in aseptic dural sinus thrombosis. *Archives of Neurology*, **38**, 431–435 (1981)

8 FOLEY, J. Benign forms of intracranial hypertension – toxic and otitic hydrocephalus. *Brain*, **78**, 1–41 (1955)

9 FORD, F. R. and MURPHY, E. L. Increased intracranial pressure. A clinical analysis of the causes and characteristics of several types. *Bulletin of the Johns Hopkins Hospital*, **64**, 369–398 (1939)

10 GETTELFINGER, D. M. and KOKMEN, E. Superior sagittal sinus thrombosis. *Archives of Neurology*, **34**, 2–6 (1977)

11 GOWERS, W. R. *A Manual of Diseases of the Nervous System*. 1st edn., Vol. 2, 416. London: Churchill (1888)

12 HARRISON, M. J. G. and TRUELOVE, S. C. Cerebral venous thrombosis as a complication of ulcerative colitis. *American Journal of Digestive Diseases*, **12**, 1025–1028 (1967)

13 HOLMES, G. and SARGENT, W. P. Injuries of the superior longitudinal sinus. *British Medical Journal*, **2**, 493–498 (1915)

14 JOHNSON, R. V., KAPLAN, S. R. and BLAILOCK, Z. R. Cerebral venous thrombosis in paroxysmal nocturnal haemoglobinuria. *Neurology*, **20**, 681–686 (1970)

15 KALBAG, R. M. and WOOLF, A. L. *Cerebral Venous Thrombosis*. London: Oxford University Press (1967)

16 KINGSLEY, D. P. E., KENDALL, B. E. and MOSELEY, I. F. Superior sagittal sinus thrombosis: an evaluation of the changes demonstrated on computed tomography. *Journal of Neurology, Neurosurgery and Psychiatry*, **41**, 1065–1068 (1978)

17 KRAYENBUHL, H. A. Cerebral venous and sinus thrombosis. *Clinical Neurosurgery*, **14**, 1–24 (1967)

18 MacEWEN, W. In *Pyogenic Infective Diseases of the Brain and Spinal Cord*, 23–28. Glasgow: James Maclehose (1893)

19 MEYERS, B. R., WORMSER, G., HIRSCHMAN, S. Z. and BLITZER, A. Rhinocerebral mucormycosis. *Archives of Internal Medicine*, **139**, 557–560 (1979)

20 PAMIR, M. N., KANSU, T., ERBENGI, A. and ZILELI, T. Papilloedema in Behçet's syndrome. *Archives of Neurology*, **38**, 643–645 (1981)

21 PATRONAS, N. J., DUDA, E. E., MIRFAKHRAEE, M. and WOLLMANN, R. L. Superior sagittal sinus thrombosis diagnosed by computed tomography. *Surgical Neurology*, **15**, 11–14 (1981)

22 PURDON MARTIN, J. and SHEEHAN, H. L. Primary thrombosis of cerebral veins (following childbirth). *British Medical Journal*, **1**, 349–353 (1941)

23 RAY, B. S. and DUNBAR, H. S. Thrombosis of the superior sagittal sinus as a cause of pseudotumour cerebri. *Transactions of the American Neurological Association*, **75**, 12–17 (1950)

24 SCHENK, E. A. Sickle cell trait and superior sagittal sinus thrombosis. *Annals of Internal Medicine*, **60**, 465–470 (1964)

25 SCOTTI, L. N., GOLDMAN, R. L., HARDMAN, D. R. and HEINZ, E. R. Venous thrombosis in infants and children. *Radiology*, **112**, 393–399 (1974)

26 SIGSBEE, B., DECK, M. D. F. and POSNER, J. B. Nonmetastatic superior sagittal sinus thrombosis complicating systemic cancer. *Neurology*, **29**, 139–146 (1979)

27 SILBERMANN, M. and FISHMAN, R. A. Primary (idiopathic) thrombosis of the superior sagittal sinus. *Transactions of the American Neurological Association*, **76**, 164–167 (1951)

28 SYMONDS, C. P. Otitic hydrocephalus. *Brain*, **54**, 55–71 (1931)

29 SYMONDS, C. P. Hydrocephalic and focal cerebral symptoms in relation to thrombophlebitis of the dural sinuses and cerebral veins. *Brain*, **60**, 531–550 (1937)

30 SYMONDS, C. P. Intracranial thrombophlebitis. *Annals of the Royal College of Surgeons of England*, **10**, 347–356 (1952)

31 TOWBIN, A. The syndrome of latent cerebral venous thrombosis: its frequency and relation to age in congestive cardiac failure. *Stroke*, **4**, 419–430 (1973)

13
Intracerebral haematoma

H. R. Müller and E. W. Radu

EPIDEMIOLOGY

Intracerebral haemorrhage (ICH) ranks second among the pathologies underlying stroke. Yet it is difficult to assess its true frequency.

According to Kurtzke[44] the prevalence of acute cerebrovascular disease (CVD) among whites is between 400 and 600, and the age-adjusted annual incidence between 100 and 200 per 100 000. The mean annual death rate of stroke was found to be 75–122 per 100 000, thus approximating half of the annual incidence. Besides thromboembolic strokes and ICH these data also include subarachnoidal haemorrhage (SAH) and any unclassifiable strokes. No reliable conclusions on the frequency of ICH can be drawn from these figures since in the surveys on which they are based there is too wide a variation in the representation of the individual subgroups of CVD.

More relevant information would appear to be available from selected community-based incidence studies. Stallones et al.[81], who based their figures on data available by 1971 on the incidence of stroke in the USA, estimated 65% of all strokes to be due to thromboembolism, 15% to ICH and 10% to SAH, a further 10% remaining ill-defined. The respective figures of Kurtzke[43], based on the weighted mean of five North American[3, 18, 38, 53, 80] and one Australian[85] community surveys, are 69%, 12%, 8% and 11%, and in a more recent estimate[43] referring to US and European studies[1, 23, 30, 93], 75%, 12%, 7% and 3%. Only in 8% was ICH reported as being the underlying cause in the 1970/74 period of the Minnesota study[23], whereas Mohr[59], in a prospective hospital survey, found this figure to be 10%.

Projecting these data on the epidemiological figures reported by Kurtzke[44] one would have to assume that the annual incidence of ICH in western countries ranges between 10 and 30 per 100 000. However, since the advent of computed tomography one has become aware that a considerable number of ICH are clinically misdiagnosed as brain infarcts (BI), resulting almost certainly in an underestimation of the incidence of ICH in any community study. In fact, Kinkel[42], reviewing

111 patients with CVD, found the ICH rate to be as high as 19%. In his material no less than 42% of the haemorrhages had been clinically diagnosed as cerebral thrombosis. It would therefore appear that the epidemiological parameters of CVD, in particular those of ICH, must be reassessed based on CT rather than clinical data.

In an attempt to determine the incidence of ICH for our own community we undertook a retrospective study on the hospital admissions in Basel, Switzerland, throughout the year of 1980. In the city of Basel (population 180 000) nearly all acute stroke patients are referred to the university hospital, and more than half of them now get a CT scan within three days after admission. This, as a rule, is also the case for a minority of stroke patients who, after initial evaluation at the university hospital, are transferred to one of the two private hospitals taking part in the in-patient care of the community. We have traced only 66 patients having acute CVD who were directly admitted to one of these hospitals. These were included in our study. Furthermore, in over 90% of the patients dying in the university hospital and in practically all cases of sudden death at home for unknown reasons a postmortem study is done. A reliable final diagnosis can therefore also be expected in those patients not surviving their stroke until an appropriate clinical evaluation has been done.

Of the 436 residents of the city of Basel admitted to hospital with a stroke in 1980, in 318 the final diagnosis was brain infarct, in 32 SAH and in 84 ICH. Forty-three of the patients with ICH were male and 41 female.

Table 13.1 Nature of strokes admitted to hospital in Basel in 1980

	n	Diagnosis based on:		Clinical grounds
		CT	Autopsy*	
BI	318	136	56 (74)	126
ICH	84	60	24 (56)	–
SAB	32	32	(5)	–

* Number refers to those autopsies where no CT scan had been done
( ) Total number of autopsies

The crude incidence rate of CVD resulting from the total of these individual categories and the population of the city of Basel is 240 per 100 000. With the assumption that the mortality rate is about half of the incidence, this value seems to be in fair accordance with the age-adjusted CVD mortality rate of Switzerland of 109 per 100 000[26].

It appears from our study that brain haemorrhage accounts for 19% of all strokes (including SAH), which is the same figure as was found by Kinkel[42]. Based on the data of Kurtzke[43], the overall age-adjusted incidence of ICH would then have to be estimated as ranging between approximately 20 and 40 rather than 10 and 30 per 100 000.

322

Table 13.2 Aetiologies of ICH according to clinical series

	Lazorthes[46] 1956 n = 354	Luessenhop[50] et al. 1967 n = 130	Grote[29] et al. 1970 n = 244	Pia[68] 1972 n = 253	Scott[78] 1975 n = 80	Personal series 1974–77 n = 200	1980 n = 84
Hypertension	25.9%	49.3%	47.9%	24.9%	53.8%	35.5%	29%
Aneurysm/AVM	33.3%	47.7%	35.2%	54.2%	16.2%	20.5%	14%
Tumor	2.8%	1.5%	–	11.0%	10.0%	–*	4%**
Anticoag. therapy	–	–	3.2%	–	–	27%	26%
Coagulopathies, blood disorders	–	–	3.2%	–	1.2%	2.5%	8%
Unknown and others	38%	1.5%	10.5%	9.9%	18.8%	14.5%	19%

* Tumour haemorrhages were excluded in our 1974/77 study.
** Only haemorrhages from tumors not diagnosed previous to the stroke.

AETIOLOGY

Excluding traumatic intracerebral bleeding, which is not considered in this chapter, there remains a wide range of aetiologies of ICH (*Table 13.2*).

Arterial hypertension

This is reported as the main cause of ICH in a number of autopsy series[7, 35, 56, 75], totalling some 57% in a compilation of 9 studies comprising over 2500 cases[35]. The frequency of hypertensive ICH varies quite considerably in clinical studies (*Table 13.2*). This presumably depends less on regional variation of incidence than on the character of the respective clinics. Thus a neurosurgical case series will obviously comprise more haemorrhages from aneurysms and a.v. malformation than from hypertension. Where anticoagulant therapy is widely used, more anticoagulant bleeds will be observed, again reducing the relative frequency of hypertensive haemorrhage.

As an example, in our personal series of 1974–77[60] comprising 200 spontaneous ICH, all diagnosed by CT, only 35.5% of the bleeds were clinically attributed to

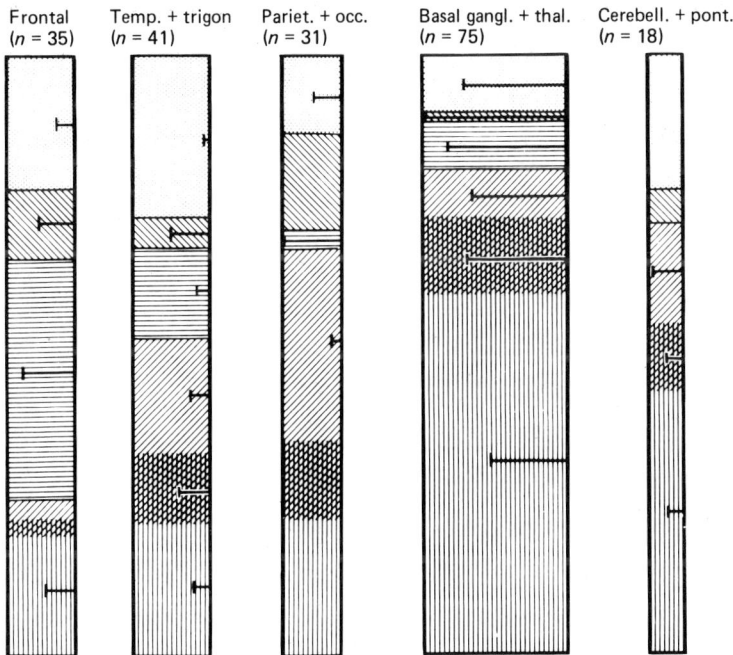

Frontal	Temp. + trigon	Pariet. + occ.	Basal gangl. + thal.	Cerebell. + pont.
(n = 35)	(n = 41)	(n = 31)	(n = 75)	(n = 18)

Figure 13.1 Localization and aetiology in 200 spontaneous ICH consecutively investigated by CT, 1974–1977. Bars coming from the right side indicate the percentage of occurrence of ventricular perforation in the individual categories. ▨ = Div.; ▧ = av malform; ▤ = aneurysms; ▨ = anticoagul. tr.; ▥ = hypertension. For abbreviations see text. (From Müller[60], courtesy of the Editor and Publishers, *Advances in Neurology*)

arterial hypertension. However, in a further 18.5% hypertension was considered as an additional risk factor in haematomas occurring under anticoagulant therapy (*Figure 13.1*).

Most of the hypertensive ICH originate in the putaminocapsular region and usually spread into the external capsule. In a considerable proportion they expand further to reach, by dissecting the white matter, the temporal or, alternatively, the frontal, parietal or occipital lobe. As a consequence, from CT evidence many ICH arising from the putaminocapsular region may be mistaken as primary lobar haematomas. This may have been the case with some lobar haematomas of our own series to be reported on in the following sections, and partly account for their relatively large proportion in our material. Expansion at the primary site and rupture into the ventricular system is an alternative evolution of putaminocapsular haemorrhages.

Other sites of predilection of hypertensive ICH are the thalamus, the pons and the cerebellum.

The majority of the thalamic haemorrhages are not limited to the primary site but rather involve the internal capsule and the basal ganglia. Not infrequently these haemorrhages also spread to neighbouring medullary layers. Ventricular perforation is as frequent as with basal ganglia haemorrhages.

The bleeding sources for basal ganglia, thalamic, pontine and cerebellar hypertensive ICH, respectively, are at the striatal branches of the middle cerebral, the thalamic branches of the posterior cerebral, the pontine branches of the basilar and those branches of the superior cerebellar artery which supply the dentate nucleus and the deep white matter of the cerebellum.

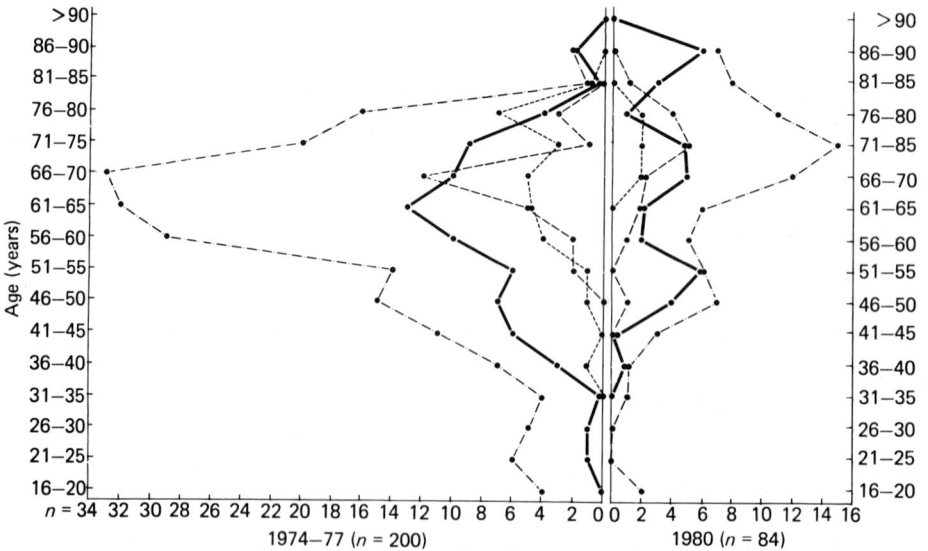

Figure 13.2 Age distribution of 200 spontaneous ICH investigated 1974–1977 and 84 spontaneous ICH admitted to the Kantonsspital Basel in 1980. ●–·–● = All aetiologies; ●——● = hypertension; ●----● = anticoagulant normotensive; ●———● = anticoagulant hypertensive

Miliary aneurysms have been claimed as the pathological substrate of many of these bleedings[9, 10] since their first description by Charcot and Bouchard[8]. Hyalinosis or fibrinoid necrosis has been identified as another underlying pathology[21, 91].

Hypertensive ICH occurs in our material with two age peaks (*Figure 13.2*). The lower one of the two is from 51–55 years, while the higher clearly shifted from 66–70 years in the case series of 1974–1977 to 71–75 years in 1980, possibly through improved antihypertensive treatment.

Aneurysms

Aneurysms are the second most frequent cause of ICH in the majority of the published case series. Aneurysm bleeds have been found to cause circumscribed haematomas around the aneurysm including ICH in 24 out of 92 CT observations of SAH[40]. They showed a clear preference for the frontal lobe in our series (*Figure 13.1*).

Angiomas and a.v. malformations

These, having the same or even a considerably higher frequency than aneurysms in some of the clinical series[29, 68], may be less than half as frequent in an unbiased material. No relationship was evident in our own case series of 1974–1977 and 1980 between the size of the malformation and the extent of the haemorrhage.

Tumours

Tumours occasionally present as ICH and thus are a possible cause of stroke[77, 92]. Glioblastomas, melanomas, hypernephromas and papillomas of the choroid plexus appear to be the most prone to cause ICH.

Microangiomas

These are believed to be the most likely underlying bleeding source in spontaneous ICH occurring in younger patients without any other aetiology being obvious on clinical and neuroradiological grounds[36, 52]. These are possibly not shown on angiograms but can sometimes be demonstrated on careful dissection.

Anticoagulant therapy

Intracranial haemorrhage as a complication of anticoagulant therapy has been increasingly reported over the last few years[47, 48, 55, 72, 79, 80]. Though subdural haematomas are more frequent than ICH, the number of the latter is not negligible. In Basel, where about 4% of the adult population has been estimated to

Table 13.3 Quick values at time of haemorrhage in 50 patients having intracerebral bleeds during anticoagulant therapy with phenprocoumon (recommended therapeutical range is 20–30% Quick)

Quick %	n	Without hypertension	With hypertension	Hypertension %
≤ 10	7	4	3	
11–15	10	6	4	36.7
16–20	13	9	4	
21–25	8	5	3	50
≥ 26	12	5	7	

be taking anticoagulants[72], ICH as a complication of this therapy has advanced to the second largest category of spontaneous intraparenchymatous bleeding in the brain[60, 61]. The commonest location of these haemorrhages is in the temporal, parietal or occipital lobes (*Figure 13.1*).

Table 13.3 shows that arterial hypertension and overdosage appear to be the important factors in producing anticoagulant ICH. Hypertension can also be recognized as a possible joint factor from *Figure 13.2*. This shows that according to the indications of this therapy, the majority of anticoagulant bleeds occur after the age of 60 years.

Coagulopathies, leukaemias

These are reported as the cause of ICH in up to 3% in clinical[29] and up to 20% in autopsy series[35]. Obviously such cases are more frequently encountered at hospitals having specialized departments with inpatient care for these types of disease.

Amphetamine abuse

More recently, amphetamine abuse has been described as a further aetiology of ICH[12, 16, 28], hypertension produced by this drug being most likely responsible for the bleeding. Further observations are needed to rule out joint factors responsible for these bleeds, for example, aneurysms or microangiomas.

SYMPTOMS AND SIGNS

Unless there is sudden loss of consciousness, as is typical for massive hypertonic basal ganglia haemorrhages, the patient will usually report a more or less sudden headache. Headache as the leading initial symptom was recorded in 43% of the cases who were admitted to our hospital in 1980, lightheadedness, experienced by 15% of the patients, being next in order among the early symptoms. Vomiting

Table 13.4 Clinical signs on emergency evaluation of 84 patients with spontaneous ICH admitted to the Kantonsspital Basel in 1980

Site of haematoma	n	Decerebration	Tetraparesis	Hemiparesis	Monoparesis	Aphasia	Homonymous hemianopia	Seizures
Lobar	34	3	–	20	2	6	6	7
Basal ganglia	35*	5	1	26	2	6	2	2
Pontine	9	6	2	1	1	–	–	3
Cerebellar	6	1	3	2	–	–	–	–
Total	84*	15 (17.8%)	6 (7.1%)	49 (58.3%)	5 (5.9%)	12 (14.2%)	8 (9.5%)	12 (14.2%)

* One patient re-admitted with fatal re-bleed

during evolution over the first hours after the onset was recorded in 13%, but according to clinical experience may be considerably more frequent. Localizing signs (*Table 13.4*) soon develop, but may be overshadowed in massive haemorrhages by coma (*Table 13.5*) and signs of decerebration. In the presence of signs of tentorial herniation, a hemiparesis has no localizing, but only a lateralizing value.

This chapter cannot deal in detail with either the specific signs or symptoms of the individual topical categories of haemorrhages. For this, the reader is referred to the concise descriptions available in current text books[32, 51, 84].

Table 13.5 State of consciousness on admission and early evolution in 84 patients with spontaneous ICH admitted to the Kantonsspital, Basel in 1980

Site of haematoma	n	Comatose		Drowsy/ stuporous	Alert
		from onset	*within 24 h*		
Lobar	34	6 (3)	6 (6)	17 (6)	5 (2)
Basal ganglia	35*	17 (15)	4 (4)	8 (7)	6 (3)
Infratent.	15	9 (9)	5 (4)	1 –	–
–					
Total	84*	32 (27)	15 (14)	26 (13)	11 (5)

* One patient re-admitted with fatal re-bleed
Parentheses indicate patients who died within 6 months

With reference to the differential diagnosis of cerebral infarction, which is now widely done by CT, Harrison[31] has re-assessed a number of clinical criteria which have traditionally been used to differentiate haemorrhagic from ischaemic stroke. According to his findings in 62 patients having ICH and 81 having cerebral infarction, a history of transient ischaemic attacks (reported by 14 ischaemic stroke patients and none of the ICH group) would appear to be a strong argument for ischaemic stroke. Headache and vomiting, being recorded in 43% of brain infarct patients and 56% of those having ICH, seems to have been of little help in separating the two groups. Ocular and facial pain was present in a small number of either group and has been reported as a frequent sign of occipital ICH by Ropper and Davis[74], which in our own clinical experience is as frequent in posterior cerebral artery infarction. Neck stiffness was present in 48% of ICH but in 4% of brain infarct. Seizures, observed in 14.2% of our own cases, were present in 9% of ICH compared with 6% in brain infarction.

According to Walker *et al.*[86] coma or unconsciousness, occurring in about one third of all stroke patients, is twice as frequently observed in haemorrhagic stroke (including SAH) as in ischaemic stroke.

In acute and especially in subacute progressive brain-stem syndromes, not primarily referrable to the medulla oblongata, ICH must always be considered and accordingly CT be performed. The same is true for acute or subacute cerebellar syndromes.

CONTRIBUTION OF COMPUTERIZED TOMOGRAPHY TO CLINICAL DIAGNOSIS

Much of the present knowledge of ICH has been contributed by computerized tomography. This is particularly true for deeply situated hemispheric as well as brain-stem and cerebellar haemorrhages.

While before the era of CT many of the smaller paracapsular haematomas were certainly misdiagnosed as brain infarcts, we have learnt from CT that in the absence of signs indicating raised intracranial pressure and ventricular perforation, these haematomas may perfectly imitate the clinical picture of a middle cerebral artery brain infarct. If located in the dominant hemisphere not only thalamic[21] but also putaminal haemorrhages[33] may produce aphasia. In a recent study of 15 patients having spontaneous deep intracerebral haemorrhages an aphasia was present in both of these groups, and classified as being of the transcortical type. Writing was moderately impaired in eight, and severely impaired in six patients. More than just slight disturbances in reading were found in seven[2].

CT not only allows the straightforward diagnosis of brain-stem and cerebellar haematomas and their differentiation from brain infarcts, but it has also shown that even patients with larger brain-stem haematomas may survive. In fact, in a recently published series[13] consisting of four pontine and four mesencephalic haemorrhages demonstrated on CT, no less than seven survived, though in six of them the largest diameter of the haemorrhage was more than 1.5 cm. In addition to the *topical*

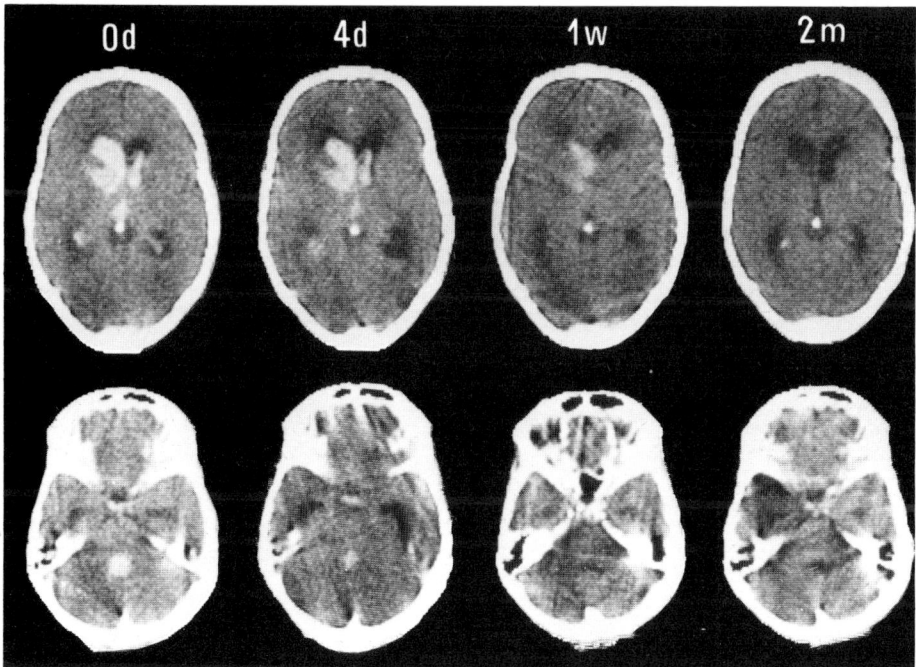

Figure 13.3 Follow-up of left hypertensive caudato-capsular haemorrhage with ventricular perforation. Spontaneous clearance of ventricles from blood coagula with good clinical recovery

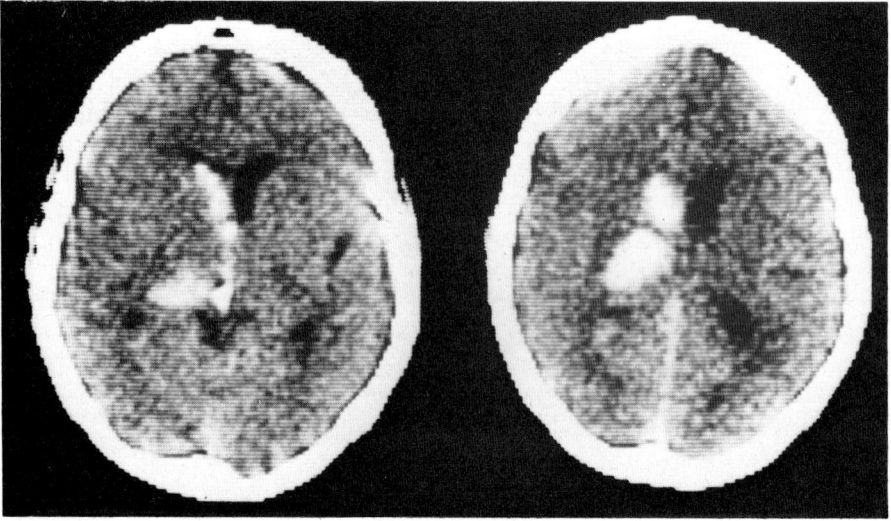

Figure 13.4 Left thalamic hypertensive haemorrhage with ventricular perforation in a 60-year-old patient presenting with aphasia and right hemiparesis. Near to full recovery. Patient working part-time as a dentist at follow-up 5½ years after event

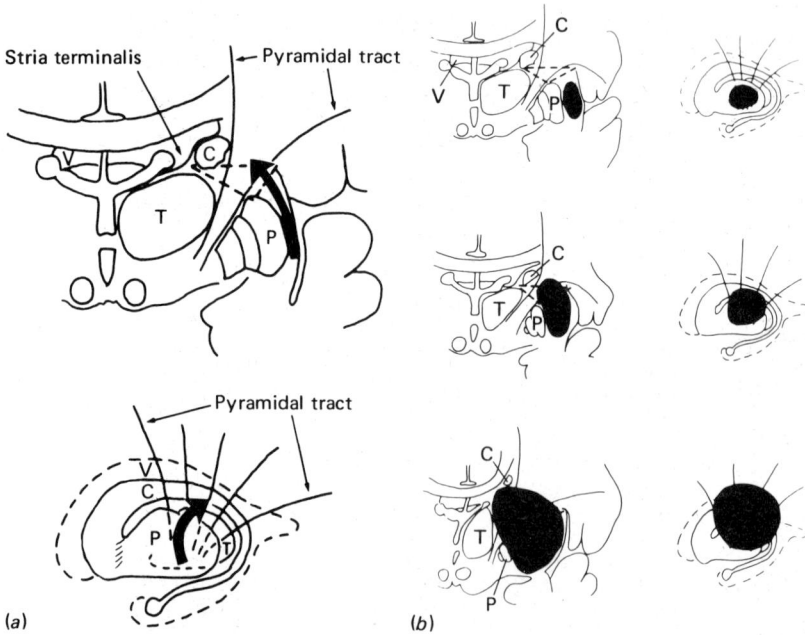

Figure 13.5 (*a*) Schematic drawing of internal capsule, ventricle and basal ganglia. The triangle indicated by dotted lines is vulnerable by putamino-capsular haemorrhages. (*b*) Correlation of 'vulnerable triangle' with various extension of putamino-capsular haematomas. (From Mizukami *et al.*[58], courtesy of the Editor and Publishers, *Stroke*)

diagnosis including the demonstration of multiple haematomas[88], CT allows early detection of *occlusive hydrocephalus* requiring arterioventricular shunting in both cerebellar and brain-stem haemorrhages[63].

Ventricular perforation can be readily detected on CT scans, and its impact on CSF circulation can be assessed. We have learnt from this method that ventricular perforation is far more frequent than was believed in the pre-CT era. In a series of 200 cases (*Figure 13.1*), two thirds of the basal ganglial and thalamic haemorrhages and almost half of those located in other regions showed blood contamination of the ventricular system, and even considerable blood content of the lateral, third and fourth ventricles (*Figure 13.3*) proved to be compatible with survival[60].

From the location of the haemorrhage and from other features displayed on the CT scans, such as the presence of subarachnoid blood and its pattern, tentative conclusions as to aetiology can be drawn. Thus haematomas in the region of the basal ganglia are mostly hypertensive in nature. Near to 40% of the frontal lobe haematomas in our material were from aneurysms and almost half of the haematomas located in the parietal and occipital lobes had occurred under anticoagulant treatment[60] (*Figure 13.1*).

CT also allows *prognostic assessments*. Small basal ganglia and thalamic hypertensive haemorrhages in general have a good prognosis for survival and

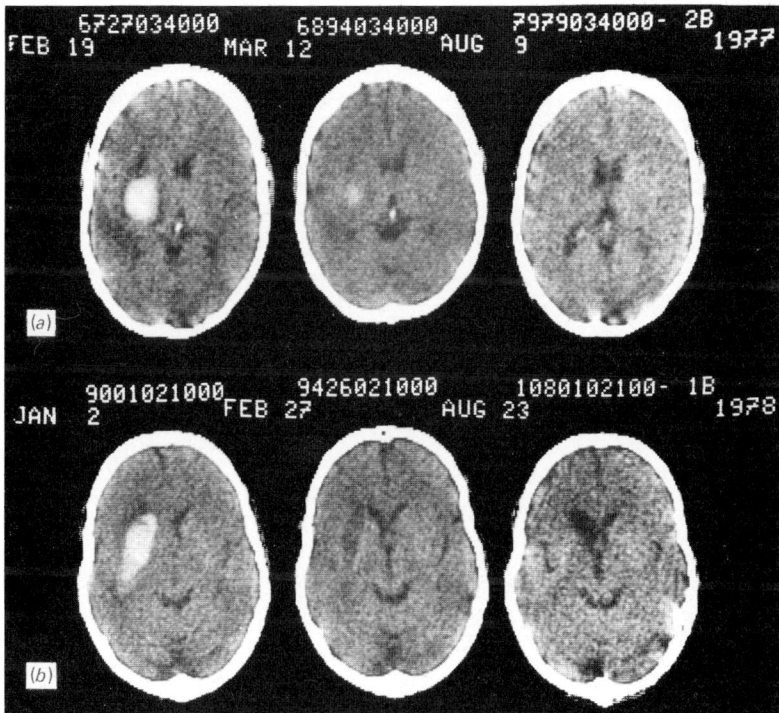

Figure 13.6 (a), (b) Follow-up in two cases of conservatively treated left putaminal haemorrhages. Initially aphasia in both cases. Patient (*a*), having a sensorimotor hemiparesis, reported a full recovery. Patient (*b*), suffering from a hemiplegia on admission, made a near to full recovery

occasionally patients having quite sizeable bleeds may make a full or near to full recovery (*Figure 13.4*). Even with large lobar ICH in the temporal, parietal or occipital lobes a survival under medical treatment can be expected if there is no massive displacement of the midline structures.

In hypertensive putaminal haemorrhages, extension of the lateral ventricle to the level of the body seems to be an adverse prognostic sign (*Figure 13.5*). None of 17 patients, in whom an initial hemiplegia had almost subsided within one month after

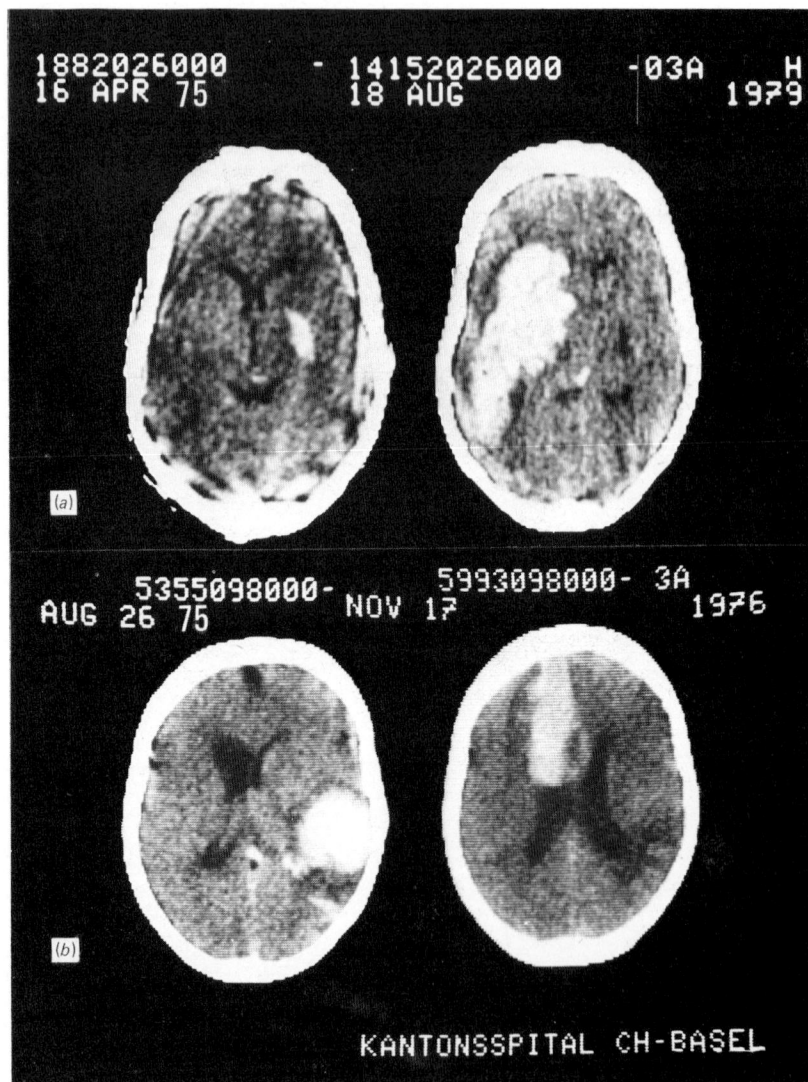

Figure 13.7 Re-bleeds in two cases of hypertensive ICH. (*a*) Massive left putaminal haemorrhage 4 years after small haemorrhage in the right putamino-capsular region with near to full recovery within 1 week following the first bleeding. (b) Left frontal haemorrhage 15 months after right temporoparietal haematoma with fair spontaneous recovery

onset, displayed the haematoma at this level. On the other hand, blood extending to this site was imaged in 18 out of 28 patients showing only little clinical improvement.[58].

Finally, CT enables us to study the evolution in time of ICH. It has been demonstrated that the region of high absorption, which is largely attributed to the haemoglobin content of the bleed[64], decreases in diameter by an average of 0.65 mm per day[14] but that the space occupying effect of the lesion may remain considerable over weeks. Even larger haematomas may resolve almost entirely, leaving lacunae too small to be detected on a CT scan (*Figure 13.6*). Secondary increase in size of a haematoma through a re-bleed is an extremely rare occurrence. On the other hand, with hypertensive ICH, late recurrences at other sites than the one of the primary bleeding are sometimes observed (*Figure 13.7*). As a rare

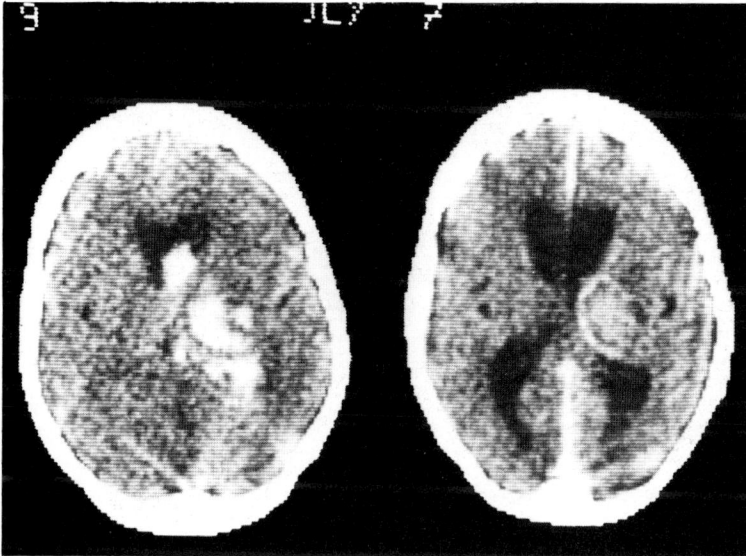

Figure 13.8 Right thalamic hypertensive haemorrhage with ventricular perforation. Picture on the right shows contrast enhanced control CT-scan 1 month after the event. Still high density zone in haematoma centre. Haematoma capsule contrast enhanced

occurrence a haematoma capsule may be formed prematurely in relation to the natural degradation of the clot. Such encapsulated haematomas may persist as space occupying lesions and on the CT pictures give rise to the differential diagnosis of a tumour (*Figure 13.8*)[62].

ANGIOGRAPHY

Angiography has long been the method of choice for the diagnosis of ICH, but now CT is widely available there is hardly a place any more for this method as a primary diagnostic tool. Angiography should, however, always be used, when from CT and clinical evidence an aneurysm or an a.v. malformation enters into the differential diagnosis, and if the patient's condition is such that surgical treatment can be considered.

It is important to know that a larger haematoma may compress an a.v. malformation[87] which consequently may not be demonstrable even on a contrast-enhanced CT scan. Even without compression through a haemorrhage, a smaller vascular malformation may easily escape the diagnosis by CT because of similar density and partial volume effect.

In younger patients suffering from ICH not obviously due to hypertension, anticoagulant therapy or any other known aetiology, the deliberate use of angiography is advisable.

TREATMENT

In spite of the advantages offered by CT[12], the treatment of ICH has remained a continuous issue of debate.

As a first result of the capability of this technique to exactly determine the site and size of the haemorrhages and thus facilitate planning of an optimal surgical approach, a general tendency to operate on larger haematomas of any site was observed more frequently. CT, on the other hand, also allowed the study of the anatomo-pathological evolution of conservatively treated haemorrhages[14, 41, 62] and their correlation with the clinical course. From the evidence of such observations, which included almost traceless resorption of haemorrhages of a considerable size (*Figure 13.6*), many centres returned to a primarily conservative strategy.

At a recent neurosurgically oriented symposium[69] there was agreement that patients with smaller ICH who are alert, stable or improving should be treated conservatively. *Surgical treatment* was generally advocated for patients having larger clots but who are stable and with a reasonable level of consciousness. Some of the participants pleaded for early operation and others for evacuation of the clot on or about the third day[25].

In our hospital a similar stategy has been adopted for the last few years, with a tendency to keep stable patients even with larger lobar haematomas under a primarily conservative regime and on the other hand to more deliberately evacuate putaminal haemorrhages[82], particularly those of more than 20 ml volume as estimated from the CT scans (*Figure 13.9*) and being either stuporous or in superficial coma. In most instances the operation is performed during the first two days. In the case of progressive neurological deficit on admission, the haematoma is evacuated immediately after the initial CT scan. Signs of early tentorial herniation are not rigidly considered as a contraindication to emergency operation; however, in the presence of bilateral signs of decerebration, surgery is not done. When deciding on surgical treatment in an individual case, the patient's age and the persistent deficit to be expected mainly with lesions in the dominant hemisphere is duly considered. Only exceptionally are patients over 70 years of age operated upon.

Lobar haematomas, if operated according to the criteria mentioned, are evacuated transcortically through a small cortical incision. This is planned according to

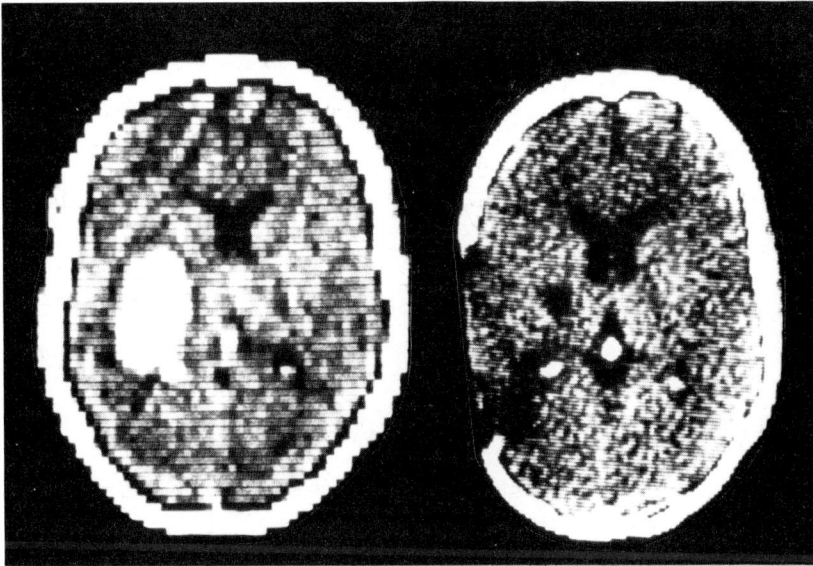

Figure 13.9 Left putaminal hypertensive haemorrhage in a 38-year-old patient before, and 7 months after, emergency operation with initial signs of tentorial herniation. Patient was reported 6 years after operation to walk indoors without a cane, walk outdoors with one, and to have a minor grade of dysphasia

the maximal extension of the haemorrhage to the surface on CT in order to minimize the brain damage. The use of a large formal craniotomy rather than a trephine opening allows patients with severely raised intracranial pressure to benefit from an efficient decompression.

Open transcortical operation of *thalamic haematomas* is generally regarded as contraindicated because of high morbidity. Stereotactic aspiration after a few days has been suggested as a possible approach[25]. Methods have been developed using CT information to calculate the co-ordinates, but to date their use for surgery of ICH has only been reported describing case examples of larger lobar haematomas[4, 34].

A stereotactic approach may also be rewarding for *putaminal haemorrhages*. Medium size and larger lesions of this site fulfilling the general criteria for operation are now frequently evacuated[37, 82], the optimal approach for conventional surgery appearing to be through the Sylvian fissure[83].

In a Japanese collaborative study[37], which compared the outcome in 145 surgically and 196 medically treated putaminal haemorrhages, no significant difference in the mortality was found in those patients remaining either alert or confused to somnolent. However, stuporous and semicomatose patients without and with signs of tentorial herniation did significantly better with surgery, the mortalities in this group being 17.8%, 28.2% and 57.1% against 52.7%, 58.2% and 100%. Forty-seven per cent of the patients operated on while being semicomatous, but showing no herniation signs, returned to full work or were left with only minimal disability. Considering further the extension of the haematoma to the external and internal capsules, it was concluded that surgical treatment should be adopted in stuporous and semicomatous patients having no herniation signs, and in whom the haematoma is localized outside the internal capsulas or extends only to its anterior limb.

In *cerebellar haematomas* prompt operation by formal suboccipital craniectomy is indicated in most instances[73]. Evacuation of the haematoma has to be done as an emergency in any case where there is CT evidence of an occlusive hydrocephalus[63]. In this condition surgical treatment should not be limited to ventricular drainage because of the risk of upward herniation[57]. Though patients having smaller cerebellar haemorrhages may fully recover under conservative treatment[65], it has been recommended to evacuate all those clots having a maximal diameter of more than 3 cm[49].

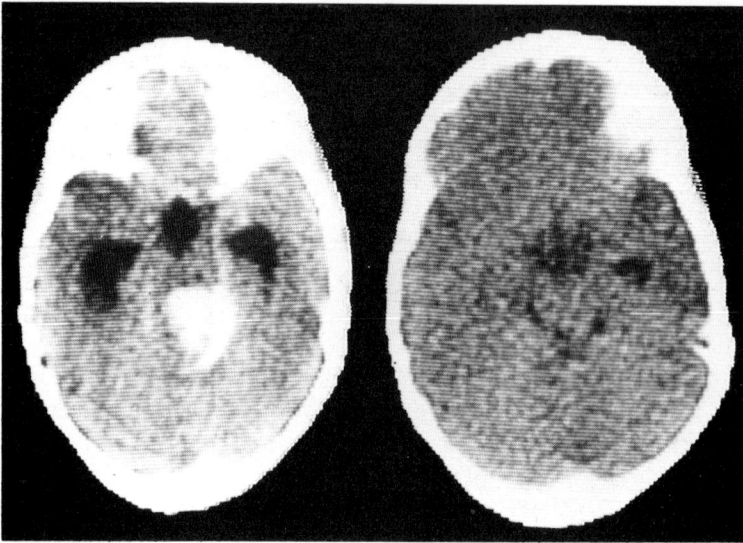

Figure 13.10 Pontine haematoma, presumably from angiographically and histologically undemonstrated vascular malformation, in a 6-year-old girl. CT before and 1 year after evacuation of haematoma and ventriculoatrial shunt (Prof. A. Lévy). Recovery to minimal neurological deficit

Evacuation of *pontine haematomas* (*Figure 13.10*) must be considered in younger normotensive patients where a vascular malformation is likely to be the underlying cause[66,76,78]. Hypertensive haemorrhages within the brain stem will usually not be operated on, although successful evacuations have been reported[54]. Patients with an occlusive hydrocephalus on CT may need ventricular drainage[76]. This is true even for those patients clinically presenting with a locked-in syndrome in order to spare them, as they are unable to communicate, possible severe headache. Patients with small pontine haemorrhages occasionally survive under conservative treatment but only one case showing a full recovery is reported in the literature[45].

If a patient is assigned to medical management, he should be treated in the vicinity of a neurosurgical service in order to allow emergency operation in case of the onset of tentorial herniation, progressive neurological deficit or evolution of an occlusive hydrocephalus. Treatment of any ICH of more than minor size and of all haemorrhages within the posterior fossa should be done in an intensive care unit.

Immediate measures are directed towards the maintenance of an adequate pulmonary ventilation. Patients in coma must be intubated and may need tracheostomy if remaining unconscious after a few days, or if long term assisted or controlled respiration is needed. Periodical suction of tracheobronchial secretions and change of the patient's position are vital in order to avoid atelectasis and bronchopneumonia. Pao_2 and $Paco_2$ and pH have to be regularly monitored.

Fluid and caloric feeding is initially done intravenously under careful control of electrolytes and fluid balance. In order to maintain the caloric requirements and to avoid a negative nitrogen balance, feeding by tube should be started after the third day[15].

Arterial hypertension must be treated with clonidine or, if necessary, sodium nitroprusside. Arterial pressure should be monitored by an indwelling catheter. Reduction of the systolic pressure below 160 mmHg has to be avoided in order to assure an optimal perfusion in spite of disturbed autoregulation. Cardiac failure and arrhythmias should be treated according to current cardiological standards. As a measure for lowering intracranial pressure, a 20–30° head-up tilted position of the patient's bed is recommendable.

Glucocorticoids, of doubtful effect in strokes due to brain infarcts[5, 39], seem to reduce brain oedema more efficiently in patients with ICH. This is based, however, on clinical observation only, and no confirmation by controlled studies using CT and measurement of intracranial pressure have been published to date.

With critically raised intracranial pressure 200 ml mannitol 20% are given as a rapid intravenous infusion over 20 min. A single dose of 100 g together with 100 mg methylenenisolone has been recommended as standard initial therapy for patients

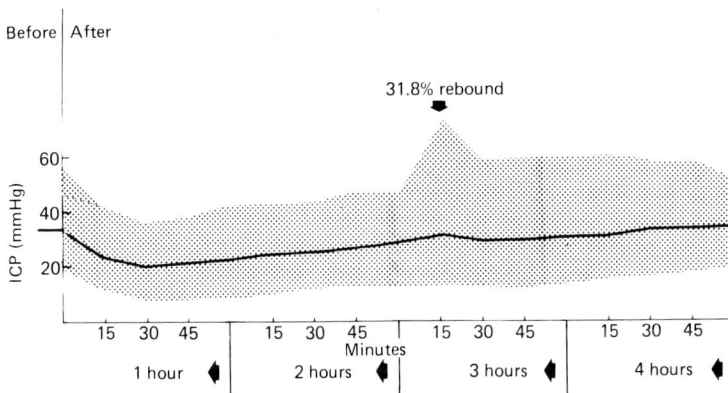

Figure 13.11 Responses obtained in 22 patients with intracranial tumour or brain injury on measuring intracranial pressure after rapid infusion of Mannitol 20% (1g/kg in 15 cases, 0.5g/kg in 4 cases, 0.25g/kg in 2 cases, 2 g/kg in one case). Continuous line represents mean values of mean intracranial pressures. Shadowed area includes all the values from the different responses. (From Ferrer *et al.*[20], courtesy of the Editor and Publishers, *Intracranial Pressure*, Vol. IV)

getting emergency surgery[11]. For repeated applications, the recommended interval between the infusions is 4 hours. Even a closer spacing, with proportional reduction of the individual doses, may be required to minimize the risk of a rebound effect. In 22 patients suffering from brain tumors or head injury, in whom the intracranial pressure was monitored after a 5–10 min rapid mannitol infusion (*Figure 13.11*), the minimal pressure was reached after between 20 and 35 min, and the mean total time of effectiveness was 130 min[20]. Controlling the osmolarity of the blood and lowering it to a value of 340 mosmol/l allows the individualize this therapy. Repeated application of mannitol, following whatever treatment schedule, requires a regular 4 hourly assessment of the electrolyte and fluid balance.

The value and practicability of monitoring intracranial pressure as a parameter for antioedematous treatment[17] is still a matter of debate. In a series of 66 patients having ICH in whom intracranial pressure was measured either continuously or periodically, it was found that the proportion of alert patients decreased with increasing level of intracranial pressure. Patients lying in deepest coma with evidence of vegetative dysregulation all showed very high pressures. However, the majority of cases with intermediate disturbances of consciousness showed no definite correlation between the clinical condition and intracranial pressure[67]. It would therefore appear that some of the patients will be overtreated when basing antioedematous therapy solely on clinical grounds. On the other hand, when CT findings are used as an additional parameter, the indication for corticosteroids and hyperosmolar agents appears to be well justified in most instances.

It is questionable whether antiepileptic drugs should be given as a measure of seizure prevention. If fits do occur, phenobarbital, 200–300 mg/day, or diphenylhydantoin, 300 mg per day, are given. A combination of both of these drugs with clonazepam intravenously is used for the management of status epilepticus.

Appropriate nursing care, physiotherapy and early mobilization are important for preventing venous thrombosis, decubitus ulcers and contractures. Patients recovering from ICH should be involved in a rehabilitation programme as early as possible after the acute phase, and in any case before leaving the hospital.

COURSE AND PROGNOSIS

Various types of clinical evolution have been described in ICH[71]. They are partly related to the site of the haemorrhage, partly to its size and the way of spreading into the surroundings.

Hyperacute course

A hyperacute course is mainly seen with massive hypertensive haemorrhages into the basal ganglia, resulting in marked destruction of brain tissue, ventricular perforation with tamponade and consequently rapidly rising intracranial pressure (Beneš's[6] type 1 of hypertensive ICH). These patients who may have experienced a headache and then rapidly lost consciousness, almost regularly are deeply comatous on hospital admission and soon show signs of decerebration due to brain stem compression and secondary haemorrhages within the pons. Survival is rarely longer than 48 hours.

Subacute course

A subacute course appears to be typical for lobar haematomas including type 2 of hypertensive ICH according to Beněs[6]. These bleeds are less destructive and result in a true haematoma rather than a widely spreading haemorrhage. Though initial coma occurs in some instances, this is far from being a regular feature. The patient may merely experience a sudden headache and then get confused, show a more or less rapidly progressing neurological deficit and, in many instances, sweat and vomit. This first phase of the subacute course lasts up to 48 hours and is followed by a period where disturbance of consciousness gradually subsides and the neurological deficit becomes stable. This phase may last from a few hours until about 3 weeks, whereafter gradual recovery or, alternatively, a deterioration takes place which in untreated cases may lead to decerebration and death.

A triphasic variant of this course has been described[71] and is particularly attributed to the lateral putaminal haemorrhages. With this course, instead of a stable phase after the initial one, a continuous evolution of the neurological signs is seen, the third phase being characterized by a rapidly progressive disturbance in consciousness and eventually coma.

Paretic course

Some of the small paraputaminal, thalamic and lobar haematomas may be associated with a solely paretic course. The neurological deficit develops as a stroke in progression over minutes to hours. Headache and disturbed consciousness may be lacking even later in the evolution, and the neurological deficit may be reversible within a few days. Focal epileptic seizures may occur with location of the lesion near the cortex.

Hydrocephalic course

This type of course may be observed in cerebellar haematomas, where after an initial attack of dizziness and vertigo the symptoms of acute occlusive hydrocephalus with severe headache and vomiting may dominate the picture. Upward and downward herniation may develop within hours, and unless the haematoma is evacuated the patient may die on the first day after onset of symptoms. According to a review of the literature[71], even with cerebellar haemorrhages a biphasic evolution is quite common. The initial symptoms are followed by a phase of one to ten days during which the patient's condition is stabilized and the cerebellar

Table 13.6 Discharges from hospital and deaths in 84 patients with spontaneous ICH admitted to the Kantonsspital Basel in 1980

Site of haematoma	n	Discharges from hospital by (months)					Deaths by 24 hours	1 week	1 month	6 months
		1	2	3	6					
1 lobe	15	6 (40%)	8	8	9 (60%)		2	4	6	6 (40%)
≥ 1 lobe	19	5 (26%)	7	8	8 (42%)		5	9	10	11 (58%)
Basal ganglia	35	4 (11%)	5	5	6 (17%)		6	20	27	29 (83%)
Pons	9	–	–	–	–		8	9	9	9 (100%)
Cerebellum	6	–	1	2	2 (33 %)		4	4	4	4 (67%)
Total	84*	15 (18%)	21	23	25 (30%)		25	46	56	59 (70%)

* One patient with basal ganglia haemorrhage included in this table, who was discharged at one month, was subsequently re-admitted with a basal ganglia re-bleed on the contralateral side, and died within 24 hours

syndrome dominates the picture. An acute deterioration with signs of brain stem compression or decompensated occlusive hydrocephalus may occur only after this interval.

Early mortality

High early mortality of ICH has long been known[22, 53, 90]. According to a recent literature review[71] only one out of five patients having an ICH would be alive one month after the event. Even fewer survivors (8%) were recorded in the 1945–1976 Minnesota study[23]. However, Gänshirt and Keuler[24], on analyzing 110 patients with ICH of different aetiologies, location and size, found a six weeks' survival rate of 54.5%. Similarly in our own case series observed in 1974 through 1977[60] the overall mortality at one month was 42%, while a mortality as high as 71.6% was found in our 1980 study comprising also patients in whom the diagnosis was only made at autopsy. Thirty to fifty per cent seems therefore to be a realistic estimate of early mortality in patients getting appropriate treatment.

The particularly high early mortality of basal ganglia and pontine haemorrhages is demonstrated in *Table 13.6*, referring to our 1980 case series.

Short term prognosis

Among the criteria for short term prognosis, the state of consciousness is undoubtedly the most important[11, 19, 51, 71]. In our case series of 1980 the chance of survival of a patient admitted in coma proved to be about half of that for a patient who was alert or had only a lesser degree of disturbed consciousness (*Table 13.6*). Signs of tentorial herniation have a particularly bad prognostic significance. But even at this stage, emergency surgery may save the patient's life. Such an example is referred to in *Figure 13.9*.

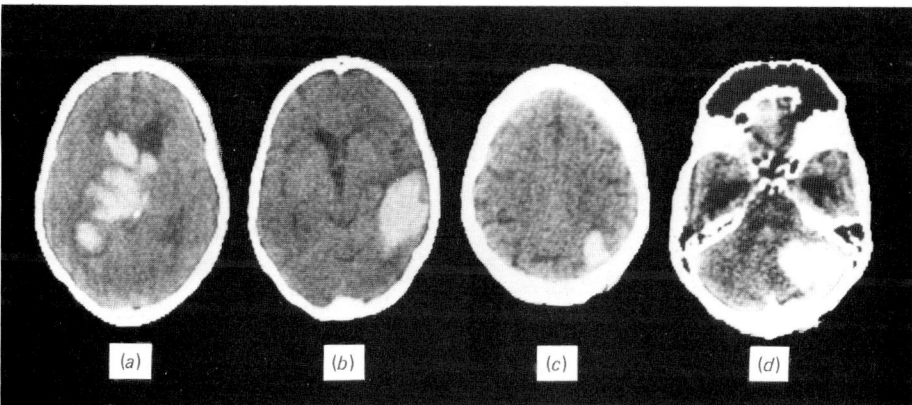

Figure 13.12 CT scans of four patients showing different types of clinical evolution. (*a*) Massive hypertensive basal ganglia haemorrhage with hyperacute course. (*b*) Lobar haematoma with biphasic course. (*c*) Small cortico-subcortical haemorrhage with right parietal lobe signs and seizures. (*d*) Cerebellar haematoma with acute 'hydrocephalic' course

The value of CT for the assessment of the prognosis has been discussed on pp. 331–332. Elements of this assessment are the location and size of the haematoma, and its extent in relation to the surrounding anatomical structures. Further prognositc criteria are the grade of midline shift and interference of the haematoma with the CSF circulation.

Ventricular perforation has much less relevance for prognosis, as one would anticipate from traditional teaching. Unless this complication arises through massive tissue disruption, as is the case with large hypertensive basal ganglia haemorrhages, the patient may survive, even when CT indicates that the whole ventricular system is clotted out with blood (*Figure 13.3*). Though such observations are rare, the concept of ventricular tamponade has to be clinically reassessed on their evidence and, with regard to fatal prognosis, limited to those cases, where an acute dilation of the blood filled ventricles can be seen on CT.

Long term prognosis

Relatively few data are available on long term prognosis in ICH. It is obvious that, apart from the location and extension of the lesion, determining the residual deficit, the patient's age and the underlying cause are the main factors determining the late outcome. Thus a young normotensive patient suffering from an ICH due to microangioma, and whose haematoma has been operated on, can be considered as cured, apart from any persistent neurological deficit and possible late epilepsy. On the contrary, with an unoperated aneurysm or a.v. malformation as a bleeding source, the patient will remain at a high risk for a possibly fatal re-bleed. Similarly in a patient surviving a hypertensive ICH, arterial hypertension will remain the adversely determining factor for the late prognosis. Not only early but also late prognosis must therefore be assessed for individual aetiological categories rather than being based on patient material that includes a variety of aetiologies.

In an attempt to get more precise data for prognoses for the two main aetiological groups in our case material of ICH we conducted a retrospective survey. This included all patients with ICH attributed to either arterial hypertension or anticoagulant therapy who were admitted to our hospital and investigated by CT in 1974 through 1977.

This study comprises a total of 125 patients of whom 41 had survived by the time of the study and had been either discharged from hospital or transferred to other institutions. Assessments of the late outcome was carried out by a questionnaire despatched in February 1981 to the family doctors and to the surviving patients. This yielded the data compiled in *Figure 13.13* and *Figure 13.14*.

Correlation of the clinical results with the size of the haemorrhages was estimated on the initial CT scans by using a stencil technique, grading the lesions into three categories. Haematomas of less than 2 ml were classified as small, lesions of an estimated volume between 2 and 20 ml as medium sized, and lesions over 20 ml volume as large.

A review of the case material showed that 17 of the 71 hypertensive haemorrhages (24%) and 18 of the 54 haemorrhages attributed to anticoagulant therapy

343

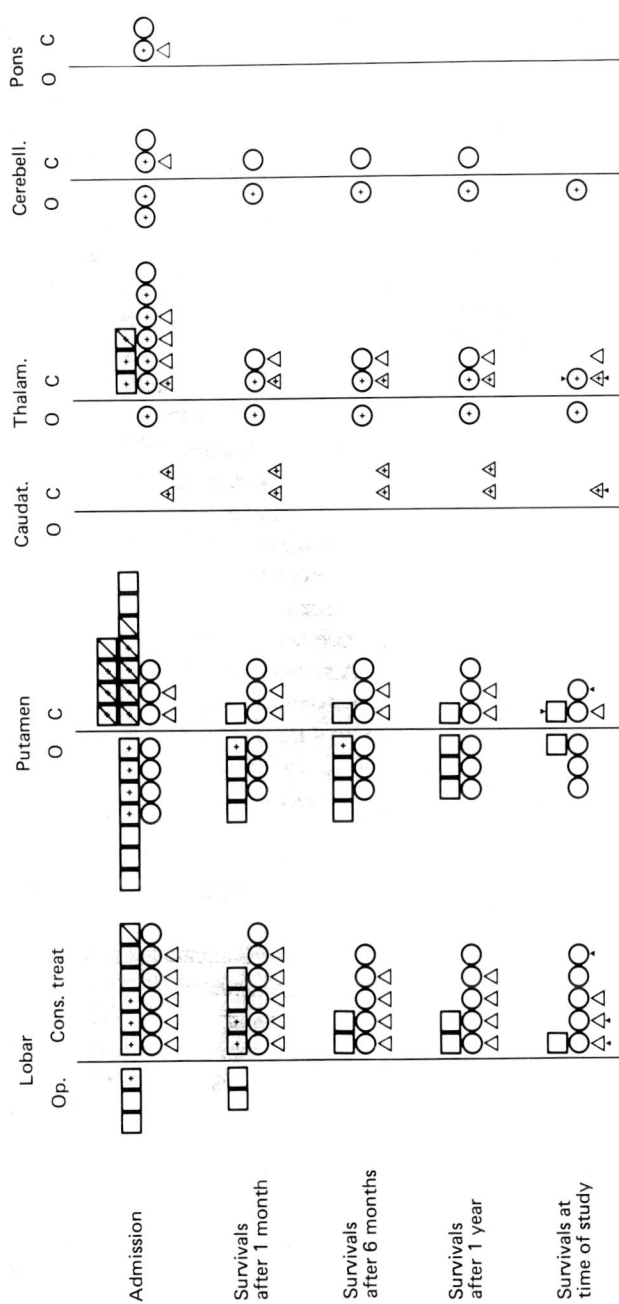

Figure 13.13 Outcome in 71 hypertensive intracerebral haemorrhages. Haematoma size as estimated from CT measurements: □ = over 20 ml; ○ = 2–20 ml; △ = less than 2 ml; + = ventricular perforation; / = decerebrated or in deep coma on admisssion; ▲ = full recovery according to self-evaluation

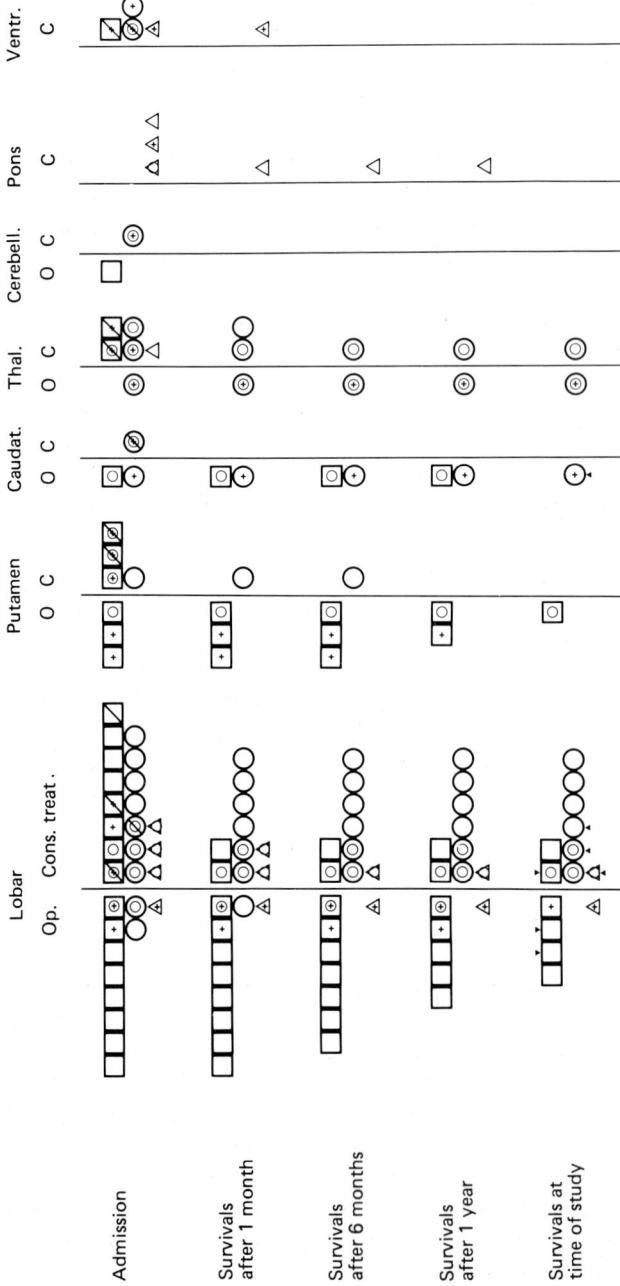

Figure 13.14 Outcome in 54 intracerebral and primary ventricular haemorrhages due to anticoagulant therapy. Haematoma size as estimated from CT measurements: □ = over 20 ml; ○ = 2–20 ml; △ = less than 2 ml; ⊙ indicates hypertension; + = ventricular perforation; / = decerebrated or in deep coma on admission; ▲ = full recovery according to self-evaluation

(33%) were operated on. In the conservatively treated groups of either category about half of the patients were not considered for operation because of the presence of deep coma and signs of decerebration. No randomization was made in the allocation of operable patients to surgical or medical treatment. The study therefore does not allow any comparison of the efficiency of the two types of management.

With a mean follow up of 5¼ years, the survival rate in both groups of aetiology proved to be approximately one third. The best immediate prognosis for survival was in lobar hypertensive haemorrhages, 85% of which were treated conservatively. In this category almost half of all patients were admitted to hospital, and 73% of those having medium sized or small haemorrhages survived the follow-up period. One third of these estimated that their recovery was practically complete.

Compared with the hypertensive intracerebral haemorrhages, lobar haematomas which occurred under anticoagulant treatment showed a higher early mortality. Large haematomas due to anticoagulant treatment definitely seemed to profit from surgery. However, by the end of the follow-up, similar to the hypertensive haemorrhages, half of the patients had died and only 62% of those with medium and small haematomas survived. Forty-two per cent of the survivors reported a full recovery.

Hypertensive putaminal haemorrhages of the large size category showed a 43% one year survival if operated on the basis of the accepted criteria, while all but one of the 11 non-operated patients of this group died within one month. In most instances the fatal prognosis had been evident from the beginning.

A quite high survival rate, 75% for the operated and 60% for the non-operated group, was observed in the cohort of medium and small putaminal haemorrhages. Only one of these patients, however, reported a full recovery. In another one, whose haematoma just entered in the large size group, neurological examination revealed minor dysphasia and dyslexia as the only persisting deficits.

CONCLUSIONS

Since the advent of CT spontaneous ICH has been recognized as being more frequent than suggested by earlier surveys. Its incidence in the western countries, as estimated from available epidemiological stroke data and from a hospital admission study in Basel, Switzerland, appears to be 20–40 per 100 000 per annum.

In most series, while hypertension remains the most common cause and bleeding from aneurysms and vascular malformations takes second place, ICH occurring as a complication of anticoagulant therapy is increasingly reported. The most rewarding approach to the problem of ICH would therefore appear to be prophylaxis through early recognition and treatment of arterial hypertension, and the critical use and careful control of anticoagulant therapy.

Not only the diagnosis of ICH, now readily made by CT, but also medical and surgical treatment of this condition has made considerable progress over the last few years. However, a critical review of the literature leaves no doubt that we are still far from an optimal use of the technical facilities available. The following primary question remains unanswered for most categories of ICH: Under which clinical and radiological conditions has an ICH to be operated on, and how long after onset has this to be done? The need for controlled multicentre studies is therefore obvious.

References

1 AHO, K. Incidence, profile and early prognosis of stroke. Epidemiology and clinical study of the 286 persons with onset of stroke in 1972 and 1973 in a South-Finnish urban area. Academic Dissertation, University of Helsinki (1975)

2 ALEXANDER, M. P. and LO VERME, S. R. Aphasia after left hemispheric intracerebral hemorrhage. *Neurology*, **30**, 1193–1202 (1980)

3 ALTER, M., CHRISTOFERSON, L., RESCH, J., MYERS, G. and FORD, J. Centrovascular disease: frequency and population selectivity in an upper midwestern community. *Stroke*, **1**, 454–465 (1970)

4 BACKLUND, E. O. Controlled subtotal evacuation of intracerebral hematomas by stereotactic technique. *Surgical Neurology*, **9**, 99–101 (1979)

5 BAUER, R. B. and TELLEZ, H. Dexamethasone as treatment in cerebrovascular disease. II. A controlled study in acute cerebral infarction. *Stroke*, **4**, 547–555 (1973)

6 BENÉS, V., KOUKOLIK, F. and OBROVSKA, D. Two types of spontaneous intracerebral hemorrhage due to hypertension. *Journal of Neurosurgery*, **37**, 509–513 (1972)

7 BREWER, D. B., FAWCET, F. J. and HORSFIELD, G. I. A necropsy series of non-traumatic cerebral haemorrhages and softenings, with particular reference to heart weight. *Journal of Pathology and Bacteriology*, **96**, 311–320 (1968)

8 CHARCOYT, J. M. and BOUCHARD, C. Nouvelles recherches sur la pathogénie de l'hémorrhagie cérébrale. *Archives de Physiologie Normale et Pathologique (Paris)*, **1**, 110–127, 643–675, 725–734 (1868)

9 COLE, F. M. and YATES, P. O. Pseudo-aneurysms in relationship to massive cerebral haemorrhage. *Journal of Neurology, Neurosurgery and Psychiatry*, **30**, 61–66 (1967)

10 COLE, F. M. and YATES, P. O. The occurrence and significance of intracerebral microaneurysms. *Journal of Pathology and Bacteriology*, **93**, 393–411 (1967)

11 CROWELL, R. M. and OJEMANN, R. G. Surgery for brain hemorrhage. In *Cerebrovascular Disease*, edited by J. Moossy and M. Reinmuth, 233–254. New York: Raven Press (1981)

12 DELANEY, P. and ESTES, M. Intracranial hemorrhage with amphetamine abuse. *Neurology*, **30**, 1125–1128 (1980)

13 DHOPESH, V. P., GREENBERG, J. O. and COHEN, M. M. Computed tomography in brainstem hemorrhage. *Journal of Computer Assisted Tomography*, **4**, 603–607 (1980)

14 DOLINSKAS, C. A., BILANIUK, L. T., ZIMMERMAN, R. A. and KUHL, D. E. Computed tomography of intracerebral hematomas. I. Transmission CT observations of hematoma resolution. *American Journal of Roentgenology, Radium Therapy and Nuclear Medicine*, **129**, 681–688 (1977)

15 DORNDORF, W. The immediate care of stroke. In *Spontaneous Intracerebral Haematomas. Advances in Diagnosis and Therapy*, edited by H. W. Pia, C. Langmaid and J. Zierski, 223–227. Berlin: Springer-Verlag (1980)

16 D'SOUZA, T. and SHRABERG, G. Intracranial hemorrhage associated with amphetamine use. Letter to the Editor, *Neurology*, **31**, 922–923 (1981)

17 DUFF, T. A., AYENI, S., LEVIN, A. B. and JAVIN, M. Nonsurgical management of spontaneous intracerebral hematoma. *Neurosurgery*, **9**, 387–392 (1981)

18 EISENBERG, H., MORRISON, J. T., SULLIVAN, P. and FOOTE, F. M. Cerebrovascular accidents. Incidence and survival in a defined population, Middlesex County, Connecticut. *Journal of the American Medical Association*, **189**, 883–888 (1964)

19 FEINDEL, W. Management of intracerebral hemorrhage. In *Advances in Neurology*, Vol. 25, edited by M. Goldstein, L. Bolis, C. Fieschi, S. Gorini and C. H. Millikan, 293–300. New York: Raven Press (1979)

20 FERRER, E., VILA, F. and ISAMAAT, F. Mannitol response and histogram analysis in raised ICP. In *Intracranial Pressure*, Vol. IV, edited by K. Shulman, A. Marmarou, J. D. Miller, D. P. Becker, G. M. Hochwald and M. Brock, 647–649. Berlin: Springer Verlag (1980)

21 FISHER, C. M. The pathological and clinical aspects of thalamic hemorrhage. *Transactions of the American Neurological Association*, **84**, 56–59 (1959)

22 FURLAN, A. J., WHISNANT, J. P. and ELVERBACK, L. R. The decreasing incidence of primary intracerebral hemorrhage, a population study. *Annals of Neurology*, **5**, 367–373 (1979)

23 GARRAWAY, W. M., WHISNANT, J. P., FURLAN, A. J., PHILLIPS, L. H., KURLAND, L. T. and O'FALLON, W. M. The declining incidence of stroke. *New England Journal of Medicine*, **300**, 449–452 (1979)

24 GÄNSHIRT, H. and KEULER, R. Intrazerebrale Blutungen. Ursachen, Klinik, Verlauf, Spätprognose. *Der Nervenarzt*, **51**, 210–206 (1980)

25 GILLINGHAM, F. J. Conservative and surgical management. In *Spontaneous Intracerebral Haematomas. Advances in Diagnosis and Therapy*, edited by H. W. Pia, C. Langmaid and J. Zierski, 391–392. Berlin: Springer-Verlag (1980)

26 GOLDBERG, I. D. and KURLAND, L. T. Mortality in 33 countries from diseases of the nervous system. *World Neurology*, **3**, 444–465 (1962)

27 GOLDSTEIN, R. J., BLEICH, H. L., CAPLAN, L. R., MELSKI, J. W., MOHR, J. P., PESSIN, M. and DUNCAN, G. W. Computer stroke registry and diagnosis program. *Neurology*, **25**, 356 (1975)

28 GOODMAN, S. J. and BECKER, D. P. Intracranial hemorrhage associated with amphetamine abuse. Letter to the Editor, *Journal of the American Medical Association*, **212**, 480 (1970)

29 GROTE, E., GELETNEKY, L., ROMPEL, K., ZORBAS, K., MEYER, E., PRILL, A. and HEENE, D. Atypische intrazerebrale Massenblutung. *Deutsches Zentralblatt für Nervenheilkunde*, **197**, 66–76 (1970)

30 HANSEN, B. S. and MARQUARDSEN, J. Incidence of stroke in Frederiksberg, Denmark. *Stroke*, **8**, 663–665 (1977)

31 HARRISON, M. J. G. Clinical distinction of cerebral haemorrhage and cerebral infarction. *Postgraduate Medical Journal*, **56**, 629–632 (1980)

32 HAYMAKER, W. *Bing's Local Diagnosis in Neurological Disease*, 15th Ed. 600 pp. St. Louis, Mosby (1969)

33 HIER, D. B., DAVIS, K. R., RICHARDSON, E. P. Jr. and MOHR, J. P. Hypertensive putaminal hemorrhage. *Annals of Neurology*, **1**, 152–159 (1977)

34 JAQUES, S., SHELDEN, H., McCANN, G. D., FRESHWATER, D. B. and RAND, R. Computerized three-dimensional stereotaxic removal of small central nervous system lesions in patients. *Journal of Neurosurgery*, **53**, 816–820 (1980)

35 JELLINGER, K. Pathology and aetiology of intracerebral haematoma. In *Spontaneous Intracerebral Haematoma, Advances in Diagnosis and Therapy*, edited by H. W. Pia, C. Langmaid and J. Zierski, 13–29. Berlin: Springer-Verlag (1980)

36 JENSEN, H. P. Microangiomas and intracerebral haematoma. In *Spontaneous Intracerebral Haematomas. Advances in Diagnosis and Therapy*, edited by H. W. Pia, C. Langmaid, and J. Zierski, 41–48. Berlin: Springer-Verlag (1980)

37 KANAYA, H., YUKAWA, H., ITOH, Z., KUTSUZAWA, H., KAGAWA, M., KANNO, T., KUWABARA, T., MIZUKAMI, M., ARAKI, G. and IRINO, T. Grading and the incications for treatment in ICH of the basal ganglia (Co-operative study in Japan). In *Spontaneous Intracerebral Haematomas. Advances in Diagnosis and Therapy*, edited by H. W. Pia, C. Langmaid, and J. Zierski, 268–274. Berlin: Springer-Verlag (1980)

38 KANNEL, W. B., DAWBER, T. R., COHEN, M. E. and McNAMARA, P. M. Vascular disease of the brain – epidemiological aspects: the Framingham study. *American Journal of Public Health*, **55**, 1355–1366 (1965)

39 KATZMANN, R. Treatment of cerebral oedema in brain infarction. In *Cerebrovascular Diseases*. Eleventh Princeton Conference, edited by T. R. Price and E. Nelson, 199–207. New York: Raven Press (1979)

40 KAZNER, E. and LANKSCH, W. CAT findings in cerebral aneurysms and subarachnoid haemorrhage. In *Cerebral Aneurysms. Advances in Diagnosis and Therapy*, edited by H. W. Pia, C. Langmaid and J. Zierski, 184–190. Berlin: Springer-Verlag (1980)

41 KENDALL, B. E. and RADUE, E. W. Computed tomography in spontaneous intracerebral haematomas. *British Journal of Radiology*, **51**, 563–573 (1978)

42 KINKEL, W. R. and JACOBS, L. Computerized axial transverse tomography in cerebrovascular disease. *Neurology*, **26**, 924–930 (1976)

43 KURTZKE, J. F. An introduction to the epidemiology of cerebrovascular disease. In *Cerebrovascular Diseases*. Tenth Princeton Conference, edited by P. Scheinberg, 239–253. New York: Raven Press (1976)

44 KURTZKE, J. F. Epidemiology of cerebrovascular disease. In *Cerebrovascular Survey Report for the Joint Subcommittee on Cerebrovascular Disease, National Institute of Neurological and Communicative Disorders and Stroke and National Heart and Lung Institute*, edited by R. G. Siekert, 135–176 (1980)

45 LAVI, E., ROTHMAN, S. and RECHES, A. Primary pontine hemorrhage with complete recovery. *Archives of Neurology*, **38**, 320 (1981)

46 LAZORTES, G. *L'hémorrhagie cérébrale vue par le neurochirurgien*. Paris: Masson (1956)

47 LÉVY, A. and STULA, D. Neurochirugische Aspekte bei Antikoagulantien-Blutungen im Zentralnervensystem. *Deutsche Medizinische Wochenschrift*, **96**, 1043–1048 (1971)

48 LIEBERMANN, A., HASS, W. K., PINTO, R., ISOM, W. O., KUPERSMITH, M., BEAR, G. and CHASE, R. Intracranial hemorrhage and infarction in anticoagulated patients with prosthetic heart valves. *Stroke*, **9**, 18–24 (1978)

49 LITTLE, J. R., TUBMAN, D. E. and ETHIER, R. Cerebellar hemorrhage in adults: diagnosis by computerized tomography. *Journal of Neurosurgery*, **48**, 575–579 (1978)

50 LUESSENHOP, A. J., SHEVLIN, W. A., FERRERO, A. A., McCULLOUGH, D. C. and BARONE, B. M. Surgical management of primary intracerebral hemorrhage. *Journal of Neurosurgery*, **27**, 419–427 (1967)

51 LUYENDIJK, W. Intracerebral haematoma. In *Handbook of Clinical Neurology*, Vol. 11, edited by F. G. Vinken and G. W. Bruin, 660–719. Amsterdam: North Holland (1972)

52 MARGOLIS, G., ODOM, G. L., WOODHALL, B. and BLOOR, B. M. The role of small angiomatomas and malformations in the production of intracerebral hematomas. *Journal of Neurosurgery*, **8**, 564–575 (1951)

53 MATSUMOTO, N., WHISNANT, J. P., KURLAND, L. T. and OKAZAKI, H. Natural history of Stroke in Rochester, Minnesota, 1955 through 1969: an extension of a previous study, 1945 through 1954. *Stroke*, **4**, 20–29 (1973)

54 MATTOS PIMENTA, L. H., MATTOS PIMENTA, A. and ZUCKERMAN, E. Pontine haematoma: successful removal of two cases with review of 22 cases previously described in accessible literature. *Neurosurgical Review*, **4**, 139–142 (1981)

55 MAZARS, G., RIBADERO-DUMAS, C. and ROGE, R. Accidents hémorrhagiques cérébraux au cours des traitements anticoagulants. *Marseille Médicine*, **104**, 27–30 (1967)

56 McCORMICK, W. F. and ROSENFIELD, D. B. Massive brain hemorrhage: a review of 144 cases and an examination of their causes. *Stroke*, **4**, 946–954 (1973)

57 McKISSOCK, W., RICHARDSON, A. and WALSH, L. Spontaneous cerebellar haemorrhage. A study of 34 consecutive cases treated surgically. *Brain*, **83**, 1–9 (1960)

58 MIZUKAMI, M., NISHIJIMA, M. and KIN, H. Computed tomographic findings of good prognosis for hemiplegia in hypertensive putaminal hemorrhage. *Stroke*, **12**, 648–652 (1981)

59 MOHR, J. P., CAPLAN, L. R. and MELSKI, J. W. The Harvard Co-operative stroke registry: a prospective registry. *Neurology*, **28**, 754–762 (1978)

60 MÜLLER, H. R. The place of computerized tomography and carotid Doppler sonography in cv episodes. In *Advances in Neurology*, Vol. 25, edited by M. Goldstein, L. Bolis, C. Fieschi, S. Gorini and C. H. Millikan, 181–197. New York: Raven Press (1979)

61 MÜLLER, H. R. Zerebrale arterielle Thrombosen, heutige Ansichten zur Prophylaxe, insbesondere mit klassischen Antikoagulantien. In *Basler Antikoagulatien-symposium*, edited by F. Duckert and F. Gruber, 39–46. Basel: Editiones Roche (1980)

62 MÜLLER, H. R. and WIGGLI, U. Cerebral, cerebellar and pontine haemorrhages. In *Computerized Axial Tomography in Clinical Practice*, edited by G. H. Du Boulay and I. F. Mosely, 249–254. Berlin: Springer Verlag (1977)

63 MÜLLER, H. R., WÜTHRICH, R., WIGGLI, U., HÜNIG, R. and ELKE, M. The contribution of computerized axial tomography to the diagnosis of cerebellar and pontine hematomas. *Stroke*, **6**, 467–475 (1975)

64 NEW, P. J. and ARONOW, S. Attenuation measurements of whole blood fractions in computed tomography. *Radiology*, **121**, 635–640 (1976)

65 OTT, K. H., KASE, C. S., OJEMANN, R. G. and MOHR, J. P. Cerebellar hemorrhage: diagnosis and treatment. *Archives of Neurology*, **31**, 160–167 (1974)

66 PAK, H., PATEL, S. C., MALIR, G. M. and AUSMAN, J. I. Successful evacuation of a pontine hematoma secondary to rupture of a venous angioma. *Surgical Neurology*, **15**, 164–167 (1981)

67 PAPO, I., JANNY, P., CARUSELLI, G., COLNET, G. and LUONGO, A. Intracranial pressure time course in primary intracerebral hemorrhage. *Neurosurgery*, **4**, 504–510 (1979)

68 PIA, H. W. The surgical treatment of intracerebral and intraventricular haematomas. *Acta Neurochirurgica (Wien)*, **27**, 149–164 (1972)

69 PIA, H. W., LANGMAID, C. and ZIERSKI, J. (Editors). *Spontaneous Intracerebral Haematomas. Advances in Diagnosis and Therapy*. Berlin: Springer Verlag (1980)

70 PIEPGRAS, U. and RIEGER, P. Thalamic bleeding. *Neuroradiology*, **22**, 85–91 (1981)

71 REGLI, F. and JEANMONOD, D. Ursachen, Spontanverlauf und Prognose der Hirnblutungen. *Aktuelle Neurologie*, **6**, 155–170 (1979)

72 REINHARDT, H. and HUBER, E. Intracranial haemorrhages under anticoagulant therapy. In *Advances in Neurosurgery*, Vol. 9 edited by H. P. Jenssen, M. Brock and M. Klinger. Berlin: Springer-Verlag (in press)

73 RICHARDSON, A. Spontaneous intracerebral haemorrhage. In *Cerebral Arterial Disease*, edited by R. W. R. Russell, 210–230. Edinburgh: Churchill Livingstone (1976)

74 ROPPER, A. H. and DAVIS, K. R. Lobar cerebral hemorrhages: acute clinical syndromes in 26 cases. *Annals of Neurology*, **8**, 141–147 (1980)

75 RUSSEL, D. S. The pathology of spontaneous intracerebral haemorrhages. *Proceedings of the Royal Society of Medicine*, **47**, 489–704 (1954)

76 SANO, K. and OCHIAI, C. Brain stem haematomas, clinical aspects with reference to indications for treatment. In *Spontaneous Intracerebral Haematomas. Advances in Diagnosis and Therapy*, edited by H. W. Pia, C. Langmaid and J. Zierski, 366–371. Berlin: Springer Verlag (1980)

77 SCOTT, M. Spontaneous intracerebral haematoma caused by cerebral neoplasms. Report of eight verified cases. *Journal of Neurosurgery*, **42**, 338–342 (1975)

78 SCOTT, B. B., SEEGER, J. F. and SCHNEIDER, R. C. Successful evacuation of a pontine hematoma secondary to rupture of a pathologically diagnosed 'cryptic' vascular malformation: case report. *Journal of Neurosurgery*, **39**, 104–108 (1973)

79 SILVERSTEIN, A. Neurological complications of anticoagulation therapy. *Archives of Internal Medicine*, **139**, 217–220 (1979)

80 SNYDER, M. and RENAUDIN, J. Intracranial hemorrhage associated with anticoagulation therapy. *Surgical Neurology*, **7**, 31–40 (1977)

81 STALLONES, R. A., DYKEN, M. L., FANG, H. C. H., HEYMAN, A., SELTSER, R. and STAMLER, J. I. Epidemiology for stroke facility planning. *Stroke*, **3**, 360–371 (1972)

82 STULA, D., MÜLLER, H. R. and LÉVY, A. CT guided surgical removal of basal ganglia hemorrhages. In *Cerebral Vascular Disease*. (Proceedings of the 8th International Salzburg Conference, September 22–25, 1976), edited by J. S. Meyer, H. Lechner and M. Reivich, 164–169. Amsterdam: Excerpta Medica (1977)

83 SUZUKI, J. and TAKAKU, A. Trans-Sylvian approach to putaminal haematomas. In *Spontaneous Intracerebral Haematomas. Advances in Diagnosis and Therapy*, edited by H. W. Pia, C. Langmaid and J. Zierski, 384–386. Berlin: Springer Verlag (1980)

84 UTTERBACK, R. A. Haemorrhagic cerebrovascular disease. In *Clinical Neurology*, Vol. 1, edited by A. B. Baker and L. H. Baker, Chapter 11, 1–31. Philadelphia: Harper and Row (1981)

85 WALLACE, D. C., CLARKE, M. C. and COLES, J. H. A study of the natural history of cerebral vascular disease. *Medical Journal of Australia*, **1**, 90–95 (1967)

86 WALKER, A. E., ROBINS, M. and WEINFELD, F. D. Clinical findings. In *The National Survey of Stroke*, edited by F. D. Weinfeld. *Stroke*, **12** (Suppl. 1), 13–31 (1981)

87 WEBER, J. Das intrazerebrale Hämatom. *Schweizer Archiv für Neurologie und Psychiatrie*, **91**, 510–552 (1963)

88 WEISBERG, L. Multiple spontaneous intracerebral haematomas: clinical and computed tomographic correlation. *Neurology*, **31**, 897–900 (1981)

90 WHISNANT, J. P., FITZGIBBONS, J. P., KURLAND, L. T. and SAYRE, G. P. Natural history of stroke in Rochester, Minnesota, 1945 through 1954. *Stroke*, **2**, 11–22 (1971)

91 ZIMMERMANN, H. M. Cerebral apoplexy: mechanism and differential diagnosis. *New York State Journal of Medicine*, **49**, 2153–2157 (1949)

92 ZUCCARELLO, M., PARDATSCHER, K., ANDRIOLI, G. C., FIORE, D. L. and IAVICOLI, R. Brain tumors presenting as spontaneous intracerebral haemorrhage. *Zentralblatt für Neurochirurgie*, **42**, 1–6 (1981)

93 ZUPPING, R. and ROOSE, M. Epidemiology of cerebrovascular disease in Tartu, Estonia, USSR, 1970 through 1973. *Stroke*, **7**, 198–190 (1976)

14
Subarachnoid hemorrhage

A. L. Sahs

In recent publications there has been a tendency to equate nontraumatic subarachnoid hemorrhage with ruptured saccular aneurysm of the circle of Willis and its adjacent branches. In the majority of instances this approach will be correct, but the clinician must be prepared to entertain a differential diagnosis to accommodate those instances in which other diseases are responsible for the bleeding[206]. Furthermore, it is recognized that in some cases no cause can be pinpointed.

Walton[314] was cognizant of the multiple causes of subarachnoid hemorrhage when he published his detailed review of the subject in 1953. He stated that '. . . although aneurysmal or angiomal rupture undoubtedly accounts for the majority of cases, from time to time numerous other pathologic conditions may underlie a brisk attack of subarachnoid bleeding'. In the 1950s the etiology of one-third of the cases of nontraumatic subarachnoid hemorrhage was not discovered[193]. Before the advent of computed axial tomography many examples of parenchymal hemorrhage with extravasation into the ventricle or into the subarachnoid space were undoubtedly included in this group. This accounts for the relatively large number incorporated in the 'general survey of cases' in the Central Registry by Locksley, Sahs and Knowler[175] in 1969. In this report 2092 of 5834 cases of subarachnoid hemorrhage (36%) were attributed to causes other than aneurysm or arteriovenous malformation. Stehbens[277] has commented that the finding of blood in the subarachnoid space is not a diagnosis in itself but merely a sign or indication of another pathological state, which is frequently a ruptured aneurysm. In 1967 Pakarinen[224] tried to make this point clear in his detailed review of the subject by indicating that subarachnoid hemorrhage is not a disease *sui generis*, but only a syndrome. Pakarinen referred to this condition as 'primary subarachnoid hemorrhage' to separate it from the traumatic group.

A detailed review of the subject of subarachnoid hemorrhage can be found in the chapter produced by Richard Heidrich[120]. He has covered the spectrum of causes of subarachnoid hemorrhage, devoted proper coverage to the role of intracranial aneurysms and included an impressive list of other etiological factors. Inevitably, however, most publications will concentrate on intracranial saccular aneurysms and some do not elaborate upon the other causes[6, 50, 292].

With the advent of computed tomography and sophisticated cerebral angiography (especially with visualization of both the carotid and vertebrobasilar circulations), the employment of multiple views, subtraction techniques, and a tendency to repeat angiographic surveys, if indicated, the numbers categorized as 'unknown etiology' are being reduced appreciably. Thus, one now encounters reports of 80% and sometimes as high as 96% yield[286]. This means, however, that there is still a small group of patients with definite, sometimes devastating, subarachnoid hemorrhage in whom no cause for the bleeding is found.

In most instances subarachnoid hemorrhage is a serious disorder which carries a high mortality and morbidity. Both Peerless[228] and Drake[64] indicated that the numbers of patients dying, plus those with neurological disability resulting from the rupture of intracranial aneurysms, remain unacceptably high and are a major problem facing all neurologists and neurosurgeons in spite of the remarkable advances made in the diagnosis and treatment of this disorder.

HISTORICAL NOTE

According to McHenry[192], mention of subarachnoid hemorrhage can be found in the Hippocratic writings. A probable reference to this disorder can be found in the Old Testament[127, 177]. A detailed historical review is available in the publication by Walton[316], who reported that the deaths of King Henry II of France and of Crown Prince Charles of Sweden were most certainly due to subarachnoid hemorrhage; that of the Duke of Aurelia possibly was due to a similar cause[60]. The early contributions of Jakob Wepfer[321] and Thomas Willis[75, 325] deserve recognition. The widely-illustrated circle was published by the latter in his famous *Cerebri Anatome* in 1664. Morgagni of Padua[201] implied that aneurysms existed in the brain. The first authentic description of an unruptured intracranial aneurysm is credited to Francisci Biumi[25] (1765), and the first detailed description of a ruptured intracranial aneurysm appears to have originated from Blackall[26], according to James Bull[34]. Notable advances in the diagnosis and treatment of subarachnoid hemorrhage have appeared from various sources[74]. Quincke[239] (1891) is credited with the clinical application of the lumbar puncture. Egaz Moniz[200] (1927) and his assistant, Lima, performed the first angiograms in humans. Notable advances in surgical therapy were carried out by Dott[62] (1930) and by Dandy[56] (1944). The article by Hounsfield[128] on computed tomography appeared in 1973.

Dandy[56] credited Brinton[32] (1851) with collecting 40 pathologically verified intracranial aneurysms. Gull[105] reported 51 cases in 1859 and is responsible for the adage that 'Whenever young persons die with symptoms of ingravescent apoplexy and after death large effusion of blood is found, especially if the effusion be over the surface of the brain in the meshes of the pia mater, the presence of an aneurism is probable.' Lebert[167] collected 86 cases in 1866 and Beadles[22] 555 in 1907. A classical paper was published by Symonds[291] in 1924. The report of McDonald and Korb[190] in 1939 was an outstanding review of the literature. Richardson and Hyland[244] followed with a detailed review of the subject in 1941.

Contributions to the pathology of aneurysms were made by Virchow[309] in 1851 and by Hutchinson[136] in 1875. More recently such pathological changes have been studied and reported by Forbus[85], Hassler[115], McCormick and Schochet[188] as well as Stehbens[277].

Efforts to classify vascular malformations of the brain were made by Luschka[178] (1854) and by Virchow[310] (1863). Later, Dandy[55] as well as Cushing and Bailey[52] became interested in these lesions. The first surgical exposure of a cerebral arteriovenous malformation is credited to Giordano[96] in 1890. Priority for the first surgical removal of a cerebral hemispheric vascular malformation belongs to Olivecrona[220] in 1932.

EPIDEMIOLOGY

So far as the general subject of stroke and its many ramifications are concerned a number of excellent reviews are available. Marquarden[181], for example, has indicated an incidence rate for all types of stroke as averaging 200 per 100 000 per year in the European population and has listed subarachnoid hemorrhage as accounting for 10% of the strokes. He has also stated that subarachnoid hemorrhage appears to be the most reliable type of diagnosis. Kurtzke[161] placed the figure at about 8% of all strokes. There is considerable variation in the incidence, however. One of the best-known and most often quoted studies on primary subarachnoid hemorrhage is that of Pakarinen[224], who cited an incidence rate of 16.8 cases per 100 000 population per year. Fogelholm's[83] figure was 19.4 per 100 000 per year. Phillips *et al.*[232] reported an annual incidence of aneurysmal subarachnoid hemorrhage at 11 per 100 000. They noted that while there was a declining incidence of other types of stroke, there was a virtually constant average incidence of subarachnoid hemorrhage during the last 30 year period. In 1956 Walton[316] made an analysis of 173 cases diagnosed clinically as spontaneous subarachnoid hemorrhage and reported that at autopsy intracranial aneurysms accounted for approximately 72%; angioma 3%; no bleeding point discovered (possible aneurysm) 8%; primary cerebral hemorrhage 5%; primary intraventricular hemorrhage 3%; miscellaneous 9%.

Modern calculations, excluding trauma and primary parenchymal hemorrhage, give the following incidence of hemorrhage. Subarachnoid hemorrhage is estimated to occur in 16 per 100 000 population in the USA per year. And this figure is only slightly lower than the figure of Sypert[292] of 17 per 100 000 per year. Thus, the estimate of 34 000 new cases of subarachnoid hemorrhage yearly in the USA can be broken down as follows: 26 000 aneurysms; 2000 angiomas; 2000 disorders of hemostasis and 4000 'other' and unidentified conditions.

The statistics on the natural history and the results of treatment of subarachnoid hemorrhage are often developed at tertiary referral centers where attrition and careful selection have screened out a number of poor risk patients. There is a significant percentage (estimated at 8%) of patients who die acutely at home or at work, while others become seriously ill and die en route to a hospital or expire in a local hospital. Still others survive long enough to reach a tertiary referral center only to expire there. It is estimated that 25% of all patients die within 24 hours. A certain number are considered too ill for surgery, have complicating diseases, or refuse operation. Binder *et al.*[23] made an effort to study such a group of 18 seriously ill patients. Seventeen died, five with an acute bulbar syndrome and cardiac arrest and 12 with an 'irreversible breakdown of brain function'.

Alvord *et al.*[13] calculated the survival rates for patients seen at different time intervals following aneurysmal subarachnoid hemorrhage. They also commented on the fact that many patients die before they reach the hospital. Once they arrive at the hospital the 'natural history' would indicate an additional mortality rate of 40–50% in two months.

ETIOLOGY AND PATHOGENESIS

Intracranial aneurysms

Saccular type aneurysms

There are a number of books on the subject of intracranial aneurysms, dating from the monograph by Dandy[56] in 1944 and continuing with those by Hamby[107], Pool and Potts[235], Walton[316], Sahs *et al.*[254] and Suzuki[287]. The neurosurgical and neurological journals are replete with publications in this field.

This type constitutes the majority of instances of nontraumatic subarachnoid hemorrhage, as already indicated. For many years there has been controversy over the etiology as to whether they are congenital or acquired. Most writers recognize that certain deficiencies exist at points of bifurcation in the circle of Willis. This phenomenon was emphasized by Forbus[85] in 1930, and gaps in the media at points of bifurcation are sometimes called 'Forbus gaps'. This does not constitute the entire picture, however. Additional changes apparently must take place before an aneurysm forms. Degeneration of the elastic layer is part of this process. Some investigators suggested that occlusion of the vasa vasora of the cerebral arteries caused by atherosclerosis weakens the elastic layer[312]. Attention has also been directed to hydrodynamic factors[144], perhaps as a result of the development of intimal pads[268]. Stehbens[277] has devoted a chapter in his book to this subject and has discussed possible etiological factors in detail. Cajander and Hassler[35] focused on possible enzymatic destruction of the elastic lamella at the mouth of a cerebral berry aneurysm. Pope *et al.*[236] indicated that some patients with cerebral aneurysms are deficient in Type III collagen. Campbell and Roach[38] demonstrated fenestrations in the internal elastic lamina at bifurcations of human cerebral arteries. Sheffield and Weller[268] have revived the idea that inelastic intimal pads form as a result of hemodynamic stress and that the presence of such pads may enhance stresses and strains at vessel bifurcations. Stehbens[278] suggests that the term 'medial defect' be abandoned, and that the term 'medial raphe' would be more appropriate because it appears to be active as a sheet anchor during vasoconstriction.

Aneurysms were produced experimentally in rats by Hashimoto, Handa and Hazama[114]. The animals were fed β-aminopropionitrile, they were unilaterally subjected to carotid ligation, and they were made hypertensive by deoxycortico-sterone and salt treatment. Aneurysms appeared on the anterior cerebral-anterior communicating artery complex in 11 of 30 rats. Suzuki and Ohara[288] postulated that the water hammer effect of the pulse causes ballooning of the normal gap at the arterial bifurcation. McCormick and Schmalstieg[189] presented evidence that questions the widely held belief that systemic arterial hypertension is a major factor either in the genesis of saccular aneurysms or in their subsequent rupture.

Considerable attention has been directed to the incidence of intracranial aneurysms. The detailed report by Hassler[115] showed a surprising yield of over 17% minute defects and 1% major berry aneurysms in a 'normal' autopsy series. The figure reported by McCormick and Schochet[188] showed an incidence of 8% of the autopsy population above one year of age. Only 25% of such aneurysms had ruptured; thus 6% of the autopsy population had incidental aneurysms. About 25% of patients with intracranial saccular aneurysms have multiple aneurysms[187].

There is little doubt that certain saccular aneurysms will increase in size with the passage of time. This phenomenon was demonstrated angiographically by Allcock and Canham[11]. Proliferation of the adventia thickens the neck of the aneurysm but the fundus, poorly bolstered by adventitia, expands and can eventually give way.

Associated or contributory disorders include the following.

(1) Coarctation of the aorta[331].
(2) Ehlers-Danlos syndrome[197].
(3) Fibromuscular dysplasia[221].
(4) Hereditary hemorrhagic telangiectasia[4, 238].
(5) Marfan's syndrome[183].
(6) Moyamoya disease[204].
(7) Polycystic kidney disease[53].
(8) Progeria[102].
(9) Pseudoxanthoma elasticum[140].

SPECIAL CONSIDERATIONS

Infancy and childhood
On rare occasions aneurysms are encountered in the newborn[168], but these are usually giant aneurysms. They are also infrequent in infancy and childhood[12, 14, 94]. Their rarity in this age group has been used to support the concept that the 'acquired' factors in the production of aneurysms accumulate over many decades. These aneurysms are managed the same as those in the adult population.

Familial aneurysms
Familial incidence is encountered occasionally. For example, Hashimoto[113] reported a family in which four members had aneurysms and one additional member was suspect. An abundant number of references in the literature has accumulated on this subject.

Multiple aneurysms

Multiple aneurysms occur in 25% of the cases. In instances of rupture there may be some difficulty in identifying the aneurysm which has bled. Generally the largest aneurysm, the one with the greatest adjacent accumulation of blood on the CT scan, or the one with the most conspicuous spasm, is the offending aneurysm. The presence of focal neurological symptoms, and evidence of one or more bulging areas as seen in the aneurysm by angiography, will provide additional information. These data are important from the standpoint of planning definitive surgery[245].

Vertebral-basilar aneurysms

Considerable attention is now being directed in the neurosurgical literature to management of vertebral-basilar aneurysms, the majority of which occur at the bifurcation of the basilar artery into the posterior cerebral arteries[283, 332]. Drake[64] has indicated that experience with over 650 patients suggests that if they are ordinary size they can be treated as safely as those on the anterior circulation. In a series of large vertebral-basilar aneurysms the surgical mortality was 5%.

Giant aneurysms

These are aneurysms which are arbitrarily defined as 2.5 cm in size or larger. These aneurysms can often be seen directly in the CT scan and sometimes are much larger than they appear at angiography because the lumen often contains a variable amount of clot. Drake[64] reported on 100 such aneurysms of the anterior circulation and 161 on the posterior circulation and indicated that they can now be treated with relative safety. The posterior circulation aneurysms, in particular, may present as space-occupying lesions[300].

Combination of aneurysm and arteriovenous malformation

Aneurysm and arteriovenous malformation will occur in combination in 2% of these cases of subarachnoid hemorrhage. Generally the aneurysm will have bled and will be the one to require priority treatment[245].

Unruptured aneurysms

These lesions are included in this chapter because, if identified, they offer an excellent opportunity to prevent a subarachnoid hemorrhage and thus to avoid many of the disastrous complications to be detailed later. Samson, Hodosh and Clark[258] reported no deaths in 50 elective craniotomies in such cases. Three patients, however, had permanent deficits. Unruptured aneurysms have been implicated as the nidus for recurrent transient neurological deficits[126, 281].

Dissecting aneurysms

Hypertension is the most frequent accompaniment of this condition and the aorta is most frequently involved. Stehbens[277] cited 35 examples of dissecting aneurysms of the cerebral arteries. In six there was evidence of subarachnoid hemorrhage. The intima is torn and is dissected away from the media. Blood may flow through true and false lumens or flow may end abruptly at the point of dissection. In certain instances the result can be infarction of the brain distal to the obstruction.

Fusiform aneurysms

Other types of aneurysmal dilatations include the so-called ectasias, dolicho-ectatic intracranial arteries, fusiform enlargements, or fusiform aneurysms[172,250]. They are said to constitute approximately 5% of all intracranial aneurysms. This lesion involves the basilar artery more frequently than the other vessels of the circle of Willis. Compression of neighborhood intracranial structures is the usual cause of symptoms but subarachnoid and intracerebral hemorrhage can occur[98,123]. These, however, are not so likely to bleed as large saccular aneurysms of the base.

Aneurysms of inflammatory origin

The use of the term 'mycotic' is misleading unless the aneurysm is definitely of fungal etiology. Inflammatory aneurysms can be caused by bacteria, fungi, treponema and other organisms. Riggs in 1956 reported, in a discussion of a paper by Ray and Wahal[243], the discovery of five inflammatory aneurysms in a series of 175 cases of rupture of an intracranial aneurysm. At the present time the incidence is considered to be low as a consequence of the specific therapy of bacterial and mycotic infections. Yet they are still reported[24,27,217,246]. In a recent report by Frazee, Cahan and Winter[91] thirteen patients with bacterial intracranial aneurysms were reviewed. This number constituted 4% of all patients admitted to their service with intracranial aneurysms. α-*Streptococcus* was the most common infecting organism. Esoteric organisms such as *Cardiobacterium hominis* are occasionally encountered[164]. It is a well-known clinical axiom that subarachnoid hemorrhage from a 'mycotic' aneurysm can be the initial manifestation of bacterial endocarditis[307].

Neoplastic aneurysms

Left atrial myxoma is a rare, but potentially treatable, cause of stroke[247]. The intracranial complications are embolic infarction, intraparenchymal hemorrhage, and aneurysm formation plus subarachnoid hemorrhage. Atrial myxoma is occasionally associated with multiple intracranial aneurysms as a result of neoplastic material lodging in and destroying the vascular wall[54]. More recently Sandok *et al.*[260] reviewed 35 patients with histologically proved atrial myxoma (seven with prior neurological events); none had subsequent delayed events attributable to the atrial myxoma.

Angiomas

These are congenital lesions which arise during an early fetal stage at the time of division into the primitive arteries, capillaries and veins[279]. Approximately 2000 new cases appear in the USA yearly[279]. In the Co-operative Study[254] there were

3265 patients registered with one or more intracranial aneurysms and 507 patients with angiomas. The natural history of arteriovenous malformations has been reviewed by Wilkins[324], presenting the statistics gleaned from the reports of Michelsen[196], Pellettieri *et al.*[229] and Drake[63]. The most common presenting symptoms are subarachnoid hemorrhage and seizures. The peak incidence of symptomatic intracranial arteriovenous malformations is in the fourth decade and there is usually a lack of significant family history[225]. However, occasional familial cases can be documented[1].

A complex terminology has developed, mainly as a result of the contributions of neuropathologists[186]. Of the various types – capillary telangiectasias, cavernous angiomas, venous angiomas, varices and arteriovenous malformations – the last is the most important for purposes of this discussion. However, intracerebral venous angioma is occasionally responsible for subarachnoid hemorrhage[261,266].

Arteriovenous malformations usually occur in the cerebral hemispheres. Intracranial arterial aneurysms and arterial malformations can co-exist[17,31,122,230,279]. Bleeding into the brain can originate either from the malformation or from the aneurysm; usually the latter is at fault. Intracranial and intraspinal arteriovenous malformations may co-exist[112].

Vascular malformations of the brain are best identified by CT scanning, followed by cerebral angiography. There are a few reported cases of angiographically occult arteriovenous malformations but these are rare[226].

Other causes

Primary parenchymal hemorrhage

As a listed cause of subarachnoid hemorrhage, parenchymal lesions now constitute a smaller and smaller number. Before the advent of computed axial tomography this group occupied an important position and was often cited under 'other causes'[254]. Blood escapes into the ventricular system or a hematoma ruptures directly into the subarachnoid space via brain substance. In general, the amount of extravasated blood is not as great as one finds in the case of a ruptured aneurysm.

Primary parenchymal hemorrhage has been labeled 'hypertensive hemorrhage' by some, and represents an important facet of cerebral vascular disease. According to Kurtzke[161] approximately 12% of strokes are the result of cerebral hemorrhage. If the incidence of stroke is 200 per 100 000 per year, the incidence for cerebral hemorrhage should be approximately 20 per 100 000 per year. This condition carries a very high mortality and accounts for about 25% of all deaths from stroke.

The vascular changes in the brain in chronic hypertension consist essentially of fibrinoid degeneration of small arteries, with eventual rupture. The pathology has been of interest since the report of Charcot and Bouchard[41] in 1869 and detailed by the report of Cole and Yates[46] in 1967. A hematoma forms as a result of the rupture; the hematoma dissects through brain tissue and may rupture into the ventricle or into the subarachnoid space. Typical locations of these hemorrhages are: putamen and thalamus; deep lobar white matter; cerebellum; pons. The cerebellar location has received considerable attention lately because of the possibility of surgical intervention.

Disorders of hemostasis

Disorders of hemostasis with subarachnoid hemorrhage are usually considered under the primary diagnoses and hence constitute a small number statistically. They are of some importance, however, because the bleeding state can mimic primary intracerebral hemorrhage, aneurysmal subarachnoid hemorrhage, ruptured intracranial angioma, and occasionally can be the presenting symptoms of the hemorrhagic state.

Patients with this disorder who develop subarachnoid hemorrhage may have a primary hemostatic defect, congenital or acquired, predisposing the patient to serious bleeding intracranially[154]. The history of abnormal bleeding tendencies in the patient or his relatives is important. Quantitative or qualitative platelet defects, hemophilioid conditions and acquired platelet or coagulation problems following drug therapy, immunological mechanisms or systemic disease will be encountered occasionally in patients who present with subarachnoid hemorrhage.

The following tests are indicated to identify possible hemorrhagic conditions: platelet count; prothrombin time; bleeding time; and partial thromboplastin time. If any of these tests yield abnormal results more elaborate studies can be carried out[124]: bleeding profile; consumption-fibrinolysis profile; and platelet profile.

Examples of several of the bleeding disorders which can result in intracranial hemorrhage are as follows. (1) Hemophilioid disorder; classical hemophilia (factor VIII deficiency); Christmas disease (factor IX deficiency). (2) Platelet disorders: predominantly thrombocytopenia. This may be caused by conditions such as decreased marrow production, increased peripheral destruction, increased sequestration of platelets in the spleen, or dilution of the blood. (3) Changes in the thrombin cascade which result in vitamin K abnormalities. These appear during liver failure or as a reaction to the use of coumarin anticoagulants[308]. As early as 1969 Barron and Fergusson[21] recorded five cases and found specific reference to 58 instances of intracranial hemorrhage during anticoagulant administration. (4) Disseminated intravascular coagulation. This condition is a complication of Gram-negative sepsis and a number of other conditions[191]. The patient bleeds into many organs in association with thrombocytopenia, hypofibrinogenemia, a prolonged prothrombin time and positive tests for fibrin misnomer and fibrin split products.

Leukemia

There is an extensive body of literature on the intracranial complications of leukemia. The figure usually cited is 15 to 45%. Groch, Sayre and Heck[103] found examples of cerebral hemorrhage in 46 of 93 autopsied cases of leukemia; 15 of these cases had subarachnoid hemorrhage. Silverstein[273] noted the importance of bleeding tendencies in leukemia in reviewing the records of 58 patients with a hemorrhagic diathesis and intracranial bleeding. Twenty-seven of these patients had acute blastic leukemia, or subacute or chronic myelogenous leukemia.

Unusual causes

There are many possible etiological factors to be considered in this broad category. This subject was reviewed in detail by Walton[314] (1953) at a time when routine angiography was not employed and computed tomography had not yet been developed. In his series 16 of 312 cases (5%) were of unusual etiology. The report of the Co-operative Aneurysm Study[254] in 1969 indicated a 33% figure of 'other causes', many of which were parenchymal hemorrhages.

The literature contains an interesting collection of various and infrequent causes of subarachnoid hemorrhage.

Brain tumors

Brain tumors may be a cause of intracranial hemorrhage. Tumors may be of many types, primary or metastatic[97]. They can range from astrocytoma[274] to meningioma[72, 100, 249, 275], pituitary adenoma (pituitary apoplexy[333]), subependymoma[40], neurilemmoma/hemangioma[148] and metastatic tumor[179]. Very rarely an aneurysm will rupture into a brain tumor and thence into the subarachnoid space.

Intracranial venous thrombosis

Estanol *et al.*[70] reported on 20 patients seen during a period of two years. Thirteen of these developed during the postpartum period. A short review of the subject is provided by Iob *et al.*[139], and by Toole and Patel[299]. The classical monograph by Kalbag and Woolf[146] describes the spinal fluid findings in cerebral venous thrombosis. These may range from clear fluid to xanthochromic staining to grossly bloody.

Arteritis

Occasionally infectious diseases of the nervous system will present with subarachnoid hemorrhage. Meningococcal septicemia is such an example[135]. Tuberculous meningitis has been known to be associated with blood in the spinal fluid[99, 311].

Cerebral arteritis can be responsible for occasional instances of intracerebral and subarachnoid bleeding[68]. One important cause is drug abuse, particularly the amphetamines[58]. Hemorrhage may appear during the course of collagen vascular disease, especially disseminated lupus erythematosus and polyarteritis nodosa.

Hereditary hemorrhagic telangiectasia

This is an autosomal dominant inherited disorder, characterized by telangiectasia of the mucous membranes, skin and viscera. Subarachnoid hemorrhage may be an unusual complication of this condition[4, 238].

Spinal subarachnoid hemorrhage

The spinal region is a rare source of subarachnoid bleeding, but should be considered when intracranial sources have been excluded[160]. This subject has been reviewed in detail by Aminoff[16], with a complete list of references. The most common etiology is a spinal angioma[334], but rupture of a spinal aneurysm is possible[306]. Tumor[121, 205], collagen vascular disease[82] and anticoagulant therapy are occasional causes. Sometimes an extremely rare condition such as endometriosis with spread to the subarachnoid space will be encountered[176]. Occasionally the cause is not found[233].

Etiology undetermined

Walton[316] encountered an 8% incidence of 'etiology undetermined' in an autopsy series. Levy[170] made an attempt to study this problem in 1960. At that time the yield of 'no vascular abnormality' was encountered in 46% of 164 cases of proven subarachnoid hemorrhage. Other figures included 39% aneurysm and 14% angioma. Bilateral carotid angiography was performed but vertebral angiography was not done. The 13% figure of 'cause unknown' by Locksley, Sahs and Sandler[174] in an autopsy population is remarkable; it is partially explained by the fact that the CT scan was not yet in use, and vertebral angiography was not routinely employed. In the modern era enough examples are encountered to continue to perplex the clinician. The convenient explanation in a case of obvious nontraumatic subarachnoid hemorrhage is that a clot has formed in the lumen of the aneurysmal sac and is responsible for isolated or repeated non-visualization of the lesion by angiography. In the instance of parenchymal hemorrhage in which no cause is found, the theory is invoked that a small arteriovenous malformation has been compressed or destroyed by the hemorrhage and is now escaping detection by arteriography, surgery or autopsy[177]. Other more remote possibilities remain, such as bleeding from fragile minute vessels in moyamoya disease[147, 156].

PATHOLOGY

After a hemorrhage the subarachnoid space is filled with a variable amount of blood admixed with cerebrospinal fluid (*Figure 14.1*). In severe cases the blood resembles a solid cast surrounding the brain in the formalin-fixed preparation. One can sometimes obtain a clue as to the source of the bleeding by observing a greater

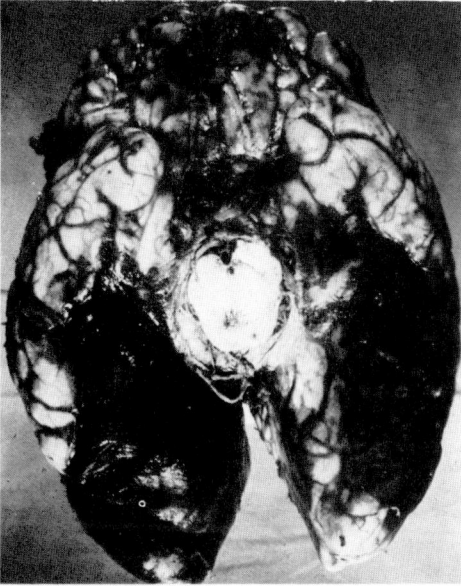

Figure 14.1 Extensive subarachnoid hemorrhage caused by ruptured saccular aneurysm

concentration of blood in one area of the subarachnoid space than in another. Blood extravasates into the distant recesses of the subarachnoid space, including the basal cisterns (*Figure 14.2*) and the spinal subarachnoid space, plus retrograde extension into the ventricular system. Arteriovenous malformations are frequently related to the middle cerebral artery complex, but bleeding into the subarachnoid space is usually not so extensive as one encounters in aneurysms. A massive intracerebral hemorrhage can rupture into the ventricular system and eventually stain the subarachnoid space generally. Head position may have some influence on

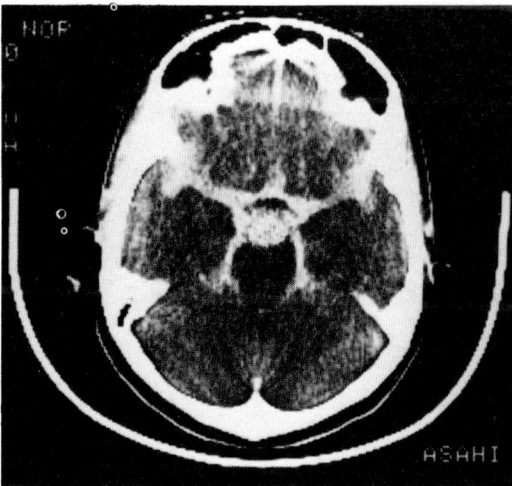

Figure 14.2 Computed tomographic scan showing accumulated blood in the subarachnoid space and basal cisterns

the amount of blood which gravitates into the posterior fossa, a situation which may have a bearing on the prognosis. In cats the greatest amount of blood was found in the posterior fossa with the animal placed in the supine position[116].

When hemorrhage occurs as a result of one of the rarer disorders the location is often atypical, the lesions are frequently multiple and the amount of subarachnoid hemorrhage is usually not so great as that seen after rupture of a saccular aneurysm. As the blood is absorbed the meninges eventually take on an orange or rust color. This is particularly evident in the fibrotic capsule surrounding an aneurysm.

The immediate reaction of the subarachnoid space has been designated hemogenic meningitis[143], eventually evolving to aseptic meningitis. The successive changes in the cellular reaction have been reviewed by Stehbens[277]. Following fresh bleeding several stages can be found: infiltration of polymorphonuclear leukocytes (4–16 hours); lymphocytes (1–3 days); macrophages (2 days); fibrosis (10 days). It has been suggested that the last of these events is responsible for the late development of hydrocephalus, and that the obstruction to the flow of cerebrospinal fluid occurs principally in the arachnoid villi[69].

Intrinsic lesions can consist of hemorrhages large enough to act as space-occupying masses. These can be present in the parenchyma, in the fissure of Sylvius or in the inter-hemispheric region. Occasionally blood will break through the pia-arachnoid and collect as a subdural hematoma. Intraventricular hemorrhage of variable degree is a common observation (*Figure 14.3*).

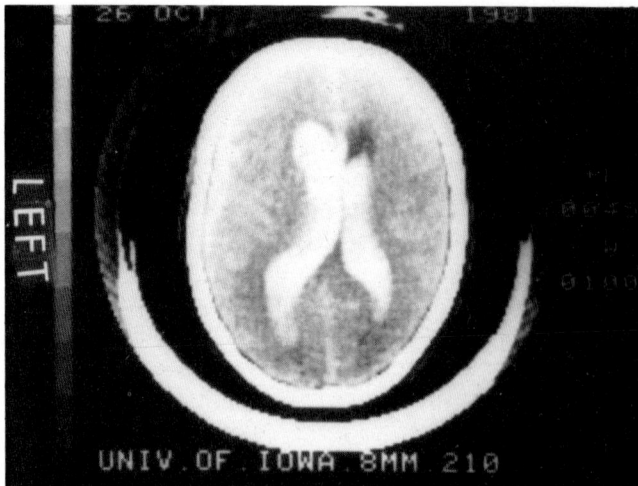

Figure 14.3 CT scan demonstrating intraventricular hemorrhage

Vascular changes are encountered frequently. This phenomenon is said to be responsible for spasm which reduces cerebral blood flow and which can be responsible for ischemic lesions in many areas of the brain. The extent and significance of these lesions were pointed out by Crompton[49] and by Schneck and Kricheff[263] many years ago. Certain areas appear to be particularly vulnerable.

Crompton[48] has recorded the hypothalamic lesions following aneurysmal rupture as ischemic and hemorrhagic in 61% of 106 consecutive cases examined. Doshi and Neil-Dwyer[61] studied 54 patients, 42 of whom had both hypothalamic and myocardial lesions. They suggested that involvement of the autonomic nervous system was responsible for some of the deleterious effects of subarachnoid hemorrhage.

An infrequent but late sequel of recurrent subarachnoid hemorrhage is the development of a condition known as superficial siderosis, in which iron pigment is deposited in the sub-pial and subependymal layers of the brain[108, 130, 158].

SYMPTOMS

Premonitory symptoms

A number of authors have attempted to identify warning signals[95, 138]. Calvert[37] found an incidence of 38.5% of patients who apparently had a significant history preceding the hemorrhage. Headache led the list. Money and Vanderfield[199] described premonitory headache in 17 of 93 aneurysm cases. Okawara's figure for warning symptoms was 48.2%[218]. Attempts have been made to associate migraine with aneurysms[90] and with arteriovenous malformations[36]. Crowell and Zervas[50] reported that premonitory features may precede rupture in as many as 60% of patients. It has been the writer's experience that separating the headache from an incipient rupture of an aneurysm or arteriovenous malformation from the maze of headaches, or other types (vascular, toxic-febrile, inflammatory, tension) may be a herculean task. Localized periorbital pain and a third nerve palsy will certainly alert the physician; a headache of sudden onset described as the worst ever experienced, especially if associated with a brief loss of consciousness, a convulsion, nausea and vomiting, photophobia, neck and back pain, should raise a strong suspicion of subarachnoid hemorrhage until proven otherwise. Unfortunately some presentations are so anomalous as to be misleading and to delay the diagnosis. The appearance of focal neurological deficit such as the third nerve palsy mentioned above, or hemiparesis, aphasia or hemianopsia should signal that a potentially ominous event is developing.

Once a rupture has occurred the succeeding events can vary appreciably. In the case of an aneurysm there may be only a tiny rent in the dome; the defect becomes sealed after the extravasation of a minimal amount of blood. One encounters this in certain cases of internal carotid-posterior communicating junctional aneurysms which are capable of producing the syndrome of 'painful ophthalmoplegia'. A more common event is the major extravasation of a considerable quantity of blood into the subarachnoid space, which produces the full-blown picture of subarachnoid hemorrhage: severe headache; nausea; vomiting and impairment of the state of consciousness, with or without a convulsion.

OTHER CLINICAL FEATURES

Central nervous system

The onset of subarachnoid hemorrhage is usually identifiable. The patient suddenly develops a severe headache, has alteration of consciousness, vomits and then complains of stiffness of the neck. Some patients will have one or more convulsions; others will remain confused or unconscious for variable periods of time. Except for those instances in which the third or sixth cranial nerves are involved[20], or those in which a hematoma develops in the fissure of Sylvius or in the interhemispheric fissure frontally, focal signs are usually not conspicuous in aneurysmal subarachnoid hemorrhage. Focal signs are more likely to be present in a ruptured arteriovenous malformation or an intracerebral hematoma from a ruptured aneurysm.

More severe examples are encountered when there is a massive extravasation of blood into the subarachnoid space, into the basal cisterns and into the ventricular system, as well as into the brain substance itself[253]. Such patients quickly lapse into coma and many of them expire. Hubschmann and Kornhauser[129] indicated that an acute subarachnoid hemorrhage over the cerebral cortex causes single or multiple waves of cellular depolarization. There is massive K^+ release and transient depression of electrocortical activity.

The complications and reactions to subarachnoid hemorrhage were reviewed by Mathew, Meyer and Hartmann[182]. They listed intracerebral hematoma, hydrocephalus and cerebral swelling (edema) with intracranial hypertension as the ones to produce the most concern in the immediate post-hemorrhagic period.

Intracerebral hematoma

Intracerebral hematoma is a well-known complication. The clinician should suspect an intracerebral bleed when there are outstanding focal signs such as hemiparesis, hemianesthesia, hemianopsia and/or aphasia. The accessibility of CT scanning will verify the diagnosis, and evacuation of the hematoma may be indicated.

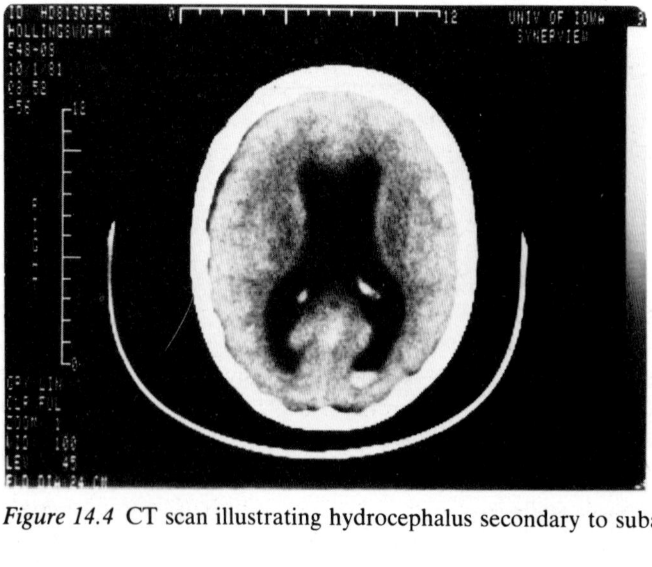

Figure 14.4 CT scan illustrating hydrocephalus secondary to subarachnoid hemorrhage

Hydrocephalus

Hydrocephalus is also a phenomenon that is well recognized[303]. Ventricular dilatation soon after subarachnoid hemorrhage is not always clinically significant but delayed ventricular enlargement (communicating hydrocephalus) occurs in about 7% of these patients and can be responsible for deterioration in the patient's condition. The findings on the CT scan (repeated) should alert the clinician to this complication which may require shunting (*Figure 14.4*).

Brain swelling and intracranial hypertension

The immediate reaction of some patients to the sudden gush of blood into the subarachnoid space has been attributed to increased intracranial pressure that approaches or equals the systemic arterial pressure[165, 166]. Hayashi *et al.*[117] have shown that imparied consciousness is secondary to increased intracranial pressure. There may be an associated initial vasospasm which contributes to cerebral ischemia. Nornes and Magnaes[216], and Nornes[214, 215] made observations on changes of intracranial pressure after a 'bleed' and verified a secondary rise in intracranial pressure. Langfitt[165] indicated that rerupture of the aneurysm may be partly the result of increase in the transmural pressure associated with the decline in intracranial pressure.

Several studies indicate that the majority of patients with significant neurological deficit and diminished levels of consciousness have associated increased intracranial pressure. The causes are varied: intracerebral and intraventricular hemorrhage; cerebral edema; infarction; hydrocephalus and intracerebral blood volume or a combination of these factors. The subsequent neurological status and intracranial pressure gradients are determined by such factors as the site and volume of extravasated blood, the vasomotor reaction, and intracranial pressure compensatory buffering capacity.

One can find numerous references to the relationship of the blood supply to the brain in the face of increasing intracranial pressure[104]. As the intracranial pressure increases moderately there is a decrease in intracranial perfusion pressure. Cerebral blood flow remains constant and cerebral blood volume increases as a result of vasodilatation. As the intracranial pressure increases or as perfusion pressure drops autoregulation becomes ineffective and there is a decrease in cerebral blood flow with subsequent ischemia.

Cerebral ischemia and vasospasm

This particular complication has been studied extensively[84]. For example, Crompton[49] reported that of 159 cases of ruptured berry aneurysm coming to autopsy, 119 (75%) had significant infarction. Vasospasm appears usually 3 to 10 days after subarachnoid hemorrhage and is heralded by a decrease in alertness and sometimes by the gradual appearance of focal neurological deficits. The vascular disorder is responsible for decreased cerebral blood flow and decreased cerebral perfusion.

Credit is given to Ecker and Riemenschneider[67] for demonstrating this phenomenon angiographically in 1951. Six of 29, or 21%, were thus identified. Reports by Fletcher, Taveras and Pool[81]; DuBoulay[66]; Schneck and Kricheff[263] and Allcock and Drake[10] followed, and the percentages ranged from 21% to 62%. Kwak *et al.*[163] indicated the presence of vasospasm prior to operation in 189 of 797 cases (23.7%). The incidence of vasospasm varies with the time of angiography, and may reach 90% or more if angiography is performed between the 8th and 12th day following the bleed.

The subject of spasm has occupied much attention in recent years[282, 323]. It is generally believed that such focal narrowing can cause neurological deterioration in the form of impairment of the state of consciousness and/or focal signs[77]. This is a progressive phenomenon which manifests itself clinically in approximately one-quarter of patients with aneurysmal subarachnoid hemorrhage and which begins insidiously toward the end of the first week[64]. The net result is a reduction in cerebral blood flow to dangerous levels (below $20\,ml\ 100\,gm^{-1}/min^{-1}$)[284] and production of cerebral infarction of variable degree. The presence of spasm can usually be established by angiography (*Figure 14.5*). Fox and Ko[89] indicated that vasospasm may be preceded by a period of relative dilatation. The identification of spasm may be a powerful deterrent to operative treatment at that particular time.

The studies of Fisher, Kistler and Davis[79] showed that there is a relationship between the amount and distribution of blood as seen in the CT scan and the development of vasospasm. They reported that blood localized in the subarachnoid

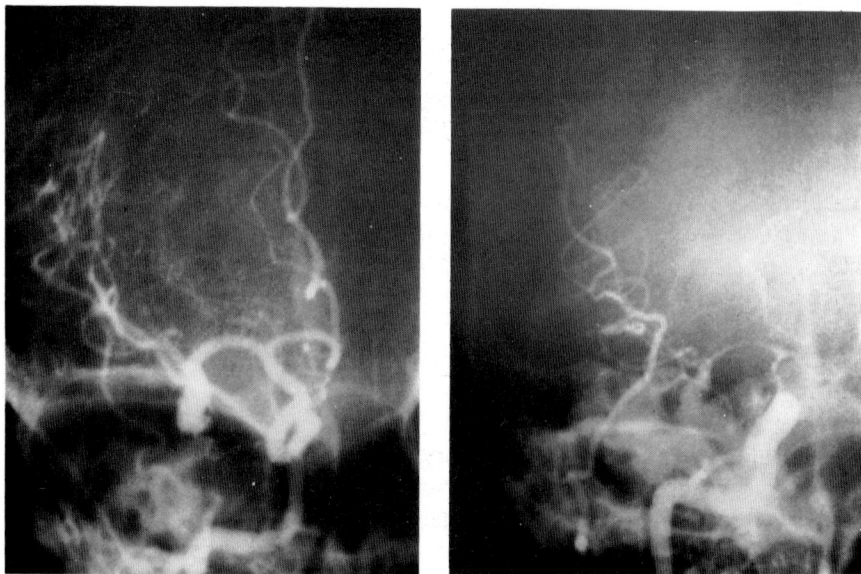

Figure 14.5 Approximately equivalent areas shown by angiography. Photograph to left shows vascular tree three days after an aneurysmal rupture. Photograph to right demonstrates severe spasm nine days after the original angiograms were performed

space in sufficient amounts at specific sites is *the* important etiological factor in vasospasm.

Results from animal experimentation[45] would suggest that in animals hemorrhaged by vascular rupture, subintimal thickening of the arteries was minimally present by three days. Progressive changes then occurred: severe subintimal proliferation, fibrosis of the smooth muscle layer and interruption of the internal elastic membrane. The agent which induces spasm is not known, but there is some evidence to indicate that it may be a product of disintegration of the erythrocytes[223], resulting in a pathological contraction of smooth muscle cells in the vascular walls.

Recent studies by Schumacher and Alksne[264] suggest that the contraction appears to involve at least two vasoactive elements: a substance, presumably serotonin, which seems to play a role in the rapid initiation of short-lived contraction; and a substance, presumably thrombaxane A_2, which induces a slower contraction, maintained for a longer period of time. Hasegawa, Watanabe and Ishii[111] indicated that cerebral vasospasm brings about systemic platelet hyperactivity and a hypercoagulable state. Cerebral ischemia could result from increased blood viscosity due to an elevated fibrinogen level, formation of microthrombosis and reduced deformability of red cells.

Histological changes can be demonstrated at necropsy[131]. The main changes involve necrosis of the tunica media and concentric intimal thickening by subendothelial fibrosis.

Seizures

Seizures as a complication of acute subarachnoid hemorrhage are mentioned frequently in the literature but most ictal activity is not witnessed by a physician because it often takes place immediately after the onset of the original hemorrhage.

Hart *et al.*[110] studied the records of 100 consecutive cases of subarachnoid hemorrhage resulting from ruptured aneurysm. Seizures occurred in 26% of the patients. They reported that seizures at the onset of subarachnoid hemorrhage were not predictors of prognosis or useful indicators of the location of aneurysms. Seizures are a nonspecific reaction to the cerebral oligemia resulting from the abrupt increase in intracranial pressure.

Rebleeding

Even if the patient survives an acute aneurysmal rupture he remains at risk for a subsequent hemorrhage. The highest probability is during the first ten days to two weeks after the initial rupture. Recurrent hemorrhage is to be feared at any time, however. If another hemorrhage occurs it is likely to be lethal because blood will now dissect through brain substance in second or third episodes because of the scarring which has now caused the aneurysm to be adherent to the meninges. If a patient survives beyond the six-month period the probability for a recurrent hemorrhage in nonsurgically managed aneurysms is approximately 3% per year[327]. Thus the patient always remains at risk to the hazards of rebleeding if his aneurysm is not corrected surgically.

Associated findings

Fever is seen in the majority of instances of subarachnoid hemorrhage. Rousseaux *et al.*[248] studied this sign in 107 cases of arterial aneurysm and indicated that the fever usually appeared on the fifth day at the latest and lasted an average of nine days. They suggested that fever of this type was related to cerebral vasospasm. Leukocytosis of variable degrees is encountered.

It is not unusual for patients to present as puzzling diagnostic problems[9] largely because of the presence of severe hypertension, pulse abnormalities, chest pain, gastrointestinal bleeding, low back pain and leg pain. These pitfalls have been emphasized by Adams *et al.*[5]. Probably the most confusing of all are the elevated blood pressure and cardiac abnormalities which can accompany subarachnoid hemorrhage. Marked hypertension and an altered state of consciousness may lead to the diagnosis of hypertensive encephalopathy. Aneurysmal patients do not ordinarily have hypertensive changes in the heart, kidney and retina. Cardiac arrhythmias and changes in the electrocardiogram are frequent complications[51], supposedly the aftermath of the sudden release of catecholamines. The most common rhythm disturbances are: ventricular tachycardia; tachycardia–bradycardia syndrome; A–V conduction defects and sinus bradycardia. The changes evident in the electrocardiogram include: U waves; prolonged Q–T interval; depression or elevation of the S–T segment or flattened T waves. Sudden death caused by a cardiac arrhythmia is a sequel of subarachnoid hemorrhage[262, 304]. Estanol Vidal *et al.*[71] found a 20% incidence of life-threatening arrhythmias occurring during the first 48 hours after subarachnoid hemorrhage. Neil-Dwyer *et al.*[208] indicated that there was an association between the necrotic lesions of the myocardium and abnormalities in the electrocardiograms and that propranolol had a cardioprotective effect.

Other possibilities should be added to the list of associated conditions. Fluid and electrolyte disturbances were found in approximately 9% of the cases reported by Takaku *et al.*[294]. The most common location of the aneurysm for this complication would appear to be the anterior communicating region and the most common electrolyte disturbance is hyponatremia[294]. Hypovolemia resulting from a number of causes such as bed rest, diuresis and pooling in the peripheral vascular bed is also very common[180]. To this list one should add pulmonary edema[101, 298, 317], which may occur rapidly[44] or be delayed[78]. Gastrointestinal bleeding appears in about 2% of patients with subarachnoid hemorrhage caused by cerebral aneurysms[295]. Hormonal imbalance has been reported in the form of abnormal levels of hydroxycorticosteroids[222]. Intraocular hemorrhages are seen in approximately 25% of patients with primary subarachnoid hemorrhage. They are said to be most commonly associated with aneurysms of the anterior communicating artery[73]. Retinal hemorrhages appear soon after the subarachnoid bleeding. The causes have been attributed to sudden increase in intracranial pressure, or extension of blood from the subarachnoid space to the lamina cribrosa, then to the fundus oculi. They can be small, punctate or subhyloid. The appearance of fundal hemorrhages adds to the gravity of the prognosis[240]. Occasionally there will be subconjunctival ecchymoses closely resembling those observed after trauma[119]. In patients presenting with coma of unknown etiology the presence of retinal hemorrhages usually gives an important clue as to the presence of subarachnoid hemorrhage.

DIAGNOSIS

The diagnosis of subarachnoid hemorrhage may be very easy in the straightforward case, or very difficult in the atypical one. Although the warning episodes, previously discussed, are said to be relatively frequent, often they are recognized only in retrospect[177]. Unfortunately, localized and diffuse headaches are very common in the population generally, so that it is not feasible to subject all headache patients to spinal puncture, CT scanning and/or angiography.

The sudden onset of violent headache has already been discussed. Sudden loss of consciousness occurs in approximately one-fifth of the patients[316], and convulsions occur in about 4% of patients. Vomiting is a sequel to the severe headache. Malaise and photophobia are commonly encountered. The neck usually becomes stiff within a few hours, and other meningeal signs appear soon thereafter. If unconsciousness continues and if coma deepens the prognosis is grave. Such patients are so seriously ill that transfer to a referral center may be futile. This group may account for at least 15% of the cases of subarachnoid hemorrhage. If the patient begins to respond after the initial insult the outlook is improved. The physician can then look for focal signs, such as cranial nerve palsies (especially the third nerve), hemiparesis, dysphasia and hemianopsia. An occasional patient will have weakness of both legs and disturbances of bladder function following rupture of an aneurysm of the anterior cerebral-anterior communicating complex.

Changes in mentation deserve comment. Mental confusion is often encountered early. Some patients will exhibit a typical Korsakoff's syndrome[315]. Sequelae include the 'organic brain syndrome', such as memory disturbances (particularly recent memory impairment), affective disturbances, irritability and decline in efficiency.

GRADING SYSTEMS

It has been known for a long time that the prognosis was dependent to a considerable degree on the state of consciousness (alertness) of the patient[19]. For many years the Botterell grading scale[29] was in common usage, listing five grades from fully awake and alert to the moribund state (*Table 14.1*). The system proposed by Hunt and Kosnik[132] has also been used extensively. Others have used that proposed by the Co-operative Aneurysm Study[213] and that suggested by the Glasgow Group[297] for trauma. The main purpose of any grading system is to

Table 14.1 Grading systems

	Botterell (1956)		Hunt and Kosnik (1974)
Grade 1	Conscious, with or without signs of blood in subarachnoid space	Grade 0	Aneurysms which have not ruptured
		Grade I	Those patients with ruptured aneurysms and with little or no reaction
Grade 2	Drowsy, without significant neurological deficit	Grade Ia	Stable with residual neurological deficit such as hemiparesis
		Grade II	Patient with headache and meningeal reaction. Mild vasospasm
Grade 3	Drowsy, with a neurological deficit and probably an intracerebral clot	Grade III	Drowsy or confused. Severe vasospasm
Grade 4	Major neurological deficit and deteriorating because of large intracerebral clot, or older patient with less severe neurological deficit but with pre-existing cerebrovascular disease	Grade IV	Severely ill, with drowsiness and focal signs
Grade 5	Moribund or near moribund with failing vital centers and extensor rigidity	Grade V	Comatose, decerebrate

evaluate the patient's neurological status, particularly his state of awareness. Unfortunately, placing a number on a patient's clinical condition does not tell the entire story. The Botterell and the Hunt and Kosnik grading systems appear in abbreviated form in *Table 14.1*.

DIFFERENTIAL DIAGNOSIS

The differential diagnosis includes a large number of possible disorders, so that arriving at a prompt and accurate diagnosis may not be a simple matter (Adams *et al.*[5]). Diagnostic pitfalls were also pointed out by De Long[59]. He reported a series of patients in whom the diagnostic difficulties were maximal, and placed particular emphasis on the importance of not confusing hypertensive headache with the rise in blood pressure which often accompanies spontaneous subarachnoid hemorrhage.

When the clinician is faced with a list of possibilities, he should consider the following. This is only a partial list.

Trauma

Is this an instance of unrecognized trauma?[106] On rare occasions the patient will be found unconscious,with no external marks of violence and with bloody spinal fluid as a result of a severe head trauma. Some patients may sustain a head injury after the hemorrhage as a result of the abrupt development of unconsciousness or as a sequel to a convulsion. The lack of witnesses further complicates the problem, and extensive studies may be indicated.

Meningoencephalitis

Differentiation is not always possible on clinical grounds alone. Some patients with subarachnoid hemorrhage will present with headache, alteration of consciousness, fever, leukocytosis and signs of meningeal irritation. Careful examination of the spinal fluid should determine the correct diagnosis.

Migraine

Migraine usually follows characteristic repetitive course, but occasionally the headache will develop in explosive fashion and the patient will be so ill as to generate concern about the possibility of subarachnoid hemorrhage. Pearce and Foster[227] reported four examples of 'complicated migraine' in 40 patients studied. In these four there were signs of meningeal irritation; the authors concluded that a lumbar puncture was a justifiable examination under such circumstances. Salloum, Lebel and Reiher[256] encountered seven such cases in three years. These patients had a clinical course suggesting subarachnoid hemorrhage but were found to have complicated migraine. When the clinician is in doubt he should carry out necessary tests to exclude subarachnoid bleeding.

Toxic/metabolic states

The difficulties in this area seem to arise when the patient is discovered comatose or when he presents as a confusional case without obvious stiffness of the neck or focal signs. Then a number of possibilities such as drug or alcohol overdosage or withdrawal, diabetic ketoacidosis and uremia present themselves.

DIAGNOSTIC PROCEDURES

Computed tomography

The computed axial tomographic (CT) scan has become an essential element in the diagnosis of subarachnoid hemorrhage[57] (*see Figure 14.2*). In fact, some authors indicate that CT scanning can eliminate the need for lumbar puncture[296]. When available, the CT scan should precede the lumbar puncture. If the CT scan shows intracranial bleeding a spinal puncture is usually unnecessary. However, if no blood is apparent and there is no mass effect, then lumbar puncture is indicated.

Aneurysms above 1.5 cm in size can usually be demonstrated with this technique. The usual finding is the demonstration of blood in the subarachnoid spaces with extravasation into the basal cisterns. Blood is occasionally seen in the lateral ventricles, in the fissure of Sylvius or within brain substance.

Sometimes one can obtain a clue as to the source of the bleeding by observing the concentration of blood in various areas about the circle of Willis[265]. The CT scan should reveal blood in at least 70% of ruptured aneurysm cases[198]. To be most effective, the CT scan should be done as soon as possible[171] because the washout diminishes chances of positive scan after the first several days. Van Gijn and Van Dongen[301] called attention to the presence of blood in the basal cisterns as almost certainly indicative of ruptured aneurysm. Kendall, Lee and Claveria[152] reported a high yield using the CT scan in the diagnosis of arteriovenous malformations, provided enhancement with contrast medium was used.

Wirth[329] has reported that CT scanning will not detect all instances of subarachnoid hemorrhage. The available estimates are as follows: aneurysm will be visible in 10% of cases; hemorrhage in 87% (provided scanning is performed within 5 days); ischemic lucency secondary to spasm in 10%; hydrocephalus in 54%.

The CT scan has been extremely valuable in aiding in the solution of the enigma of parenchymal hemorrhage versus subarachnoid hemorrhage[209]. Yet occasionally such differentiation is still not possible[272]. Repeating the CT scan as indicated will usually provide information regarding the size of the ventricles, the appearance of new blood in the subarachnoid space (cases of suspected rebleeding) and the development of ischemic zones in brain substance.

Spinal puncture

Although diagnostic lumbar puncture has been available since the time of Quincke[239] (1891) there appear to be uncertainties about the indications and contraindications for this procedure as well as the methods of examination of the spinal fluid once it has been obtained. Petito and Plum[231] in 1974 pointed out that the lumbar puncture has its greatest value in the identification of non-neoplastic processes. Hence, the possible presence of subarachnoid hemorrhage constitutes an important indication for spinal puncture if a mass lesion is not present. This is where the CT scan performs a valuable service in advance of the spinal fluid examination.

Once the spinal puncture is attempted, one certain way to cause confusion and consternation is to report uniformly bloody spinal fluid, when, in fact, the spinal puncture was a traumatic one. Thus, improper evaluation of the results at this point can lead to uncomfortable situations along the diagnostic pathway. Petito and Plum[231] emphasized the importance of distinguishing intrinsic from traumatically induced bleeding. If bloody spinal fluid is encountered, the operator should note closely as more fluid is withdrawn. In subarachnoid hemorrhage subsequent tubes of fluid will be as bloody as the first, while traumatic bleeding will tend to clear. Cell counts on the several specimens removed will verify this fact. In addition, the supernatant fluid of a centrifuged specimen should be examined as soon as possible. In subarachnoid hemorrhage the xanthochromic staining will be evidence. Shuttleworth *et al.*[271] have utilized the elevation of lactate values in the spinal fluid to indicate subarachnoid hemorrhage.

The physician should be reminded that various types of cellular response will be present during the first few weeks. After three weeks, if there is no further bleeding, the fluid may present the picture of aseptic meningitis, thus adding confusion to a meningeal syndrome if an earlier puncture was not performed. Such patients have been known to carry the diagnosis of 'viral meningitis' until another rupture occurs. Ito and Inaba[142] have described a method capable of detecting subarachnoid hemorrhage 15 to 17 weeks after its occurrence, through the demonstration of iron-positive cells in the spinal fluid. The physician should be reminded that hypoglycorrhachia sometimes occurs after subarachnoid hemorrhage. Vincent[305] reported an unusually high incidence of 70%. Attempts have been made to monitor fibrinolytic activity in the cerebrospinal fluid by means of serial assay of fibrin degradation products as a possible guide to rebleeding[185].

Cerebral angiography

The value of cerebral angiography has been documented and the procedure is now used universally as an important, moderately safe method of identifying the usual source of intracranial bleeding (*Figure 14.6*). However, identification of aneurysms and arteriovenous malformations is not always accomplished, as indicated previously. The incidence of normal cerebral angiography in patients with proven

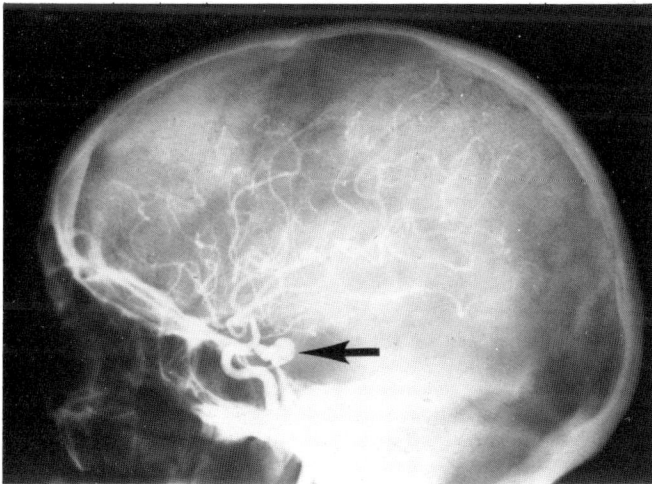

Figure 14.6 Carotid angiogram showing saccular aneurysm (arrow) arising from the junction of the internal carotid and posterior communicating arteries

subarachnoid hemorrhage is steadily declining. Levy[170] at one time reported a series of negative results totalling 46%. Figures of 22% to 27% were reported by Forster et al.[86] and Hayward[118]. The value of repeated studies[86] is illustrated by the remarkable report of Bohmfalk and Story[28] in which an aneurysm was visualized intermittently through five angiographic examinations. Previous observations of this nature had been made by Spetzler et al.[276] Subtraction techniques and multisection angiotomography[184] add to the diagnostic armamentarium. Occasionally a cerebral aneurysm will rupture during angiography[65, 157, 159].

Angiography is presently the most reliable method for identifying an intracranial aneurysm or arteriovenous malformation and for determining the presence or absence of vasospasm. This last item has become an important matter for the timing of surgery in aneurysmal patients. Carmody et al.[39] have called attention to the introduction of a new technique, intravenous angiography. The patient risk is said to be low though it is not yet known how often aneurysms may be missed[43].

Cerebral blood flow determinations

Considerable information is now available regarding cerebral blood flow after aneurysmal rupture. Kelly et al.[151] identified those patients with normal perfusion and those in whom perfusion was decreased and in whom operation should be delayed by radionuclide brain scanning.

Determination of cerebral blood flow after surgery[195], using the non-invasive ^{133}Xe clearance technique, indicated that the presence or absence of a postoperative rise in cerebral flow was correlated with the patient's level of consciousness after surgery. Ishii[141] also reported that abnormalities in the degree of flow correlated well with the clinical severity of the neurological defects.

Electroencephalography

Electroencephalography has not gained acclaim as a diagnostic procedure in subarachnoid hemorrhage. A moderate amount of literature has accumulated in this area[194a]. Nau and Bock[207] reported on 35 cases of subarachnoid hemorrhage which showed generalized slowing and focal abnormalities, due apparently to spasm.

Other methods

Olinger and Wasserman[219] reported on the use of an electronic stethoscope for the detection of cerebral aneurysms, vasospasm and arterial disease.

The role of positron emission tomography is being studied[76].

Central conduction time has been used as an index of ischemia in subarachnoid hemorrhage[290].

TREATMENT

General measures

As already indicated, patients with subarachnoid hemorrhage vary as to the severity of their illness. Many are critically ill, with several life-threatening complications. They are managed best in a major medical center where neurosurgeons, neurologists, radiologists and other experts are available and where careful monitoring can be carried out. The importance of skilled nursing care cannot be overemphasized[134, 210]. Plans should be made to transfer these patients to such a center, as soon as their condition permits, if there is a probability of survival for the next few hours. In a number of areas transfer by helicopter is now feasible.

During the acute phase in seriously ill patients, three objectives should take precedence[165]: (1) Recognition and treatment of those patients with a space-occupying intracranial hematoma. In the past the proper identification of this group of patients was very difficult and sometimes uncertain, even with the utilization of cerebral angiography. However, with the advent of computerized tomography this problem has been simplified. One should re-emphasize that in the presence of a mass lesion a spinal puncture should not be performed. (2) Identification of the cause of the stupor or coma and instituting necessary supportive measures to try to improve the patient's status. (3) Prevention of rebleeding. Many clinicians favor the use of antifibrinolytic therapy during this period following aneurysmal rupture, and some combine antifibrinolytic with antihypertensive therapy (p. 379).

The aim also is to preserve residual brain function and to prevent systemic complications. Very little tangible information is available on the true 'natural history' of subarachnoid hemorrhage, but the available figures indicate a drop-out of at least 50% up to this stage.

An impressive list of medical complications can be anticipated in this group of acutely ill patients. Weir[318] encountered 54% respiratory, 23% cardiovascular, 26% genitourinary, 3% gastrointestinal and 3% other complications in a series of 100 patients with ruptured aneurysms.

The usual monitoring procedures instituted in an intensive care unit or stroke unit are employed. The following conditions are monitored: arterial blood pressure; temperature; electrocardiogram and ventilatory measurements. Central venous pressure and pulmonary artery wedge pressures as well as intracranial pressure measurements may be indicated at times. Vital signs are recorded every hour.

The patient should be placed at absolute bed rest and visitors should be restricted. The patient may need protection so that he does not fall out of bed. Anti-embolic stockings are used.

The laboratory studies should include, in addition to the CT scan, an X-ray examination of the chest. Hematological and biochemical studies are indicated, and should include serum and urinary osmolality[320].

Seriously ill patients will require an indwelling catheter. Stool softeners are indicated as part of the care of the bowels. Headache will require codeine or other analgesics. An efficient sedative is phenobarbital or diazepam. Convulsions can usually be controlled with phenytoin or phenobarbital. Appropriate antibiotics will be indicated if infection occurs. For special situations antiedema agents such as dexamethasone or mannitol are used. Volume expanders may also be indicated.

Respiratory management

During the state of severe depression of consciousness respiratory support is essential; if the patient is in coma, proper attention to the airway is mandatory. There is always the possibility that the patient may have aspirated vomitus. If there are ventilatory problems the patient may be hypoxic and hypocapnic. The therapeutic goals should be the prevention of progressive respiratory complications (accumulation of secretions, aspiration atelectasis, pneumonia), and the maintenance of an arterial PO_2 of 70 mmHg or more.

Blood pressure

Fluctuations in blood pressure have already been discussed. The usual course is in the direction of hypertensive levels after the bleeding episode. The therapeutic objective would be to maintain systemic arterial pressure of such grade that blood flow to the brain is optimal in the presence of vasospasm and/or increased intracranial pressure, yet not be so high as to increase the chance of re-rupture of the aneurysm or other lesion producing the hemorrhage. Most clinicians prefer to maintain blood pressure at an average or 'nearly normal' value, with the knowledge that there is an unpredictable relationship between intracranial pressure and systemic arterial pressure[33]. Antihypertensive therapy is best performed with rapidly acting and reversible preparations such as parenterally administered hydralazine hydrochloride. Extreme measures such as the use of intravenous nitroprusside may be necessary, but usually treatment of pain, agitation and intracranial pressure will induce reduction in the blood pressure.

Fluids and electrolytes

Whenever fluid intake is limited, especially when the level of consciousness is impaired, fluids will have to be given by the intravenous route and alimentation provided by nasogastric tube. Dextrose and sodium chloride are administered in doses of 30 to 50 ml kg 24 hours. The caloric intake should be at least 2000 calories daily. Care must be taken to identify and treat the hyponatremia associated with inappropriate secretion of antidiuretic hormone[88, 330]. Such inappropriate secretion probably occurs in a high percentage of cases of subarachnoid hemorrhage. Careful attention to fluid intake and electrolyte balance will prevent hyponatremia from occurring in many. Joynt, Feibel and Sladek[145] studied a group of stroke patients, including four with subarachnoid hemorrhage, and found the antidiuretic hormone levels significantly elevated, but hyponatremia was not observed. They cautioned that fluid intake and electrolyte levels should be closely monitored. Treatment of this condition involves careful water restriction.

In contrast to inappropriate secretion of antidiuretic hormone, diabetes insipidus occurs in less than 5% of patients following subarachnoid hemorrhage. In most instances it is transient. The treatment of this condition consists of replacement of fluids and electrolytes and the administration of aqueous pitressin[269].

Blood volume

Hypovolemia is not an uncommon complication of subarachnoid hemorrhage. Maroon and Nelson[180] found a decrease in red blood cell mass and total blood volume. Replacement therapy should be considered in such cases.

Antifibrinolytic therapy

The possible effectiveness of antifibrinolytic therapy in reducing the incidence of early rebleeding from ruptured aneurysms was first reported in the 1960s[3]. In spite of a number of favorable reports concerning the use of aminocaproic acid and tranexamic acid, the use of these preparations remains controversial because some studies have shown no benefit from antifibrinolytic therapy while other reports indicate complications from this form of treatment.

Following the encouraging report by Mullan and Dawley[202] in 1968, the Co-operative Aneurysm Group embarked on a randomized treatment program[211] which at first yielded a death rate of 5.8% from the use of antifibrinolysins during the two-week period following a rupture, compared to those on drug induced hypotension with a death rate of 28.9%. In a later study[212] the death rate was found to be 11.6% within the 14-day period. A subsequent report by Adams *et al.*[8] placed the rebleeding rate at 10% among the treated patients and the overall mortality at 10.7%. Serious complications from the use of this drug were infrequent. Favorable reports have come from Chowdhary *et al.*[42]. A recent report by Hasegawa, Watanabe and Ishii[111] indicated that recently, due to advances made in monitoring the effect of antifibrinolytic therapy, the incidence of rebleeding while the patient is awaiting surgery has been reduced to 2.8%.

Not all reports are favorable, however[93, 150, 270]. One of the latest reviews is that of Ameen and Illingworth[15] who reported they could find no significant difference in recurrent bleeding between treated cases and controls. The comprehensive review by Ramirez-Lassepas[241] concludes with the statement that 'the data do not support the contention that antifibrinolytic therapy has a favourable influence on the natural history of aneurysmal SAH.'

Brain swelling and intracranial hypertension

One of the main objectives in the management of patients with a space-occupying hematoma is early diagnosis and surgical treatment. Reference has already been made to the value of the CT scan and cerebral angiography in this condition.

Various methods have been utilized to reduce increased intracranial pressure[154]. There is a greater availability and safety of devices for the continuous recording of pressure than formerly. Several methods of therapy can be utilized: corticosteroids in large doses; or hyperosmolar agents, such as mannitol; hyperventilation and ventricular drainage. Kenning, Toutant and Saunders[153] monitored intracranial pressure and found a marked diminution in intracranial pressure when the patient was placed in a sitting or semi-sitting position. Van Gilder and Torner[302] reported that patients with persistently elevated intracranial pressure had a 58% mortality over a 28-day period.

Vascular spasm

It is well known that rupture of an intracranial aneurysm is followed by cerebral vasospasm in a significant percentage of cases. The implications and ramifications of spasm are many. One very important matter is the proper identification of spasm before operation on an aneurysm is contemplated. For example, Cooper *et al.*[47] found that in 35 Grade I patients, only one of 28 patients in whom spasm was absent or mild had an unsatisfactory outcome, while four of seven Grade I patients with moderate to severe angiographic spasm had an unsatisfactory outcome.

Reports on attempts to prevent and treat vasospasm are legion[149, 237, 322]. Therapeutic approaches have been recently reviewed by Boullin[30] and by Fleisher and Tindall[80]. There is presently no specific therapy for this condition. After the aneurysm has been clipped attention can be directed to the use of volume expanders and drugs which elevate blood pressure.

Surgical treatment

Aneurysms

Present methods of surgical therapy have brightened the outlook for the good-risk patient with aneurysmal subarachnoid hemorrhage and for certain poor-risk patients who require emergency surgery for evacuation of a life threatening hematoma, for example. The objective of surgical intervention is usually prophylactic – to reduce the possibility of rebleeding and death[285, 326].

Drake[64] has made note of the fact that in a Japanese study only 1.6 aneurysmal cases/100 000 population per year were treated surgically. The figure for Ontario in 1977 was estimated as 3.6/100 000 per year. This means that there is a conspicuous fall-out of patients who do not come under the care of the surgeon. It is well known that surgery does little to save the 40% or more of patients who die from the first recognized hemorrhage. In the Rochester, Minnesota, study 32% were Grade 4 or 5 among those who survived long enough to receive medical attention[232].

The technical advances, however, have been outstanding, particularly through the use of the operating microscope and improvements in anesthesia. At the present time surgical treatment for patients in good-risk status carries a mortality of no more than 5% in experienced hands[64]. When less selection is exercised the 14-day mortality from surgery may approach 18%. Both of these figures are encouraging in terms of operative results when comparison is made with the past[194]. For example, in the 851 aneurysmal cases studied in the period 1970–1974 in Denmark[242], 16% corresponded to Hunt's Grades 4 and 5, and 76% were found suitable for surgery. Five hundred and sixty-seven patients underwent surgery, with a mortality of 32%. In another report, that of the Co-operative Aneurysm Study[7], 249 patients underwent surgery during the period 1974–1977. There was a 36.2% mortality. The surgical complications in 1000 cases of intracranial aneurysms were reviewed by Takaku *et al.*[293].

EARLY SURGERY VERSUS LATER SURGERY

The optimal timing for intracranial surgery to correct a ruptured aneurysm of the circle of Willis is one of the major controversies in neurosurgery today. There are presently a number of reports in the literature to the effect that neurosurgeons are taking another look at the possibility of surgery within the first few days after the bleeding episode[173]. Drake[64] has discussed the various options in his excellent 1981 review and warns against indiscriminate early operation. Advocates of early surgery have also presented their case. As early as 1961 Pool[234] indicated that the mortality from early operation need not be prohibitively high in young patients in good condition, but under the other circumstances too early an operation could lead to a forbiddingly high mortality rate. Hunt and Miller[133] in 1976 suggested that 'Early intervention is justified in a small percentage of cases with aneurysmal hemorrhage' and indicated that careful selection of good-risk patients was essential. Suzuki, Onuma and Yoshimoto[289] called attention to their results, namely that mortality rates resulting from operation on the first and second days were low in comparison with those done in the remaining days of the week. Samson *et al.*[259] found no significant difference in mortality rates in early or late operation in good grade patients. Adams[2] reported that in 100 cases in which surgery was done within one week after the bleed the mortality was 22%. Operations during the second week carried a mortality of 5% and in the third week none died from the operation. The report by Weir and Aronyk[319] analyzed retrospectively a group of 224 patients with supratentorial aneurysm admitted on the day following their subarachnoid hemorrhage. Seventy-five (34%) died without a definitive operation. There was no significant difference in the postoperative and management mortality rates when patients were categorized by time of operation, except for the increased management mortality for the more seriously ill patients who were operated upon late. An international co-operative study has been initiated to try to cast light on this controversial subject[251, 252].

ENDOVASCULAR METHODS

According to Mullan, Duda and Patronas[203] the use of balloon catheters in medicine is not new. They discussed various applications of this technique in the treatment of giant aneurysms and fistulas. Serbinenko[267] reported the use of balloon techniques in 600 examples of vascular pathology such as arteriovenous and arterial aneurysms. This technique has not received wide application.

Arteriovenous malformations

As a general rule, arteriovenous malformations will become symptomatic before the age of 40, either through rupture or the production of convulsions. The hemorrhage occurs abruptly and is usually into the parenchyma with 'spillage' into the subarachnoid space. This accounts for the fact that focal signs are usually much more evident with this disorder than with aneurysm, and the amount of subarachnoid hemorrhage is usually much less than one encounters in ruptured saccular aneurysm. If the patient has a combination of aneurysm and arteriovenous malformation, and if the aneurysm is proximal to the arteriovenous malformation, the aneurysm should be corrected prior to therapy of the malformation. Otherwise the stress placed on the aneurysm will cause it to rupture.

Seizures are almost as common as hemorrhage. The convulsions may be generalized, focal or a combination. Another phenomenon is a slowly progressing neurological deficit such as a homonymous hemianopsia. Headaches can be associated but are usually difficult to single out as being indicative of an arteriovenous malformation. Sometimes the patient is aware of a cranial bruit.

The diagnosis may be suspected by inspection of plain skull films, in which one finds areas of abnormal calcification. The dynamic scan will usually demonstrate the lesion. The CT scan will usually show a high-density enhancing lesion with or without calcification. Intracerebral hemorrhage will be demonstrable readily in the

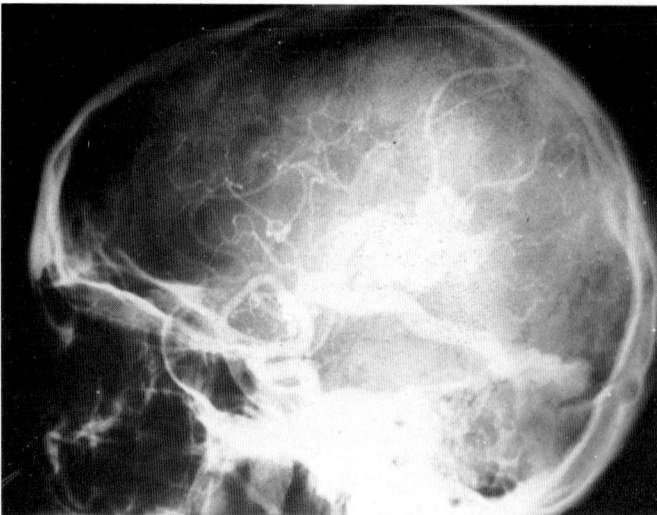

Figure 14.7 Angiogram showing a large arteriovenous malformation

CT scan. The most informative diagnostic test will be cerebral angiography (*Figure 14.7*); the complete study would include the malformation itself and a demonstration of the afferent and efferent vascular supply, as well as the rapid circulation time.

In the case of the patient who has bled, the medical management and grading of clinical status are similar to those for aneurysms. There is not the urgency for surgery that one encounters in intracranial aneurysms, unless there is a large intracerebral hematoma which requires urgent evacuation.

The objective of surgery is to eliminate the malformation. Total excision is now possible in approximately 75% of cases, and the mortality rate from surgery is now quoted at 5%.

Embolization with sialastic spheres has been proposed as a method of treatment, with or without eventual surgery. Kvam, Michelson and Quest[162] indicated that 157 patients had undergone artificial embolization at one institution. The intravascular use of a rapidly polymerizing acrylic compound such as isobutyl-2-cyanocrylate (IBC) has also been reported[257].

The employment of radiotherapy, including conventional and proton-beam types, has been utilized in the treatment of vascular malformations, particularly those deemed inoperable. Stereotactic radiosurgery has been utilized[18], stemming from the original reports of Leksell[169] in 1951. Stein and Wolpert[280] cite radio-necrosis and mortality from recurrent hemorrhage as the chief disadvantages of this form of therapy.

Primary intracerebral hemorrhage

The outstanding feature of this disorder is the rapid development of a focal neurological defect, often preceded by a headache and resulting in rapid impairment or loss of consciousness in an individual who has a history of hypertension. Thalamic and putaminal hemorrhages can rupture into the adjacent ventricle, pontine hemorrhage rapidly destroys vital functions and hemorrhage into the cerebellum can become rapidly fatal because of pressure on brain stem structures as well as a production of hydrocephalus.

The diagnosis of intracranial hemorrhage has been revolutionized by the use of the CT scan. The location and extent of the lesions are evident on the unenhanced views. In the modern era it is often unnecessary to perform a spinal fluid examination because one is dealing with a mass lesion. The spinal fluid is not always bloody. One recent report (Harrison[109]) indicated that in 30 cases of cerebral hemorrhage in which the spinal fluid was examined, 18 showed gross blood, nine revealed xanthochromia or microscopic evidence of bleeding and three (10%) had clear spinal fluid.

For the most part, the management of such patients follows the pattern suggested for aneurysms. Surgery is utilized for special situations such as acute cerebellar hemorrhage[92, 125] and certain hematomas in the subcortex of the non-dominant cerebral hemisphere (Hoff[125]) and rarely in the putamen of the non-dominant side.

PROGNOSIS

Reference has been made several times in this chapter to the high mortality of subarachnoid hemorrhage. In 1950 Hyland[137] indicated that there was a mortality of slightly over 50% in the attacks which brought patients to the hospital. Winn *et al.*[328] reported on the survival statistics after six months in a follow-up of 213 patients, 37 of whom died from recurrent hemorrhage during the 20 years of follow-up. An additional 25 patients died of causes unassociated with late rebleeding.

Drake[64] has indicated that 25 000 aneurysms rupture yearly in the United States, and 3000 yearly in Canada. About 8500 of this group of 28 000 are operated upon. Of the 8500 some 5000 per year can be considered recovered and protected from further bleeding.

It is most difficult to obtain accurate figures on morbidity. For example, Fortuny and Prieto Valiente[87] reported that only 40% of their surgically treated patients claimed to be feeling as well as before the operation. In the Rasmussen *et al.*[242] report follow-up studies showed 52% of the survivors to be fully capacitated, 20% partially capacitated and 28% were incapacitated.

CONCLUSIONS

(1) Nontraumatic subarachnoid hemorrhage remains a serious disease, with high mortality and morbidity rates.
(2) In spite of the remarkable advances in surgical treatment of aneurysms, only one-fifth of these patients are presently protected against further rebleeding.
(3) Means should be developed to identify the person who is 'at risk' before the subarachnoid hemorrhage occurs.
(4) The profession should be made alert to the necessity for prompt attention to those patients who have experienced minor episodes or warning symptoms.

References

1 ABERFELD, D. C. and RAO, K. R. Familial arteriovenous malformation of the brain. *Neurology*, **31**, 184–186 (1981)
2 ADAMS, C. B. T., LOACH, A. B. and O'LAOIRE, S. A. Intracranial aneurysms: analysis of results of microsurgery. *British Medical Journal*, **2**, 607–609 (1976)
3 ADAMS, H. P. Jr. Current status of antifibrinolytic therapy for treatment of patients with aneurysmal subarachnoid hemorrhage. *Stroke*, **13**, 256–259 (1982)
4 ADAMS, H. P. Jr., SUBBIAH, B. and BOSCH, E. P. Neurologic aspects of hereditary hemorrhagic telangiectasia. *Archives of Neurology*, **34**, 101–104 (1977)
5 ADAMS, H. P. Jr., JERGENSON, D. D., KASSELL, N. F. and SAHS, A. L. Pitfalls in the recognition of subarachnoid hemorrhage. *Journal of the American Medical Association*, **244**, 794–796 (1980)
6 ADAMS, H. P. Jr., KASSELL, N. F. and SAHS, A. L. Intracranial aneurysms and subarachnoid hemorrhage. *Journal of the Iowa Medical Society*, **70**, 19–21 (1980)
7 ADAMS, H. P. Jr., KASSELL, N. F., TORNER, J. C., NIBBELINK, D. W. and SAHS, A. L. Early management of aneurysmal subarachnoid hemorrhage. A report of the Co-operative Aneurysm Study. *Journal of Neurosurgery*, **54**, 141–145 (1981)

8 ADAMS, H. P. Jr., NIBBELINK, D. W., TORNER, J. C. and SAHS, A. L. Antifibrinolytic therapy in patients with aneurysmal subarachnoid hemorrhage. A report of the Co-operative Aneurysm Study. *Archives of Neurology*, **38**, 25–29 (1981)

9 ADAMS, H. P. Jr. and SAHS, A. L. Aneurysmal subarachnoid hemorrhage. *Modern Concepts of Cardiovascular Disease*, **50**, 47–52 (1981)

10 ALLCOCK, J. M. and DRAKE, C. G. Ruptured intracranial aneurysms – the role of arterial spasm. *Journal of Neurosurgery*, **22**, 21–29 (1965)

11 ALLCOCK, J. M. and CANHAM, P. B. Angiographic study of the growth of intracranial aneurysms. *Journal of Neurosurgery*, **45**, 617–621 (1976)

12 ALMEIDA, G. M., PINDARO, J., PLESE, B., BIANCO, E. and SHIBATA, H. K. Intracranial arterial aneurysms in infancy and childhood. *Child's Brain*, **3**, 193–199 (1977)

13 ALVORD, E. C. Jr., LOESER, J. D., BAILEY, W. L. and COPASS, M. K. Subarachnoid hemorrhage due to ruptured aneurysms. A simple method of estimating prognosis. *Archives of Neurology*, **27**, 273–284 (1972)

14 AMACHER, A. L. and DRAKE, C. G. Cerebral arterial aneurysms in infancy, childhood and adolescence. *Child's Brain*, **1**, 72–80 (1975)

15 AMEEN, A. A. and ILLINGWORTH, R. Anti-fibrinolytic treatment in the preoperative management of subarachnoid hemorrhage caused by ruptured intracranial aneurysm. *Journal of Neurology, Neurosurgery and Psychiatry*, **44**, 220–226 (1981)

16 AMINOFF, M. G. Spinal subarachnoid hemorrhage and haematomyelia. In *Spinal Angiomas*, edited by M. J. Aminoff, 43–53. Oxford: Basil Blackwell and Mott Ltd. (1976)

17 ANDERSON, R. M. and BLACKWOOD, W. The association of arteriovenous angioma and saccular aneurysm of the arteries of the brain. *Journal of Pathology and Bacteriology*, **77**, 101–110 (1959)

18 BACKLUND, E.-O. Stereotactic radiosurgery in intracranial tumours and vascular malformations. In *Advances and Technical Standards in Neurosurgery*, Volume 6, edited by H. Krayenbühl, *et al.*, 1–37. New York: Springer-Verlag (1979)

19 BARNES, A. D. Subarachnoid haemorrhage. *British Journal of Hospital Medicine*, **19**, 414 (1978)

20 BARNETT, H. J. M. Some clinical features of intracranial aneurysms. *Clinical Neurosurgery*, **16**, 43–71 (1969)

21 BARRON, K. D. and FERGUSSON, G. Intracranial hemorrhage as a complication of anticoagulant therapy. *Neurology*, **9**, 447–455 (1959)

22 BEADLES, C. F. Aneurisms of the larger cerebral arteries. *Brain*, **30**, 285–336 (1907)

23 BINDER, H., GERSTENBRAND, F., JELLINGER, K., KRENN, J. and WATZEK, C. The symptomatology with the most severe clinical course of spontaneous subarachnoid hemorrhage. *Journal of Neurology*, **222**, 119–129 (1979)

24 BINGHAM, W. F. Treatment of mycotic intracranial aneurysms. *Journal of Neurosurgery*, **46**, 428–437 (1977)

25 BIUMI, F. Observationes Anatomicae. Observation V. Carotis ad Receptaculum Vieussenii Aneurysmatica, etc. In *Thesarus Dissertationum, Ludguni Batavorum*, Volume 3, edited by E. Sandifort, 373–379. S. and J. Luchtmans (1778)

26 BLACKALL, J. Observations on the Nature and Cure of Dropsies. London, 1813. Cited by Bull, J. A Short History of Intracranial Aneurysms. *London Clinic Medical Journal*, **3**, 47–62 (1962)

27 BOHMFALK, G. L., STORY, J. L., WISSINGER, J. P. and BROWN, W. E. Jr. Bacterial intracranial aneurysm. *Journal of Neurosurgery*, **48**, 369–382 (1978)

28 BOHMFALK, G. L. and STORY, J. L. Intermittent appearances of a ruptured cerebral aneurysm on sequential angiograms. Case report. *Journal of Neurosurgery*, **52**, 263–265 (1980)

29 BOTTERELL, E. H., LOUGHEED, W. M., SCOTT, J. W. and VANDEWATER, S. L. Hypothermia, and interruption of carotid, or carotid and vertebral circulation, in the surgical management of intracranial aneurysms. *Journal of Neurosurgery*, **13**, 1–42 (1956)

30 BOULLIN, D. J. *Cerebral Vasospasm*, 337 pp. New York: John Wiley and Sons (1980)

31 BOYD-WILSON, J. S. The association of cerebral angiomas with intracranial aneurysms. *Journal of Neurology, Neurosurgery and Psychiatry*, **22**, 218–223 (1958)

32 BRINTON, W. Cases of cerebral aneurysms. *Transactions of the Pathological Society of London*, **3**, 49 (1850–1852)

33 BRUCE, D. A., LANGFITT, T. W., MILLER, J. D., SCHUTZ, H., VAPALAHTI, M. P., STANEK, A. and GOLDBERG, H. I. Regional cerebral blood flow, intracranial pressure, and brain metabolism in comatose patients. *Journal of Neurosurgery*, **38**, 131–144 (1973)

34 BULL, J. A. A short history of intracranial aneurysms. *London Clinic Medical Journal*, **3**, 47–62 (1962)

35 CAJANDER, S. and HASSLER, O. Enzymatic destruction of the elastic lamella at the mouth of cerebral berry aneurysm? *Acta Neurologica Scandinavica*, **53**, 171–181 (1976)

36 CALDWELL, A. and KENNEDY, R. Migraine headache with preheadache retinal and visual disturbances in a case of congenital vascular anomaly and subarachnoid hemorrhage. *Archives of Neurology and Psychiatry*, **69**, 397–398 (1953)

37 CALVERT, J. M. Premonitory symptoms and signs of subarachnoid hemorrhage. *Medical Journal of Australia*, **1**, 651–657 (1966)

38 CAMPBELL, G. J. and ROACH, M. R. Fenestrations in the internal elastic lamina at bifurcations of human cerebral arteries. *Stroke*, **12**, 489–496 (1981)

39 CARMODY, R. F., SMITH, J. R. L., SEEGER, J. F. and WEINSTEIN, P. R. Intravenous cerebral angiography: early clinical experience. *Arizona Medicine*, **38**, 349–350 (1981)

40 CHANGARIS, D. G., POWERS, J. M., PEROT, P. L. Jr., HUNGERFORD, D. and NEAL, G. B. Subependymoma presenting as subarachnoid hemorrhage. Case report. *Journal of Neurosurgery*, **55**, 643–645 (1981)

41 CHARCOT, J. M. and BOUCHARD, C. Nouvelles recherches sur la pathogénie de l'hémorrhagie cérébrale. *Archives de Physiologie* (Paris), **1**, 110–127, 643–665, 725–754 (1868)

42 CHOWDHARY, U. M., CAREY, P. C. and HUSSEIN, M. M. Prevention of early recurrence of spontaneous subarachnoid hemorrhage by ε-aminocaproic acid. *Lancet*, **1**, 741–743 (1979)

43 CHRISTENSON, P. C., OVITT, T. W., FISCHER, H. D. III, FROST, M. M., NUDELMAN, S. and ROEHRIG, H. Intravenous angiography using digital video subtraction: intra-

venous cervicocerebrovascular angiography. *American Journal of Roentgenology*, **135**, 1145–1152 (1980)

44 CIONGOLI, A. K. and POSER, C. M. Pulmonary edema secondary to subarachnoid hemorrhage. *Neurology*, **22**, 867–870 (1972)

45 CLOWER, B. R., SMITH, R. R., HAINING, J. L. and LOCKARD, J. Constrictive endarteropathy following experimental subarachnoid hemorrhage. *Stroke*, **12**, 501–508 (1981)

46 COLE, F. M. and YATES, P. O. The occurrence and significance of intracerebral micro-aneurysms. *Journal of Pathology and Bacteriology*, **93**, 393–411 (1967)

47 COOPER, P. R., SHUCART, W. A., TENNER, M. and HUSSAIN, S. Preoperative arteriographic spasm and outcome from aneurysm operation. *Neurosurgery*, **7**, 587 –592 (1980)

48 CROMPTON, M. R. Hypothalamic lesions following the rupture of cerebral berry aneurysms. *Brain*, **86**, 301–314 (1963)

49 CROMPTON, M. R. Cerebral infarction following the rupture of cerebral berry aneurysms. *Brain*, **87**, 263–280 (1964)

50 CROWELL, R. M. and ZERVAS, N. T. Management of intracranial aneurysm. *Medical Clinics of North America*, **63**, 695–713 (1979)

51 CRUICKSHANK, J. M., NEIL-DWYER, G. and STOTT, A. W. Possible role of catecholamines, cortiocosteroids and potassium in production of electrocardiographic abnormalities associated with subarachnoid haemorrhage. *British Heart Journal*, **36**, 697–706 (1974)

52 CUSHING, H. and BAILEY, P. *Tumors Arising from the Blood Vessels of the Brain. Angiomatous Malformations and Hemangioblastomas*, 219 pp. Springfield, Illinois: Charles C. Thomas (1928)

53 DALGAARD, O. Z. Bilateral polycystic disease of the kidneys. Aneurysms of the basal arteries of the brain in persons with polycystic kidneys. *Acta Medica Scandinavica*, **158** (Suppl. 328) 186–190 (1957)

54 DAMASIO, H., SEABRA-GOMES, R., daSILVA, J. P., DAMASIO, A. R. and ANTUNES, J. L. Multiple cerebral aneurysms and cardiac myxoma. *Archives of Neurology*, **32**, 269–270 (1975)

55 DANDY, W. E. Arteriovenous aneurysm of the brain. *Archives of Surgery*, **17**, 190–243 (1928)

56 DANDY, W. E. *Intracranial Arterial Aneurysms*, 147 pp. Ithaca, New York: Comstock Publishing Company, Inc. (1944)

57 DAVIS, J. M., DAVIS, K. R. and CROWELL, R. M. Subarachnoid hemorrhage secondary to ruptured intracranial aneurysm: prognostic significance of cranial CT. *American Journal of Roentgenology*, **134**, 711–715 (1980)

58 DELANEY, P. and ESTES, M. Intracranial hemorrhage with amphetamine abuse. *Neurology*, **30**, 1125–1128 (1980)

59 DELONG, W. B. The diagnostic pitfalls of subarachnoid hemorrhage from intracranial aneurysms. *Western Journal of Medicine*, **123**, 92–100 (1975)

60 DIONIS, M. *Dissertation sur la Mort Subite et sur la Catalepsie*, 2nd edition. Paris: Laurent D'Houry (1718)

61 DOSHI, R. and NEIL-DWYER, G. A clinicopathological study of patients following a subarachnoid hemorrhage. *Journal of Neurosurgery*, **52**, 295–301 (1980)

62 DOTT, N. Intracranial aneurysmal formations. *Clinical Neurosurgery*, **16**, 1–16 (1969)

63 DRAKE, C. G. Cerebral arteriovenous malformations: considerations for and experience with surgical treatment in 166 cases. *Clinical Neurosurgery*, **26**, 145–208 (1979)

64 DRAKE, C. G. Management of cerebral aneurysm. *Stroke*, **12**, 273–283 (1981)

65 DUBLIN, A. B. and FRENCH, B. N. Cerebral aneurysmal rupture during angiography with confirmation by computed tomography: a review of intra-angiographic aneurysmal rupture. *Surgical Neurology*, **13**, 19–26 (1980)

66 DU BOULAY, G. Distribution of spasm in the intracranial arteries after subarachnoid haemorrhage. *Acta Radiologica: Diagnosis*, **1**, 257–266 (1963)

67 ECKER, A. and RIEMENSCHNEIDER, P. A. Arteriographic demonstration of spasm of the intracranial arteries. With special reference to saccular arterial aneurysms. *Journal of Neurosurgery*, **8**, 660–667 (1951)

68 EDWARDS, K. R. Hemorrhagic complications of cerebral arteritis. *Archives of Neurology*, **34**, 549–552 (1977)

69 ELLINGTON, E. and MARGOLIS, G. Block of arachnoid villus by subarachnoid hemorrhage. *Journal of Neurosurgery*, **30**, 651–657 (1969)

70 ESTANOL, B., RODRIGUEZ, A., CONTE, G., ALEMAN, J. M., LOYO, M. and PIZZUTO, J. Intracranial venous thrombosis in young women. *Stroke*, **10**, 680–684 (1979)

71 ESTANOL, B. V., BADUI DERGEL, E., CESARMAN, E., MARIN SAN MARTIN, O., LOYO, M., VARGAS LUGO, B. and PEREZ ORTEGA, R. Cardiac arrhythmias associated with subarachnoid hemorrhage: prospective study. *Neurosurgery*, **5**, 675–680 (1979)

72 EVERETT, B. A., KUSSKE, J. A. and PRIBRAM, H. W. Anticoagulants and intracerebral hemorrhage from an unsuspected meningioma. *Surgical Neurology*, **11**, 233–235 (1979)

73 FAHMY, J. A., KNUDSEN, V. and ANDERSEN, S. R. Intraocular haemorrhage following subarachnoid haemorrhage. *Acta Ophthalmologica*, **47**, 550–559 (1969)

74 FEARNSIDES, E. G. Intracranial aneurysms. *Brain*, **39**, 224–296 (1916)

75 FEINDEL, W. Thomas Willis (1621–1675) the founder of neurology. *Canadian Medical Association Journal*, **87**, 289–296 (1962)

76 FEINDEL, W., YAMAMOTO, Y. L., THOMPSON, Ch., LITTLE, J. and MEYER, E. Positron emission tomography. A new method for examination of the circulation and metabolism of the brain in man. *Acta Neurochirurgica (Wien)*, **46**, 307–308 (1979)

77 FISHER, C. M., ROBERSON, G.H. and OJEMANN, R. G. Cerebral vasospasm with ruptured saccular aneurysm – the clinical manifestations. *Neurosurgery*, **1**, 245–248 (1977)

78 FISHER, A. and ABOUL-NASR, H. T. Delayed nonfatal pulmonary edema following subarachnoid hemorrhage. Case report. *Journal of Neurosurgery*, **51**, 856–859 (1979)

79 FISHER, C. M., KISTLER, J. P. and DAVIS, J. M. The relation of cerebral vasospasm to subarachnoid blood visualized by computerized tomographic scanning. *Neurosurgery*, **6**, 1–9 (1980)

80 FLEISCHER, A. S. and TINDALL, G. T. Cerebral vasospasm following aneurysm rupture. A protocol for therapy and prophylaxis. *Journal of Neurosurgery*, **52**, 149–152 (1980)

81 FLETCHER, T. M., TAVERAS, J. M. and POOL, J. L. Cerebral vasospasm in angiography for intracranial aneurysms. Incidence and significance in one hundred consecutive angiograms. *Archives of Neurology*, **1**, 38–47 (1959)

82 FODY, E. P., NETSKY, M. G. and MRAK, R. E. Subarachnoid spinal hemorrhage in a case of systemic lupus erythematosus. *Archives of Neurology*, **37**, 173–174 (1980)

83 FOGELHOLM, R. Subarachnoid hemorrhage in Middle-Finland: incidence, early prognosis and indications for neurosurgical treatment. *Stroke*, **12**, 296–301 (1981)

84 FORBES, H. S. The cerebral circulation. I. Observation and measurement of pial vessels. *Archives of Neurology and Psychiatry*, **19**, 751–761 (1928)

85 FORBUS, W. D. On the origin of miliary aneurysms of the superficial cerebral arteries. *Bulletin of the Johns Hopkins Hospital*, **47**, 239–284 (1930)

86 FORSTER, D. M. C., STEINER, L., HAKANSON, S. and BERGVALL, U. The value of repeat pan-angiography in cases of unexplained subarachnoid hemorrhage. *Journal of Neurosurgery*, **48**, 712–716 (1978)

87 FORTUNY, L. A. I. and PRIETO-VALIENTE, L. Long-term prognosis in surgically treated intracranial aneurysms. Part 2: morbidity. *Journal of Neurosurgery*, **54**, 35–43 (1981)

88 FOX, J. L., FALIK, J. L. and SHALHOUB, R. J. Neurosurgical hyponatremia: the role of inappropriate diuresis. *Journal of Neurosurgery*, **34**, 506–514 (1971)

89 FOX, J. L. and KO, J. P. Cerebral vasospasm: a clinical observation. *Surgical Neurology*, **10**, 269–275 (1978)

90 FRANKEL, K. Relation of migraine to cerebral aneurysm. *Archives of Neurology and Psychiatry*, **63**, 195–204 (1950)

91 FRAZEE, J. G., CAHAN, L. D. and WINTER, J. Bacterial intracranial aneurysms. *Journal of Neurosurgery*, **53**, 633–641 (1980)

92 FREIDBERG, S. R. Treatment of intracranial hemorrhage. *Primary Care*, **6**, 805–812 (1979)

93 GELMERS, H. J. Prevention of recurrence of spontaneous subarachnoid hemorrhage by tranexamic acid. *Acta Neurochirurgica*, **52**, 45–50 (1980)

94 GEROSA, M., LICATA, C., FIORE, D. L. and IRACI, G. Intracranial aneurysms of childhood. *Child's Brain*, **6**, 295–302 (1980)

95 GILLINGHAM, F. J. The management of ruptured intracranial aneurysm. *Annals of the Royal College of Surgeons of England*, **23**, 89–117 (1958)

96 GIORDANO, D. Contributo alla cura delle lesione traumatiche ed al trepanzione del cranio. *Osservatore, Torino*, **41**, 5–15 (1890)

97 GLASS, B. and ABBOTT, K. H. Subarachnoid hemorrhage consequent to intracranial tumors: review of literature and report of seven cases. *Archives of Neurology and Psychiatry*, **73**, 369–379 (1955)

98 GOLDSTEIN, S. J. and TIBBS, P. A. Recurrent subarachnoid hemorrhage complicating cerebral arterial ectasia. Case report. *Journal of Neurosurgery*, **55**, 139–142 (1981)

99 GOLDZIEHER, J. A. and LISA, J. R. Gross cerebral hemorrhage and vascular lesions in acute tuberculous meningitis and meningo-encephalitis. *American Journal of Pathology*, **23**, 133–141 (1947)

100 GORAN, A., CIMINELLO, V. J. and FISHER, R. G. Hemorrhage into meningiomas. *Archives of Neurology*, **13**, 65–69 (1965)

101 GRAF, C. J. and ROSSI, N. P. Pulmonary edema and the central nervous system: a clinico-pathological study. *Surgical Neurology*, **4**, 319–325 (1975)

102 GREEN, L. N. Progeria with carotid artery aneurysms. Report of a case. *Archives of Neurology*, **38**, 659–661 (1981)

103 GROCH, S. N., SAYRE, G. P. and HECK, F. J. Cerebral hemorrhage in leukemia. *Archives of Neurology*, **2**, 439–451 (1960)

104 GRUBB, R. L. Jr., RAICHLE, M. E., PHELPS, M. E. and RATCHESON, R. A. Effects of increased intracranial pressure on cerebral blood volume, blood flow, and oxygen utilization in monkeys. *Journal of Neurosurgery*, **43**, 385–398 (1975)

105 GULL, W. Cases of aneurism of the cerebral vessels. *Guy's Hospital Reports*, **5**, (Series 3) 281–304 (1859)

106 GURDJIAN, E. S. and WEBSTER, J. E. *Head Injuries. Mechanisms, Diagnosis and Management.* Boston: Little, Brown and Co. (1958)

107 HAMBY, W. B. *Intracranial Aneurysms*, 564 pp. Springfield, Illinois: Charles C. Thomas (1952)

108 HAMILL, R. C. Report of a case of melanosis of the brain, cord and meninges. *Journal of Nervous and Mental Disease*, **35**, 594 (1908)

109 HARRISON, M. J. Clinical distinction of cerebral haemorrhage and cerebral infarction. *Postgraduate Medical Journal*, **56**, 629–632 (1980)

110 HART, R. G., BYER, J. A., SLAUGHTER, J. R., HEWETT, J. E. and EASTON, J. D. Occurrence and implications of seizures in subarachnoid hemorrhage due to ruptured intracranial aneurysms. *Neurosurgery*, **8**, 417–421 (1981)

111 HASEGAWA, T., WATANABE, H. and ISHII, S. Studies of intravascular components in cerebral vasospasm following subarachnoid hemorrhage. *Neurosurgical Review*, **3**, 93–100 (1980)

112 HASH, C. J. GROSSMAN, C. B. and SHENKIN, H. A. Concurrent intracranial and spinal cord arteriovenous malformations. Case report. *Journal of Neurosurgery*, **43**, 104–107 (1975)

113 HASHIMOTO, I. Familial intracranial aneurysms and cerebral vascular anomalies. *Journal of Neurosurgery*, **46**, 419–427 (1977)

114 HASHIMOTO, N., HANDA, H. and HAZAMA, F. Experimentally induced cerebral aneurysms in rats: part II. *Surgical Neurology*, **11**, 243–246 (1979)

115 HASSLER, O. Morphological studies on the large cerebral arteries with reference to the aetiology of subarachnoid haemorrhage. *Acta Psychiatrica et Neurologica Scandinavica*, **36** (Suppl. 154) 1–145 (1961)

116 HAYAKAWA, T. and WALTZ, A. G. Influence of head position on the prognosis of experimental subarachnoid hemorrhage. *Archives of Neurology*, **35**, 206–212 (1978)

117 HAYASHI, M., MARUKAWA, S., FUJII, H., KITANO, T., KOBAYASHI, H. and YAMAMOTO, S. Intracranial hypertension in patients with ruptured intracranial aneurysm. *Journal of Neurosurgery*, **46**, 584–590 (1977)

118 HAYWARD, R. D. Subarachnoid haemorrhage of unknown aetiology. A clinical and radiological study of 51 cases. *Journal of Neurology, Neurosurgery and Psychiatry*, **40**, 926–931 (1977)

119 HECK, A. F. Manifestations of spontaneous subarachnoid hemorrhage in the orbit and bulbus oculi. Report of previously undescribed hemorrhagic phenomena in the conjunctivae. *Neurology*, **11**, 701–709 (1961)

120 HEIDRICH, R. Subarachnoid Haemorrhage. In *Vascular Diseases of the Nervous System*, Part 2, edited by P. H. Vinken and G. W. Bruyn, 68–204. Amsterdam: North-Holland Publishing Company (1972)

121 HENSON, R. A. and CROFT, P. B. Spontaneous spinal subarachnoid haemorrhage. *Quarterly Journal of Medicine*, **25**, 53–66 (1956)

122 HIGASHI, K., HATANO, M., YAMASHITA, T., INOUE, S. and MATSUMURA, T. Coexistence of posterior inferior cerebellar artery aneurysm and arteriovenous malformation fed by the same artery. *Surgical Neurology*, **12**, 405–408 (1979)

123 HIRSH, L. F. and GONZALEZ, C. F. Fusiform basilar aneurysm simulating carotid transient ischemic attacks. *Stroke*, **10**, 598–601 (1979)

124 HOAK, J. C. Hemostatic defects and bleeding: diagnosis and treatment. In *Synopsis of Surgery*, edited by R. D. Liechty and R. T. Soper, 55–64. St. Louis: C. V. Mosby Company (1976)

125 HOFF, J. T. Intracerebral hemorrhage. In *Current Surgical Management of Neurologic Disease*, edited by C. B. Wilson and J. T. Hoff, 215–222. New York: Churchill Livingstone (1980)

126 HOFFMAN, W. F., WILSON, C. B. and TOWNSEND, J. J. Recurrent transient ischemic attacks secondary to an embolizing saccular middle cerebral artery aneurysm. *Journal of Neurosurgery*, **51**, 103–106 (1979)

127 Holy Bible, II Kings, **4**, 18–20

128 HOUNSFIELD, G. N. Computerized transverse axial scanning (tomography) 1. Description of system. *British Journal of Radiology*, **46**, 1016–1022 (1973)

129 HUBSCHMANN, O. R. and KORNHAUSER, D. Cortical cellular response in acute subarachnoid hemorrhage. *Journal of Neurosurgery*, **52**, 456–462 (1980)

130 HUGHES, J. T. and OPPENHEIMER, D. R. Superficial siderosis of the central nervous system. *Acta Neuropathologica*, **13**, 56–74 (1969)

131 HUGHES, J. T. and SCHIANCHI, P. M. Cerebral artery spasm. A histological study at necropsy of the blood vessels in cases of subarachnoid hemorrhage. *Journal of Neurosurgery*, **48**, 515–525 (1978)

132 HUNT, W. E. and KOSNIK, R. J. Timing and perioperative care in intracranial aneurysm surgery. *Clinical Neurosurgery*, **21**, 79–89 (1974)

133 HUNT, W. E. and MILLER, C. A. The results of early operation for aneurysm. *Clinical Neurosurgery*, **24**, 208–215 (1976)

134 HUNTER, C. Nursing problems of patients undergoing aminocaproic acid treatment for subarachnoid hemorrhage due to aneurysm. *Journal of Neurosurgical Nursing*, **11**, 160–165 (1979)

135 HUSKISSON, E. C. and HART, F. D. Fulminating meningococcal septicaemia presenting with subarachnoid haemorrhage. *British Medical Journal*, **2**, 231–232 (1969)

136 HUTCHINSON, J. Aneurysm of the internal carotid within the skull diagnosed eleven years before the patient's death. Spontaneous cure. *Transactions of the Clinical Society of London*, **8**, 127–131 (1875)

137 HYLAND, H. H. Prognosis in subarachnoid hemorrhage. *Archives of Neurology and Psychiatry*, **63**, 61–78 (1950)

138 ILLINGWORTH, R. Surgical treatment of ruptured intracranial aneurysms. *American Heart Journal*, **98**, 269–271 (1979)

139 IOB, I., SCANARINI, M., ANDRIOLI, G. C. and PARDDATSCHER, K. Thrombosis of the superior sagittal sinus associated with idiopathic thrombocytosis. *Surgical Neurology*, **11**, 439–441 (1979)

140 IQBAL, A., ALTER, M. and LEE, S. H. Pseudoxanthoma elasticum: a review of neurological complications. *Annals of Neurology*, **4**, 18–20 (1978)

141 ISHII, R. Regional cerebral blood flow in patients with ruptured intracranial aneurysms. *Journal of Neurosurgery*, **50**, 587–594 (1979)

142 ITO, U. and INABA, Y. Cerebrospinal fluid cytology after subarachnoid hemorrhage. *Journal of Neurosurgery*, **51**, 352–354 (1979)

143 JACKSON, I. J. Aseptic hemogenic meningitis. An experimental study of meningeal reactions due to blood and its breakdown products. *Archives of Neurology and Psychiatry*, **62**, 572–589 (1949)

144 JAIN, K. K. Mechanism of rupture of intracranial saccular aneurysms. *Surgery*, **54**, 347–350 (1963)

145 JOYNT, R. J., FEIBEL, J. H. and SLADEK, C. M. Antidiuretic hormone levels in stroke patients. *Annals of Neurology*, **9**, 182–184 (1981)

146 KALBAG, R. M. and WOOLF, A. L. *Cerebral Venous Thrombosis*, 280 pp. London: Oxford University Press (1967)

147 KARASAWA, J., KIKUCHI, H. and FURUSE, S. Subependymal hematoma in 'moyamoya' disease. *Surgical Neurology*, **13**, 118–120 (1980)

148 KASANTIKUL, V. and NETSKY, M. G. Combined neurilemmoma and angioma. Tumor of ectomesenchyme and a source of bleeding. *Journal of Neurosurgery*, **50**, 81–87 (1979)

149 KASSELL, N. F., PEERLESS, S. J., DRAKE, C. G., BOARINI, D. J. and ADAMS, H. P. Jr. Treatment of ischemic deficits from cerebral vasospasm with high dose barbiturate therapy. *Neurosurgery*, **7**, 593–597 (1980)

150 KASTE, M. and RAMSAY, M. Tranexamic acid in subarachnoid hemorrhage. A double-blind study. *Stroke*, **10**, 519–522 (1979)

151 KELLY, P. J., GORTEN, R. J., ROSE, J. E., GROSSMAN, R. G. and EISENBERG, H. M. Radionuclide cerebral angiography and the timing of aneurysm surgery. *Neurosurgery*, **5**, 202–207 (1979)

152 KENDALL, B. E., LEE, B. C. P. and CLAVERIA, E. Computerised tomography and angiography in subarachnoid haemorrhage. *British Journal of Radiology*, **49**, 483–501 (1976)

153 KENNING, J. A., TOUTANT, S. M. and SAUNDERS, R. L. Upright patient positioning in the management of intracranial hypertension. *Surgical Neurology*, **15**, 148–152 (1981)

154 KERR, C. B. Intracranial haemorrhage in haemophilia. *Journal of Neurology and Psychiatry*, **27**, 166–173 (1964)

155 KLAFTA, L. A. Jr. and HAMBY, W. B. Significance of cerebrospinal fluid pressure in determining time for repair of intracranial aneurysms. *Journal of Neurosurgery*, **31**, 217–219 (1969)

156 KODAMA, N., MINEURA, K., SUZUKI, J., KITAOKA, T., KURASHIMA, Y. and TAKAHASHI, S. Cerebrovascular moyamoya disease associated with aneurysm at the peripheral

portion of the posterior choroidal artery. *Neurological Surgery (Tokyo)*, **4**, 985–991 (1976)

157 KOENIG, G. H., MARSHALL, W. H. Jr., POOLE, J. and KRAMER, R. A. Rupture of intracranial aneurysms during cerebral angiography: report of ten cases and review of the literature. *Neurosurgery*, **5**, 314–324 (1979)

158 KOEPPEN, A. H. W. and BARRON, K. D. Superficial siderosis of the central nervous system: a histological, histochemical and chemical study. *Jornal of Neuropathology and Experimental Neurology*, **30**, 448–469 (1971)

159 KOGA, H., KANEKO, M. and HOSAKA, Y. Extravasation from aneurysms during angiography. *Surgical Neurology*, **12**, 453–456 (1979)

160 KORMOS, R. L., TUCKER, W. S., BILBAO, J. M., GLADSTONE, R. M. and BASS, A. G. Subarachnoid hemorrhage due to a spinal cord hemangioblastoma: case report. *Neurosurgery*, **6**, 657–660 (1980)

161 KURTZKE, J. F. Epidemiology of cerebrovascular disease. In *Cerebrovascular Survey Report*, edited by R. G. Siekert, 135–176. Rochester, Minnesota: Whiting Press, Inc. (1980)

162 KVAM, D. A., MICHELSON, W. J. and QUEST, D. O. Intracerebral hemorrhage as a complication of artificial embolization. *Neurosurgery*, **7**, 491–494 (1980)

163 KWAK, R., NIIZUMA, H., TAGATSUGU, O. and SUZUKI, J. Angiographic study of cerebral vasospasm following rupture of intracranial aneurysms. Part I. Time of the appearance. *Surgical Neurology*, **11**, 257–262 (1979)

164 LAGUNA, J., DERBY, B. M. and CHASE, R. *Cardiobacterium hominis* endocarditis with cerebral mycotic aneurysm. *Archives of Neurology*, **32**, 638–639 (1975)

165 LANGFITT, T. W. Conservative care of intracranial hemorrhage. *Advances in Neurology*, **16**, 169–180 (1977)

166 LANGFITT, T. W., KASSELL, W. F. and WEINSTEIN, J. D. Cerebral blood flow with intracranial hypertension. *Neurology*, **15**, 761–773 (1965)

167 LEBERT, H. Ueber die Aneurysmen der Hirnaterien. *Berliner Klinische Wochenschrift*, **3**, 209–212 (1866)

168 LEE, Y. J., KANDALL, S. R. and GALI, V. S. Intracerebral arterial aneurysm in a newborn. *Archives of Neurology*, **35**, 171–172 (1978)

169 LEKSELL, L. The stereotaxic method and radiosurgery of the brain. *Acta Chirurgica Scandinavica*, **102**, 316–319 (1951)

170 LEVY, L. F. Subarachnoid haemorrhage without arteriographic vascular abnormality. *Journal of Neurosurgery*, **17**, 252–258 (1960)

171 LILIEQUIST, B. and LINDQVIST, M. Computer tomography in the evaluation of subarachnoid hemorrhage. *Acta Radiologica Diagn (Stockholm)*, **21**, 327–331 (1980)

172 LITTLE, J. R., ST. LOUIS, P., WEINSTEIN, M. and DOHN, D. F. Giant fusiform aneurysm of the cerebral arteries. *Stroke*, **12**, 183–188 (1981)

173 LJUNGGREN, B., BRANDT, L., KAGSTRÖM, E. and SUNDBARG, G. Results of early operations for ruptured aneurysms. *Journal of Neurosurgery*, **54**, 473–479 (1981)

174 LOCKSLEY, H. B., SAHS, A. L. and SANDLER, R. Subarachnoid hemorrhage unrelated to intracranial aneurysm and A-V malformation. In *Intracranial Aneurysms and Subarachnoid Hemorrhage*, edited by A. L. Sahs, G. E. Perret, H. B. Locksley and H. Nishioka, 223–244. Philadelphia: J. B. Lippincott Company (1969)

175 LOCKSLEY, H. B., SAHS, A. L. and KNOWLER, L. General survey of cases in the central registry and characteristics of the sample population. In *Intracranial Aneurysms and Subarachnoid Hemorrhage*, edited by A. L. Sahs, G. Perret, H. B. Locksley and H. Nishioka, p. 20. Philadelphia: J. B. Lippincott Company (1969)

176 LOMBARDO, L., MATEOS, J. H. and BARROETA, F. F. Subarachnoid hemorrhage due to endometriosis of the spinal canal. *Neurology*, **18**, 423–426 (1968)

177 LOUGHEED, W. M. and BARNETT, H. J. M. Lesions producing spontaneous hemorrhage. In *Neurological Surgery*, Volume 2, edited by J. R. Youmans, 709–723. Philadelphia: W. B. Saunders Company (1973)

178 LUSCHKA, H. Cavernöse Blutgesechwulst des Gehirnes. *Virchows Archives*, **6**, 458–470 (1854)

179 MANDYBUR, T. I. Intracranial hemorrhage caused by metastatic tumors. *Neurology*, **27**, 650–655 (1977)

180 MAROON, J. C. and NELSON, P. B. Hypovolemia in patients with subarachnoid hemorrhage: therapeutic implications. *Neurosurgery*, **4**, 223–226 (1979)

181 MARQUARDSEN, J. The epidemiology of cerebrovascular disease. *Acta Neurologica Scandinavica*, **57** (Suppl. 67) 57–75 (1978)

182 MATHEW, N. T., MEYER, J. S. and HARTMANN, A. Diagnosis and treatment of factors complicating subarachnoid hemorrhage. *Neuroradiology*, **6**, 237–245 (1974)

183 MATSUDA, M., MATSUDA, I., HANDA, H. and OKAMOTO, K. Intracavernous giant aneurysm associated with Marfan's syndrome. *Surgical Neurology*, **12**, 119–121 (1979)

184 MASUZAWA, H., KOBAYASHI, M., INOYA, H., KAMITANI, H., SATO, J. and SATO, O. Multisection angiotomography of intracranial aneurysms. *Acta Neurochirurgica*, **28** (Suppl.) 550–553 (1979)

185 MAURICE-WILLIAMS, R. S., GORDON, Y. B. and SYKES, A. Monitoring fibrinolytic activity in the cerebrospinal fluid after aneurysmal subarachnoid hemorrhage: a guide to the risk of rebleeding? *Journal of Neurology, Neurosurgery and Psychiatry*, **43**, 175–181 (1980)

186 McCORMICK, W. F. The pathology of vascular ('arteriovenous') malformations. *Journal of Neurosurgery*, **24**, 807–816 (1966)

187 McCORMICK, W. F. The natural history of intracranial saccular aneurysms. *Weekly Update: Neurology and Neurosurgery*, **1** (3), 1–8 (1978)

188 McCORMICK, W. F. and SCHOCHET, S. S. Jr. *Atlas of Cerebrovascular Disease*, 422 pp. Philadelphia: W. B. Saunders Company (1976)

189 McCORMICK, W. F. and SCHMALSTIEG, E. J. The relationship of arterial hypertension to intracranial aneurysms. *Archives of Neurology*, **34**, 285–287 (1977)

190 McDONALD, C. A. and KORB, M. Intracranial aneurysms. *Archives of Neurology and Psychiatry*, **42**, 298–328 (1939)

191 McGAULEY, J. L., MILLER, C. A. and PENNER, J. A. Diagnosis and treatment of diffuse intravascular coagulation following cerebral trauma. *Journal of Neurosurgery*, **43**, 374–376 (1975)

192 McHENRY, L. C. Jr. *Garrison's History of Neurology*, 522 pp. Springfield, Illinois: Charles C. Thomas (1969)

193 McKISSOCK, W. and PAINE, W. K. E. Subarachnoid haemorrhage. *Brain*, **82**, 356–366 (1959)

194 McKISSOCK, W., PAINE, K. W. E. and WALSH, L. S. An analysis of the results of treatment of ruptured intracranial aneurysms. *Journal of Neurosurgery*, **17**, 762–776 (1960)

194a MARGERISON, J. H., BINNE, C. D. and McCAUL, I. R. Electroencephalographic signs employed in the location of ruptured intracranial arterial aneurysms. *Electroencephalography and Clinical Neurophysiology*, **28**, 296–306 (1970)

195 MERORY, J., THOMAS, D. J., HUMPHREY, P. R. D., DU BOULAY, G. H., MARSHALL, J., ROSS RUSSELL, R. W., SYMON, L. and ZILKHA, E. Cerebral blood flow after surgery for recent subarachnoid haemorrhage. *Journal of Neurology, Neurosurgery and Psychiatry*, **43**, 214–221 (1980)

196 MICHELSEN, W. J. Natural history and pathophysiology of arteriovenous malformations. *Clinical Neurosurgery*, **26**, 307–313 (1979)

197 MIRZA, F. H., SMITH, P. L. and LIM, W. N. Multiple aneurysms in a patient with Ehlers-Danlos syndrome: angiography without sequelae. *American Journal of Roentgenology*, **132**, 993–995 (1979)

198 MODESTI, L. M. and BINET, E. F. Value of computed tomography in the diagnosis and management of subarachnoid hemorrhage. *Neurosurgery*, **3**, 151–156 (1978)

199 MONEY, R. A. and VANDERFIELD, G. K. Premonitory symptoms and signs of subarachnoid haemorrhage. *Medical Journal of Australia*, **1**, 859–860 (1966)

200 MONIZ, E. L'encephalographie artérielle, son importance dans la localisation des tumeurs cérébrales. *Revue Neurologique*, **34**, 72–90 (1927)

201 MORGAGNI, J. B. De sedibus et causis morborum per anatomen indagatis. In *The Seats and Causes of Disease*, book I, letter II, article 20 (1761) translated by B. Alexander, p. 31. New York: Hafner Publishing Company (1960)

202 MULLAN, S. and DAWLEY, J. Antifibrinolytic therapy for intracranial aneurysms. *Journal of Neurosurgery*, **28**, 21–23 (1968)

203 MULLAN, S., DUDA, E. D. and PATRONAS, N. J. Some examples of balloon technology in neurosurgery. *Journal of Neurosurgery*, **52**, 321–329 (1980)

204 NAGAMINE, Y., TAKAHASHI, S. and SONOBE, M. Multiple intracranial aneurysms associated with moyamoya disease. *Journal of Neurosurgery*, **54**, 673–676 (1981)

205 NASSAR, S. I. and CORRELL, J. W. Subarachnoid hemorrhage due to spinal cord tumors. *Neurology*, **18**, 87–94 (1968)

206 NATHANSON, M., ROBINS, A. L. and GREEN, M. A. Blood in the subarachnoid space. A clinical evaluation of its occurrence in 190 consecutive cases. *Neurology*, **3**, 721–724 (1953)

207 NAU, H.-E. and BOCK, W. J. Value of electroencephalography (EEG) before and after surgery of intracranial aneurysms. *Acta Neurochirurgica*, **47**, 45–52 (1979)

208 NEIL-DWYER, G., WALTER, P., CRUICKSHANK, J. M., DOSHI, B. and O'GORMAN, P. Effect of propranolol and phentolamine on myocardial necrosis after subarachnoid haemorrhage. *British Medical Journal*, **2**, 990–992 (1978)

209 NEW, P. F. J. Computed tomography in the diagnosis of hemorrhagic stroke. *Advances in Neurology*, **16**, 145–168 (1977)

210 NEWMAN, J. Nursing care study. Cerebral aneurysm. *Nursing Times*, **72**, 1156–1161 (1976)

211 NIBBELINK, D. W. Antihypertensive and antifibrinolytic therapy following subarachnoid hemorrhage from ruptured intracranial aneurysm. In *Aneurysmal*

Subarachnoid Hemorrhage, edited by A. L. Sahs, D. W. Nibbelink and J. C. Torner, 287–296. Baltimore: Urban and Schwarzenberg (1981)

212 NIBBELINK, D. W., TORNER, J. C. and HENDERSON, W. G. Antifibrinolytic therapy in recent onset subarachnoid hemorrhage. In *Aneurysmal Subarachnoid Hemorrhage*, edited by A. L. Sahs, D. W. Nibbelink and J. C. Torner, 297–306. Baltimore: Urban and Schwarzenberg (1981)

213 NISHIOKA, H. Report on the co-operative study of intracranial aneurysms and subarachnoid hemorrhage. Evaluation of the conservative management of ruptured intracranial aneurysms. *Journal of Neurosurgery*, **25**, 574–592 (1966)

214 NORNES, H. The role of intracranial pressure in the arrest of hemorrhage in patients with ruptured intracranial aneurysm. *Journal of Neurosurgery*, **39**, 226–234 (1973)

215 NORNES, H. Monitoring of patients with intracranial aneurysms. *Clinical Neurosurgery*, **22**, 321–331 (1974)

216 NORNES, H. and MAGNAES, B. Intracranial pressure in patients with ruptured intracranial aneurysm. *Journal of Neurosurgery*, **36**, 537–547 (1972)

217 OJEMANN, R. G., NEW, P. F. J. and FLEMING, T. C. Intracranial aneurysms associated with bacterial meningitis. *Neurology*, **16**, 1222–1226 (1966)

218 OKAWARA, S.-H. Warning signs prior to rupture of an intracranial aneurysm. *Journal of Neurosurgery*, **38**, 575–580 (1973)

219 OLINGER, C. P. and WASSERMAN, J. F. Electronic stethoscope for detection of cerebral aneurysm, vasospasm and arterial disease. *Surgical Neurology*, **8**, 298–312 (1977)

220 OLIVECRONA, H. and RIIVES, J. Arteriovenous aneurysms of the brain. Their diagnosis and treatment. *Archives of Neurology and Psychiatry*, **59**, 567–602 (1948)

221 OSBORN, A. G. and ANDERSON, R. E. Angiographic spectrum of cervical and intracranial fibromuscular dysplasia. *Stroke*, **8**, 617–626 (1977)

222 OSTERMAN, O. Hypothalamo-pituitary-adrenal function following subarachnoid hemorrhage. *Acta Neurologica Scandinavica*, **52**, 56–62 (1975)

223 OZAKI, N. and MULLAN, S. Possible role of the erythrocyte in causing prolonged cerebral vasospasm. *Journal of Neurosurgery*, **51**, 773–778 (1979)

224 PAKARINEN, S. Incidence, aetiology and prognosis of primary subarachnoid haemorrhage. *Acta Neurologica Scandinavica*, **48** (Suppl. 29) 1–128 (1967)

225 PARKINSON, D. and BACHERS, G. Arteriovenous malformations. Summary of 100 consecutive supratentorial cases. *Journal of Neurosurgery*, **53**, 285–299 (1980)

226 PATIL, A. A. Angiographically occult arteriovenous malformation of the brain. A case report. *Acta Neurochirurgica*, **58**, 99–104 (1981)

227 PEARCE, J. M. S. and FOSTER, J. B. An investigation of complicated migraine. *Neurology*, **15**, 333–340 (1965)

228 PEERLESS, S. J. Pre- and postoperative management of cerebral aneurysms. *Clinical Neurosurgery*, **26**, 209–231 (1979)

229 PELLETTIERI, L., CARLSSON, C. A., GREVSTEN, S., NORLEN, G. and UHLEMANN, C. Surgical versus conservative treatment of intracranial arteriovenous malformations: a study in surgical decision-making. *Acta Neurochirurgica*, **29** (Suppl.) 1–86 (1979)

230 PERRET, G. and NISHIOKA, H. Report on the co-operative study of intracranial aneurysms and subarachnoid hemorrhage. Section IV. Arteriovenous-malformations. *Journal of Neurosurgery*, **25**, 467–490 (1966)

231 PETITO, F. and PLUM, F. The lumbar puncture. *New England Journal of Medicine*, **290**, 225–227 (1974)

232 PHILLIPS, L.H. II, WHISNANT, J.P., O'FALLON, M. and SUNDT, T. M. Jr. The unchanging pattern of subarachnoid hemorrhage in a community. *Neurology*, **30**, 1034–1040 (1980)

233 PLOTKIN, R., RONTHAL, M. and FROMAN, C. Spontaneous spinal subarachnoid haemorrhage. Report of 3 cases. *Journal of Neurosurgery*, **25**, 443–446 (1966)

234 POOL, J. L. Timing and techniques in the intracranial surgery of ruptured aneurysms of the anterior communicating artery. *Journal of Neurosurgery*, **19**, 378–388 (1962)

235 POOL, J. L. and POTTS, D. G. *Aneurysms and Arteriovenous Anomalies of the Brain*, 463 pp. New York: Harper and Row (1965)

236 POPE, F. M., NICHOLLS, A. C., NARCISI, P., BARTLET, T., NEIL-DWYER, G. and DOSHI, B. Some patients with cerebral aneurysms are deficient in type III collagen. *Lancet*, **1**, 973–975 (1981)

237 PRITZ, M. B., GIANNOTTA, S. L., KINDT, G. W., McGILLICUDDY, J. F. and PRAGER, R. L. Treatment of patients with neurologic deficits associated with cerebral vaso-spasm by intravascular volume expansion. *Neurosurgery*, **3**, 364–368 (1978)

238 QUICKEL, K. E. Jr. and WHALEY, R. J. Subarachnoid hemorrhage in a patient with hereditary hemorrhagic telangiectasia. *Neurology*, **17**, 716–719 (1967)

239 QUINCKE, H. Die Lumbalpunction des Hydrocephalus. *Berliner Klinische Wochenschrift*, **38**, 929–933 (1891)

240 RACZ, P., BOBEST, M. and SZILVASSY, I. Significance of fundal hemorrhage in predicting the state of the patient with ruptured intracranial aneurysm. *Ophthalmologica*, **174**, 61–66 (1977)

241 RAMIREZ-LASSEPAS, M. Antifibrinolytic therapy in subarachnoid hemorrhage caused by ruptured intracranial aneurysms. *Neurology*, **31**, 316–322 (1981)

242 RASMUSSEN, P., BUSCH, H., HAASE, J., HANSEN, J., HARMSEN, A., KNUDSEN, V., MARCUSSEN, E., MIDHOLM, ST., OLSEN, R. B., ROSENORN, J., SCHMIDT, K., VOLDBY, B. and HANSEN, L. Intracranial saccular aneurysms. Results of treatment in 851 patients. *Acta Neurochirurgica*, **53**, 1–17 (1980)

243 RAY, H. and WAHAL, K. Subarachnoid hemorrhage associated with subacute bacterial endocarditis. *Archives of Neurology and Psychiatry*, **76**, 623–624 (1956)

244 RICHARDSON, J. C. and HYLAND, H. H. Intracranial aneurysms. *Medicine*, **20**, 1–83 (1941)

245 RISH, B. L. Treatment of intracranial aneurysms associated with other entitities. *Southern Medical Journal*, **71**, 553–557, 560 (1978)

246 ROACH, M. R. and DRAKE, C. G. Ruptured cerebral aneurysms caused by micro-organisms. *New England Journal of Medicine*, **273**, 240–244 (1965)

247 ROELTGEN, D. P., WEIMER, G. R. and PATTERSON, L. F. Delayed neurologic complications of left atrial myxoma. *Neurology*, **31**, 8–13 (1981)

248 ROUSSEAUX, P., SCHERPEREEL, B., BERNARD, M. H., GRAFTIEAUX, J. P. and GUYOT, J. F. Fever and cerebral vasospasm in ruptured intracranial aneurysms. *Surgical Neurology*, **14**, 459–465 (1980)

249 ROZARIO, R., ADELMAN, L., PRAGER, R. J. and STEIN, B. M. Meningiomas of the pineal region and third ventricle. *Neurosurgery*, **5**, 489–495 (1979)

250 SACKS, J. G. and LINDENBURG, R. Dolicho-ectatic intracranial arteries: symptomatology and pathogenesis of arterial elongation and distention. *Johns Hopkins Medical Journal*, **125**, 95–106 (1969)

251 SAHS, A. L. History of the co-operative aneurysm study and central registry. In *Aneurysmal Subarachnoid Hemorrhage*, by A. L. Sahs, D. W. Nibbelink and J. C. Torner, 3–16. Baltimore: Urban and Schwarzenberg (1981)

252 SAHS, A. L. Phase VII: timing of surgery. In *Aneurysmal Subarachnoid Hemorrhage*, 12–13. Baltimore: Urban and Schwarzenberg (1981)

253 SAHS, A.L. and KEIL, P. G. Subarachnoid hemorrhage caused by ruptured intracranial aneurysm. *American Heart Journal*, **26**, 645–661 (1943)

254 SAHS, A. L., PERRET, G. E., LOCKSLEY, H. B. and NISHIOKA, H. *Intracranial Aneurysms and Subarachnoid Hemorrhage. A Cooperative Study*, 296 pp. Philadelphia: J. B. Lippincott Company (1969)

255 SAKAKI, S., MATSUO, Y., KUWABARA, H. and MATSUOKA, K. Rupture of an aneurysm into a parasellar epidermoid cyst. Case report. *Journal of Neurosurgery*, **55**, 629–632 (1981)

256 SALLOUM, A., LEBEL, M. and REIHER, J. Accès céphalagiques simulant une hémorragie méningée. *Revue Neurologique*, **133**, 131–138 (1977)

257 SAMSON, D., DITMORE, Q. M. and BEYER, C. W. Jr. Intravascular use of isobutyl-2-cyanoacrylate. Part I. Treatment of intracranial arteriovenous malformations. *Neurosurgery*, **8**, 43–51 (1981)

258 SAMSON, D. S., HODOSH, R. M. and CLARK, W. K. Surgical management of unruptured asymptomatic aneurysms. *Journal of Neurosurgery*, **46**, 731–734 (1977)

259 SAMSON, D. S., HODOSH, R. M., REID, W. R., BEYER, C. W. and CLARK, W. K. Risk of intracranial aneurysm surgery in the good grade patient. Early versus late operation. *Neurosurgery*, **5**, 422–426 (1979)

260 SANDOK, A., VON ESTORFF, I. and GIULIANI, E. R. Subsequent neurological events in patients with atrial myxoma. *Annals of Neurology*, **8**, 305–307 (1980)

261 SARWAR, M. and McCORMICK, W. F. Intracerebral venous angioma. *Archives of Neurology*, **35**, 323–325 (1978)

262 SCHAAL, S. F., WALLACE, A. G. and SEALY, W. C. Protective influence of cardiac denervation against arrythmias of myocardial infarction. *Cardiovascular Research*, **3**, 241–244 (1969)

263 SCHNECK, S. A. and KRICHEFF, I. I. Intracranial aneurysm rupture, vasospasm, and infarction. *Archives of Neurology*, **11**, 668–681 (1964)

264 SCHUMACHER, M. A. and ALKSNE, J. F. Mechanisms of whole blood-induced cerebral arterial contraction. *Neurosurgery*, **9**, 275–282 (1981)

265 SCOTTI, G., ETHIER, R., MELANCON, D., TERBRUGGE, K. and TCHANG, S. Computed tomography in the evaluation of intracranial aneurysms and subarachnoid hemorrhage. *Radiology*, **123**, 85–90 (1977)

266 SCOTTI, L. N., GOLDMAN, R. L., RAO, G. R. and HEINZ, E. R. Cerebral venous angioma. *Neuroradiology*, **9**, 125–128 (1975)

267 SERBINENKO, F. A. IV. Balloon techniques. Six hundred endovascular neuro-surgical procedures in vascular pathology. *Acta Neurochirurgica*, **28** (Suppl.) 310–311 (1979)

268 SHEFFIELD, E. A. and WELLER, R. O. Age changes at cerebral artery bifurcations and the pathogenesis of berry aneurysms. *Journal of the Neurological Sciences*, **46**, 341–352 (1980)

269 SHUCART, W. A. and JACKSON, I. Management of diabetes insipidus in neurosurgical patients. *Journal of Neurosurgery*, **44**, 65–71 (1976)

270 SHUCART, W. A., HUSSAIN, S. K. and COOPER, P. R. Epsilon-aminocaproic acid and recurrent subarachnoid hemorrhage. A clinical trial. *Journal of Neurosurgery*, **53**, 28–31 (1980)

271 SHUTTLEWORTH, E. C., PARKER, J. M., WISE, G. R. and STEVENS, M. E. Differentiation of early subarachnoid hemorrhage from traumatic lumbar puncture. *Stroke*, **8**, 613–617 (1977)

272 SILVER, A. J., PEDERSON, M. E. Jr., GANTI, S. R., HILAL, S. K. and MICHELSON, W. J. CT of subarachnoid hemorrhage due to ruptured aneurysm. *American Journal of Neuroradiology*, **2**, 13–22 (1981)

273 SILVERSTEIN, A. Intracranial hemorrhage in patients with bleeding tendencies. *Neurology*, **11**, 310–317 (1961)

274 SIMA, A. A. F. and ROBERTSON, D. M. Subependymal giant-cell astrocytoma. Case report with ultrastructural study. *Journal of Neurosurgery*, **50**, 240–245 (1979)

275 SKULTETY, F. M. Meningioma simulating ruptured aneurysm. Case report. *Journal of Neurosurgery*, **29**, 380–382 (1968)

276 SPETZLER, R. F., WINESTOCK, D., NEWTON, H. T. and BOLDREY, E. B. Disappearance and reappearance of cerebral aneurysm in serial arteriograms. Case report. *Journal of Neurosurgery*, **41**, 508–510 (1974)

277 STEHBENS, W. E. *Pathology of the Cerebral Blood Vessels*, 661 pp. St. Louis: C. V. Mosby Company (1972)

278 STEHBENS, W. E. Aetiology of cerebral aneurysms. *Lancet*, **2**, 524–525 (1981)

279 STEIN, B. M. and WOLPERT, S. M. Arteriovenous malformations of the brain. I. Current concepts and treatment. *Archives of Neurology*, **37**, 1–5 (1980)

280 STEIN, B. M. and WOLPERT, S. M. Arteriovenous malformations of the brain. II. Current concepts and treatment. *Archives of Neurology*, **37**, 69–75 (1980)

281 STEWART, R. M., SAMSON, D., DIEHL, J., HINTON, R. and DITMORE, Q. M. Unruptured cerebral aneurysms presenting as recurrent transient neurologic deficits. *Neurology*, **30**, 47–51 (1980)

282 STORNELLI, S. A. and FRENCH, J. D. Subarachnoid hemorrhage – factors in prognosis and management. *Journal of Neurosurgery*, **21**, 769–780 (1964)

283 SUGITA, K., KOBAYASHI, S., SHINTANI, A. and MUTSUGA, N. Microneurosurgery for aneurysms of the basilar artery. *Journal of Neurosurgery*, **51**, 615–620 (1979)

284 SUNDT, T. M. Jr. Cerebral vasospasm following subarachnoid hemorrhage: evolution, management, and relationship to timing of surgery. *Clinical Neurosurgery*, **24**, 228–239 (1977)

285 SUNDT, T. M. Jr. and WHISNANT, J. P. Subarachnoid hemorrhage from intracranial aneurysms. *New England Journal of Medicine*, **229**, 116–122 (1978)

286 SUTTON, D. and TRICKEY, S. E. Subarachnoid haemorrhage and total cerebral angiography. *Clinical Radiology*, **13**, 297–303 (1962)

287 SUZUKI, J. *Cerebral Aneurysms*, 751 pp. Tokyo: Neuron Publishing Co. (1979)

288 SUZUKI, J. and OHARA, H. Clinicopathological study of cerebral aneurysms. Origin, rupture, repair, and growth. *Journal of Neurosurgery*, **48**, 505–514 (1978)

289 SUZUKI, J., ONUMA, T. and YOSHIMOTO, T. Results of early operations on cerebral aneurysms. *Surgical Neurology*, **11**, 407–412 (1979)

290 SYMON, L., HARGADINE, J., ZAWIRSKI, M. and BRANSTON, N. Central conduction time as an index of ischaemia in subarachnoid haemorrhage. *Journal of the Neurological Sciences*, **44**, 95–103 (1979)

291 SYMONDS, C. P. Spontaneous subarachnoid haemorrhage. *Quarterly Journal of Medicine*, **18**, 93–122 (1924)

292 SYPERT, G. W. Intracranial aneurysms: natural history and surgical management. *Comprehensive Therapy*, **4**, 64–73 (1978)

293 TAKAKU, A., TANAKA, S., MORI, T. and SUZUKI, J. Postoperative complications in 1000 cases of intracranial aneurysms. *Surgical Neurology*, **12**, 137–144 (1979)

294 TAKAKU, A., SHINDO, K., TANAKA, S., MORI, T. and SUZUKI, J. Fluid and electrolyte disturbances in patients with intracranial aneurysms. *Surgical Neurology*, **11**, 349–356 (1979)

295 TANAKA, S., MORI, T., OHARA, H., TAKAKU, A. and SUZUKI, J. Gastrointestinal bleeding in cases of ruptured cerebral aneurysms. *Acta Neurochirurgica*, **48**, 223–230 (1979)

296 TARLOV, E. Subarachnoid hemorrhage. *Primary Care*, **6**, 791–803 (1979)

297 TEASDALE, G., MURRAY, G., PARKER, L. and JENNET, B. Adding up the Glasgow coma score. *Acta Neurochirurgica*, **28** (Suppl.) 13–16 (1979)

298 THEODORE, J. and ROBIN, E. D. Speculations on neurogenic pulmonary edema (NPE). *American Review of Respiratory Disease*, **113**, 405–411 (1976)

299 TOOLE, J. F. and PATEL, A. N. *Cerebrovascular Disorders*, 2nd edition, 412 pp. New York: McGraw Hill Book Company (1974)

300 TULLEKEN, C. A. F. Giant aneurysms of the posterior fossa presenting as space occupying lesions. *Clinical Neurology and Neurosurgery*, **79**, 161–186 (1976)

301 VAN GIJN, J. and VAN DONGEN, K. J. Computerized tomography in subarachnoid hemorrhage: difference between patients with and without an aneurysm on angiography. *Neurology*, **30**, 538–539 (1980)

302 VAN GILDER, J. C. and TORNER, J. C. Subarachnoid hemorrhage: patients with severe neurologic defect. In *Aneurysmal Subarachnoid Hemorrhage*, by A. L. Sahs, D. W. Nibbelink and J. C. Torner, 349–361. Baltimore: Urban and Schwarzenberg (1981)

303 VASSILOUTHIS, J. and RICHARDSON, A. E. Ventricular dilatation and communicating hydrocephalus following spontaneous subarachnoid hemorrhage. *Journal of Neurosurgery*, **51**, 341–351 (1979)

304 VIDAL, B. E., DERGAL, E. B., CESARMAN, E., SAN MARTIN, O. M., LOYO, M., LUGO, B. V. and ORTEGA, R. P. Cardiac arrhythmias associated with subarachnoid hemorrhage: prospective study. *Neurosurgery*, **5**, 675–680 (1979)

305 VINCENT, F. M. Hypoglycorrhachia after subarachnoid hemorrhage. *Neurosurgery*, **8**, 7–9 (1981)

306 VINCENT, F. M. Anterior spinal artery aneurysm presenting as a subarachnoid hemorrhage. *Stroke*, **12**, 230–232 (1981)

307 VINCENT, F. M., ZIMMERMAN, J. E., AUER, T. C. and MARTIN, D. B. Subarachnoid hemorrhage – the initial manifestation of bacterial endocarditis. *Neurosurgery*, **7**, 488–490 (1980)

308 VINTERS, H. V., BARNETT, H. J. M. and KAUFMANN, J. C. E. Subdural hematoma of the spinal cord and widespread subarachnoid hemorrhage complicating anticoagulant therapy. *Stroke*, **11**, 459–464 (1980)

309 VIRCHOW, R. Ueber der Erweiterung kleinerer Gefässe. *Archiv für pathologische Anatomie und Physiologie*, **3**, 427–462 (1851)

310 VIRCHOW, R. Die krankhaften Geschwülste. Berlin: A Hirschwald, **3**, 456–463 (1863)

311 VIRMANI, V., RANGAN, G. and SHRINIWAS, G. A study of the cerebrospinal fluid in atypical presentations of tuberculous meningitis. *Journal of the Neurological Sciences*, **26**, 587–592 (1975)

312 WALKER, A. E. and ALLEGRE, G. W. The pathology and pathogenesis of cerebral aneurysms. *Journal of Neuropathology and Experimental Neurology*, **13**, 248–259 (1954)

313 WALTON, J. N. The electroencephalographic sequelae of spontaneous subarachnoid haemorrhage. *Electroencephalography and Clinical Neurophysiology*, **5**, 41–52 (1953)

314 WALTON, J. N. Subarachnoid haemorrhage of unusual aetiology. *Neurology*, **3**, 517–543 (1953)

315 WALTON, J. N. The Korsakov syndrome in spontaneous subarachnoid haemorrhage. *Journal of Mental Science*, **99**, 521–530 (1953)

316 WALTON, J. N. *Subarachnoid Haemorrhage*, 350 pp. Edinburgh: E. and S. Livingstone (1956)

317 WEIR, B. K. Pulmonary edema following fatal aneurysm rupture. *Journal of Neurosurgery*, **49**, 502–507 (1978)

318 WEIR, B. Medical aspects of the preoperative management of aneurysms: a review. *Canadian Journal of Neurological Sciences*, **6**, 441–450 (1979)

319 WEIR, B. and ARONYK, K. Management mortality and the timing of surgery for supratentorial aneurysms. *Journal of Neurosurgery*, **54**, 146–150 (1981)

320 WELT, L. G. Disorders of fluids and electrolytes. In *Harrison's Principles of Internal Medicine*, 7th edition, Chapter 264, 1343–1355. New York (1974)

321 WEPFER, J. J. Observationes anatomicae ex cadaveribus eorem quos sustulit apoplexia. Schaffhusii, Impensis Onophrii a Waldkirch, typis A Riedingii (1675)

322 WILKINS, R. H. Attempted prevention or treatment of intracranial arterial spasm: a survey. *Neurosurgery*, **6**, 198–210 (1980)

323 WILKINS, R. H. The role of intracranial arterial spasm in the timing of operations for aneurysm. *Clinical Neurosurgery*, **24**, 185–207 (1977)

324 WILKINS, R. H. Update – Subarachnoid hemorrhage and saccular intracranial aneurysms. *Surgical Neurology*, **15**, 92–101 (1981)

325 WILLIS, T. Cerebri anatome cuiaccessit nervorum descriptio et usus. London: J. Flesher (1664)

326 WILSON, C. B., PITTS, L. and SPETZLER, R. F. Cerebral aneurysms. In *Current Surgical Management of Neurologic Disease*, edited by C. B. Wilson and J. T. Hoff, 123–143. New York: Churchill Livingstone (1980)

327 WINN, H. R., RICHARDSON, A. E. and JANE, J. A. The long-term prognosis in untreated cerebral aneurysms. I. A 10-year evaluation of 364 patients. *Annals of Neurology*, **1**, 358–370 (1977)

328 WINN, H. R., RICHARDSON, A. E., O'BRIEN, W. and JANE, J. A. The long-term prognosis in untreated cerebral aneurysms. II. Late morbidity and mortality. *Annals of Neurology*, **4**, 418–426 (1978)

329 WIRTH, F. P. Computerized tomography and subarachnoid hemorrhage. *Journal of the American Medical Association*, **241**, 563–564 (1979)

330 WISE, B. L. Syndrome of inappropriate antidiuretic hormone secretion after spontaneous subarachnoid hemorrhage: a reversible cause of clinical deterioration. *Neurosurgery*, **3**, 412–414 (1978)

331 WOLTMAN, H. W. and SHELDEN, W. D. Neurologic complications associated with congenital stenosis of the isthmus of the aorta. *Archives of Neurology and Psychiatry*, **17**, 303–316 (1927)

332 WRIGHT, D. C. and WILSON, C. B. Surgical treatment of basilar aneurysms. *Neurosurgery*, **5**, 325–333 (1979)

333 WRIGHT, R. L., OJEMANN, R. G. and DREW, J. H. Hemorrhage into pituitary adenomata. Report of two cases with spontaneous recovery. *Archives of Neurology*, **12**, 326–331 (1965)

334 WYBURN-MASON, R. *The Vascular Abnormalities and Tumours of the Spinal Cord and its Membranes,* 196 pp. London: H. Kimpton (1943)

Index

Note: For consistency English spelling is used throughout.